Cobert's Manual of Drug Safety and Pharmacovigilance

Second Edition

Barton Cobert, MD, FACP, FACG, FFPM
President
BLCMD Associates LLC
Westfield, New Jersey

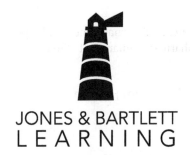

JONES & BARTLETT
LEARNING

World Headquarters

Jones & Bartlett Learning
40 Tall Pine Drive
Sudbury, MA 01776
978-443-5000
info@jblearning.com
www.jblearning.com

Jones & Bartlett Learning
Canada
6339 Ormindale Way
Mississauga, Ontario L5V 1J2
Canada

Jones & Bartlett Learning
International
Barb House, Barb Mews
London W6 7PA
United Kingdom

Jones & Bartlett Learning books and products are available through most bookstores and online booksellers. To contact Jones & Bartlett Learning directly, call 800-832-0034, fax 978-443-8000, or visit our website, www.jblearning.com.

Substantial discounts on bulk quantities of Jones & Bartlett Learning publications are available to corporations, professional associations, and other qualified organizations. For details and specific discount information, contact the special sales department at Jones & Bartlett Learning via the above contact information or send an email to specialsales@jblearning.com.

The authors, editor, and publisher have made every effort to provide accurate information. However, they are not responsible for errors, omissions, or for any outcomes related to the use of the contents of this book, and take no responsibility for the use of the products and procedures described. Treatments and side effects described in this book may not be applicable to all people; likewise, some people may require a dose or experience a side effect that is not described herein. Drugs and medical devices are discussed that may have limited availability controlled by the Food and Drug Administration (FDA) for use only in a research study or clinical trial. Research, clinical practice, and government regulations often change the accepted standard in this field. When consideration is being given to use of any drug in the clinical setting, the healthcare provider or reader is responsible for determining FDA status of the drug, reading the package insert, and reviewing prescribing information for the most up-to-date recommendations on dose, precautions, and contraindications, and determining the appropriate usage for the product. This is especially important in the case of drugs that are new or seldom used.

Production Credits
Executive Publisher: Christopher Davis
Associate Editor: Laura Burns
Associate Production Editor: Jill Morton
Marketing Manager: Rebecca Rockel
V.P., Manufacturing and Inventory Control: Therese Connell
Composition: Abella Publishing Services
Cover Design: Scott Moden
Cover Image: © ajt/ShutterStock, Inc.
Printing and Binding: Courier
Cover Printing: Courier

Library of Congress Cataloging-in-Publication Data
Cobert, Barton L.
  Cobert's manual of drug safety and pharmacovigilance / by Barton Cobert. — 2nd ed.
     p. cm.
  Rev. ed. of: Manual of drug safety and pharmacovigilance / Barton L. Cobert. c2007.
  Includes bibliographical references and index.
  ISBN-13: 978-0-7637-9159-9
  ISBN-10: 0-7637-9159-8
  1. Drugs—Side effects—Handbooks, manuals, etc. 2. Pharmacoepidemiology—Handbooks, manuals, etc.
I. Barton L. Cobert. Manual of drug safety and pharmacovigilance. II. Title.
  RM302.5.C63 2012
  615'.7042—dc22

                                        2011002097

6048

Printed in the United States of America
15 14 13 12   10 9 8 7 6 5 4 3 2

Thank You

My thanks to Dr. Marc Berthiaume of Health Canada and his colleagues for reviewing and assisting with the chapter on Health Canada. Thanks also to Mr. Mick Foy of the United Kingdom Medicines and Healthcare products Regulatory Agency for his assistance on some of the United Kingdom matters. Thanks also to the contributors for the chapters that I did not feel comfortable writing.

Thanks to Chris Davis and the team at Jones & Bartlett Learning who saw enough merit in the first edition to publish a second edition.

Thanks to my many colleagues in the drug safety world for their advice and clarification.

And to my loving and lovely wife for tolerating my hours in front of the computer.

Contents

Mano Murty, MD, CCFP, FCFP, Kevin Bernardo, ND, BHsc, and Alison Ingham, PhD

Introductions

■ Introduction to the First Edition

This manual is a practical instruction book on drug safety. It is aimed at newcomers, old-timers, and outsiders to the field who would like a demystification and explanation of what adverse events are and how drug safety departments work. Hopefully, readers, especially those not in the field, will understand that drug safety, like all other areas of medicine, is as much an art as it is a science.

For newcomers, this is a "Drug Safety 101" course giving a broad overview of how adverse events are handled from start to finish. For old-timers, this book will fill in gaps in knowledge on drug safety. For outsiders not working directly in this field, this book will explain how "side effects" are handled by the industry and by health authorities.

This book is not meant to be an encyclopedia. There are other such books already available. Rather, it is my hope that this will be an approachable book that will give a global overview of the field.

It is expected that, after carefully reading and absorbing the contents, the reader will be able to begin work in a drug safety department, or, if an outsider, understand what happens in such a department and where listings or adverse events come from.

I have attempted to avoid excess jargon ("This spontaneous SAE is expeditable since it is unlisted") and make the book approachable for those with limited or no knowledge of medicine or pharmacology.

Housekeeping: In this age of high technology, the references in the text are primarily websites rather than published citations. After much discussion, it was felt that putting URLs directly in the text would be distracting and of little use. Thus, they are noted in an appendix at the back of the book. In addition, accompanying this text is a CD-ROM with the entire contents of the book. This allows for rapid and easy searching for any topics the reader wishes. The URLs are "active" so that with a click or two the reader will be able to jump to that website when using the CD-ROM. All of the links were active and correct when this book was prepared but they cannot be guaranteed to be so in the future. Also, copying and pasting links into your browser may solve errors that you encounter.

I wish you well in the world of drug safety.

■ Introduction to the Second Edition

The first edition of this book was written about 4 years ago, and since that time, much has changed in the world of drug safety. The use of technology, which exploded in other areas of medicine over the past 30 or 40 years, has now hit drug safety (EDC, E2B, CDISC, HL-7, DSUR, PPR, ICSR—if you don't know what these mean, read the rest of this book). This is and will be a "game changer." It is likely that our current systems will look prehistoric or at best medieval in 10, 20, or 30 years, as everyone's medical life (if not entire life) is digitalized and readily available for review, study, analysis, correlation, tweeting, social media, and so on. Whether one likes this or not, it is necessary to keep up to date to remain employable and to conduct quality drug safety work. This book attempts to help the reader wade through the theory and methodology of drug safety and pharmacovigilance to high quality work.

Many changes in the field are heartening, but many are disheartening. On the heartening side, we are starting to understand pharmacology better. We are starting to develop methodology that will allow us to hopefully predict potential and likely drug toxicity in an individual. Perhaps genomics will allow us to truly tailor drug therapy to the individual. But we are not there yet, and genomics is barely mentioned in this book. With luck, we will see significant contributions to public health as our medical knowledge increases. The paradigms (sorry for the use of that word, but it fits) are changing: it is now "benefit–risk," "quality management systems," and "risk aversion." These words and concepts were hardly used in medicine 50 years ago. Next, drug safety has gone global. It is quaint to think that the International Conference on Harmonization, which began in 1989, included all the major players in the field: the United States, Europe (actually just three or four major western European countries), and Japan, with a few silent observers. Drug safety is now global, in large part because of the Uppsala Monitoring Centre, with new and vibrant ideas coming from all over the world.

On the disheartening side, we see corporatization, digitalization, depersonalization, politicization, commoditization, and other "-izations" in drug safety and medicine in general. Medicine is now a mass-market commodity, and drug safety is following that path too. We see laxity and bad behavior on the part of industry, healthcare practitioners, patients, consumers, government, universities, and nongovernmental organizations. We see politics and money continue to play a big role in the world of pharmacology. We also see the downside of globalization, with enormous fragmentation and duplication of efforts, and little upside. Add to this the "human condition" of wanting a magic pill to allow us to eat, drink, smoke, and do other things to our heart's content without damage to our health.

A suggestion: There are two major uses for this manual. The first is as a textbook for those who wish to learn the field or review their knowledge of drug safety. Those folks may wish to read the book cover to cover (on their own or as part of a course) or the parts they need to brush up on. The second is as a reference. For this, I would highly suggest loading the manual onto your PC, Mac, iPhone, iPad, Android, or other techno-marvel and using a PDF search tool (e.g., in Adobe) for the key word or concept you are looking for. Although I have attempted to keep concepts in their dedicated chapters, many ideas (e.g., causality determinations) must be discussed in multiple chapters. Using a PDF search will quickly get you to the right place in the text.

There it is. I hope you find the book useful, accurate, and easy to read and absorb. Best of luck. You'll need it.

Contributors

Kevin Bernardo, ND, BHsc
Marketed Health Products Directorate
Health Canada
Ottawa, Ontario
Canada

Barton Cobert, MD, FACP, FACG, FFPM
President
BLCMD Associates LLC
Westfield, New Jersey

Lisa Beth Ferstenberg, MD
Chief Medical Officer
Accelovance, Inc.
Rockville, Maryland

Alison Ingham, PhD
Natural Health Products Directorate
Health Canada
Ottawa, Ontario
Canada

Ana T. Menendez, PhD
Senior Director of Biotechnology
Catalent Pharma Solutions
Somerset, New Jersey

Mano Murty, MD, CCFP, FCFP
Marketed Health Products Directorate
Health Canada
Ottawa, Ontario
Canada

Contributors

Notice

This book is not meant to be used in the practice of medicine or for the prescription of medicines, drugs, biologics, over-the-counter medications, health foods, supplements, and so forth. The medications described do not necessarily have specific approval by the U.S. Food and Drug Administration, European Medicines Agency, Health Canada, or any other regulatory or health agency for use in the diseases, patients, or dosages discussed. The approved labeling in the United States and other countries and regions must be consulted for that jurisdiction before any product is used or prescribed. Because standards for usage change, it is advisable to keep abreast of revised recommendations, precautions, safety warnings, and adverse events, particularly those concerning new products.

This book is not intended to express opinions about the value of specific products or their comparative value within a drug class, even when a specific product is used to provide examples of adverse reactions. The content of this book is not meant to be used in choosing therapies in medical practice by healthcare practitioners or consumers. As with all medications and therapies, the official approved product labeling should be consulted before prescribing or using.

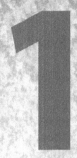

The Theory and Definitions of Drug Safety (Pharmacovigilance)

What is an adverse event (AE)? A serious AE? An adverse drug reaction (ADR)? A suspected adverse drug reaction (SADR)? A suspected, unexpected, serious adverse reaction (SUSAR)? A suspected, expected, serious adverse reaction? What do expected and unexpected mean?

Note: Unless otherwise noted, the words "drug" or "drug product" should be taken in this book to include "biologics" and "vaccines" too.

■ The Theory

There have been many variants on the terms and definitions used to talk about safety issues over the years. The terminology is somewhat confusing and is explained below.

The "official" and accepted definitions in most countries are based on the International Conference on Harmonization (ICH) E2A Guideline and are as follows:

Adverse Event—ICH

Any untoward medical occurrence in a patient or clinical investigation subject administered a pharmaceutical product and which does not necessarily have to have a causal relationship with this treatment (ICH E2A).

Any unfavorable and unintended sign (including an abnormal laboratory finding, for example), symptom, or disease temporally associated with the use of any dose of a medicinal product, whether or not considered related to the medicinal product (ICH E2A).

Adverse Event/Adverse Experience—EMA

Any untoward medical occurrence in a patient or clinical-trial subject administered a medicinal product and which does not necessarily have to have a causal relationship with this treatment (Article 2(m) of Directive 2001/20/EC). An adverse event can therefore be any unfavourable and unintended sign (e.g. an abnormal laboratory finding), symptom, or disease temporally associated with the use of a medicinal product, whether or not considered related to the medicinal product (EMA, Volume 9A).

Adverse Experience/Event—FDA

The FDA uses the term *adverse event/experience* and defines it as follows for postmarketing cases:

Any adverse event associated with the use of a drug in humans, whether or not considered drug related, including the following: An adverse event occurring in the course of the use of a drug product in professional practice; an adverse event occurring from drug overdose whether accidental or intentional; an adverse event occurring from drug abuse; an adverse event occurring from drug withdrawal; and any failure of expected pharmacological action (21CFR314.80(a)).

For clinical trial cases, FDA revised the definition effective March 2011 to read as follows (21CFR312.32):

Any untoward medical occurrence associated with the use of a drug in humans, whether or not considered drug-related.

In practice most people use the term *adverse event* (AE) to refer to any "bad thing" that occurs during the use of a drug without implying that the bad thing is due to the drug. The bad thing may be due to the drug substance, excipients, packaging, or storage issues, and may or may not be due to the active ingredient.

Adverse Reaction

In the preapproval (i.e., not yet marketed, experimental) phase of a product, the definition is as follows: "All noxious and unintended responses to a medicinal product related to any dose should be considered adverse drug reactions." This means "that a causal relationship between a medicinal product and an adverse event is at least a reasonable possibility, i.e. the relationship cannot be ruled out" (ICH E2A).

For postapproval (i.e., marketed) products, the definition is as follows: "A response to a drug which is noxious and unintended and which occurs at doses normally used in man for prophylaxis, diagnosis, or therapy of disease or for modification of physiological function" (ICH E2A).

Note that this is one of the few areas where the preapproval definition is different from the marketed definition. The issue here revolves around implied causality (see Chapter 13).

Serious Adverse Event and Serious Adverse Reaction

A serious adverse event (experience) or serious adverse reaction is any untoward medical occurrence that at any dose:

■ Results in death
■ Is life-threatening

   Note: The term *life-threatening* in the definition of *serious* refers to an event in which the patient was at risk of death at the time of the event; it does not refer to an event that hypothetically might have caused death if it were more severe:

■ Requires inpatient hospitalization or prolongation of existing hospitalization
■ Results in persistent or significant disability/incapacity or
■ Is a congenital anomaly/birth defect

Medical and scientific judgment should be exercised in deciding whether expedited reporting is appropriate in other situations, such as important medical events that may not be immediately life-threatening or result in death or hospitalization but may jeopardize the patient or may require intervention to prevent one of the other outcomes listed in the definition above. These should also usually be considered serious.

Examples of such events are intensive treatment in an emergency room or at home for allergic bronchospasm; blood dyscrasias or convulsions that do not result in hospitalization; or development of drug dependency or drug abuse (ICH E2A).

The Food and Drug Administration (FDA) (21CFR312.32, 21CFR314.80(a)) and EMA (Volume 9A and 10) definitions are similar but do differ somewhat. Note that an event or reaction may meet one or more of the criteria for seriousness simultaneously. Only one is needed, however, to consider the event or reaction to be serious. For an individual case safety report (ICSR) to be serious, it takes only one serious AE out of all the AEs present. To be a nonserious ICSR, all the AEs must be nonserious.

FDA's definition of "serious" for clinical trials (21CFR312.32(a)):

An adverse event or suspected adverse reaction is considered "serious" if, in the view of either the investigator or sponsor, it results in any of the following outcomes: Death, a life-threatening adverse event, inpatient hospitalization or prolongation of existing hospitalization, a persistent or significant incapacity or substantial disruption of the ability to conduct normal life functions, or a congenital anomaly/birth defect. Important medical events that may not result in death, be life-threatening, or require hospitalization may be considered serious when, based upon appropriate medical judgment, they may jeopardize the patient or subject and may require medical or surgical intervention to prevent one of the outcomes listed in this definition. Examples of such medical events include allergic bronchospasm requiring intensive treatment in an emergency room or at home, blood dyscrasias or convulsions that do not result in inpatient hospitalization, or the development of drug dependency or drug abuse.

Note that this now includes both the investigator and the sponsor. Either may declare an event/reaction to be serious. FDA also moved the idea of "disability" directly into the definition in the section on incapacity.

A *suspected* adverse reaction is defined by FDA for clinical trials is:

Any adverse event for which there is a reasonable possibility that the drug caused the adverse event. For the purposes of IND safety reporting, "reasonable possibility" means there is evidence to suggest a causal relationship between the drug and the adverse event. Suspected adverse reaction implies a lesser degree of certainty about causality than adverse reaction, which means any adverse event caused by a drug.

Nonserious

An event or reaction that is nonserious (does not meet any of the criteria for seriousness).

Suspected Adverse Drug Reaction (SADR)

A noxious and unintended response to any dose of a drug or biologic product for which there is a reasonable possibility that the product caused the response. In this definition, the phrase "a reasonable possibility" means that the relationship cannot be ruled out (ICH E2A).

The point here is the word *suspected*, which means some level of causality with the drug in question, is present. It may be serious or nonserious.

Serious, Unexpected, Adverse Drug Reaction

An SADR that is serious and unexpected. See the definitions for serious and unexpected. The FDA does not use this definition formally for cases, though the concept is similar.

Serious, Expected, Adverse Drug Reaction

An SADR that is serious and expected. See the definitions for serious and expected. The FDA does not use this definition formally for cases, though the concept is similar.

Suspected Adverse Reaction—FDA

Any adverse event for which there is a reasonable possibility that the drug caused the adverse event. For the purposes of IND safety reporting, "reasonable possibility" means there is evidence to suggest a causal relationship between the drug and the adverse event.

Suspected adverse reaction implies a lesser degree of certainty about causality than adverse reaction, which means any adverse event caused by a drug (21CFR312.32).

Suspected, Unexpected, Serious Adverse (Drug) Reaction (SUSAR)—EMA

An SADR suspected of being due to the drug in question (causality) and unexpected. See the definitions for serious and unexpected.

Unexpected—FDA

FDA issued new final rules effective March 2011 in which they change and explain their concept of unexpected. Previously the idea was that an adverse event would be unexpected if it was possibly associated with or related to the use of the drug. FDA has now changed this definition for clinical trial (IND) reporting to read as follows:

For a pre-marketed product: An adverse event or suspected adverse reaction is considered "unexpected" if it is not listed in the investigator brochure or is not listed at the specificity or severity that has been observed….For example, under this definition, hepatic necrosis would be unexpected (by virtue of greater severity) if the investigator brochure referred only to elevated hepatic enzymes or hepatitis. Similarly, cerebral thromboembolism and cerebral vasculitis would be unexpected (by virtue of greater specificity) if the investigator brochure listed only cerebral vascular accidents. "Unexpected," as used in this definition, also refers to adverse events or suspected adverse reactions that are mentioned in the investigator brochure as occurring with a class of drugs or as anticipated from the pharmacological properties of the drug, but are not specifically mentioned as occurring with the particular drug under investigation (21CFR312.32(a)).

For marketed products: Any adverse drug experience that is not listed in the current labeling (Package Insert or Summary of Product Characteristics (SPC)) for the drug product. This includes events that may be symptomatically and pathophysiologically related to an event listed in the labeling, but differ from the event because of greater severity or specificity. For example, under this definition, hepatic necrosis would be unexpected (by virtue of greater severity) if the labeling only referred to elevated hepatic enzymes or hepatitis (21CFR314.80(a)).

Note that AEs that are "class related" (i.e., allegedly seen with all products in this class of drugs) and are mentioned in the labeling (Package Insert or SPC) or investigator brochure but are not specifically described as occurring with this product are considered unexpected.

Unexpected Adverse Reaction—EMA

An adverse reaction, the nature, severity or outcome of which is not consistent with the Summary of Product Characteristics (SPC) (Article 1(13) of Directive 2001/83/EC67). This includes class-related reactions which are mentioned in the SPC but which are not specifically described as occurring with this product. For products authorised nationally, the relevant SPC is that approved by the Competent Authority in the Member State to whom the reaction is being reported. For centrally authorised products, the relevant SPC is the SPC authorised by the European Commission. During the time period between a CHMP Opinion in favour of granting a marketing authorisation

and the Commission Decision granting the marketing authorisation, the relevant SPC is the SPC annexed to the CHMP Opinion (Volume 9A).

These adverse reactions, when the SPC is used as the reference document, are referred to as *unlabeled*. This is quite different from *unlisted* (see below).

Unlisted Adverse Reaction—EMA

An adverse reaction that is not specifically included as a suspected adverse effect in the Company Core Safety Information (CCSI). This includes an adverse reaction whose nature, severity, specificity or outcome is not consistent with the information in the CCSI. It also includes class-related reactions which are mentioned in the CCSI but which are not specifically described as occurring with this product. (Volume 9A)

Expected

As opposed to "unexpected," an event that is noted in the investigator brochure or labeling (Package Insert or SPC). The complication in the European Union (EU) is that two different reference documents (labels) are used for marketed drugs for expectedness. One is the global EU-level label (SPC) and the other is the company's core safety labeling (CCSI). Usually, these are quite similar if not identical, but not always. An event/reaction may be found in one, the other, or both. If it is not found in the SPC, it is considered unlabeled. If it is not found in the core labeling of each member state, it is unlisted.

Thus, an event in the United States is expected or unexpected depending on whether it is found in the reference document: the investigator's brochure for unapproved products and the approved labeling for marketed products. In the Eurpean Union, it is the same for unapproved products, but for marketed products an unexpected event/reaction may be unlabeled (not in the SPC) or unlisted (not in the CCSI).

■ The Practice

In practice, these definitions are rather murky and confusing. It is not clear that FDA's recent attempts to clarify the pre-marketing definitions have improved the situation. Attempts have been made to standardize this nomenclature around ICH/Council for International Organizations of Medical Sciences (CIOMS) definitions. This may succeed at some point in the future but all these terms will be used in various ways and places for some time to come.

AEs are unintended "bad things" that occur when taking a drug (or biologic or vaccine, etc.). They may or may not be due to the drug itself (the "active moiety," or "active pharmacological ingredient" [API]), the formulation, excipients in the product (e.g., the inactive ingredients, fillers), the packaging (e.g., leaching of products from a container into the liquid drug product), a contaminant, manufacturing problems, the underlying disease, or some other unknown cause or causes. Thus, an AE does not imply that the drug (i.e., the active component) caused the bad thing to occur.

An ADR or AR is an AE in which there is "reasonable possibility" of a causal relationship between the drug and the AE. Some interpret this to mean that the relationship cannot be ruled out. This is probably too extreme as it implies that unless causality can be absolutely, positively ruled out, it is "possibly related" or that there is a "reasonable possibility" of causality. FDA in its guidance on IND Safety Reporting of September 2010 (http://www.fda.gov/downloads/Drugs/GuidanceComplianceRegulatoryInformation/Guidances/UCM227351.pdf) discussed this at length and indicated that they do not want to see cases reported as expedited reports if there is "not enough evidence to suggest that there was a reasonable possibility that the drug caused the AE." This is done to increase the likelihood that the information sent to FDA will be "interpretable and will meaningfully contribute to the developing safety profile of the investigational drug and improve the overall quality of safety reporting." The notion of causality is discussed in much greater detail in Chapter 13. Thus, an AE possibly or probably due to the drug is an ADR or AR.

These terms are being replaced in practice by "suspected adverse drug reaction" (SADR), which emphasizes the suspicion that the drug is *a* possible cause of the bad thing or is *the* possible cause of the bad thing. Following logically from this, we now have the term *suspected, unexpected, serious adverse reaction* (SUSAR). The addition of the words "serious" and "unexpected" to the SADR term represents the criteria for submission as expedited reports (see Chapters 15 and 16) to government health agencies in many countries of serious reactions from clinical trials.

Suspected, expected, serious adverse reactions usually do not have to be submitted as expedited reports

Table 1.1	
AE	Adverse event or adverse experience
AR	Adverse reaction
ADE	Adverse drug event
ADR	Adverse drug reaction
SAE	Serious adverse event
SAR	Serious adverse reaction
SADR	Suspected adverse drug reaction
SUSAR	Suspected, unexpected, serious adverse reaction
NSAE	Nonserious adverse event
NSAR	Nonserious adverse reaction

to governmental agencies. They are usually submitted periodically (e.g., yearly) or at the end of the study in the final study report (Table 1.1).

Expectedness represents an often highly subjective area. An event or reaction is expected if it is found in the product reference document (IB for clinical trials and the postmarketing labeling for approved drugs). More specific or more severe events or reactions, however, are considered to be unexpected. Thus, if "pneumonia" is in the brochure or product labeling and the patient has "streptococcal pneumonia," this is considered unexpected because the "streptococcal" designation is more specific. Similarly, "fatal pneumonia" is considered unexpected if only pneumonia is labeled. See Chapter 13 on expectedness.

The bottom line here is that there are multiple definitions and variants floating around. They all more or less add up to the same cases being "expeditable" in the United States, European Union, and elsewhere. There are nuanced differences in the definitions of related/unrelated, but fundamentally what they come down to is that cases that are serious (death, life-threatening, hospitalization, disability/incapacity, birth defect) and related ("reasonable possibility" that the AE is due to the drug) and unexpected (not in the IB or only included in the class labeling section) are expeditable in the clinical trial setting. In general, one should be conservative in applying the definitions, and if one has to discuss or debate whether something is serious and/or related and/or unexpected, then it is. That is, if there is any doubt about any of these three definitions, choose the more conservative approach (serious, related, unexpected).

2

Clinical Trials, Clinical Research Organizations, Phases I–IV, and Investigator-Initiated Trials

To obtain approval to market a new drug in the United States, Canada, the European Union, and most other countries, a series of clinical trials on patients is required. The extent of the trials depends on the drug (already approved for other uses or formulations, a new breakthrough product, expected to be very toxic, etc.), the disease or indication treated (severe diseases such as advanced cancer vs. mild allergies, diseases with no known treatments, rare diseases with few patients afflicted, etc.), the nature of the patients studied (healthy, very ill, young, old, etc.), experience in other countries where it is already sold, and other factors.

After the appropriate pharmacology and toxicology testing in vitro and in animals, development of small-scale and sometimes (even at this early stage) larger-scale manufacturing procedures, and other preparatory testing, the drug is ready to be used in humans in the so-called first in man, or first in humans, study. In the United States, a company (sometimes an individual or an academic center) submits an Investigational New Drug Application (IND) to the Food and Drug Administration (FDA) (or the equivalent to a health authority outside the United States) containing the preparatory data. This is, in most cases, data that are proprietary and not available to the public. In addition, the submitter includes in the package a protocol for a clinical trial in humans.

Drug trials are heavily regulated, and multiple layers of protections and precautions have been developed to protect the subjects. These include investigational review boards, data safety monitoring boards, sponsor and health authority scrutiny, and some level of public notification and publicizing of the study on the internet (clinical trial registries). Trials are divided into four phases, although there is usually some overlap.

■ Phase I

Phase I trials actually belong to human pharmacology, in contrast to animal pharmacology. These are the first steps in determining the profile of both the beneficial and the untoward effects in humans. They are designed mainly to find the maximum tolerated dose and the pathways for metabolizing and eliminating the drug. Safety is more important in this phase than efficacy. The first study is often a single-dose trial in a small number (e.g., a dozen) of healthy, often male (to avoid any possible pregnancy issues), volunteers. If tolerated, a multiple-dose study and a rising-dose study follow. The aim of phase I trials is to study absorption, distribution in the body, metabolism, and excretion (so-called ADME studies) as well as safety and toxicity.

Other things that may be examined include the proposed formulation to be used in subsequent trials and marketing (as they may be different) and the dosing frequency or schedule. Drug interaction studies may be done in phase I or later in phase II. If the drugs are known to be toxic or have severe and predictable ADRs, these studies are often done for ethical reasons in patients with the disease to be treated rather than in healthy volunteers (e.g., cancer chemotherapy or AIDS). Each study is short, often running no more than a few days to a few weeks at most. The trial design is usually simple and open label. They may or may not be controlled. Several phase I studies often take a year or so and may include around 100 patients in total.

There is usually no benefit to the subjects in the trial, and they participate either because of generosity of spirit or because they are paid. Because there is no gain to the individual subjects, all efforts are made to minimize the risk of toxicity. Serious adverse events are usually rare in phase I trials. Subjects are often "housed" for these studies in special clinical research centers run by academic medical centers or clinical research organizations (CROs). Note that the term *subjects* in this context usually refers to "normal people," not patients. The term *patients* is usually used to refer to people with the disease in question and not "normal" people. Hence, phase I trials usually involve healthy subjects, and phase II, III, and IV trials involve patients. This distinction is not always followed, and some use the terms interchangeably.

Adverse events seen in phase I trials are always noteworthy because the subjects are usually normal and a low starting dose of the drug in question is usually used. Because few subjects are studied in phase I, any AE should be investigated thoroughly. SAEs and the rare death seen in phase I trials should be looked at immediately, and if the event is severe, stopping further dosing or enrollment should be considered. Note that the FDA now requires all serious AEs (whether labeled or not, whether felt to be due to the drug or not) to be submitted as expedited reports. In addition to the toxicity of the drug preparation, subjects have been known to hide serious medical problems or medical history to participate in the study, especially if the subjects are compensated.

■ Phase II

Phase II trials are done after the drug has successfully passed through all or parts of phase I trials. Phase II trials are usually performed in patients afflicted with the disease for which that drug was developed. Whereas phase I trials are usually done for safety, phase II trials are done for both efficacy and safety. The goal is to find the minimal effective dose that retains efficacy with the minimum of AEs. These studies may also continue the ADME investigations of phase I as well as develop safety and efficacy markers and tests for subsequent larger phase III trials. The studies may include up to hundreds of patients and are usually double blinded. They may run several weeks or months.

Sponsors and investigators participating in phase II trials must pay particular attention to toxicity because unexpected SAEs and even deaths may occur. Severe and unexpected toxicity may force the immediate stopping of the study or a midstream alteration of the protocol and informed consent to decrease toxicity. Patients in phase II trials usually are not compensated for their participation.

Special studies may be done in phase I, II, III, or IV, such as drug-interaction studies (sometimes in healthy volunteers, sometimes in patients with the disease), food or alcohol interaction studies, and evaluation studies in renal failure or liver failure patients. These special studies, however, are usually required for the MA or NDA submission and so must be done at some point.

Some drugs or products (e.g., oncology drugs or herbals) may not fully undergo phase I and phase II testing as is classically done and as described above. Oncology drugs, which are often very toxic, are rarely studied in normals but are used directly in patients with malignancy. Similarly, "orphan drugs," which are drugs developed for rare diseases, may undergo abbreviated testing.

■ Phase III

Phase III is often divided into phases IIIA and IIIB. Phase III trials include hundreds to thousands of patients, and the whole phase may take several years to complete, depending on the treatment duration and outcomes of the disease studied. Each individual trial may include multiple sites on one or more continents and run months to a year or more. (Survival studies may take even longer because the study does not end until the last patient dies.) The goal is regulatory approval to market the drug.

Phase IIIA trials are usually the key (the old term is "pivotal") studies to be submitted for regulatory approval, and they are incorporated in the NDA submission or "MA dossier." The design used in these trials is usually double blind, but many other varieties are used. Depending on the drug and disease under study, the comparator is either the known and accepted therapy called the "standard of care" (e.g., obligatory in almost all cancer, infection, severe pain trials) or placebo (e.g., in treating mild headache or nasal congestion). In some cases, the FDA and other agencies may require a placebo-controlled trial. This is becoming more and more controversial in terms of the ethics of using placebo. Many health agencies often prefer trials against the standard of care rather than placebo. Although both have a place in drug development, placebo trials are felt to be less and less acceptable.

Phase IIIB trials are additional (usually) large-scale studies that may be started during the examination of the initial dossier by the health agency (the reviewing process) and may end before or after the approval for marketing (NDA or MA). Because the total elapsed review time by the health agency may take a year or more, sponsors may continue studies during this review period. These studies may focus on pharmacoeconomic or risk evaluation issues as well as cost-effectiveness and studies against competitor drugs. Sometimes surprising or unexpected results of phase IIIA studies force late changes in phase IIIB studies. As most products now have full life cycle risk evaluation and management programs in place, additional testing may be added to phase III trials to evaluate risks that are unclear or that need further evaluation. By doing such testing in phase III, it may be possible to achieve more rapid marketing approval though postmarketing studies, and other commitments for risk evaluation, management, and mitigation may continue in phase IV.

■ Phase IV

Phase IV studies include different types of studies. They are done after the approval and marketing of the drug. Note that a drug may not always be marketed immediately after approval. Sometimes the company receiving the approval may choose to sell or out-license the drug, or timing may make it wiser to wait (e.g., new seasonal allergy drugs should be marketed near the time for the allergy season to hit). The health authority may require that certain phase IV studies be done as "commitments" immediately after marketing as a requirement of marketing approval. This may be done to clarify some safety and efficacy issues that remained after phase III but which the health agency believed were not sufficient to prevent or delay marketing of the drug. In the United States, the FDA now has the legal authority to require

phase IV commitments, including Risk Evaluation and Mitigation Strategies (REMS) and formal clinical or observational studies. Similarly, the EMA and member states may require further studies in their Risk Management Plans (RMPs). Failure to perform such tasks may result in penalties to the company or even withdrawal or limitation of the marketing approval.

Phase IV studies may also be marketing or pharmacoeconomic studies to aid in selling the product by studying head-on comparisons with competitor drugs. They may be studies looking at subgroups of the approved group and indication (e.g., testing a drug approved for diabetes on diabetics who are elderly or are also in heart failure). They may be done in children, not only to evaluate the usefulness and safety but also to obtain, in various markets, additional patent exclusivity.

Phase IV studies may be done for specific safety reasons to investigate an AE or a signal that has unexpectedly occurred after marketing. Such studies may be classical clinical trials or they may be observational or epidemiologic studies done in large databases. The design and size are very variable, ranging from small open-label trials to massive, multicenter, double-blind comparator trials or "large simple safety studies" with simple protocols and minimal record-keeping. Sometimes patients are compensated for participation.

So-called market-driven phase IV "seeding studies" are now forbidden in most parts of the world. These were pure marketing projects designed to encourage physicians to prescribe a particular product in place of a competitor's product. A protocol was usually written (to justify calling the endeavor a study) but was often of poor quality. Results were not always collected by the sponsor and, if collected, were often not analyzed. Prescribers were sometimes compensated. In a more subtle way, postmarketing trials for entirely legitimate purposes may include elements aimed at getting physicians to use the new drug in place of another product ("stealth seeding trials"). By doing this, the prescriber becomes familiar with the product, and the company hopes he or she will prescribe it for other patients after the trial is completed.

■ Late Phase Studies

A term that has appeared in the last few years is *late phase studies*, referring to the grab bag of requirements that agencies and companies are doing both for registration, risk, and marketing reasons. They include registries (product, disease, safety/ADR), postmarketing observational studies, classic phase IV trials as discussed earlier, clinical effectiveness trials, OTC trials, community-based trials, health economic and outcomes studies (retrospective, prospective, observational), cost effectiveness, burden of illness, patient reported outcome (PRO, quality of life [QoL], chart review, survey (physicians, patients), health economic piggyback trials, risk management, expanded access, drug safety, and others.

■ Investigator-Initiated Trials or Studies

Investigator-initiated trials (IITs) or studies (IISs), also called investigator-sponsored trials (ISTs), are usually new ideas thought up by researchers in the academic world or occasionally suggested by the pharmaceutical company. New uses or ways of administering drugs are frequently proposed by academic researchers to pharmaceutical companies. Many companies actually have physicians, PhDs, or pharmacologists on staff (often called "medical liaisons") who travel to academic medical centers and seek out such clever new uses. Such trials are usually done at single centers. Sometimes the investigator will come up with the idea and approach the company (sponsor or patent holder) for assistance with either a grant or product supply (especially if the product is costly).

This type of study can be instrumental in the scientific development of a drug. The advantages of IITs are that new ideas are found and explored, costs are usually fairly small, and the studies can be done fairly quickly. The disadvantage is that many details that should be determined before the trials are not addressed (e.g., effective dose and safety in this population). An IIT that fails usually ends that idea. Thus, if too low a dose is chosen, one might never know that a higher dose would produce positive results. Funding is usually from the pharmaceutical company in the form of a grant-in-aid, drug supply, protocol, or case report form support. A contract or agreement is usually signed by both parties. The legal sponsor of the study is not the pharmaceutical company but rather the investigator. It is he or she who opens the IND with the FDA or the equivalent in other countries (often with the help of the pharmaceutical company). The usual safety provisions are followed: Good Clinical Practices, investigational review boards, and SAE reporting to the health agency by the investigator. Note that FDA in its 2011 IND regulatory rules requires the investigator/sponsor to handle safety reporting to the FDA, IRB etc. as if he/she were a sponsor such as a pharmaceutical company. Most pharmaceutical companies also require the investigator

to report SAEs to the company (in addition to the health authority) so that the company maintains a full safety database for all uses of a product. It is less clear from FDA regulations whether the pharmaceutical company should also submit the cases if the company receives them from the investigator of an IIT who is required to submit them directly to FDA. These trials would technically be phase I if a new indication, formulation, or delivery is being studied. If not, they would most probably be considered phase IV trials. Not all studies require an IND (if the use of the drug is fully covered within the approved labeling). Such studies usually have to be registered with the appropriate health authority and clinical trial database (e.g., clinicaltrials.gov in the United States and EudraCT in the European Union).

In earlier years, disputes occurred over ownership of data and the publication (or rather lack of publication) of negative results. These are resolving, in general, with both parties retaining "ownership" of data and with the right to publish retained by the investigator regardless of the results.

■ Other Study Related Issues

Study phases are often hazier than the "official" schema described above. Phase I studies that go beyond the initial dose finding and escalation studies are often done throughout the phases over several years. If a drug does not go beyond phase II because of lack of efficacy (i.e., the company "kills" it), there is little point in doing drug, food, or alcohol interaction studies early in the course of development.

Some companies have been known to try to speed up development (and lower costs) by doing somewhat larger phase II trials that, should they succeed, are submitted to the health agencies as combined phase II–III trials for approval. For critical drugs, this may be advantageous as long as it does not compromise the safety and efficacy evaluations. In general, the more patients who are studied, the more comfortable one is with the safety profile of the drug. Smaller safety databases obtained in phases I–III may require larger postmarketing safety study commitments to obtain additional information to adequately evaluate the benefit/risk profile as larger numbers of disparate patients use the drug.

Phase I studies are created and supervised in most pharmaceutical companies by a dedicated phase I group (e.g., the pharmacokinetics/pharmacodynamics group) usually run by pharmacologists (PhDs, PharmDs) and physicians. The actual study is often outsourced to CROs or academic centers (clinical research units), where the patient enrollment and dosing occur.

Phases II and III are usually run by "high power" clinical or medical research groups within the company led by physicians (often subspecialists such as cardiologists, oncologists, etc.). These studies are complex and have large infrastructures supporting them in biostatistics, study-site monitoring, in-house data monitoring, clinical research, regulatory affairs, safety monitors, quality control, quality assurance, external data monitoring committees, and so on. Many companies, particularly smaller ones, also outsource the trials (or parts of the trials) to one or more CROs and other vendors. These studies are rigorously done and are likely to be audited by the health authority before marketing approval. These studies may run into tens of millions of dollars and require complex organization, project management, and information technology support.

Phase IV studies may be done by the phase II–III group or by a separate postmarketing group. If phase IV studies are done in the clinical research department, the rigor of the earlier phases usually carries over to these phase IV studies. If the phase IV studies are done by the marketing department in isolation from the clinical research group, these studies may be somewhat more variable in quality and rigor. Some companies now have separate Safety/Epidemiology/Risk Management departments that handle postmarketing clinical and epidemiologic trials (but not the marketing studies). Many of these are now outsourced to CROs or firms specializing in "late phase" trials.

Some company executives have argued that small phase IV marketing studies or IITs are dangerous because they might discover some safety "problem" and might fail to show efficacy, thus doubly hurting the drug. Safety officers often argue just the reverse: these studies may uncover a previously unknown safety issue that can now be added to the product labeling to better inform prescribers and patients.

Clinical trial registries have been set up by health authorities and governments (clinicaltrials.gov in the United States and EudraCT in Europe) as well as by pharmaceutical companies and others in which all or almost all research trials are now posted, in detail, on a website. It has been felt by some that this will raise the standards for all trials and allow for easier data comparisons. That is not yet clear. Several things have happened, though. Patients and disease support groups are now more easily able to find and track studies involving their disease by simply searching through the databases. There is also a new industry that mines the databases for information on patient and investigator availability, enrollment, completion dates, and so forth.

IITs have traditionally posed problems. IITs are usually encouraged by companies by having roving medical liaisons visit academic medical centers to seek out new trials. These visiting medical liaisons may or may not be trained in classic clinical research methodology. They may also do "in-service" teaching or training on the company's new products in the medical centers. Thus, this role combines a medical and a marketing function. In well-structured pharmaceutical companies, protocols submitted by academics are reviewed by the clinical research department, the statisticians, and the pharmacovigilance group to ensure good quality. A formal contract requiring completion, a final report within a finite period (e.g., 1 year), and SAE reporting must be done under good clinical practices. Pharmacovigilance departments in companies usually submit the SAEs to their own MAs, NDAs, and INDs, as the case may be, even if the investigator has said he or she has also done so. In less well-structured companies, the medical marketing group may be less well-connected to the other research groups and details may slip.

Other types of outreach programs (sometimes in combination with registries) are also used by companies for various reasons:

- To help patients finish the course of therapy when they are already taking the drug
- As part of a REMS/RMP as an ETASU (an "element to assure safe use of the drug")
- To help sell the drug

In particular, for chronic therapy diseases such as cancer, hepatitis, and hypertension, companies have found that it is good medicine and good marketing to encourage patients to stay on their therapy to the end (until the cancer is in remission or cured, the viral titers drop, etc.). This means continued sales of the drug as well as successful patient treatment. The usual reasons for stopping therapy are AEs, dosing problems, or convenience reasons. Outreach programs that use nurses or pharmacists to contact patients every week or month on how to handle AEs and other issues are now common. When the therapy is done well, the patient's physician is kept informed of issues and progress and is able to work with the patient and the outreach staff to get the patient over rough patches in the treatment regimen. AE data must be collected by the company, kept in the safety database, and reported to the health authority as required.

■ Frequently Asked Questions

Q: Does the company have to collect all AEs from all trials?

A: Basically yes, in one form or another. First, it is good medicine to collect all serious and nonserious AEs so that one fully understands the safety profile of the product. Second, it is legally required. In practice, in clinical trials only SAEs must be collected by the drug safety group and reported either in 7 or 15 days, or periodically in yearly reports. Nonserious AEs and some SAEs (e.g., expected SAEs that the sponsor and health authority agree will be reported only at the end of the study) do not get reported until the final study report.

What this means is that in many pharmaceutical companies two databases contain safety information. There is the drug safety database maintained by the drug safety group for expedited and periodic regulatory reporting and the clinical research database for marketing authorization and NDA submissions. The safety database contains all serious clinical trial AEs (as well as all serious and nonserious postmarketing AEs) but not nonserious clinical trial AEs. This database is dynamic and always up to date. The clinical research database contains the (paper or electronic) case report form information, including all serious and nonserious AEs.

Sometimes data are not entered into the clinical research database rapidly but rather only when paper case report forms arrive in the research department, perhaps monthly or even less frequently. In other cases, where electronic data capture is used instead of paper CRFs, the data entry at the site may be delayed or incomplete. Some companies using electronic data capture also require an e-mail, fax, or direct download of EDC data into the safety department's database. Nonetheless, the use of electronic case records should make data available more rapidly than in paper-based studies.

Having two databases produces various problems. To get a full picture of the safety in the trial, one must obtain the SAEs from the safety group (their database is usually up to date) and the nonserious AEs from the clinical research group's database (which may not be up to date). The data outputs must then be combined (a problem if the two database outputs are not compatible or normalized) to have a full data set. In addition, the SAEs in the two safety databases must be reconciled if the same SAE safety data are collected in two different places or in two different ways (e.g., EDC and e-mail/fax of the case to the sponsor's drug safety group).

Signaling investigations should be done using all serious and nonserious clinical trial data no matter where they are stored or how they are obtained. This may mean the creation of a "data warehouse" to allow access to the data contained in both databases. It is likely that, as EDC and health data standardization advance, clinical trial safety data will be collected in one place without the need for double collecting systems. Modernizing clinical trial data collection will have many implications:

- Safety data (serious and nonserious AEs) would be received in real time.
- Electronic data entry would be done remotely at each study site rather than centrally at the company or CRO. This takes the data entry out of the direct control of the company or CRO and put into the hands of employees (of variable skill levels and oversight) at each investigational site. Issues with training, personnel turnover, and quality maintenance at each site now become critical.
- The company drug safety database may not be linked electronically to the EDC database, and new procedures would have to be developed to get the safety data to the safety group for entry into the safety database in an accurate and timely manner.
- Source documents (e.g., laboratory tests, x-ray reports) might not be sent to the company now that studies are "paperless." In fact, source documents may now be electronic, because the classic case report form no longer exists. Where paper source documents exist, they may need to be scanned and added to the EDC, clinical trial, or safety databases.
- Getting follow-up information, which was always a challenge, would still remain difficult.

One can envisage the day when the United States, the European Union, and other medical systems are standardized and online. All data, including study data and safety data, will be sent electronically in real time and simultaneously to all needed databases at the company, the health agencies, the hospital, the insurance companies, and so on. Safety data will be accurate and rapidly received everywhere they are needed. Maybe.

Q: Are phase IV study SAEs reportable as clinical trial AEs (to the IND in the United States) or as postmarketing AEs (to the NDA in the United States), or as both?

A: If a study is done under an IND or a similar premarketing situation, then the SAEs that meet reporting criteria are reported to the IND. Many companies believe that the NDA/MA takes precedence over the IND and would report those SAEs to the NDA/MA also. This may vary from country to country, so local rules and regulations must be checked. SAEs from studies not done under an IND should be reported to the NDA and in most jurisdictions treated as postmarketing AEs. The FDA published a summary of the United States requirements in its September 2010 Guidance:

Drug marketed or approved* in U.S.?	Under U.S. IND?	Trial site location	Must report to IND?	Must report per postmarket requirements?
Yes	Yes	U.S. or Foreign	Yes	Yes
Yes	No	U.S. or Foreign	No	Yes
No	Yes	U.S. or Foreign	Yes	
No	No	Foreign		

*If a drug is approved in the United States, but is not currently being marketed in the United States, the postmarket requirements would still apply.

Q: If multiple companies or investigators are involved in a trial (whether it is an IIT or a formal company sponsored trial), should there be double (or even triple) reporting just to be sure the cases are not missed?

A: No. There is no reason for duplicate reporting in general. If more than one company is involved, the protocol or other formal written document should contain an agreed-upon mechanism for a single company to handle safety reporting. In such situations, both companies may keep the AEs in their respective databases, but only one company should submit the cases to the regulatory authorities both as expedited and aggregate (annual) reports.

In some situations, however, companies request that the investigator doing an IIT send a copy of each SAE ICSR to the company. The investigator, as the sponsor, must report such cases to the regulatory authority. The company, in many cases, will also report the case to the regulatory authority "just to be sure," noting in the transmission that this is an IIT and that the investigator is the sponsor and should be submitting the case.

Q: Should AEs be reported from observational or epidemiologic trials or registries?

A: This again may vary from country to country, but in general, if a case meets the four validity criteria, then it should be submitted even if it is not from a classic clinical trial. In its September 2010 Guidance the FDA clarified this issue by saying that such cases must be reported. For large amounts of data (e.g., "data dumps" from poison control centers), the sponsor may wish to discuss with the agency how such large numbers of cases should be handled.

Q: I thought most of the reporting requirements for clinical trial SAE cases have been harmonized, so why does it seem so complex?

A: To a degree, there has been harmonization. Clinical trial deaths and life-threatening SAEs that are unlabeled and possibly related to the study drug are reportable in 7 and 15 days, respectively. However, there are many exceptions or other requirements (e.g., review of similar cases for the FDA and others), local language requirements if the case is a domestic case, nonexpedited reporting if the case is not domestic, and so forth. Some countries want or require electronic reporting and others still take or require paper reports (e.g., CIOMS I forms). It is likely things will harmonize eventually, but they are not yet at the level of harmonization for postmarketing reports. Note that there are different requirements for devices, and, in some countries, there are different requirements for over-the-counter products, neutraceuticals, biologics, and herbals. Finally, a drug may be in clinical trials and not yet approved for marketing in one country, and approved and marketed in another country with different reporting requirements. Keep in mind also that the United States spells "harmonization" with a "z" (pronounced "zee" in the United States and "zed" elsewhere) and the UK and others as "harmonisation" with an "s." So we have not yet even harmonized spelling and pronunciation!

3

Spontaneous Postmarketing Adverse Events

Their pivotal and irreplaceable role in providing safety information when a wider population is exposed to a new product.

Before a drug comes to market, it is studied in patients in clinical trials that aim to show efficacy of the product for a particular selected disease in a highly selected sample of the population. The clinical trials may be large, covering up to 10,000 patients, or very small, covering dozens to hundreds of patients (e.g., for orphan drugs). The clinical trials also aim to define the safety profile of the drug, at least in this selected population with this selected disease.

These studies, which are (usually) carried out with rigorous and highly regulated methodology, have significant limitations in defining the safety profile. They generally only find frequently occurring AEs. For example, if in studying 10,000 patients not a single patient has a particular AE, such as a heart attack, we can be only 95% confident that the chance of having a heart attack based on the data from this trial is less than 1 in 3,333. If we raise the safety threshold to be 99% confident that a heart attack has an incidence of only 1 in 10,000 with this drug, we would need to have no heart attacks in

46,000 patients studied. In other words, studying even 5000 or 10,000 patients does not give a warm enough or fuzzy enough feeling that the major or rare safety issues have been identified before the drug goes on the market for large-scale use.

This means that the uncommon AEs and even the fairly common AEs (e.g., an incidence of 1 in 500) will not be picked up until the drug is extensively used in the general population after marketing. When, say, a million people start using a new drug in the months after a product launch, a "rare" AE with a 1 in 10,000 incidence rate could be expected in about 100 patients. Should the AE in question be dramatic and rapidly discovered, such as torsades de pointes, aplastic anemia, or rhabdomyolysis (a severe skeletal muscle injury), there will be a torrent of recriminations about why this was not discovered earlier during the clinical testing. The correct response is that the testing of only 5,000 to 10,000 patients could not pick up such a rare event because this is the way the drug approval system is designed. This response is usually lost in the clamor. There are now attempts under way to get a better handle on the safety profile before marketing and to follow the safety (and benefit) profile after marketing in a much more rigorous manner.

Also of note is that the clinical trials are often done in a narrow group of patients. For example, an antihistamine may be tested in otherwise healthy adults between 18 and 60 years of age with allergies. Even if the drug is only approved for use in this population, physicians in most jurisdictions have the right (which they freely exercise) to prescribe the drug for anyone and for any disease. Thus, many people with other diseases and at the extremes of the age range (the very old and young) receive the drug and may have AEs that the healthy 18- to 60-year-old study population did not experience in the clinical trials. The elderly, for example, are particularly sensitive to certain AEs (e.g., swallowing disorders) or to certain classes of psychotropic drugs.

Polypharmacy and drug interactions, among other things, cannot be adequately studied in the preapproval setting. Although food interaction studies and some drug interaction studies are done before approval, it is not possible to study "real world" patients (often elderly) who take many drugs and have peculiar or irregular eating and drinking habits. Even after marketing, it is difficult or even impossible to predict or know how the use of three, four, or more drugs given at the same time will act or interact.

Hence, particular attention must be paid to the time just after a product is first marketed to fully understand the drug's safety profile and minimize risks. In a sense, the first 500,000 to 1,000,000 patients prescribed the drug after launch are doing the large-scale safety testing.

What this means then is that the entire edifice of the drug safety system as it now stands depends on the good will and energy of nurses, pharmacists, physicians, and consumers to report AEs. Without them, no one would know of the AEs that are appearing as individual cases in isolated areas around the country or the world. These people must take time out of their day to report such events. The report will inevitably lead to a request for supplementary data (laboratory reports, cardiograms, hospital records, etc.) that are time- and effort-consuming. There is no evident or immediate gain to the reporter. The gain rather is to society at large, which is largely unaware of this noble effort.

Health authorities and regulators well understand the weakness of this system. Major efforts are now under way to look at how the spontaneous reporting system has worked in the past. That is, although we think it is useful and appropriate to rely on this system, did it, in fact, lead to early pick-up of serious problems, leading to a change in the product labeling and its use in clinical practice?

Various health agencies, particularly in North America and Europe, are looking at this question.

There is a lot more data sitting in various computers on drug safety that are not being looked at in a systematic manner. Obtaining these data on an ongoing basis and using them for safety analysis is an obvious way to identify a drug's safety profile. However, the devil is in the details. The databases around the world must be identified and the data extracted in a valid and consistent way. This is a very difficult task since data collection is not yet standardized. Multiple efforts (both nationally and globally) are under way to standardize and normalize data so that they are easily collected, databased, retrieved, and analyzed in a useful, valid, and rapid manner. If every encounter a patient has with the healthcare system is digitalized, we should be able to retrieve excellent safety data rapidly. This, however, will take years to achieve on a national level, let alone a global level. When this does occur, the spontaneous reporting system may then decrease in importance. The fundamental system now in place to discover AEs with marketed products remains the spontaneous reporting system. This system is used, in one form or another, in more than 50 countries around the world, including the United States, Canada, the European Union, Japan, Australia, New Zealand, and South Africa. The WHO and Uppsala Monitoring Centre are actively working with other countries to set up PV (pharmacovigilance) systems.

The principles of the system are simple. All healthcare professionals (and consumers in most countries, including the United States, the European Union, and Canada) are encouraged to spontaneously report AEs to either the manufacturer or the governmental healthcare agency or a third party. Standardized forms have been developed (the MedWatch form in the United States, the CIOMS I form elsewhere) specifically for this purpose and are available online, in publications (e.g., the *Physicians' Desk Reference* in the United States), as apps on the iPhone and other smartphones, and elsewhere. The form can be folded up and mailed (postage-free), faxed, or filled in online and uploaded to the healthcare agencies. Phone reports and faxes to the manufacturer and most health agencies are also possible.

The forms are one or two pages in length and include the expected information requests: patient demographics; the AEs that occurred; medical history; drugs taken, including the one or more drugs suspected of causing the AE in question; comedications; dose and timing; a narrative summary of the case; and reporter information. In most cases, confidentiality is guaranteed by law, regulation, or policy regarding the patient's identity and the reporter's identity. In online systems, the "forms" may be intelligent in the sense that the context determines which questions are asked. For example, if the patient is a male, the pregnancy questions will be eliminated from the online form.

In the United States, the United Kingdom, and other countries, information submitted spontaneously to the health authority is available for free or for a small fee to anyone in the public under Freedom of Information Acts. The cases are redacted before being released by the health agency to avoid identifying the patient or reporter. In the United States, in 2008 approximately 33,000 reports were sent directly to FDA (6% of the total reports received) with the remaining approximately 493,000 (94%) to the manufacturers, who then forward them to the FDA. Most reporters tend to be pharmacists. In 2004, the FDA's Office of Drug Safety noted in its annual report (Web Resource 3-1) that the breakdown of the sources of reports was as follows:

Pharmacists, 37%

Physicians, 12%

Nurses, 11%

Dentists, <1%

Unknown, 23%

Consumers, 17%

The requirements for AE reporting have largely been standardized through the International Conference on Harmonization (ICH). Reporting for healthcare professionals (and consumers in most places) is usually voluntary and is highly encouraged by agencies, although there is some skepticism about the utility and value of consumer reports, particularly those for OTC products and those not validated by a healthcare professional.

There is no time frame for reporting by a consumer or healthcare professional after the occurrence of the AE, but obviously rapid reporting is preferred for public health reasons; in some cases, it may save lives. For manufacturers, reporting is obligatory in almost all jurisdictions. Any AE that comes into a company, whether through sales representatives, phone calls, internet and e-mail, literature reports (which must be actively searched for by the company), or other media must be rapidly reviewed by qualified medical personnel.

For marketed drugs in most countries, all serious AEs that are unexpected (i.e., that do not appear in the approved product labeling) must be reported to the health authority by the company within 15 calendar days. In the United States, most of the remaining serious and nonserious cases must be reported to the FDA in NDA periodic reports (PADERs) or PSURs (quarterly for newer drugs and yearly for older drugs). In the European Union, Canada, and elsewhere (and soon perhaps in the United States), periodic reporting is done as PSURs, which are prepared every 6 months, yearly, or every 2.5, 3, or 5 years, depending on the age of the drug and the country receiving the report. Periodic reporting is not yet obligatory in Canada.

These reports contain line listings of various cuts of the data as well as medical analyses prepared by the company's medical team, usually headed by a physician. They look at AEs that are expected and unexpected and indicate which need to be added to the drug labeling as new ADRs, warnings, precautions, and so forth, and which AEs/ADRs need to be watched with heightened vigilance. These reports are then scrutinized by the regulatory agencies who may agree or disagree with the company analysis and who decide on changes to the drug labeling, conditions of marketing of the drug, and so forth. There is usually dialogue between the health agency and the company before an action is taken, though health authorities are empowered to act immediately and unilaterally if the public health is at risk. At the health agency, the data are then entered into a database and reviewed. Analysis of individual AE cases and of aggregates of AE cases is done.

Many countries send extracts from their spontaneous databases of local AE reports to the Uppsala Monitoring Centre (UMC) in Sweden (Web Resource 3-2). There are 96 full and 32 associate member countries that supply AE reports to the Centre, which has more than 5,000,000 cases. About half are from the United States, 10% from Canada, and 5% each from Germany, France, and Australia. Further information is available from the UMC describing the details of the database and the international monitoring system on its website (Web Resource 3-3). Extracts of the database are available for a fee from the UMC or from private vendors who have access to the database. Specifically regarding spontaneous reports, a company must set up a failure-proof system to receive, process, report, and analyze AEs. Time is of the essence, because some of the reports must be sent to the health authorities within 15 days. The clock for reporting starts counting down from the moment the first person anywhere in the company (or a partner, comarketer, etc.) hears about a "valid" AE.

For phone reports, this means that any phone number in the company is a potential source of AE reports, and anyone who answers the phone in the company must be instructed in what to do if an AE report comes into a place where it is not normally expected. A rapid and painless (to the caller) transfer system must be set up if the information is not immediately written down by the company employee first answering the call. No one wants to be kept on hold or to repeat the same story for the third or fourth time. No AE may be lost, so all efforts must be directed to the proper handling of the call. Because some AEs may need to be reported to one or more healthcare agencies within 15 days, time cannot be lost. The company must be ready to accept calls 24 hours a day, 7 days a week and in multiple languages if that is the normal custom in the country. Many companies do not maintain 24-hour coverage in their company, preferring to outsource this function to private companies (sometimes abroad, often in India). Many companies, even those maintaining a call center during business hours, outsource after-hours calls to poison control centers or private companies. Many companies also use this number (e.g., a toll-free number) for other functions, including product information, queries, and marketing.

Similarly, any e-mail or website in which an outsider can send a message or key in free text is a source of AEs. Many companies, much to their chagrin, receive complaints and AEs on job-posting websites, free sample websites, survey websites, message boards, and so forth.

Sales representatives must also be aware that a physician, pharmacist, or other healthcare worker they call on may be the source of an AE. Even innocuous off-the-cuff remarks about a possible AE ("Oh, by the way one of my patients took your other drug XXXX and had a heart attack the next day.") made to a company representative constitute a report to the company that must be acted on. Even offhand remarks over the barbecue on a Sunday afternoon in which a neighbor casually relates an AE to a company employee must be reported to the drug safety department!

Many companies have media services that review transcripts of newspapers, television shows, websites, blogs, and so forth, looking for anything about their products. Should AEs be noted, they must be sent to the safety department. There is no obligation to scan the Web, trawling for AEs, but anything found in the course of surfing is a reportable AE.

Lawsuits often represent the point of entry of AEs. The legal department must be aware that they must also report the AE noted in the suit to the safety department usually within 48 hours.

Some people still write "snail mail" letters, and the company mail room or mail screeners must be aware that AEs received in the mail are to be sent to the drug safety group immediately (usually by PDF/e-mail or fax and not interoffice mail).

One of the more complex problems companies face is the phone call or letter that notes a product complaint ("the pill was the wrong color"), an AE ("and then I took it and had violent stomach pains"), and then requests restitution ("I want my money back now!"). These cases must be handled by three or more departments in the company: (1) the drug safety group to get details and report the AE, (2) the manufacturing or quality group to see why the pill was the wrong color, and (3) the marketing/sales group to refund (or not refund) the money. Companies must set up systems to handle this.

United States Regulations

The United States reporting requirements for spontaneous reporting are found in 21CFR314.80. Serious, unlabeled (Package Insert), spontaneous, and literature events, whether felt to be causally related or not, must be reported within 15 calendar days (plus day 0) when the four minimum criteria are met. Reports from FDA, either from the MedWatch to Manufacturer Program or FOI, do not have to be sent to FDA but may need to be sent to other HAs.

European Union Requirements

The European Union regulations are far more complex in terms of sponsor reporting. Some countries require cases to be sent both electronically and on paper. Some go to the health authority and some go to a non-health-authority-designated agency. All cases should go to Eudravigilance. Reporting depends on whether the case comes from an European Union member state or from outside the European Union. See the extensive series of charts in Volume 9A (Tables 6.1.1, 6.1.2, and 6.1.3) at the Eudralex website (Web Resource 3-4). Local updates from member states should be tracked in case of changes in the regulations.

Other Regions

Many countries follow the ICH/CIOMS criteria of spontaneous unlabeled reporting within 15 calendar days of first becoming aware of a valid case (four criteria: drug, SAE, patient, reporter). Some countries have differences. These often revolve around receiving all domestic SAEs (whether labeled or not) but only some (SAEs that are unlabeled) nondomestic cases. Some countries do not want any nondomestic cases.

Australia: Interestingly, Australia only requires Australian SAEs to be reported within 15 calendar days, whether expected or not, using their "blue card" system (the official Australian system to capture AEs is akin to the US MedWatch program and the United Kingdom Yellow Card system). Nonserious Australian AEs should be reported as line listings in the PSUR. For postmarketing studies done in Australia, similarly, all SAEs are to be reported in 15 calendar days and the nonserious AEs at the end of the study. Non-Australian cases do not have to be reported. Rather "any significant safety issue or action which has arisen from any analysis of foreign reports, or which has been taken by a foreign regulatory agency, including the basis for such action" should be reported to the health authority (TGA—Therapeutic Goods Administration) within 72 hours. See Web Resource 3-5.

Canada: Health Canada requires all domestic reports of serious ARs and "unusual failure in efficacy for new drugs" be reported within 15 calendar days. Foreign unexpected serious adverse reactions must be reported in 15 calendar days. See the guidance at Web Resource 3-6.

There is now a transition by companies reporting serious AEs to health agencies from paper or fax reporting of paper forms (MedWatch or CIOMS I) to electronic reporting using a standardized electronic format and transmission known generically as "E2B transmissions" after the ICH document of that name. This reporting is either through the internet (using an electronic gateway or direct entry online into the database.). In theory, electronic case transmission of a case is the same to all agencies around the world and simplifies the multiple reporting obligations now in force from country to country. This has not turned out to be entirely the case, however, as various countries (notably the United States and Japan) want special or additional information and data in the electronic transmission.

■ Process Issues

There is also a trend toward reporting from standardized lists of drug names, medical and surgical history, AE codes, laboratory data, and demographic codes. This allows people to document AE cases in a standardized language and format that is easily translated by the computer into any other language. The only area proving resistant to this computerization is the medical narrative, where a case is summarized in prose in a few paragraphs such that the reader can get an understanding of what happened to the patient. Whether a computer-derived narrative (or no narrative at all) will prove to be as useful as a narrative prepared by a safety-trained healthcare professional remains to be seen.

Interestingly, English has become the international language of AE reporting. PSURs and E2B transmissions are written in English. Some countries require translation of some or all sections, but this is becoming less prevalent as short time frames and international harmonization are requiring that English be the language of drug safety—at least for 15-day expedited reporting and periodic reporting. Sometimes AEs occurring in a particular country must be reported to the national health authority in the language of that country rather than or in addition to English.

After the report is received or uploaded to the database in a company's safety department, it must be logged in and a unique number assigned (either before or after a search for duplicate cases). How this is done depends on whether the case arrives electronically or has to be manually entered into the safety database. A rapid determination must be made by a medical professional to see whether it is an "expedited" or "alert" report that must be sent to the health authorities within 15 calendar days of first arrival. The data must be entered into the database (if not already uploaded), coded, medically reviewed, quality-checked, and dispatched outside the company to the appropriate health authorities, subsidiaries, and business partners, as well as to others inside the company such as clinical research physicians who follow the safety profile of the drug in question. Any horrific AEs that might produce immediate regulatory or public health problems must also be identified and acted on urgently.

From a more general point of view, the wisdom of relying on spontaneous reporting of AEs, and thus trusting the goodwill and timely reporting of the healthcare community and patients, has been seriously questioned in the past few years. As many drugs have been withdrawn from the market or have had urgent labeling changes made following the reports of severe toxicity, the search for a more efficient way of rapidly identifying new safety issues is under way in many quarters. The FDA is examining its spontaneous reporting system in a special project (IMPACT: Evaluation of the Contribution of the Food and Drug Administration's Spontaneous Adverse Event Surveillance System to Support Safety-Related Regulatory Actions Throughout a Product's Life Cycle), and other health agencies around the world are also examining better mechanisms to capture SAEs.

It is highly likely that electronic healthcare records will in time supplant the spontaneous AE reporting systems now in place. With the electronic tracking of all patients' encounters with the healthcare system (prescriptions given and filled, doctor visits, hospital stays, complaints and diagnoses recorded in standardized forms, etc.), it is likely that health agencies and possibly companies will be able to "mine" the information using complex search algorithms to do real-time SAE tracking. Prospective use and epidemiology studies will become feasible. Adding genomic data, health economic information, and other data will transform the drug safety surveillance system. This is not likely to happen soon and there will surely be false starts and dead ends in the quest to obtain drug safety data, but there is little doubt that this will occur to everyone's (presumed) benefit. Note also that the regulations for the handling and reporting of postmarketing AEs are not static in spite of "harmonization." FDA is likely to change the regulations, incorporating many of the proposals from their 2003 proposed new regulations ("The Tome") as they did in late 2010 for the premarketing regulations.

■ Frequently Asked Questions

Q: Is it really worthwhile reporting another penicillin rash or some other clearly well-described adverse event? Isn't this a waste of time, money, and resources that could be better used elsewhere?

A: Yes, that is probably true. Known reactions for old drugs in the approved patient populations using the approved formulation, dose, and route of administration do not really add much to the general knowledge of drug safety. It probably is better to use limited resources looking at newer drugs or patient groups where safety is less well characterized.

This is not what most health agencies (officially) say for the understandable reason that, once they ask healthcare professionals and consumers to start making judgments about what is worth reporting and what is not, they begin the slide down the slippery slope. Their reasoning is that it is better to overreport, even known

AEs on old drugs, than underreport and risk missing something. After many years on the market, even old drugs can have new data found on AEs and in particular drug interactions. Whether enough resources will remain available for this remains to be seen.

Q: Does a doctor or other healthcare professional have the right to report a patient's medical and health information to a private company without the consent of the patient?

A: A good and troubling question. In many jurisdictions (including the United States), drug safety reporting by healthcare professionals to companies and the health agency is both legal and encouraged even without the patient's consent. Disease registries have been in place for decades (e.g., for syphilis) in which physicians and hospitals must report cases to the authorities. In other countries, however, the laws can be complex, and some level of consent may be required, particularly if lab tests, x-rays or scans, or other complementary data are also to be sent. The healthcare professional should check on the requirements and limitations in his or her country.

Q: Are consumer reports really worth collecting?

A: Clearly, the information collected from consumers is less useful and less able to be acted on than information healthcare professionals supply. Many reasons account for this: imprecise terminology, lack of complete data, misunderstanding by the patient of complex medical issues, and so forth. This is particularly true for OTC products where there is no healthcare professional intervention in most cases, as the patients self-diagnose and self-treat. Having said all that, useful information can still be obtained that will lead to a signal and further investigation. This is probably not an efficient way to do this, however. In addition, companies handling consumer information, particularly via telephone calls, note that it is time-consuming and requires great diplomatic skills from call center workers. Consumers tend to be more talkative, less precise, and more available than medical personnel who want to report the information and get on to their next patient. Again, it is hoped that electronic health records will make this system obsolete in the future.

4

The Theory of Drug Safety (Pharmacovigilance)

Why a company needs a drug safety group and how it is constituted. The mission of a drug safety group within a pharmaceutical company. A brief history of the U.S. FDA's safety duties and functions. The FDA's mission. Pressures on the corporate safety department and the FDA. An overview of the safety functions of government agencies outside the United States.

■ A Brief History of the FDA

A century or two ago, the requirements for the safety and efficacy of drug products were either nonexistent or poorly defined at best. In 1906, the Pure Food and Drugs Act prohibited interstate commerce of mislabeled and adulterated drugs and food within the United States. This covered some safety aspects of drugs but not efficacy. The FDA had, at that time, no jurisdiction or control of efficacy claims made for drugs. In 1912, the law was changed to cover false and fraudulent claims made for drugs. However, the law did not mandate safety and, in

effect, unsafe products could be and were marketed. The FDA could not seize unsafe drugs and was limited only to issuing public warnings.

In 1937, a company in the United States marketed elixir of sulfanilamide, which contained diethylene glycol (similar to antifreeze). More than 100 people (including children) died from this product. Because the law did not require safety testing for drugs, the company had done none. As a result of this, the Federal Food, Drug and Cosmetic Act was passed into law in 1938. This law required safety testing to be performed and submitted to the FDA in a New Drug Application (NDA). Additional laws were passed in the 1940s requiring testing for purity, strength, and quality of many drugs. The next major event was the thalidomide disaster of the early 1960s, when the NDA for thalidomide was valiantly opposed by Dr. Frances Kelsey at the FDA because of insufficient safety information despite strong pressure to approve it. Though never marketed in the United States, thalidomide was extensively used in the investigational setting, and by 1962, the terrible teratogenic (birth defect) aspect of the drug became known as babies were born with severely deformed arms and legs (phocomelia). In 1962, the Kefauver-Harris Amendment became law and introduced the modern era of drug regulation. Drug manufacturers now had to demonstrate to the FDA both safety and efficacy before marketing a new drug. In 1971, the National Drug Experience Reporting System was begun as was the publication of "The FDA Drug Bulletin" to alert physicians and pharmacists to drug issues. In 1985, the regulations on AE reporting for marketed drugs were strengthened, and new requirements for Investigational New Drug Applications (INDs) were introduced. Over the years, the FDA has had multiple reorganizations and alterations in its structure and function as the overseer of drug safety and efficacy in the United States. The result is the complex system of AE collection, analysis, and reporting that we know today. See a brief history of the Center for Drug Evaluation and Research (CDER) on the FDA's website (Web Resource 4-1).

■ Regulations, Laws, and Guidances

The regulations, laws, guidances, rules, and other relevant documents covering drug safety are detailed, arcane, and scattered throughout multiple places in the Code of Federal Regulations for the United States and the various venues for European Union (EU) and member state documents. Each individual country in the European Union and most others in the world have their own set of local laws, regulations, and guidances (often available only in the local language). Most are updated fairly frequently.

Most countries' regulations are fairly similar in requiring all or almost all serious AEs and some nonserious AEs to be reported quickly if there appears to be a potential impact on public health, and at periodic intervals for more routine AEs. Most countries also require some form of aggregate reporting of serious and nonserious AEs at periodic intervals (e.g., every 3 months, 6 months, yearly, every 3 years), depending up whether the drug is in clinical trials or on the market and whether it is new or old. Although the rules are similar throughout the world, they are sufficiently different in detail ("the devil is in the details") to be infuriating and well nigh impossible to track, categorize, and keep up to date without personnel in each country tracking such matters. The major documents for the United States and the European Union are listed below. Those with an asterisk should be read and digested by anyone doing drug safety for a living. The contents of these documents are topics of this book.

The United States regulations do not explicitly state that a department or group must exist to deal with drug safety. Rather, sponsor obligations are spelled out. To do this adequately, an organized system or department is necessary.

The European Union regulations are more specific and require that a formal pharmacovigilance system be put in place (from Volume 9A—*Pharmacovigilance. Rules Governing Medicinal Products in the European Union*, published by the European Commission, Directorate Enterprise, Regulatory Framework and Market Authorisations [Version September 2008]: "All Marketing Authorisation Holders are required to have an appropriate system of pharmacovigilance in place" (Section 2.2.3).

■ The United States Regulations and Guidances

Drug safety in the United States is covered under several sections of the Code of Federal Regulations. A searchable version of 21CFR is available on the FDA's website (Web Resource 4-2).

■ The United States Code of Federal Regulations, Title 2, Chapter 312 covers INDs. 21CFR312.32 covers IND safety reports, including expedited 7- and 15-day reports. Section 21CFR33 covers the IND annual reports. The NDA regulations are found in section 21CFR314.80.

Updates to regulations are published in the *Federal Register* and are viewable on its website (Web Resource 4-3). The Food, Drug and Cosmetic Act is available at Web Resource 4-4.

FDA has created several Web pages for industry:

Drugs: Web Resource 4-5.

Devices: Web Resource 4-6

Biologics: Web Resource 4-7

Dietary supplements: Web Resource 4-8

Guidance documents: Web Resource 4-9

MedWatch: Web Resource 4-10

■ In addition, MedWatch has an automatic e-mail notification system that sends out free safety updates periodically. Information is available on its website (Web Resource 4-11).

■ In August 1997, the FDA issued a short Guidance for Industry entitled "Postmarketing Adverse Experience Reporting for Human Drug and Licensed Biological Products: Clarification of What to Report." This document covers the four data elements needed for an AE report, solicited information, and nonserious labeled cases. See the CDER website (Web Resource 4-12).

■ In March 2001, the FDA published a Guidance for Industry entitled "Postmarketing Safety Reporting for Human Drug and Biological Products Including Vaccines." This document has not been formally issued as a final regulation, however. It is worth reading to better understand the FDA's more or less current thinking on safety reporting. See the CDER website (Web Resource 4-13).

- CDER has a guide for FDA field inspectors on what to look for when doing inspections on safety matters. It is worth reading (though it is a bit old) and can be found on the CDER's website. 7353.001 Chapter 53 is called "Postmarketing Surveillance and Epidemiology: Human Drugs" (Web Resource 4-14).

- In March 2003, the FDA published proposed new regulations markedly altering the reporting requirements in 21 CFR parts 310, 312, 314, 320, 600, 601, and 606. These proposals have been nicknamed "The Tome." They have been issued for clinical trials (21CFR312) but not yet for the postmarketing requirements. They are expected soon. For the complete text, see Web Resource 4-15.

For risk management documents, see Chapter 30.
For ICH documents, see Chapter 37.
For CIOMS documents, see Chapter 36.

■ The European Union Directives, Regulations, and Guidances

A summary of safety documents for the European Union can be found at the Eudravigilance website (Web Resource 4-16), the European Commission website (Web Resource 4-17), and the EMA website (Web Resource 4-18).

There are two major documents covering drug safety: Volume 9A and Volume 10.

The major document covering postmarketing safety in the European Union is a 200-plus-page document entitled, "Volume 9A—Rules Governing Medicinal Products in the European Union: Pharmacovigilance for Medicinal Products for Human Use" (Web Resource 4-19).

It is extremely well written and clear. It is downloadable as a PDF file and is thus easily searchable. It contains key documents and templates (e.g., risk management template).

The major document covering clinical trial safety in the European Union is a shorter document entitled "Volume 10—Clinical Trials Guidelines." There are many references in Volume 10 to Volume 9A, as many of the procedures are the same for clinical trial and marketed drugs.

There are several subsections devoted to drug safety also available at this website. "Volume 10—Clinical Trials Guidelines" (Web Resource 4-20) includes:

- detailed guidance on the collection, verification, and presentation of adverse reaction reports arising from clinical trials on medicinal products for human use

- detailed guidance on the European database of suspected unexpected serious adverse reactions (Eudravigilance—Clinical Trial Module)

- questions and answers specific to adverse reaction reporting in clinical trials

Pharmaceutical companies are obliged to capture AEs, analyze them, and report them to their health agency locally and to other health authorities, or to companies abroad for submission to their HAs if there are formal corporate arrangements for sales and trials outside the home country. Thus, a company needs to create or have full-time (24/7) access to a safety team or department equipped to handle spontaneous and clinical trial AEs (as required) or to outsource this function. If the company is based solely in one country, the department may be relatively small and uncomplicated and report AEs only to the HA in that country. If, however, AEs can come from subsidiaries or affiliates in other countries or from business partners with which the company has contractual relationships, the complexity of the needs and requirements grows enormously. If a single-country company is doing clinical trials outside its borders, it must be able to report AEs and handle all other safety and regulatory matters with other countries' health agency.

Different languages, time zones, ever-changing government requirements, reporting due dates, documents and formats, electronic transmission, and so forth must be taken into account. Standard operating procedures, MedDRA (Medical Dictionary for Regulatory Activities), and training systems must be in place. An electronic safety database must be built (an enormous task) or purchased (still a complex and costly endeavor). Risk evaluation and management/mitigation systems must be in place.

Healthcare personnel, including physicians, nurses, pharmacists, and support staff, must be hired. The business relationships with other concerned departments within the company, such as regulatory affairs, sales and marketing, legal, clinical research, and others, must be established. In other words, creating a safety department is a complex and expensive endeavor that must be done absolutely correctly.

After an AE report is received by the safety department, it must be entered or uploaded into the safety database, which is used for storage, retrieval, analysis, and reporting data. Although such databases may start out in small companies as spreadsheets with the data typed onto MedWatch or CIOMS 1 forms, most companies respond to this need by purchasing an expensive (up to hundreds of thousands or millions of dollars, depending on the number and location of users and information technology [IT] maintenance staff) dedicated safety database. They create complex departments with tight standard operating procedures to ensure that the company remains in full compliance with all laws, regulations, and guidelines and will withstand inspections and audits from the FDA, EMEA, and other HAs; business partners; outside auditing companies; and others.

There is usually a senior executive (typically a vice president for drug safety), who is also an experienced physician, to oversee the entire group. Within the drug safety group, there are multiple functions to handle. Depending on the size of the company, separate people or groups may handle each of the categories below. In small companies, all functions may fall on one or two people or are outsourced.

- Case receipt, triage, and processing by (nonprofessional) data entry personnel
- Case evaluation by medical professionals
- Coding of AEs in MedDRA (sometimes this group is separate from drug safety)
- Coding of drugs in WHO-Drug or another drug dictionary
- Quality review
- Medical review by physicians
- Submission to HAs, subsidiaries, business partners, and so on

To support the drug safety group, there is often a dedicated informatics (IT; computer) group, a signaling/pharmacovigilance group, a training group, a standard operating procedure group, an epidemiology group, a risk management group, and more. These groups may be within or separate from the drug safety department. Sometimes a medical report writing group also falls under drug safety to prepare aggregate reports, such as Periodic Safety Update Reports (PSURs), annual reports, NDA periodic reports, IND annual reports, and so on.

Similar groups often exist within HAs. Some authorities (FDA, MHRA, Health Canada, AFSSAPS, TGA, and others) receive reports directly from healthcare professionals and consumers. The agencies may form departments similar to those in companies to receive, enter, and evaluate data and make medical judgments on the

cases. The volumes in companies may run to the tens or even hundreds of thousands of cases per year. The FDA received more than 526,000 postmarketing reports in 2008, of which about 33,000 were sent directly to FDA. See its website (Web Resource 4-21).

This is a large task and is performed by most health agencies throughout the world. Because serious cases tend to be reported to all health agencies, there is enormous duplication of effort in creating databases in each agency and company. In practice, only HAs in large countries with advanced pharmacovigilance practices are able to maintain relatively complete databases and conduct meaningful signal analyses.

The Uppsala Monitoring Centre (UMC) in Sweden and the European Eudravigilance database are attempting to centralize data collection to create large repositories of safety information. There are four major databases with large but not total overlap for postmarketing AEs: the FDA in the United States, the Eudravigilance database in the EMA (London), the United Kingdom MHRA database, and the Vigibase at the UMC in Sweden.

Clinical trial AEs tend to be more scattered and far less transparent than AEs for marketed products because most of the information on drugs not yet on the market is proprietary and guarded as secret information by both companies and HAs. In many countries, clinical trials by pharmaceutical companies, universities, consortia, health agencies, and others must be entered into Web-based registries. The largest is the clinical trial website maintained by the U.S. National Institutes of Health (Web Resource 4-22), with nearly 90,000 trials in more than 170 countries registered. The data, however, are variable, and often there is little or no safety data and the data are not up to date. Various countries, including the United States, have mandated regularly posting and updating complete safety (and efficacy) data. These requirements, though officially in effect now, have not been fully complied with and it will likely be several years before we begin to see complete and meaningful data posted in these registries.

The mission of the drug safety group must be clearly defined and made known to all employees of the company, in particular to senior management and marketing and sales. It is also good policy to let the general public know of the company's or health agency's commitment to patient safety. For example, see FDA's Sentinel Initiative Mission Statement (Web Resource 4-23), Health Canada (Web Resource 4-24), and the United Kingdom's MHRA (Web Resource 4-25). Companies also explain their safety functions to the public; see, for example, Pfizer

(Web Resource 4-26), Merck (Web Resource 4-27), and Novartis (Web Resource 4-28).

The mission of the drug safety group, whether in a company or a health agency, is first and foremost to protect the public health by maintaining accurate, up-to-date, and complete safety information. Medical analyses must be done with patient safety in mind, not "product and sales protection." It is argued that the best product and sales protection comes from ensuring that full, unbiased, scientific, and complete safety information is available to all stakeholders: patients, medical professionals, health agencies, and the company. Secondary goals within a company's safety department relate to such corporate functions as consultation within the company on safety issues, legal matters including litigation, response to patient and healthcare professional queries, training, and supporting the sales force.

There is often enormous pressure on the safety group to minimize or wait on safety issues until they are proved beyond a shadow of a doubt. The attitude that the "drug is innocent until proven guilty" and that safety warnings should not be issued to the health agency or the public until this point is reached is not at all appropriate in the world of safety. Rather, each safety issue must be evaluated and acted on because of its own merit and criticality in a timely fashion to evaluate and minimize risk. Some problems must be addressed on Friday at 5 PM and over the weekend.

In the corporate world, this attitude runs contrary to the prevailing fiduciary obligation of a corporation ("to increase stockholder value by making more profit"). The personnel in the drug safety department needs a fair amount of masochism and a thick skin to work in this nonglorious field, unlike the world of clinical research or sales where there are congratulations (and monetary bonuses) for completing a study, getting drugs approved, or selling more product. Rather, drug safety personnel need strong backbones to be able to say to management that a product has a safety problem that must be acted on immediately or tracked until more data are in. Good and wise corporate management understands this and welcomes "straight talk" from the safety unit. Bad management buries or delays. This is becoming more dangerous as the penalties (commercial, regulatory, and legal) are becoming more severe. It is hoped that corporate executives will realize that a safety problem hidden in the short run may, in the long run, appear on the front page of the *New York Times*, on TV or the Web, or the six o'clock news. They may need to explain their actions to governmental investigation panels and to the multiple lawsuits—class action, civil, and criminal—that now pop up in the United States and, interestingly, elsewhere in the world on any safety-related issue.

Similarly, the role of drug safety in the health agency is difficult. The primary mission is similar to the corporate safety role: to protect the public health. However, the profit-making motive is not present. Instead, there are always intense budget pressures to save money as well as the need to answer to multiple demanding constituencies: in the United States, the FDA answers in one way or another to the Secretary of Health and Human Services, the U.S. Congress, the public, the press, the internet blogosphere, the health professions, and the companies (and lobbies) the HA regulates. Similar political pressures exist for other agencies around the world.

■ Frequently Asked Questions

Q: Why would anyone want to work in drug safety?

A: Good question. Once the decision is made by a healthcare professional to move out of the clinical world and into industrial/pharmaceutical medicine, it is noted that certain personality types tend to go to drug safety. Unlike the "glamour" of clinical research, where new and exciting drugs are tested, drug safety tends to have a different atmosphere, dealing with the problems of the new and exciting (and old and dull) drugs.

There is much more detective work and medical analysis in working hard to obtain all the clinical facts available, perform a defensible medical analysis, and come to a medically sound conclusion often based on incomplete data. The work can be quite academic when one is working up a complex signal or risk evaluation/mitigation plan. And as always in medicine, one never has enough information. There is always one more test or examination one could do to get closer to the truth. Like the clinician, the drug safety worker is usually dealing with uncertainty and must still make rapid and often irreversible decisions. Yet given the data available, one must come to the medically proper and defensible conclusion and convey this in a cogent way to both medical and nonmedical people. The work is challenging and fulfilling when done well.

The ethical issues come up when clear, compelling safety arguments calling for action are made and no action is forthcoming from management. This puts drug safety personnel in awkward and sometimes legally risky positions.

There is also much drama and excitement. Much can be routine, but the next e-mail or Tweet may bring a disaster with widespread consequences if the signal bears out. The adrenaline level rises and the "crisis" team mobilizes. The drug safety department is the emergency room of the company. Those who perform drug safety as a career are often passionate about it. Few decide at the outset of a pharmaceutical career that they want to "do side effects." Rather, they want to discover new drugs or do clinical research or study the pharmacology of drugs. Many come into drug safety after trying other areas in the industry and discover they love it.

Q: Is there not an inherent conflict of interest in asking a company to police itself?

A: In a sense yes, especially when money is involved. Most regulated professions have some level of self-policing, including aviation, banking and finance, the food industry, medicine, and law. The results of self-policing have not always been happy. Thus, there must be some level of outside oversight to ensure that self-policing is done correctly. Finding the right balance is always the trick. In practice, there is far too much to do and oversee in the pharmaceutical industry to have total outside oversight from health agencies. Rather, practicalities force the system to police itself with regulations, periodic reports, monitoring, reviews, audits, and other mechanisms looking over the industry's shoulder to "keep it honest." In recent times, following terrible banking and investment scandals, there is a strong tendency toward risk aversion and the demand that there be more regulation and control "to prevent another (fill in your own crisis: Vioxx, AIG, Madoff, earthquake, etc.)." Thus, we are likely to see more regulation and perhaps less risk-taking. Whether this will lead to better outcomes (safer drugs) remains to be seen.

5

Adverse Events with New Chemical Entities, Generics, Excipients, Placebos, and Counterfeits

Are some adverse events (AEs) created more equal than others? Are some AEs more important than others? Why AEs with generics and older drugs are important. What to do with other manufacturers' AEs. Why AEs with new chemical entities are critically important. Why AEs due to excipients are so hard to pick up. Why AEs with over-the-counter drugs are also important. Why AEs before taking the drug can matter.

The reporting requirements for AEs and drugs are generally thought of as being critical for the safety evaluation of new chemical entities (NCEs), also called new molecular entities (NMEs), newly approved for marketing. NCEs, by definition, have not been on the market before. Their safety profile is known only from limited laboratory, animal, and human testing under an IND or equivalent. Clearly, AE reporting is critical in this period, and companies and agencies pay particular attention to the spontaneous AE reports received shortly after launch (known as the Weber effect: a large number of AEs/ADRs

reported just after launch that decrease after some months to a lower, more steady-state number of reports). Rare AEs that were not seen in the trials are often picked up in the weeks to months after launch in major markets with good AE reporting structures, such as the United States or Europe. Regulations on AE reporting are written with this in mind.

Given the large number of AEs that drugs can produce and given the limited number of resources that health agencies, companies, and healthcare professionals can devote to reporting and processing AEs, there is an ongoing debate about what AEs are most cost-effective and medically important to collect to protect the public health. Much work is under way to either improve or add to the spontaneous reporting systems in use throughout the world. The FDA MedWatch program collects safety information about prescription and over-the-counter drugs, biologics, medical and radiation-emitting devices, and special nutritional products (e.g., medical foods, dietary supplements, and infant formulas). See the FDA's website (Web Resource 5-1). Health Canada has a similar system known as MedEffect (Web Resource 5-2). The United Kingdom's MHRA has a system known as the Yellow Card system, dating back to when yellow handwritten cards were used to submit AEs (Web Resource 5-3). The French system is described in French on the website of the French Health Authority (Web Resource 5-4). Many other countries have their systems described and available online on the health authority's website.

Generics

The current regulations from the FDA do not address generics. Any drug under an NDA or an ANDA must meet the AE reporting requirements in 21CFR314.80. This includes generics and NCEs. In the European Union, a similar requirement for generic pharmacovigilance is noted in Volume 9A:

> The pharmacovigilance obligations apply to all medicinal products authorised in the European Union, including those authorised before 1 January 1995 and whatever procedure was used for their authorisation. For example, the obligations are the same for products authorised under Articles 10(1), 10(4), 10a, 13 to 16 and 16a to 16i of Directive 2001/83/EC ("generic", "similar biological medicinal product", "well-established use", "homeopathic" and "herbal" products respectively) as for products authorised under Article 6 of the same Directive (Section 2.0, page 15).

If the manufacturer of a branded product receives an AE from a generic version of its product, it should database the AE and report it, as appropriate, as an expedited report or in the periodic report, noting that it is the generic and not the company's branded drug. If the manufacturer of the generic is known, the branded company should still database the event and may or may not send a copy of the event to the manufacturer of the generic. Volume 9A (Section 4.1. page 56) states:

> When a Marketing Authorisation Holder receives an Individual Case Safety Report (ICSR) where the invented name of the medicinal product is not specified but the active substance is included in any of the medicinal products for which a marketing authorisation is held, the Marketing Authorisation Holder should assume that the report may relate to their product.

Most other countries have similar requirements for generic drug safety reporting.

Excipients

An excipient is a theoretically inactive ingredient added to a drug to provide bulk or to give it form or consistency. In regard to excipients, there are many types, including binders, fillers, diluents, lubricants, sweeteners, preservatives, flavors, printing inks, colors, and others. The most common ones used in the United States include magnesium stearate, lactose, microcrystalline cellulose, silicon dioxide, titanium dioxide, stearic acid, sodium starch glycolate, gelatin, talc, sucrose, povidone, pregelatinized starch, hydroxyl propyl methylcellulose, shellac, calcium phosphate (dibasic), and others. Standards are set by committees of the United States Pharmacopeial Convention and published in the United States Pharmacopeia and the National Formulary.

Excipients became a major issue in the United States when a sulfonamide elixir was diluted in diethylene glycol (automobile antifreeze) and killed about 100 Americans, including children. It led in 1938 to the Food, Drug, and Cosmetic Act. An excipient for drugs is approved for use in the United States by one of three mechanisms:

1. It meets the requirements of being "Generally Recognized as Safe" under 21CFR182, 184, 186.

2. The FDA approves a petition as a food additive under 21CFR171.

3. It is referenced in an approved NDA for a particular function for that drug.

Excipients for over-the-counter products must comply with section 21CFR330.1(e) as "safe in the amounts administered and do not interfere with the effectiveness of the preparation."

Please refer to the excellent website run by the International Pharmaceutical Excipients Council (Web Resource 5-5) for further information.

The FDA definition of an adverse drug experience refers to "any AE associated with the use of a drug" (21CFR314.80a)) without indicating whether the event is associated with the active ingredient (moiety) or an excipient. Should the submitter have some reason to suspect an excipient to be the cause of the AE, this should be noted in the report and the appropriate investigations and follow-up done. Note that the FDA has revised its definitions for pre-marketing AEs (21CFR312) and is expected to do the same for the postmarketing definitions based on ICH and the proposed FDA regulations ("The Tome").

The ICH document Q8 describes in detail how excipients are handled in pharmaceuticals. See ICH's website for the document (Web Resource 5-6).

In the European Union, Volume 9A only refers to excipients in regard to altering PSUR cycles. There is no direct comment on AEs possibly related to fillers or excipients. Excipients in one country may be considered active ingredients in other countries and vice versa. As in the United States, the European Union, and elsewhere, Good Manufacturing Practices have detailed regulations and guidelines on excipients.

In general, most countries require Quality Management systems and life cycle risk management for all products. Under this general heading, excipients are included. Thus, if a signal or safety issue should arise regarding an excipient, this is expected to be handled expeditiously. Most regulations require safety reporting for the entire product, not just the active moiety. Thus, adverse events seen with the drug product, whether due presumably to the active ingredient or an excipient, must be handled in the same way as expedited reports or periodic reports as required by regulation and law. The trick is to distinguish an AE due to an excipient rather than the active ingredient. If the former, the problem should be rectifiable, if the latter, then the event is a pharmacologic property of the drug and unlikely to be diminished with manufacturing changes.

■ Placebo

As placebos are rarely used explicitly in clinical practice, this refers only to clinical trials. All AEs (whether to active drug, comparator, or placebo) must be captured and databased. The only issue is expedited reporting of placebo events.

In the United States, placebo AEs from trials do not generally have to be reported as expedited reports. However, many blinded trials do have AEs (including serious AEs) reported as blinded events during the trial either as expedited reports or in periodic or annual reports. At the end of the study, the unblinding reveals some of them to be associated with placebo and not active drugs. In addition, in preparing final study reports, integrated safety sections for NDAs, dossiers for marketing approval in the European Union and elsewhere, and comparisons of AEs on active drug and placebo must be reported if there is a placebo arm of the trial. Thus, all placebo AEs should be recorded and tracked in the safety database.

In the European Union, some countries require reporting of all AEs related to the "biomedical research," not just to taking the active study drug. In this case, placebo cases need to be reported as expedited reports and in periodic summary reports. The European Union Clinical Trial Directive (2001/20/EC of April 4, 2001) defines an "investigational medicinal product" as "a pharmaceutical form of an active substance or placebo being tested or used in a clinical trial" and requires certain serious AEs to be reported as expedited reports. Some have read this to mean a requirement for placebo reporting. Volume 9A does not expressly address placebo reporting. In the United Kingdom, the "Clinical Trials Toolkit" from the United Kingdom Department of Health/Medical Research Council (Web Resource 5-7) states:

> For blinded trials involving a placebo and an active drug, seriousness, causality and expectedness should be evaluated as though the patient was on active drug. Cases that are considered serious, unexpected and possibly, probably or definitely related (i.e. possible SUSARs) would have to be unblinded. Only those events occurring among patients on the active drug (unless thought to be due to the excipient in the placebo) should be considered to be SUSARs requiring reporting to the regulatory authority and ethics committee.

The Good Pharmacovigilance Practice Guide (MHRA Pharmaceutical Press, London, 2009, www.pharmapress.com), from the MHRA, also notes:

> For the purpose of triage of a SAR in a blinded trial, expectedness may be assessed initially using the assumption that the test drug has been given. If it is assessed as unexpected against the test drug reference document, it should be unblinded. If, following unblinding, it is seen that the clinical trial subject received the comparator drug, but the event still meets the criteria for a SUSAR, in that it is unexpected according to the comparator reference document (which should be defined in the protocol), then it should be expedited according to the requirements. . . and notified to the company that holds the marketing authorisation for the comparator drug. If, following unblinding, it is discovered that the IMP (investigational medical product) was a placebo, then this event will not require expedited reporting, unless in the opinion of the investigator or sponsor the event was related to a reaction to the placebo, for example an allergic reaction to an excipient (Section 12.3.7, page 140).

In any case, all AEs—whether seen with the study drug, comparator, or placebo—must be recorded in the case report form/EDC system and databased, as they will be used in the final study report to calculate AE occurrence rates for each arm of the study.

■ Other Manufacturers' Drugs' AEs

For the postmarketing situation, the United States regulations are not clear on this point. There is a section, 21CFR314.80(1)(iii), on how to handle 15-day expedited serious AEs a company receives whose name appears on the product as a packer, distributor, or manufacturer but who is not the applicant (holder of the NDA). This section allows the nonapplicant to submit the serious AE to the FDA or to transmit it within 5 calendar days to the applicant, who will then submit it to the FDA. Some have extrapolated from this section to mean that AE reports that are received but are clearly those of another company's product should be sent to the other company. This is a judicious way to handle the matter and represents best (and ethical) practice.

If the drug is a generic version of the branded product, see the earlier section on how this is handled.

Outside the United States, the regulations and guidelines are largely silent on this point. Most companies will immediately send an SAE report to the manufacturer of the drug if the drug and the chemical entity are not theirs. If the drug is a competitor drug with the same chemical entity, the case will be databased usually and transmitted to the other company if known. Some sponsors will report the case to the HA. In some cases, a concomitant drug is actually felt by the manufacturer to be the cause of the AE. In these cases, many companies will report the case to the HAs and forward a copy of the case to the other manufacturer with a note explaining the situation. The situations and rules are often nebulous, but fortunately, these cases are relatively rare. In the clinical trial setting, as noted, all AEs should be databased and active, and comparator SAEs (when the criteria are met) should be reported as expedited reports. The reporting company may or may not notify the manufacturer of the comparator drug.

In practice, companies collect all AEs that come to them whether the drug in question is their drug, a generic, or a placebo, or whether excipients are suspected. The data are usually handled in the usual way and entered into the database. During the workup, the issues of generic, placebo, and so forth are sorted out.

■ Placebo and Breaking the Blind in Clinical Trials

The practice for placebo is variable, depending on whether a company breaks the blind when reporting 7- and 15-day expedited reports to health authorities. If a company breaks the blind routinely for all serious, unexpected, possibly related AEs from a trial and the product in question is placebo, this case is usually not reported to the health agencies (as the case does not meet the four minimal criteria for a valid case: no drug) but kept in the company's database for listing in the final study report. If, however, the company does not unblind and thus reports blinded cases to the health authorities as 15-day reports, when the blind is broken at the end of the study, the company must submit a follow-up noting whether the patient received drug or placebo. Many agencies discourage this methodology, saying that blinded expedited reports are useless. Health authorities in the United States and in the European Union do not want blinded expedited reports.

In the European Union, as a general rule, treatment codes should be broken by the sponsor before reporting a SUSAR to the CA and the ethics committee. Once this is done for one region or agency, the case should be reported unblinded to other agencies. As a rule of thumb, all agencies should be told the same thing at the same time.

When an SAE may be an SAR (i.e., unexpected) and thus expeditable, it is recommended that the blind be broken only for that specific patient by the sponsor even if the investigator has not broken the blind. Those responsible for data analysis and interpretation of results at the study's conclusion should be kept blinded, if possible.

If the case appears to be a SUSAR and thus reportable, then the blinding should be broken. Then three possibilities resulting from the procedure of unblinding must be considered:

1. The patient took the test product: The case would be reported as a SUSAR to the relevant competent authorities and the relevant ethics committees.

2. The patient took a marketed comparator: The SAE should be reassessed for expectedness according to the SPC or labeling for that product. If it is unexpected, then the SUSAR should be reported; otherwise, it is an expected SAR and not reportable on an expedited basis.

3. The patient took placebo: Events associated with placebo will usually not satisfy the criteria for a SAR and therefore are not expeditable (Volume 10).

In the United States, for each AE, a suspect product should be identified. Reports from blinded studies should be submitted only after the code is broken. The blind should always be broken for each patient or subject undergoing a serious, unexpected adverse experience unless arrangements have been made otherwise with the responsible FDA review division. FDA clarified this situation in its final rules, which went into effect in March 2011 (Web resource 5-8). They note that serious unexpected suspected adverse reactions should be reported to FDA with the blind broken (unblinded). Placebo reports should not be submitted. The sponsor may propose alternative arrangements before the study starts and write these into the protocol after agreement is reached with FDA.

The FDA also clarified that they do not believe that it is appropriate to report study endpoints as expedited reports for trials that are designed to evaluate the effect of the drug on disease-related mortality or morbidity. However, if a serious and unexpected adverse event occurs for which there is evidence suggesting a causal relationship between the drug and the event (e.g., death from anaphylaxis), the event must be reported as an expedited report even if it is a component of the study endpoint (e.g., all-cause mortality).

Most health authorities do not want blinded expedited reports. Thus, the blinding should be broken before submission if the case is to be submitted as an expedited report. However, it is wise to verify in each country how the case should be handled. It is wise to do this before the study starts.

■ Picking up AEs due to Excipients

It is very difficult to pick up AEs due to excipients. The reasons are many. Most drug safety personnel do not pay much attention to excipients and may not even know what excipients are in which drug. Excipients often vary from formulation to formulation of the same drug and may vary in quantity from dose strength to dose strength (e.g., higher doses of the same active ingredient may be larger tablets or capsules and have more fillers and excipients) and may vary from country to country.

Manufacturers change excipients and production methods (with the appropriate Good Manufacturing Practice change control and notification to the regulatory agencies) without telling the drug safety department. Thus, there may be hundreds to hundreds of thousands of individual products with varying excipients manufactured by a large company. These are usually not easily computerized, updated, and searchable. A problem with one excipient in one or only a handful of lots or formulations may go undetected unless there is an obvious and unusual AE and a high level of suspicion on the part of the reviewer.

Manufacturers also often change vendors for excipients, and this too may produce issues if product quality or characteristics change. For companies with many products and formulations manufactured in many countries, tracking formulations is impossible for the drug safety group.

The author recalls a product that contained lactose as a filler and that had much more lactose in the United States version than in the Canadian version. When it was discovered that the incidence of diarrhea in the United States was higher than in Canada, the signal investigation revealed the lactose dose difference to be the cause. A very high level of suspicion must be maintained to keep open the possibility of an excipient causing an AE. It is particularly difficult if the AE is common, like diarrhea, or may be caused by the active ingredient itself.

■ Generics

In general, if an AE is reported and the product is identified by the reporter of the AE as a generic and the manufacturer is known, this AE is reported to that manufacturer rather than to the health authority directly. It would be the responsibility of the manufacturer of the product (the generic) to report it to the health authority. Many companies, however, would do both: report the SUSAR to the health agencies and to the other manufacturer. If the AE is not known to be from the sponsor's drug or from a generic, then the sponsor receiving the report must treat it as if it were that company's product and handle it in the usual manner for submission to the authority. Note in the report that the manufacturer is unknown. This should, nonetheless, be verified in each country where the product is marketed. It is wise to database all cases for the chemical entity no matter the manufacturer as the data will be used in signaling.

It is obviously important that the correct manufacturer of a drug be identified. Problems might occur with one company's drug and not another's. Causes could relate not just to the active compound but also to manufacturing issues (product quality complaints), different excipients, impurities, supplier issues, and so on. Thus, when a company receives a spontaneous AE for a product it must make a concerted effort to determine the manufacturer if other versions are marketed to ensure that the report is attributed to the correct drug.

■ Adverse Events with Counterfeit, Impure, and Other Nonstandard Products

In recent years, multiple new problems have arisen, leading to increased drug toxicity and adding difficulties to pharmacovigilance:

■ Counterfeits: "Drug counterfeiting is a serious public health concern," said Margaret A. Hamburg, MD, commissioner of FDA. "We look forward to working with industry to help ensure that consumers are not exposed to products containing unknown, ineffective, or harmful ingredients" (Web Resource 5-9). The FDA has issued a draft guidance on "Draft Guidance for Industry: Incorporation of Physical-Chemical Identifiers into Solid Oral Dosage Form Drug Products for Anticounterfeiting" (Web Resource 5-10). FDA has issued multiple warnings to consumers about purchasing drugs over the internet (Web Resource 5-11). The United Kingdom's MHRA has similarly warned about counterfeits (Web Resource 5-12) as has Health Canada and other agencies. The World Health Organization (Web Resource 5-13) has stated that counterfeit medications are now a global problem, affecting both developed and developing countries. The main targets are the most profitable markets where sales and demand are high. Although "lifestyle" medications were some of the first targets of counterfeiters, fake medications are now seen in cancer and cardiac products. Many countries serve as transfer points and not end-user markets. Online purchases are particularly problematic as the WHO estimates that 50% of medications sold on websites that hide or do not reveal their physical address are counterfeit. The WHO estimates that 10% of all drugs sold globally are counterfeits and may be as high as 25% in developing countries. Up to 40% of artesunate-based malaria medications are fake (News Roundup, *BMJ.* 2005;330:1044).

The counterfeits usually contain a smaller amount of the active moiety or, in some cases, none at all. In the best cases, only fillers are used that should be nontoxic (though the therapeutic benefits of the active entity are nonexistent). In the worst case, toxic substitutes are used, and no one has any idea what is in them.

The issues here are complex, as various government entities allow, if not encourage, the purchase of medicines for lower prices either online or in jurisdictions out of their legal control ("pharmacies just over the border"). Similarly, reimportation may produce issues if counterfeits enter the supply chain. One of the interesting and striking observations from experts on counterfeit drugs is that the quality of the packaging must be impeccable, but that the quality and chemicals in the drug product itself is far less important from the point of view of the counterfeiter. Suspicion by the pharmacist or patient of a counterfeit is low if the package appears legitimate, has a real lot number, and is difficult to distinguish from the genuine packaging. Once the user accepts the package as real, the contents are usually not carefully scrutinized. In addition, unlike buying a fake luxury watch or handbag for $3 on the street, where the consumer knows very well he or she is getting a counterfeit ("knock-off") and does not care, the consumer definitely does not want a counterfeit drug product.

We are thus now seeing an increased risk of ineffective and toxic medications entering the market. The counterfeits appear to be genuine, and consumers and healthcare professionals will report AEs in entirely good faith. However, unbeknown to the reporters, manufacturers, and health agencies, these AEs may be due to toxic ingredient and the safety profile of the drug will be "contaminated" as well.

Other than vigilance by all concerned, it is not clear that there is an easy or short-term answer for this problem, which is recognized but, so far, not well quantified. Pharmacovigilance personnel should keep this possibility in mind when strange new AEs or patterns start appearing. Careful questioning on the sourcing of the product should be done, though consumers may be hesitant to admit to the company or (in particular) the government that they obtained the products in a not entirely legal or appropriate manner. It is likely that this problem will worsen as the world globalizes. The source of the product, if dubious, should be noted in an AE report and in the database. Suspicion of a counterfeit should similarly be noted with the reasons stated.

■ Generics, Sourcing Issues and Manufacturing Quality, and Drug Safety:It has been estimated that 40% to 80% of generic drugs in the United States are sourced from India and China, and this number is growing (Web Resource 5-12). Similarly, active moieties in branded drugs are also outsourced from traditional sources to lower-production-cost areas. Quality scandals recently regarding contaminated heparin (branded) and manufacturing problems with generics have highlighted this issue. For example, in September 2008, the FDA issued two warning letters and instituted an Import Alert barring the entry of all finished drug products and active pharmaceutical ingredients from Ranbaxy's Dewas, Paonta Sahib, and Batamandi Unit facilities because of violations of United States cGMP requirements. That action barred the commercial importation of 30 different generic drugs into the United States (Web Resource 5-14).

The safety and quality of the supply chain of medications is now receiving much greater attention and action. See FDA's report on "FDA's Approach to Medical Product Supply Chain Safety" (Web Resource 5-15).

Thus, from the supply chain and manufacturing point of view, safety issues and AEs may arise that are not clearly due to the active moiety or may be due to problematic products. Again, there is little that the pharmacovigilance personnel can do directly to resolve or clarify this issue. Watchful vigilance is required.

■ Frequently Asked Questions

Q: So, for products with generic formulations or several branded formulations of the same chemical entity, the FDA and other health authorities receive multiple reports from multiple manufacturers at varying time points, some of which may be duplicates. This doesn't seem, shall we say, optimal. Is there not a better way to do this?

A: Another fine question. Clearly, there is multiple reporting of cases to different countries, reporting of AEs for particular chemical entities to separate and unrelated INDs and NDAs at the FDA and equivalent reporting in other countries, and then retransmission, often with recoding of AEs, to other databases (e.g., World Health Organization's Uppsala Monitoring Centre in Sweden). It is nearly impossible to sort out duplicates, excipient effects, counterfeits, and other subtle and not-so-subtle causes of AEs. There are no central or complete databases that list a product's excipients from all manufacturers. Each company keeps its own AE database, usually not linked to a formulations database.

The solutions are straightforward but not easily done. A single, enormous, worldwide database, or well-linked multiple databases or data warehouse, updated frequently, in which all drugs (generic, branded, branded generics, etc.), formulations, excipients, lot numbers, registration numbers, dose, and so on would be the optimal solution. The likelihood of this happening in the near future is nil for multiple reasons, including cost, lack of ownership, lack of a complete data set, commercial secrets, lack of a perception that this is really needed, and lack of the desire to give up national sovereignty or control of pharmaceuticals in each country. In reality, with globalization and easy access and with thousands of pharmaceutical manufacturers worldwide, it is unlikely we will ever attain a complete database. It is more likely that the major players (United States, European Union, China, Japan, India, and a handful of others), representing the large majority of manufacturers and users of drugs, will set up some degree of database linking. This will go part of the way to resolving many of these issues.

Q: If resources are limited and demand infinite, should we even bother looking at all generics and excipients? Shouldn't we concentrate on the newest or most used or most dangerous products and concede such things as excipients problems in little used products?

A: Yes, you are probably right. It is impossible to track everything. In the United States alone, some 4 billion (4×10^9) prescriptions are filled every year. Rather, a triage strategy needs to be developed to make rational use of pharmacovigilance resources and to avoid duplicative work from agency to agency and company to company. Alternatively, the pharmacovigilance of a particular product might be assigned to one national health agency, which would be responsible for worldwide safety surveillance, sort of the way the European Union works in some regards with rapporteur countries. One might wish to look at a particular excipient in only, say, five products in five countries periodically to identify safety issues. One must also decide whether to be proactive and do such investigations periodically and in anticipation of potential safety issues or whether to be reactive and start an investigation only after a problem or signal arises. Lots of solutions are possible, but none is on the horizon right now.

Q: What about generics? Shouldn't they all be grouped under one marketing authorization or NDA or something like that for AE and signaling purposes?

A: Yes, that is probably a good idea but very difficult to do under the current laws and regulations around the world. Rather, the same result could be attained (and is, in fact, done) at the database level, where data are combined or analyzed over multiple products with the same chemical entity. But this would probably require cooperation among competitors, many of whom

are in different countries. Good in theory, not easy in practice.

Q: Do counterfeit products produce more AEs than the branded products?

A: Since counterfeiters of drugs will often put into their products whatever is on hand and cheap, there are many instances of fake drugs that have been found to contain toxic ingredients. The "formulation" may vary from day to day and batch to batch. FDA reported weight-loss products that contained a chemical that could produce high blood pressure, seizures, tachycardia, palpitations, heart attack, or stroke (Web Resource 5-16). Similar reports abound. However, some counterfeits will contain no active ingredients and inactive excipients. In this case, the danger is lack of efficacy. So, there is no way, a priori, to know or predict what effects (good or bad) counterfeits produce.

Acute and Chronic (Late Occurring) Adverse Events, Adverse Events That Disappear (Bendectin), and Diethylstilbesterol

Adverse events (AEs) seen shortly after starting or stopping drugs are common and relatively easy to recognize (though if it were that easy, there would be little need for this book). There is usually a high index of suspicion, a close temporal relationship, and often biologic and pharmacologic plausibility.

This is not the case for AEs that occur weeks, months, or even years after stopping the drug ("long latency period"). There may be no medical record available, the patient's memory of using the product may be hazy, the index of suspicion is low or nonexistent, and there may be no logical, biologic, or pharmacologic reason for this AE to be associated with the drug. Examples are common in long-latency diseases or behaviors. Examples include cigarette smoking and cancer of the lung many years later, asbestos inhalation producing pleural mesotheliomas decades after exposure ended, or the classic example of vaginal cancer in the offspring of women taking diethylstilbestrol (DES). If one considers alcohol a drug, then its effects on the liver, brain, and other organs also may not be seen for many years.

It is now increasingly recognized that drug therapy as well as other therapies (radiation therapy, neutraceuticals, OTCs, etc.) can produce late AEs. Usually, it takes an insightful clinician or a good epidemiologic study to show that a particular drug caused (or is associated with) a particular AE years later. Such a finding is often first met with disbelief and even ridicule. However, public health and good science demand that all contingencies be kept in mind and examined when appropriate.

Finally, to keep us humble, an example of what looked like a clear and related AE and that turned out not to be such is presented (Bendectin).

From empirical observations, the latency period from starting or stopping of a drug to the onset of the AE is variable. AEs can be seen immediately after starting a drug, shortly thereafter, or even after weeks or months of taking the drug with no problems. AEs can also be seen long after stopping the drug. Examples that follow are of AEs seen long after starting or stopping a drug.

Bendectin: A False Alert

Market Removal

Bendectin was a fixed combination of three active ingredients used for treating nausea and vomiting during pregnancy:

1. Doxylamine, an H1 antihistamine that acts as an antinausea and antivomiting agent

2. Pyridoxine, vitamin B6

3. Dicycloverine, removed from the product shortly before market withdrawal of Bendectin

This product was incorrectly suspected of causing congenital abnormalities. Several case-control studies were performed, and their results formed the basis for the exoneration of this product. It had been on the market for about 27 years and was taken by some 33 million pregnant women in the United States, representing 20–40% of all pregnant women. It was voluntarily withdrawn from the U.S. market and never returned even after its exoneration. It was sold under the name of Debendoxin other countries (Fleming *BMJ* 1981;283:99; CSM/MCA, *Curr Problems Pharmacovigilance* 1981;6; *Lancet* 1984;2:205; *BMJ* 1985;271:918).

Return to the Market in Canada and Europe

A laboratory was authorized to sell a product containing doxylamine and pyridoxine under the name of Diclectin. To reduce the remaining suspicions held by obstetricians, it was specified in the product labeling that the therapeutic category for which this combination was approved was "anti-nausea agent for the nausea and vomiting of pregnancy." A group of Canadian experts published a statement on August 11, 1989, affirming that this fixed association was safe. The British authorities had also expressed the same opinion. The Canadian government had thus maintained a marketing authorization for this product for a Canadian manufacturer (CSM/MCA, *Curr Problems Pharmacovigilance* 1981;6; *Lancet* 1984;2:205; Medico-Legal Committee Opinion, *J Soc Obstet Gynaecol Can* 1995;17:162; Koren, *Can J Clin Pharmacol* 1995;2:38). An epidemiologic study in 2003 compared the rate of birth defects in the United States in the years 1970 to 1992 and found no change in the rate of birth defects after the cessation of Bendectin in the 1980–1984 period (Bendectin and birth defects II: Ecological analyses, Kutcher JS, Engle A, Firth J, Lamm SH, *Birth Defects Res A: Clin Mol Teratol* 67[2]:88–97).

There is an enormous literature on Bendectin, and it is maintained by some workers that this is the most-studied drug in pregnancy ever. There are several books and hundreds of references available.

Adriamycin

Examples of drugs producing late AEs include Adriamycin (doxorubicin HCl), which may produce cardiac problems years after therapy has ended.

Myocardial toxicity manifested in its most severe form by potentially fatal congestive heart failure may occur either during therapy or months to years after termination of therapy. The probability of developing impaired myocardial function based on a combined index of signs, symptoms and decline in left ventricular ejection fraction (LVEF) is estimated to be 1 to 2% at a total cumulative dose of 300 mg/m2 of doxorubicin, 3 to 5% at a dose of 400 mg/m2, 5 to 8% at 450 mg/m2 and 6 to 20% at 500 mg/m2.* The risk of developing congestive heart failure (CHF) increases rapidly with increasing total cumulative doses of doxorubicin in excess of 450 mg/m2. This toxicity may occur at lower cumulative doses in patients with prior mediastinal irradiation or on concurrent cyclophosphamide therapy or with pre-existing heart disease (Package Insert for Adriamycin, Pharmacia, 2005).

Gene Therapy

An area of increasing concern is the possibility of late-occurring AEs seen after gene therapy. The United States FDA has cited this as an issue in gene therapy:

Many of the potential adverse effects of concern in gene therapy patients are the same as those of concern for other therapies; however, gene therapy raises some concerns that are relatively unique. Perhaps the greatest area of concern is that of late-occurring toxicities. By permanently altering the genetic makeup of the recipient cells, some forms of gene therapy may cause toxicities that do not manifest themselves until years later. Additionally, some gene therapies use viral vectors with the potential to form latent infections that may emerge clinically years later (Center for

Biologics Evaluation and Research Publication: Gene Therapy Patient Tracking System, Final Document, June 27, 2002). See the FDA's website (Web Resource 6-1).

Antiretroviral Drugs

It is now well recognized that many human immunodeficiency virus drugs can produce late toxicity. The FDA has issued guidance noting that long-term follow-up should be done in clinical trials:

Because multiple adverse events have been observed with chronic administration of antiretroviral therapy, mechanisms should be used for systematically evaluating adverse events over prolonged periods following traditional approval. Controlled comparisons and prospectively evaluated cohorts may be helpful in characterizing and defining drug associations for late-occurring adverse events. Therefore, after traditional approval, the Division strongly encourages sponsors to continue to collect safety data in key randomized studies or other treatment cohorts for prolonged periods (3–5 years)" (Guidance for Industry, Antiretroviral Drugs Using Plasma HIV RNA Measurements—Clinical Considerations for Accelerated and Traditional Approval, Center for Drug Evaluation and Research, October 2002). See the FDA's website (Web Resource 6-2).

Diethylstilbestrol (DES)

Perhaps the most interesting and striking example of delayed-onset AEs is that of vaginal cancer in the offspring of women who took DES. This is examined in detail.

DES is an estrogen first synthesized in 1938. In 1941, DES was approved by the FDA for human use. In 1947, the agency approved the use during pregnancy for the treatment or prevention of spontaneous abortion (miscarriage) based largely on the work of Harvard researchers George and Olive Smith, work that eventually proved to be wrong; the drug did not prevent miscarriages.

The suspicion of a problem arose in 1970, when clinicians observed a rare vaginal cancer occurring in women aged 14 to 22 years. This cancer, clear cell adenocarcinoma (CCA), was classically seen only in women in their seventies. No explanation seemed apparent until the mother of one of the young cancer patients mentioned that she had taken DES to prevent a miscarriage. Questioning of the other mothers revealed that they too had taken DES, and Dr. Arthur Herbst confirmed the association between DES and CCA in a case-control study in 1971.

Delayed Onset of Malignancy (Long Latency)

The delay in the appearance of the adverse drug reaction after the last dose (the latency period) is among the longest ever seen. The delay in detection has several explanations:

- The AE did not occur in the women who took DES but in their female offspring exposed during the critical window of vaginogenesis.

- The AE was not visible in the female offspring at birth.

- The AE was not evident until after puberty during a gynecologic examination.

- Obstetric problems appeared only when a pregnancy occurred.

The spontaneous reporting consisted of a publication of the first series of cases and a case-control study.

The reported risk of developing CCA in DES-exposed women is approximately 1 in 1000 from birth to 34 years of age. The risk increases rapidly from the onset of puberty until the late teens and early twenties. Subsequently, the risk drops dramatically, although a few cases have been reported in women in their forties. Other less serious but more frequent obstetric and gynecologic problems in the DES-exposed progeny have also been commented on in the medical literature:

- Vaginal adenosis, cervical ectropion (normal, albeit misplaced, columnar epithelium)

- Structural anomalies, such as cervical hoods, hypoplastic, and T-shaped uterus

- Functional problems, such as decreased fertility, ectopic pregnancy, spontaneous abortions (relative risk, 92:1), and preterm births (relative risk, 5:1)

- Possible abnormalities in children of daughters whose mothers received DES (i.e., third generation)

- Benign malformations, such as small testicles and epididymal cysts in males exposed in utero

Actions Taken

In 1971, the FDA banned the use of DES in pregnant women (FDA Drug Bulletin 1971). In the same year, a registry was established with Dr. Arthur Herbst as the chairperson, and in 1978, the DESAD Project was developed to study DES-exposed women with adenosis. In 1973, the U.S. National Institutes of Health notified medical schools and gynecologic oncologists about increased cancer risk. In 1977, France withdrew the obstetric indication. A movement known as DES Action was created in the United States, Canada, France, the United Kingdom, and elsewhere. See its website (Web Resource 6-3).

In 1999, the U.S. Congress directed the National Cancer Institute to fund a 3-year DES National Educational Campaign housed at the Centers for Disease Control and Prevention (Herbst, *N Engl J Med* 1971;284;878–881; Wilcox, *N Engl J Med* 1995;332:1411; Giusti, *Ann Intern Med* 1995;122:778; DES Action VOICE, Summer 2000 [section adapted from Cobert and Biron, Pharmacovigilance from A to Z]). The third generation (offspring of DES sons and daughters) are now being followed for possible health issues related to DES use by grandmothers. CDC maintains a complete website with multiple links (Web Resource 6-4).

There are other examples of long-latency AEs, though rarely as long or as dramatic as DES. Using the Yellow Card system in the UK, it was reported that practolol, a beta-blocker withdrawn from the UK market in 1975, was associated with sclerosing peritonitis, which did not appear for an average of 201 weeks after the drug start date (range .5 to 11.5 years). (See an instructive example of a long–latency adverse drug reaction—sclerosing peritonitis due to practolol. [Mann RD, *Pharmacoepidemiol Drug Safety* 2007;16[11]:1211–1216].)

■ The Future for Long-Latency AEs

The U.S. Institute of Medicine addressed long-latency AEs seen after vaccinations in "Research Strategies for Assessing Adverse Events Associated with Vaccines: A Workshop Summary" (1994) (Web Resource 6-5); however, no particular new strategy was identified to better find such AEs.

An academic Canadian group has studied late-occurring AEs and other ill effects that occur long after stopping treatment with biotherapeutics. They have proposed the creation of a registry to track such events throughout Canada: Post-Market Surveillance of Biotherapeutics for Late Health Effects—A Systematic Review and Recommendations on Active Surveillance in Canada. See its website (Web Resource 6-5).

■ Frequently Asked Questions

Q: This seems to put the practitioner in an impossible position. How can one even begin to make a rational attempt to determine whether a particular sign, symptom, or AE is due to a drug (or drugs) taken weeks, months, or even years ago? The patient may not even remember or know precisely what he or she was taking. And how can we even approach AEs due to the drugs a parent took a generation ago?

A: A valid point. The practitioner really can't make such a determination. The finding of very long-term or skipped-generation AEs remains primarily in the domain of epidemiology and observational studies. There is a tendency to run the safety arm of clinical trials for longer periods of time after the acute study is over. However, even that will not pick up the rare AE due to the small number of patients involved and the difficulties of long-term observational studies of safety where all patients will have AEs (and will die) if you follow the patients long enough. That is, there are confounding and coincidental events that make interpretation of the long-term results very difficult. It may well be that when large populations have electronic health records, a more formal health authority-driven-review of large databases in an ongoing manner will have more sensitivity in discovering long-latency, low-frequency AEs.

Spontaneous reporting by astute clinicians remains the best current approach based on the examples seen to date. Perhaps pharmacoepidemiology and genomics will provide more answers. From the practitioner's point of view, a high level of suspicion must be maintained. The patient should be quizzed on both recent and remote drug history, including over-the-counter medications. Beyond that, we must await better techniques and methodology for tracking drugs taken and resulting AEs.

7

The Mathematics of Adverse Events and a Brief Note on Pharmacoepidemiology

This chapter is not intended to be a reference on statistics, epidemiology, or the technical mathematical aspects of data analysis. Rather, it is meant to give a very elementary and selective overview of some of the "numbers" used in pharmacovigilance and to show why, in our view, they have not been useful yet in clinical medicine and pharmacovigilance.

When a new adverse event (AE) begins to be reported in association with a new product, the two fundamental questions raised in the eyes of the regulator and the manufacturer are about rates (Will it?) and causality (Can it?).

Suppose that spontaneous reports of liver injury with drug X start coming in at the safety department or health authority. First, what is the likely causality link between the liver problem and that suspect drug? Were the patients exposed to only the suspect drug or were they simultaneously taking other products, including over-the-counters (OTCs), "natural" products, and so forth? Was the time to onset short enough to be very suggestive or was it so long that suspicion is rather low? Was there significant alcohol consumption? Was the patient in perfect health

or was he or she at high risk of developing viral hepatitis? According to these and other diagnostic criteria, the clinician will roughly assess causality: definite, probable, possible, or unlikely. When enough details are available in a case report and when the report is complete enough, these judgments are feasible and they matter. We then say these reports are valid and (it is hoped) of high quality.

The next question is the rate of occurrence of this reported AE; in other words, what is the probability of the next patient exposed to product X developing severe liver disease? One in 10, 1 in 100, 1 in 1000? It is obviously important to know.

Over the years, many attempts have been made to apply statistics and epidemiologic methods to case series of AEs, primarily with spontaneously reported AEs. The results have been largely disheartening.

It is necessary to differentiate between AEs received in clinical or epidemiologic trials and those received spontaneously or in a solicited manner. The use of statistics is well described and defined for data generated in formal clinical trials. The patient populations to some degree are under the control of the investigator or researcher. The methodology for efficacy and safety analysis is well described and largely agreed on. Placebo- and comparator-controlled trials give clear pictures of occurrence rates of AEs, and significance values and confidence intervals can be determined and used to draw conclusions (at least for the efficacy criteria since the studies are usually not of sufficient statistical power to make safety judgments). The data are usually very solid, because data integrity is good to excellent. In addition, the data collected are usually complete. As patients are seen by the investigator at periodic intervals and as the investigator and his or her staff question the patient on AEs, it is believed that few AEs are missed, especially serious or dramatic ones. Incidence rates calculated from these data are held to be believable and useful.

Spontaneous reports are a different situation entirely. The data are unsolicited in most cases and may come from consumers or healthcare professionals. Follow-up is variable, and source documents (e.g., laboratory reports, office and hospital records, autopsy reports) are not always obtained because of privacy issues, busy physicians or pharmacists unable to supply records from multiple sources, patients' not wanting to disclose information, and so on. If no healthcare professional was involved, such as when a patient uses an OTC product, the data usually cannot be verified. Hence, the data integrity is variable and inconsistent.

There are multiple biases involved in spontaneous data reporting that can produce cases that do not truly represent the situation. Two phenomena that act on spontaneously reported data are worth examining: (1) the Weber effect and (2) secular effects, described below.

■ Weber Effect

The Weber effect, also called the product life cycle effect, describes the phenomenon of increased voluntary reporting after the initial launch of a new drug. "Voluntary reporting of adverse events for a new drug within an established drug class does not proceed at a uniform rate and may be much higher in the first year or two of the drug's introduction" (Weber, *Advances in Inflammation Research*, Raven Press, New York, 1984, pages 1–7). This means that for the period of time after launch (from 6 months to as long as 2 years), there will be a large number of spontaneously reported AEs/adverse drug reactions (ADRs) that taper down to steady-state levels after this effect is over. It is to be distinguished from secular effects. This phenomenon has been seen in multiple other situations since the original report. (Replication of the Weber effect using postmarketing adverse event reports voluntarily submitted to the United States Food and Drug Administration. Hartnell NR, Wilson JP. 2004;24(6):743–749.)

■ Secular Effects

Drug safety officers live in dread of reports of celebrities or politicians using a particular product, especially if an AE is reported or if spectacular efficacy or harm is anecdotally reported. This phenomenon is also called *temporal bias* and reflects an increase in AE reporting for a drug or class of drugs after increased media attention, use of a medication by a celebrity, a warning from a health agency, and so on. There are many multipliers of this effect over the internet, blogs, and other social media. "Overall adverse drug reaction reporting rates can be increased several times by external factors such as a change in a reporting system or an increased level of publicity attending a given drug or adverse reaction" (Sachs and Bortnichak, *Am J Med* 1986;81[suppl 5B]:49).

■ Reporting Rates Versus Incidence Rates

Perhaps the most difficult problem with spontaneous and stimulated reporting is incomplete data. Ideally, one would like to calculate incidence rates for a particular AE with a particular drug, where

$$\frac{\text{Numerator}}{\text{Denominator}} = \frac{\text{AEs that occurred}}{\text{Patients exposed}}$$

However, the number of reports of an AE is always less than the true number of occurrences, because not all AEs are reported. It is estimated that in the United Kingdom only 10% of serious ADRs and 2–4% of nonserious ADRs that occur are reported (Rawlins, *J R Coll Phys Lond* 1995;29:41–49). In the United States, the FDA estimates that only 1% of serious suspected ADRs are reported (Scott, Rosenbaum, Waters, et al., *R I Med J* 1987;70:311–316). These figures are cited by the FDA in a continuing medical education article from the FDA entitled, "The Clinical Impact of Adverse Event Reporting" (October 1996) available on its website (Web Resource 7-1). In a study in Swedish hospitals, an underreporting rate of 86% for 10 selected diagnoses was found in one study (Underreporting of serious adverse drug reactions in Sweden. Bäckström, Mjörndal, Dahlqvist, *Pharmacoepidemiol Drug Safety* 2004;13(7):483–487).

The number of uncaptured AEs is therefore quite variable. This renders the numerator in the proportion quite suspect.

In addition, the denominator, patient exposure, is unknown. Although one can obtain prescription data and one can know how many tablets, capsules, or tubes were sold, it is hard to know how many people actually took the product in the manner and for the length of time prescribed. Should one count the patient who took one tablet once in the same way as someone who took three tablets a day for a month or a year?

Denominator data are reported in a number of ways including patients exposed, patient-time of exposure (number of patients times number of time units each patient took the drug such as patient-months or patient-years), tablets sold, kilograms sold, kilograms manufactured, prescriptions written or filled, and so on.

Nonetheless, by obtaining these data, crude estimates of reporting rates can be made. However, the numbers are often not terribly meaningful. The author recalls one widely used product for which 12 cardiac arrhythmia reports were received for what was calculated to be 9 billion (9,000,000,000) patient-years of exposure. This works out to 12/9,000,000,000 or a reporting rate of 0.0000000013 cardiac arrhythmia events/patient-years of exposure, which is not a meaningful number, particularly to a clinician who needs to make a decision on whether a particular patient should be given this drug. In fact, this number is so low that it is below the naturally occurring incidence of cardiac arrhythmias in the population, meaning marked underreporting of the AEs. Thus, one could argue that the drug in question actually *prevents* cardiac arrhythmias, which is clearly not the case.

The manufacturing data (kilograms manufactured) are available from the company producing the product, and the prescription information and the patient exposure data are obtained from various private companies that track such things (e.g., IMS Health Incorporated; see www.imshealth.com). Confounders include generic products in which the denominator is not included in the calculation but in which the company reporting on the branded drug receives and includes AEs (numerator cases) as well as counterfeit drugs where the denominator and numerator are compromised. Nonetheless, these data can be broken down by gender, age, and other demographic characteristics. Trends over time in usage can be observed.

In summary, as Dr. David Goldsmith has said, "the numerator is bad, the denominator is worse, and the ratio is meaningless." Hence, one cannot calculate incidence rates for a particular AE based on spontaneous data, only reporting rates. Period.

However, the spontaneous data can be somewhat useful and new techniques looking at proportional reporting are under development. These include proportional reporting rate (PRR), gamma poisson shrinker (GPS), urn-model algorithm, reporting odds ratio (ROR), Bayesian confidence propagation neural network–information component (BCPNN-IC), and adjusted residual score (ARS). The PRR is described below.

Proportional Reporting Rate (PRR), Also Known As Disproportionality

There are various methods employed, and all more or less revolve around proportional reporting techniques. They look at the AEs for a particular drug and compare the same AEs for the remaining drugs in a database.

This basic PRR is simple and uses a 2×2 table:

	Drug of Interest	All Other Drugs
AE of Interest	A	B
All other AEs	C	D

PRR = [A/C]/[B/D]

For example:

	Drug X	All Other Drugs
AE of Interest	345	291
All other AEs	6901	14556

PRR = [234/6901]/[291/14556] = 2.5

In words, the proportion of a particular AE divided by all AEs seen with the drug of interest is divided by the proportion of this AE divided by all AEs seen with all the other drugs in the database (excluding the drug of interest). In the previous example, if 5% of all AEs seen with drug X are chest pain and 2% of all AEs seen with all the other drugs in the database (excluding drug X and its AEs), then the PRR is 5%/2% or 2.5. This means that there are (dis)proportionately more chest pain AEs with drug X compared with all the other drugs in the database, and this is noteworthy as a possible signal.

Since it is unusual that the PRR will be exactly 1.0, when the PRR is calculated for all AEs in the database, every PRR will either be below 1.0 or above 1.0. In theory, values below 1.0 would suggest a protective effect (the AE is less likely with drug X), and values above 1.0 would suggest an AE that is more likely due to drug X. Thus, one must be careful not to overinterpret the data, especially since there are more than 80,000 terms in MedDRA, and one could theoretically calculate some 80,000 PRRs. In practice, one sets a threshold above which the PRR is considered noteworthy, such as a value of 3.0. Any AE that has a PRR above 3.0 will be considered a signal and will be further examined. The higher the PRR, the greater the specificity but the lower the sensitivity. Alternatively, one might simply take the 10 or 20 highest PRRs and evaluate those regardless of how high the PRR is above 1.0.

There are other issues with using this score. When the database is small, problems can occur.

- For example, adding or subtracting one case can markedly alter the PRR results. For example, if there is one myocardial infarct (MI) in the four-patient database of drug X, this gives an incidence of 1/4 or 25%. Taking away the one case or adding one more MI would change the rate to 0% (0/3) or 40% (2/5). If the database had 1000/4000 cases, adding one or taking one away would have a negligible effect.

- Another problem may occur if the databases are inappropriate. It may not be appropriate to compare the incidence of a particular AE in the population treated with drug X against the incidence of that AE in the whole AE database. If the treatment for drug X is for, say, breast cancer, and is given only to elderly women, then comparing the incidence of an AE in the elderly female population versus the whole database in which elderly women are not predominant may give misleading results.

- Another problem may occur if drug X is frequently prescribed with drug Y and drug Y is known to produce a particular AE. Unless this is accounted for, it may appear in a simple PRR that drug X caused the AE when it probably was drug Y that did it.

- Similarly, certain common comorbid conditions or diseases may produce a high number of AEs that are due to the disease and not the drug.

- Finally, if the safety database used for the denominator of the PRR is small or has a high proportion of a particular type of patient or disease this may also produce flawed PRRs.

Various other statistical methods, or filters, may be added to this calculation to refine the technique to attempt to increase sensitivity. Some have adopted a rule of thumb that signals are worth pursuing if the PRR is more than 3.0, the chi-squared value is more than 4, and that there are at least three of the particular AE in question. Thus, if one has a sufficiently large database, the PRR

could be programmed to run periodically (e.g., monthly or quarterly) using the filters as noted to generate possible signals. This method will be less useful if MedDRA coding is not crisp and correct. As always, the issue here is generating too many signals with too many false positives for the personnel available to review the signals. For a further discussion of this and other signaling matters, see Chapter 19.

■ Other Data Mining Methods

Although the disproportionality method is commonly used by companies and health agencies to generate signals, other methods are being developed to compensate for some of these problems. Some of the other approaches are found in the broad category of "Bayesian approaches." These methods account for the number of cases (cell sizes) and decrease the sensitivity of the PRR score if the cell sizes are small. One method, the Bayesian confidence propagation neural network (BCPNN), was developed by the Uppsala Monitoring Centre (see Chapter 27) and is used for signal detection in their database. Other methods, such as the gamma poisson shrinker (GPS) and the multi-item gamma poisson shrinker (MGPS), are also used to attempt to make the PRR more useful. These methods have been used by various health agencies, including the Food and Drug Administration (FDA) and Medicines and Healthcare Products Regulatory Agency (MHRA). Treatment of these methodologies in detail is beyond the scope of this book, and the reader is referred to the standard textbooks of pharmacoepidemiology. A good, approachable summary of the field is available in Signal Detection Methodologies to Support Effective Safety Management (Van Manen, Fram, DuMouchel, *Expert Opin Drug Safety* 2007;6(4):451–464). See also "Practical Aspects of Signal Detection in Pharmacovigilance," Report of the CIOMS Working Group VIII. Counsel for the International Organizations of Medical Sciences. Geneva, 2010.

A brief note on other terms you may run across:

Event rate—The number of people experiencing an AE as a proportion of the number of people in the population.

Absolute risk—The probability of occurrence of an AE in patients exposed to a drug. For example, one may say the absolute risk of a myocardial infarction with drug X is 5%. Obviously, this value is often hard or impossible to obtain and is why pharmacovigilance exists.

Absolute risk reduction—The arithmetic difference between two absolute risk rates. For example, the absolute risk of a myocardial infarction with drug X is 5% and with drug Y 2%. The risk reduction is 5%-2% = 3%.

Relative risk (or risk ratio)—In a trial or in an observational cohort, the ratio between the rate of an adverse outcome (e.g., an AE) in a group exposed to a treatment and the rate in a control group. It is a measure of the strength of a cause–effect relationship. For example, the rate of myocardial infarction in the drug X group is 5% and in the control group 2.5%. The ratio (relative risk) is 5%/2% = 2.5.

Relative risk reduction—The difference in event rates between two groups, expressed as a proportion of the event rate in the untreated group.

Odds Ratio—Also known as estimated or approximate relative risk. In case-control studies concerning drug safety, the ratio between the rate of exposure to a suspect drug in a group of cases (with the AE) and the rate of exposure in a group of noncases (controls without the AE). Like relative risk from cohort studies, the odds ratio is a useful estimation of the strength of cause–effect relationships. This parameter is often used in meta-analyses.

Risk difference or attributable risk—The difference between the rate of an adverse outcome (e.g., an AE) in a group exposed to an experimental drug and the rate in a control group.

Number needed to harm (NNH)—Also called number needed to harm one. The number of patients that must be exposed to a drug to produce an AE/ADR in one patient. Exposure may, for example, be one course or one year of treatment. For example, one could calculate based on a study that the number needed to produce one case of rhabdomyolysis with a particular statin is 3500 patients.

Number needed to benefit (NNB)—A similar concept reflecting the number needed to receive a positive effect from the drug. For example, one might need to treat three patients with a particular statin to get a positive effect (e.g., cholesterol reduction).

Benefit–Risk Ratio—Various techniques have been developed using such data as NNH and NNB to calculate an actual number for the benefit–risk ratio. For example, using the statin example above, the ratio of benefit:risk = 3/3500 is 0.0009 or, conversely, the risk:benefit ratio is 3500/3 = 1167.

In the former, the lower the number, the better. In the latter, the higher, the better, but each represents the same calculation. The use of NNB and NNH is a useful and intuitive method for clinicians: In this example, the NNB is 1 in 3 and the NNH for this AE is 1 in 3500, a favorable benefit:risk balance.

Confidence intervals—Most studies are based on samples, not entire populations, which adds an element of uncertainty and unreliability to the results because the whole population was not studied. Thus, we cannot be totally sure that the 15% of the study population that had serious AEs represents the true value for the whole population rather than just for the smaller sample. The confidence interval represents the range of the correct or true value for the whole population and gives an idea of the reliability of the data and of the estimate. One can calculate various levels of "assurance," 90%, 95%, 99%, 99.9%, and so on, for the confidence interval. Usually, the 95% level is used. The narrower or smaller the distance between the upper and lower values of the confidence interval (called the confidence limits), the better. In general, the more patients in the study, the narrower (better) the confidence interval.

■ Pharmacoepidemiology and Trials

A brief note on the types of trials you may encounter in drug safety. Some people distinguish between a study (done on normal, nondiseased people) and a trial (done on ill patients). However, in practice, these words are used synonymously.

Randomized Clinical Trial or Study

A randomized clinical trial is an experimental study (not an observational study) in which the investigator, using a written protocol, studies one drug in comparison to another drug or drugs or placebo. The trial may attempt to show the drug treatment is superior to the comparator or that it is "the same," "not worse," or "nonsuperior." This is an important distinction and will alter the design and size of the trial. The study may differ from the normal treatment ("standard of care" or SOC) and practice of medicine in an attempt to find a better treatment. Randomization means that chance will determine which patient gets which drug treatment. Most such studies are blinded:

- Single blind: the patient does not know the treatment
- Double blind: neither the patient nor the investigator knows the treatment.
- Triple blind: neither the patient, the investigator nor the evaluator of the results knows the treatment.

Note that statistical calculations are usually not done on the safety data from clinical trials, as the studies are not sufficiently powered to detect differences in safety parameters. Thus safety data are presented as listings or tables without statistical testing. Studies that are larger and designed to study safety would normally be sufficiently powered and statistics can be done.

Case-Control Study

In this type of retrospective, nonclinical epidemiologic trial, a group of patients that had the AE and another group that did not have the AE are found and compared to see how many in each group took the drug in question. This type of study determines the chance (odds, or probability) of having taken the suspect drug in a group of patients already suffering from an AE and compares that with the chance of having taken the drug in a group of patients that did not have the AE. An odds ratio is calculated from the results. A large safety database (e.g., a claims database, a hospital database) is usually used and the two groups are matched as closely as possible (e.g., age, sex, race, disease, comeds). Both groups should have the opportunity to receive the drug. This type of design is useful for studying rare AEs because one can seek out a database that has this AE in reasonable numbers. These studies are usually fast and not too expensive. There are problems in the design, including marked biases in the selection of the patients, data quality, the medical history data (especially in claims databases), and the drug exposure data.

Cohort Study

In this type of nonclinical epidemiologic trial, a group of patients that took the drug and another group (the cohort) that did not are found and compared to determine how many experienced the AE in each group. Patients' records are reviewed, and the incidence of the AE is calculated for each group. The study may be prospective or retrospective. An absolute risk and excess risk can be calculated (unlike in the case-control study).

Nested Case-Control Study

This is a type of case-control study that obtains patients (AE cases and non-AE controls) from a cohort that has already been followed over time, such as in a health database. Thus, the cohort at the beginning of the study has exposure information, and, over time, some patients will develop the adverse event in question (cases) and some will not (controls).

The investigator will then compare exposure frequencies in cases and in controls just as in a regular case-control study. This type of study decreases recall bias compared with a nonnested case-control study and is usually faster and less expensive to perform than cohort studies.

The reader is referred to the many excellent textbooks at all levels available on epidemiology, pharmacoepidemiology, and statistics in medicine and pharmacology, including the following:

Brian Strom: *Pharmacoepidemiology*. 2005. John Wiley Inc.

Ron Mann and Elizabeth Andrews: *Pharmacovigilance*. 2007. John Wiley Inc.

Brian L. Strom and Stephen E Kimmel: *Textbook of Pharmacoepidemiology*. 2007. John Wiley Inc.

John Talbot and Patrick Waller: *Stephens' Detection of New Adverse Drug Reactions*. 2004. John Wiley Inc.

David Streiner, Geoffrey Norman: *PDQ Epidemiology*. 2009. BC Decker.

David Streiner, Geoffrey Norman: *PDQ Statistics*. 2003. BC Decker.

Beth Dawson, Robert G. Trapp: *Basic and Clinical Biostatistics (LANGE Basic Science)*. 2004. McGraw-Hill.

Another interesting book is not about medicine, statistics, or pharmacology but is about the concept and history of risk, particularly financial risk. It gives a broad and well-written overview on the role of risk in society:

Peter Bernstein: *Against the Gods—The Remarkable Story of Risk*. 1996. Wiley.

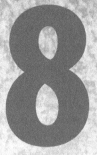

Where Data Reside

There is an enormous amount of data collected in the course of doing pharmacovigilance work. Much of it is reliable and verified but much is not. The problem is obtaining access to the data, verifying that it is real and correct, ensuring that no duplicates occur, getting it into a database accurately, and making valid clinical judgments at the individual patient level and at the aggregate (public health) level. As with everything else in drug safety, this is a moving target.

Adverse event (AE) data are collected all over the world by many people and groups. There is little standardization in the way they are collected, how they are measured and graded, how they are stored, and how they are used. Some of the data are collected as a matter of public health, and some are collected by pharmaceutical companies or other companies or nongovernmental organizations that process the data and make available or sell them to others. In theory, with the International Conference on Harmonization (ICH), Council for International Organizations of Medical Sciences (CIOMS), Medical

Dictionary for Regulatory Activities (MedDRA), and other standards, such as HL-7, we are moving toward improved standardization and use of these data.

AE data reside in several places. One main resource is the United States Food and Drug Administration.

■ AERS

The FDA has a large amount of data stored in four publicly accessible databases of primarily postmarketing safety data as well as other proprietary databases containing clinical trial information. The FDA drug database for all approved drug and therapeutic biologic products, the Adverse Event Reporting System (AERS), is discussed here.

AERS (Web Resource 8-1) collects information about AEs, medication errors, and product problems on marketed drug and therapeutic biologic products. It is ICH E2B compliant and MedDRA is used for coding. Quarterly (noncumulative) data files since January 2004 are available under the United States Freedom of Information Act for downloading as zipped SGML or ASCII files. Data include information on patient demographics, the drug(s) reported, the adverse reaction(s), patient outcome, and the source of the reports. The actual files can be downloaded directly. The data can be downloaded and manipulated (though not easily), and various companies offer services that include periodic updates, data searches, or repackaging of the data in a more user-friendly form. The database cannot be searched directly.

There is a variable lag of several months between AEs' being reported to the FDA and their making it into the quarterly data files. Should further information be desired after reviewing the data from the quarterly report, the full MedWatch form (anonymized to protect the reporter and patient) can be obtained using the unique identification number assigned to each case by the FDA. Data can be obtained directly from the FDA under the Freedom of Information Act (Web Resource 8-2) or from private companies. Using the latter ensures the anonymity of the requester, and some companies use these services to obtain information on their competitors' products.

Although getting and using the data can be difficult, it can be rewarding because large amounts of detailed data are available, particularly for newer products. The full MedWatch forms are available, and the narratives can be read to obtain clinical summaries of the cases.

This database is rather large, with some 4 million cases, and is growing by roughly half a million cases per year. About 35,000 are received directly by the FDA each year with the remainder from industry. Of the industry reports, about 300,000 are 15-day expedited reports and the rest are from periodic reporting. AERS contains primarily postmarketing data from prescription drugs, biologics, and over-the-counter drugs with an approved NDA sold in the United States, but it also contains some foreign reports of AEs for these drugs. Most of the industry reports are sent electronically, though paper reports (MedWatch 3500A forms) are still accepted at this writing. The data vary in quality, ranging from full due diligence inquiries and follow-ups with complementary data (laboratory reports, electrocardiograms, etc.) to lay consumer reports not validated by a medical professional. Note that FDA's AERS database has nothing at all to do with the commercial product from Oracle also known as AERS.

■ Clinical Trial Data

There are few clinical trial data in the FDA AERS database. The clinical trial data are proprietary and are generally not available, although some advocacy groups would like to see a change in this. FDA's new clinical trials registry will hold more data (including more safety information)

in the next few years as the FDAAA requirements come into effect (many in 2012).

Some clinical trial safety data can be found in Summary Basis of Approval documents that the FDA sometimes releases after a drug is approved. They are not easily found on the website and need to be searched for using the search box. Postmarket Requirements and Commitments may be searched for at (Web Resource 8-3).

Potential Signals of Serious Risks/New Safety Information that FDA has found in AERS is available at (Web Resource 8-4).

Approved risk evaluation and mitigation strategies (with links to PDF files containing the full REMS documents in most cases) are available at (Web Resource 8-5).

Finally, FDA was required by the Food and Drug (FDAAA) of 2007 to do a periodic review of new drugs (New Molecular Entity Postmarketing Safety Evaluation), looking at all data within 5 years of first approval. A pilot program completed the review of three products: apomorphine, aripiprazole, and duloxetine (Web Resource 8-6). Further reviews may be undertaken.

FDA has a new project under way to redo the AERS database. The agency is developing an electronic system called MedWatchPlus for receiving, processing, evaluating, and analyzing AE reports and other safety information for all FDA-regulated products. Within this system will be FAERS (FDA Adverse Event Reporting System), FDA's new database.

The FDA also has databases containing clinical trial information (Web Resource 8-7) as well as drug-specific information, including labeling for approved drugs (Web Resource 8-8).

■ The Uppsala Monitoring Centre (UMC)

The Uppsala Monitoring Centre maintains three database that safety officers should know about. Further information on the UMC's other activities can be found in Chapter 27.

■ Vigibase

Vigibase (Web Resource 8-9) is the AE database that the UMC maintains on behalf of the World Health Organization. The database has more than 5 million AE case reports from 90 countries and is growing by nearly half a million cases a year. The data are supplied by national health authorities. Much of the data are from the United States and are supplied by the FDA. The UMC does not review or assess the individual cases put into the database, but it does pharmacovigilance analyses and signaling. Not all of the supplying countries allow their data to be released. The database does not contain all the data found in the national databases (e.g., FDA's AERS) but rather contains extracts. In particular, there are no narratives. The UMC notes that the data are "available to anyone with a health professional degree-level education (physician, dentist, nurse, pharmacist)." The database contains information on drugs as well as OTC products and herbals.

Three types of reports are available. Ad hoc searches can also be done if none of the reports below are suitable. Samples of the output are available. Results are presented in WHO-ART terms but, upon request, can be presented as MedDRA terms:

- Overview Reports give numbers of reported cases with a specified reaction, a whole organ class, or all reactions listed for individual drugs. The information is grouped by reporting country or by year. Reactions are listed by preferred term. The summary gives the result as the total number of reactions for the criteria specified, listed by preferred term. In the "by year" and "by country" reports, the reactions are sorted by system organ class.

- ADR profiles provide similar information in a graphical and tabular format.

- Detail reports include further details about each individual case (date of report, case number, type of report, reporter, country, seriousness, death outcome, patient demographics, relevant medical history, AEs [MedDRA and WHO-ART terms], causality where available, suspect drugs, and concomitant drugs). Narratives are not stored in the database and are not available. The reports are available as case reports (one case per page or multiple pages if long), CIOMS line listings (.xls format), or spreadsheet (.xls format).

- Customized searches are available.

Costs of searches run roughly between $500 and $1200. Requests can be made directly to the UMC by e-mail, fax, or snail mail. Reports are returned electronically usually within a week or two (Web Resource 8-10). In addition, the UMC has arrangements with several vendors that provide Web access and tools for using the UMC (as well as FDA AERS) data (Web Resource 8-11).

The UMC's other databases (WHO Drug Dictionary Enhanced and WHO-ART for AE coding) are discussed elsewhere in this manual. See Chapter 14.

■ EMEA EudraVigilance Database

EudraVigilance is a data-processing network and management system for reporting and storing ADRs from clinical trials and in the postmarketing setting for products in the European Economic Area (EEA). It was launched in 2001.

EudraVigilance is used for the electronic exchange of SAEs among the European Medicines Agency (EMA), member states' health authorities, MA holders, and sponsors of clinical trials in the EEA; detection of possible safety signals; and the continuous monitoring and evaluation of potential safety issues.

There are two modules: The EudraVigilance Clinical Trial Module (EVCTM) and the Post-Authorisation Module (EVPM).

The database is maintained by the EMA in London. Data are not available to the public, though the EMA has been saying for some time that data will be made available to the public in the future. Companies may, in general, obtain data on their own products. Data are received from companies under obligatory reporting requirements for certain cases and from member states' health authorities.

From a practical point of view, since most data cannot be obtained from EudraVigilance, it plays little role in PV for the companies other than in the requirement to submit cases.

■ Motherisk

Motherisk is a clinical, research, and teaching program affiliated with the University of Toronto (Canada). They have many services and much valuable information on pregnancy aimed at mothers, families, and healthcare practitioners (Web Resource 8-12). In particular, in regard to drug safety, they have a website with information about the use of drugs in pregnancy (Web Resource 8-13). Their comments are based on their reviews of data from around the world. It is their view that "it is now clear that there are many drugs that are safe for use in pregnancy." They have comments and reviews of many specific drugs as well as information on herbals and breast-feeding and drugs. They do not have a database of AE cases per se.

Note that their information represents their own views and not necessarily those of the manufacturers, Health Canada or other health authorities, others in the medical community, or the author of this manual. There are other viewpoints, and some feel that some of these drugs should *not* be used in pregnancy or by women who may become pregnant. Prescribers and patients should refer to the approved labeling in their country for further information on the safety of medicines in pregnancy.

■ Health Canada

Health Canada's drug safety database is available online for immediate searches. See Chapter 25.

■ MHRA

The United Kingdom health agency has information from its Yellow Card Scheme available as Drug Analysis Prints (DAPs). DAPs contain complete listings of all suspected ADRs from the Yellow Card Scheme. They include both healthcare professional and consumer reports for a particular medicine. Products are listed by ingredient on the MHRA DAP Web page. The information is updated periodically. These listings are useful for signaling and are available as PDF files. See Web Resource 8-14 and Chapter 8 for further information.

■ Teratology Data

The Teratogen Information System (TERIS) and the online version of Shepard's Catalog of Teratogenic Agents is available at Web Resource 8-15. TERIS is an online database containing a series of agent summaries, each of which is based on a thorough review of published clinical and experimental literature. Summaries may be accessed using either generic or brand names. Each summary includes a risk assessment derived by consensus of an advisory board comprising authorities in clinical teratology.

An updated, automated version of Shepard's Catalog of Teratogenic Agents is distributed with TERIS. Users can access both systems simultaneously.

■ General Practice Research Database (GPRD)

The GPRD (formerly called VAMP) is a large database of anonymized longitudinal medical records from primary care practitioners linked with other healthcare data. Currently data are collected on more than 4 million active patients of research standard from around 500 primary care practices throughout the United Kingdom. It is used for drug safety, clinical epidemiology, pharmacoeconomics, and many other subjects in healthcare. Data can be obtained via the internet or on CD-ROM. Linked GPRD is only available through the GPRD Division of the MHRA in London and is the ONLY source of regularly updated, validated GPRD data. It is controlled and managed by the United Kingdom MHRA. See Web Resource 8-16.

■ Other Registries and Databases

There are many registries around the world containing safety data related to drugs. It is often quite difficult to find these databases, especially those that would be useful for obtaining safety data when preparing Risk Management Plans (RMPs) or Risk Evaluation and Mitigation Strategies (REMS). One organization that has collected many useful databases is B.R.I.D.G.E. TO DATA, with more than 75 databases from 15 countries. Databases can be located with information on exposure or outcomes of pharmacoepidemiology and pharmacoeconomic studies, as well as other studies of drug safety. A (paid) subscription is required. See its website for further information (Web Resource 8-17).

It is likely that drug safety databases will grow explosively in the near future as various efforts in the United States and the European Union to create data warehouses, linked databases, and electronic medical records databases move to fruition. The collection, standardization, normalization, transmission, and validation of the data, including HL-7 (Web Resource 8-18), are moving ahead. When large amounts of good data become available, the world of drug safety will change markedly.

Regulations, Directives, Guidances, and Laws

Pharmacovigilance (PV) is governed by a large body of requirements. Some are written and rigid. Others are written and far less rigid. Others are not requirements but only guidances or guidelines, and still others are unwritten customs and (best) practices. Obviously, laws and regulations vary from country to country. The sections that follow summarize briefly the obligations in the United States and the European Union (EU) for drugs and over-the-counter (OTC) products.

■ United States

Legal requirements for drug safety come from multiple areas. There are laws, regulations, and guidances issued by the United States federal government. These are the predominant formal requirements governing drug safety. In the United States, a "law" is a written statute, requirement, or ordinance that has been passed by a legislature and then signed into law (where required) by the executive. That is, a federal law is passed by Congress in Washington, D.C., and signed by the president. Laws may be created at multiple levels of government (federal, state, and local).

The law governing investigational drugs ("New Drugs") is found in Section 505(i) [21 U.S.C. 355], and the law governing marketed drugs is found in Section 505(k) of the Food Drug and Cosmetic Act (Web Resource 9-1).

In addition to laws, the United States Food and Drug Administration (FDA) is empowered to create regulations. Regulations are rules issued by government authorities under the power of laws. Regulations thus have the force of law. To create a regulation, the FDA publishes the proposed version of the new or amended regulation in the *Federal Register* (Web Resource 9-2). A period is defined during which time the public may send written comments on the proposal to the FDA. After review, a final regulation is published in the *Federal Register* and in the *Code of Federal Regulations* (Web Resource 9-3). A long period may elapse between publishing the draft and the final regulation; also, the draft regulation may be withdrawn.

Finally, the FDA issues guidances that contain the FDA's preferences on laws and regulations. As the FDA states on its Center for Drug Evaluation and Research Guidance website (Web Resource 9-4): "Guidance documents represent the Agency's current thinking on a particular subject. They do not create or confer any rights for or on any person and do not operate to bind FDA or the public. An alternative approach may be used if such approach satisfies the requirements of the applicable statute, regulations, or both." However, it is generally held in practice in the industry to be a wise course of action to follow FDA guidances.

Many of the applicable pharmacovigilance guidances can be found at Web Resource 9-5. Clinical trial guidances may be found at Web Resource 9-6. A more complete listing of FDA guidances can be found at Web Resource 9-7.

■ European Union

The European Union situation is different from the United States', in particular because the European Union is composed of 27 separate member states (countries) and 3 affiliated states that are different from the 50 United States. The European Union member states are sovereign countries; the United States are not. The member states are Austria, Belgium, Bulgaria, Cyprus, the Czech Republic, Denmark, Estonia, Finland, France, Germany, Greece, Hungary, Ireland, Italy, Latvia, Lithuania, Luxembourg, Malta, the Netherlands, Poland, Portugal, Romania, Slovakia, Slovenia, Spain, Sweden, and the United Kingdom.

The European legislation often refers to and applies to the European Economic Area (EEA), which consists of the 27 European Union member states plus Iceland, Liechtenstein, and Norway, which are not European Union member states but which participate in much of the European Union single market and adopt the European Union legislation. To complicate matters further, one sometimes sees reference to the European Free Trade Association (EFTA), which was set up originally for countries not in the European Union (then called the Common Market). The EFTA now includes only Iceland, Norway, Switzerland, and Liechtenstein. The Committee for Medicinal Products for Human Use (CHMP), which handles drug regulation for the European Union, includes members from the 27 countries and Iceland and Norway.

European Union "primary legislation" derives from treaties and agreements among the member states. This includes the Single European Act (1987), the Maastricht Treaty (1992), the Treaty of Amsterdam (1997), and the Lisbon Treaty (2009). "Secondary legislation" derives from the treaties. There are several types. The ones that touch most on pharmacovigilance are as follows:

- Regulations: Directly applicable and binding in all European Union member states without the need for any additional national implementation legislation. That is, the regulation as it is published is, word for word, the law in each of the member states. Note that this is different from the use of the word *regulation* in the United States.
- Directives: This legislation binds member states to the objectives of the legislation within a certain time period but allows each member state to create its own form of national law to achieve it. That is, each member state may modify the wording and requirements of the directive as long as the objectives of the directive are met.
- Recommendations, guidelines, and opinions: nonbinding and similar to FDA guidances.

The main European Union website is Web Resource 9-6, and the website covering European Union legislation can be found at Web Resource 9-8.

The key European Union regulatory and procedural documents relating to pharmacovigilance can be found at Web Resource 9-9. This site contains Volume 9A, Volume 10, The Rapid Alert System document, Eudravigilance and risk, and management documents. Additional guidelines for Marketing Authorization (MA) holders, health authorities, and PV practices are found at Web Resource 9-10.

The European Union situation regarding drug safety is, in many ways, far more complex than the United States'. In the United States, the requirements for drug safety come primarily from the FDA. A few state and local requirements apply to pharmacovigilance for companies, but in practice, these do not touch on drug safety as much as reimbursement, formularies, health insurance, dispensing, and other non-PV areas. There are, at rare times, requirements for registries or other safety obligations imposed by other governmental entities such as the National Institutes of Health (NIH) and the National Cancer Institute (NCI) for clinical trials. In contrast, the European Union has the supranational body of directives, regulations, and such from the European Medicines Agency (EMA) (empowered by the European Commission, Parliament, Council of Ministers in Brussels), as well as legal requirements in each member state, which may differ from or add onto the European Union-level requirements. European Union documents are generally available in many of the European Union languages (of which there are 23 official ones). Member state documents are published in the language of the member state but are not consistently published in other languages. Most, if not all, European Union-level documents are available in English. Summaries of Product Characteristics (SPCs), for example, are usually available in the official language of each country where the product is approved. National documents may only be available in that country's language.

Any company dealing in the European Union must obtain expertise at the European and member state level to stay in compliance with all safety obligations. In practice, this usually means the creation of affiliates or subsidiaries or the hiring of local companies or agents in the European countries where the drug is sold or studied.

In particular, the European Union requires the presence of a "Qualified Person" (Directive 2001/83/EC and Volume 9A). This person must be physically in one of the European Union member states and is responsible for pharmacovigilance. The person is responsible for "the establishment and maintenance of a system which ensures that information about all suspected adverse reactions which are reported to the personnel of the company, and to medical representatives, is collected and collated in order to be accessible at least at one point in the Community" (i.e., the European Union) as well as for preparing reports and responding to questions on safety matters, including the risk–benefit analyses of the products. See the directive (articles 103 and 104 in particular) and Volume 9A (see Chapter 23).

■ The Practice

In practice, the laws and regulations often leave areas of ambiguity. No law or regulation is ever able to predict or account for every conceivable circumstance that may arise. Where feasible, a guidance is issued to clarify issues. However, it is a complex, time-consuming, and difficult bureaucratic process to create laws, guidances, and regulations, and there is always a time lag between the need for a clarification and the publication of such.

For example, the definition of *serious* (see Chapter 1) would seem fairly clear:

> Any adverse drug experience occurring at any dose that results in ... death, a life-threatening adverse drug experience, inpatient hospitalization or prolongation of existing hospitalization, a persistent or significant disability/incapacity or congenital anomaly/birth defect. Important medical events that may not result in death, be life-threatening, or

require hospitalization may be considered a serious adverse drug experience when, based upon appropriate medical judgment, they may jeopardize the patient or subject and may require medical or surgical intervention to prevent one of the outcome listed in this definition.

In fact, several areas are unclear, and there is a long series of dialogues, publications, and meetings to address such ambiguities:

■ Is staying in a hospital emergency room overnight considered inpatient hospitalization (and thus a serious adverse event)? The consensus: No.

■ Is a preplanned inpatient hospitalization that occurs after an adverse event but perhaps for a totally separate condition considered inpatient hospitalization (and thus a serious adverse event)? The consensus: No.

■ What is an "important medical event"? Is thrombocytopenia, if the count is 5,000? Yes. 50,000? Probably yes. 350,000 (where the normal is up to 400,000)? Probably no.

■ What is "medically important" or "significant"? There is no clear consensus on this. It is left to individual reviewers' and reporters' judgments.

Thus, in circumstances where there is no clear answer, the best approach is to take the most conservative course of action and "overcall": if the question is between serious and nonserious, prefer serious; if the question is between reporting and not reporting a case to the health authority, prefer reporting. Calls to the agencies are possible to ask such questions, but it is not always possible to reach the right person to have a policy question answered. In such cases, try to get a written confirmation. If that is not possible, write detailed minutes of the telephone call and file them with the case. For cases submitted to multiple health authorities around the world, it is not practical to call each authority to get an answer, and it is possible the answers would be contradictory. Again, the best course of action is the most conservative course.

■ Over-the-Counter Drugs

Reporting requirements vary from country to country.

United States

In the United States, an OTC product is sold based on whether it got to market via (1) an approved New Drug

Application (NDA) (Rx to OTC switch) or an Abbreviated New Drug Application (ANDA), or (2) the OTC drug monograph process.

The safety obligations depend on which method is used to get the product to market. If an OTC product has an approved NDA, the requirements are the same as for a prescription product (expedited reports, periodic reports, etc.). For monograph products, the situation is different. Until 2007, there were no obligatory safety reporting requirements, though many manufacturers voluntarily reported serious adverse events (SAEs) to the FDA.

The regulations and guidances changed when FDA put forth the:

- Dietary Supplement and Nonprescription Drug Consumer Protection Act, December 2006 (Web Resource 9-11)
- Guidance for Industry Postmarketing Adverse Event Reporting for Nonprescription Human Drug Products Marketed Without an Approved Application, July 2009 (Web Resource 9-12)

These documents changed the reporting requirements for the monograph products:

- Manufacturer, packer, or distributor whose name is on the label (called the "responsible person") must submit to FDA all SAEs with a copy of the label within 15 business days.
- All follow-up information received within 1 year of the initial report must be submitted within 15 business days.
  - Law says 1 year but FDA wants no time limit. That is, report all follow-ups forever.
- Use MedWatch (3500A) form or E2B.
- Use NDA definitions for minimum criteria, reportability, and so forth.
  - For brand families need to know the active ingredient to have a reportable drug.
  - If multiple suspect drugs, submit Individual Case Safety Report (ICSR) to FDA and to other manufacturers.
- No aggregate reporting requirements.

Reporting requirements for NDA/ANDA products are unchanged.

European Union

In the European Union, in general, there are no OTC products without MAs. Thus, all prescription (Rx) requirements (expedited reporting, PSURs, signaling, etc.)

are the same as for Rx products. Agencies collect AEs on OTC products (e.g., the Medicines and Healthcare Products Regulatory Agency [MHRA] collects them under its Yellow Card Scheme).

If a product is sold in the United States and the European Union, in practice, the product is handled as a drug with expedited reporting, PSURs, and so forth, for global use.

Canada: There is no difference between OTC and prescription pharmaceuticals for expedited or periodic reporting of adverse reactions in Canada. OTC pharmaceuticals are included in the industry guidance document for AR reporting (Web Resource 9-13).

■ Staying Up to Date

As noted in multiple places throughout this manual, the world of drug safety is changing almost daily. Personnel handling drug safety and PV must stay up to date with changes that occur both in the scientific and medical world (new SAEs, new interactions, etc.) for drugs they handle and in the regulatory–operational world. The best way to do both is through journals, meetings and conferences, and the internet.

Scientific/Medical Literature

New and important medical information on areas that involve drug safety are found in many medical journals throughout the world, including major pharmacology and medical publications such as the *New England Journal of Medicine*, the *Lancet*, the *Annals of Internal Medicine*, and specialized drug safety journals, including:

- *Drug Safety*, the official journal of the International Society of Pharmacovigilance (ISoP) published by Adis (Web Resources 9-14 and 9-15).
- *Expert Opinion on Drug Safety* (Web Resource 9-16) covers medical issues on particular drugs.
- *Pharmacoepidemiology and Drug Safety*, the official journal of the International Society for Pharmacoepidemiology (Web Resources 9-17 and 9-18).
- *Drug Information Journal*, published by the Drug Information Association. This journal carries articles on the whole field of pharmaceuticals, including sections on drug safety (Web Resource 9-19).
- *Applied Clinical Trials*. This journal sometimes has articles on drug safety in clinical trials (Web Resource 9-20).

■ The Regulatory Affairs Professionals Society publishes a magazine for members that has occasional articles on drug safety. It is also a good resource for staying up to date on regulatory changes in general (Web Resource 9-21).

Meetings and Conferences

Many conferences cover drug safety only or have sections dedicated to drug safety.

■ Drug Information Association: DIA holds many conferences in the United States, Europe, and Asia, as well as sessions before and during annual meetings. Each January, conferences on drug safety are held in Washington, D.C., and there are annual conferences in the European Union (Web Resource 9-22).

■ Other private (nonprofit) organizations offer training, including the Pharmaceutical Education and Research Institute (PERI) (Web Resource 9-23), the Uppsala Monitoring Centre (see Chapter 27) (Web Resource 9-24), and the Drug Safety Research Unit (Web Resource 9-25). The EMA and MHRA do occasional training sessions.

■ The International Society for Pharmacovigilance holds meetings and training courses (Web Resource 9-26).

■ International Society for Pharmacoepidemiology has conferences, meetings, and training courses (Web Resource 9-27).

■ The FDA and certain other agencies hold advisory committee meetings and public hearings that are open to the public. Some are also transmitted online or are available as podcasts or webinars on the respective websites.

■ The Regulatory Affairs Professionals Society (Web Resource 9-28) has training sessions and conferences on the general field of regulatory affairs and sometimes addresses drug safety.

■ Many private, for-profit organizations train in drug safety on all continents. They are best found by doing a Google search on drug safety conferences.

The Internet

There are many resources on the internet. They are ever changing, with new ones appearing, old ones disappearing, and current ones changing:

■ Government e-mail alerts, e-newsletters, and RSS feeds. The FDA, EMA, MHRA, Health Canada, TGA, and many other governmental agencies issue periodic alerts as either e-mail or, more commonly now and replacing e-mail alerts, RSS feeds. See the chapters in this manual on these agencies for the URLs.

■ The Drug Information Association has excellent daily and weekly alerts on hot issues (*DIA Daily*, Web Resource 9-29), advisory committee meetings (*DIA Dispatch*, Web Resource 9-30), and regulatory changes (*DIA Global Regulatory Activity Digest*, Web Resource 9-31).

■ *Fierce Pharma* (Web Resource 9-32) is a set of daily publications on various areas of the industry.

■ Pharmalot is a blog that covers the industry with hot topics, news, and excellent links to primary sources (Web Resource 9-33).

■ Blogs. There are many blogs on the pharma industry, some serious, some outrageous, some outraged, all opinionated. They change frequently and their credibility varies. Best found by a periodic Google search. Caveat emptor.

■ Google Alerts. An excellent Google function is called Google Alerts. This is an automated mechanism that can be set up on Google to deliver, as it becomes available, daily or weekly information found on the net. The use of key words such as "pharmacovigilance" and "drug safety" will bring interesting news, press releases, blog addresses, and sites (Web Resource 9-34).

It is easy to spend one's entire day just reading blogs and news on the internet. A good compromise would be to find one or two sources that provide the updates the reader needs for his or her work. Attending a conference on drug safety once or twice a year is also valuable for both updates and networking.

10

Children, Elderly, and Other Special (Vulnerable) Groups

◾ Background

Similar to the testing of new drugs in pregnant women, the testing of drugs in special ("vulnerable") groups poses issues. Special groups include children, neonates, and the elderly as well as other groups with specific disease states, genetic conditions, and, sometimes controversially, various ethnic, racial, or religious backgrounds. The question here is whether the presence of the "special" condition alters the effects of the drug and produces more or different adverse events (AEs).

◾ The Theory

Children

Children are a special group because they are not simply "small adults" but rather are (depending on age and other factors) biologic beings who absorb, distribute, metabolize, and excrete drugs differently from adults.

A key document on pediatric drug development is the International Conference on Harmonization (ICH) E11 "Guidance on Clinical Investigation of Medicinal Products in the Pediatric Population," which can be found at Web Resource 10-1. This guidance notes in regard to safety that children differ from adults in having still-developing body systems and that additional considerations may be involved.

> Long term studies or surveillance data, either while patients are on chronic therapy or during the post-therapy period, may be needed to determine possible effects on skeletal, behavioral, cognitive, sexual and immune maturation and development.... Normally the pediatric (safety) database is limited at the time of approval. Therefore, post-marketing surveillance is particularly important. In some cases, long term follow-up studies may provide additional safety and/or efficacy information for subgroups within the pediatric population or additional information for the entire pediatric population.

The guidance also addresses the definition of a "child," noting the following possible categories and describing the issues in safety and efficacy of each:

- Preterm newborn infants
- Term newborn infants (0–27 days)
- Infants and toddlers (28 days to 23 months)

- Children (2–11 years)
- Adolescents (12–16 or –18 years, depending on region)

In the United States

In the United States, the FDA has been encouraging pediatric pharmaceutical research by companies for many years, but these efforts generally met with little success because of the hesitancy to test new chemical entities in children and babies.

In December 1998, the FDA issued a final rule entitled "Regulations Requiring Manufacturers to Assess the Safety and Effectiveness of New Drugs and Biological Products in Pediatric Patients," which is available at Web Resource 10-2. This rule required that every new product contain a pediatric assessment or a deferral or waiver of this assessment. It also allowed the FDA to require pediatric studies and required a pediatric section in New Drug Application (NDA) periodic reports.

In September 1999, the FDA issued a Guidance for Industry entitled "Qualifying for Pediatric Exclusivity Under Section 505A of the Food, Drug and Cosmetic Act," which is available at Web Resource 10-3. This guidance allowed the FDA to request, before approval of a drug, that pediatric clinical trials be done. As an industry incentive to do this, a 6-month additional period of "exclusivity" (patent protection) could be granted. This was followed up by additional FDA actions, including a draft guidance in 2000 on pediatric oncology studies, and other guidances on complying with this rule, including one in 2000 on complying with the Pediatric Rule (21 CFR314.55(a) and 601.27(a). See Web Resource 10-4.

However, major changes occurred with the 2007 PDUFA/FDAAA legislation. Two sections of the FDA Amendments Act (entitled the Pediatric Research Equity Act (PREA) concerned children:

- Title IV reaffirmed FDA's authority to require a manufacturer to submit an NDA for a new chemical entity, indication, dosage form, dosing regimen, or route of administration to submit a pediatric assessment. Sponsors may be given waivers from this for appropriate reasons (e.g., no pediatric formulation).
- Title V allows FDA to give an additional 6 months of marketing exclusivity to a manufacturer of a drug who submits data on pediatric use.

An internal FDA review committee was established in 2007 and has been meeting frequently and issuing reviews, assessments, and label changes and has requested various studies. A Pediatric Advisory Committee (Web Resource 10-5) has issued many product-specific safety reviews (see Web Resource 10-6). Labeling changes for safety that relate to children are available at Web Resource 10-7.

There has been much discussion and movement regarding pediatric safety and labeling. One major area of controversy revolved around the use of cough and cold products (usually over-the-counter, or OTC) in children, especially young children. After much discussion, FDA and the manufacturers agreed on a labeling change, noting that the products should not be used in children younger than 4 years of age. New measuring devices and child proof packaging changes were also introduced. See Web Resource 10-8.

Another area that has produced and continues to produce controversy is the use of psychiatric drugs in children. In particular, the FDA has issued an advisory about the use of selective serotonin reuptake inhibitors (SSRIs) and suicidality, notably about their use in children and adolescents. See Web Resource 10-9. A similar advisory was issued by the European Medicines Agency (EMA) (Web Resource 10-10).

In the European Union

New legislation, Regulation (EC) No 1901/2006 (see Web Resource 10-11), covering children aged 0 to 17 years was passed in 2007.

The key elements of the legislation include:

- Creation of a Pediatric Committee in the EMA.
- A requirement for pediatric data based on a Pediatric Investigation Plan (PIP) for new products and certain products already on the market and still under patent. If this is done,
    - An additional 6 months of patent protection may be granted for "regular" products and a 2-year extension for orphan products.
    - A new Marketing Authorization (called the pediatric use marketing authorization) may be granted, giving a 10-year period of market protection.
- A European database of pediatric clinical trials is to be created.
- Data from pediatric clinical trials must be submitted to the regulatory authorities.
- A European Pediatric Clinical Trials Network was set up along with new funding for off-patent drug studies.

- Use of an identifying symbol on the package of all products approved for children.

For further information see the EMA website (Web Resource 10-12) and the MHRA website (Web Resource 10-13). The latter site has extensive information on the history and status of pediatric drug issues as well as drug-specific assessment reports.

Bottom Line: Nevertheless, despite aggressive initiatives in the United States, the European Union and elsewhere, the status, knowledge, and safety of drugs for use in children still remains unsatisfactory and largely unknown. In practice, children are often treated as "small adults" because the initiatives still do not get around the fact that most companies, physicians, and parents are loath to perform clinical trials on children. Much of the safety data comes from postmarketing reports of AEs seen in children given drugs aimed primarily at adults. It is not clear how this situation can be resolved. Similarly, the other key safety issues, such as drug–drug, drug–food, and other safety matters are largely unknown in children, and most recommendations in these areas are based on extrapolations from adult data (much of which is also unsatisfactory).

The Elderly

The elderly, like children, also represent a special group in pharmacology for several reasons. There are certain diseases that are seen only or primarily in the elderly (e.g., Alzheimer's disease or osteoporosis). The elderly tend to have more diseases than the young, especially those that are related to chronic conditions (osteoarthritis, hyperlipidemia) or habits (smoking, alcohol use, obesity). As a consequence, the elderly consume more drugs and for longer durations. Hence, the risk of drug–drug interactions may increase, particularly if there is a decrease in renal or hepatic function. Finally, pharmacokinetics and pharmacodynamics may also be altered in the elderly, producing different effects from those that would occur in younger patients.

Swallowing disorders and dysfunction are often worse in the elderly than in the young. A tablet or other oral preparation that is large, sticky (e.g., having a hydroxycellulose outer layer), or oddly shaped may be difficult to swallow and could even get stuck or cause obstruction in the pharynx or esophagus.

Drug–drug, drug–food, drug–alcohol, and drug–disease interactions also may be different in the elderly, but these areas are largely unexplored.

As long ago as 1996, it was clearly noted that 21.3% of community-dwelling elderly patients in the United States received at least 1 of 33 potentially inappropriate medications (Zhan, Sangl, Bierman, Miller, et al., Potentially inappropriate medication use in the community-dwelling elderly. *JAMA* 2001;286:2823–2829). This led to the creation of a list of medications that should not be used in the elderly (see Fick, Cooper, Wade, Waller, Maclean, Beers, updating the Beers criteria for potentially inappropriate medication use in older adults. *Arch Intern Med* 2003;163:2716–2724). This is based on the so-called Beers criteria for medication use in the elderly:

- Always to be avoided
- Rarely appropriate
- Sometimes indicated but often misused

See also an excellent review and update in the Merck Manual (Web Resource 10-14).

The ICH and FDA Guideline

The ICH guideline E7 entitled "Studies in Support of Special Populations: Geriatrics" of 1993 was published by the FDA in August 1994. It is directed primarily at drugs expected to have significant use in diseases of the elderly (e.g., Alzheimer's disease) or at drugs that are used in large numbers by the elderly (e.g., antihypertensives). The guideline takes an arbitrary definition of geriatric as 65 years or older but recommends seeking out patients 75 years and older for studies. In general, there should be no upper age limit. Nor should the elderly with concomitant diseases specifically be excluded, because these are frequently the patients that most need to be studied.

The guideline recommends that geriatric patients be included in phase III and, at the sponsor's option, phase II studies in "meaningful numbers." For diseases "not unique to but present in the elderly," a minimum of 100 patients studied is recommended. For studies of diseases of the elderly, it is obviously expected that most of the patients studied will be elderly.

Pharmacokinetic studies should be done to determine whether the drug is handled differently in the elderly compared with younger patients. Studies in patients with renal or hepatic insufficiency should be done, although often studies involving the young suffice, and separate studies in the elderly may not be needed. Pharmacodynamic dose-response studies usually do not have to be conducted except for sedative/hypnotic agents and other psychoactive drugs, or where phase II/III studies suggest age-associated issues. Drug–drug interaction studies should be done when appropriate and do not necessarily have to be limited to the elderly.

FDA Guideline and Rule

In 1997, the FDA (62 FR 45313) established the "Geriatric Use" section in drug labeling. In October 2001, the FDA issued a guidance on this rule (Web Resource 10-15). It reviews the requirements for geriatric information in the various sections of approved labeling such as "Indications and Usage" and "Clinical Pharmacology, Warnings, Precautions." In regard to safety specifically, the FDA states that the labeling should include the following: "A statement describing a specific hazard with use of the drug in the elderly that references appropriate sections (e.g., 'Contraindications, Warnings, Precautions') in the labeling for more detailed discussion."

The FDA also issued a document aimed at consumers entitled "Medicines and You: A Guide for Older Adults," available at Web Resource 10-16, which summarizes some of the issues in geriatric use of medications.

Reporting requirements for AEs that occur in the elderly are the same as those for other age groups. Data on particular issues for a drug in the elderly should be included in the product labeling.

The elderly present a different picture from that seen with children. There are generally more data available about drugs in the elderly and about conditions more commonly seen in the elderly, such as renal or hepatic insufficiency, diabetes, and alcohol use. It is, in general, easier to study drugs in the elderly than in children, since with children there are often issues of informed consent. Thus, if there are not actual data from studies in the elderly, there are often data on these conditions that allow the healthcare professional to alter doses, change duration of therapy, order special tests, and so on to suit the elderly patient in question with some degree of medical science and data behind the decision. Drug–drug interactions pose a particular risk in the elderly, and much has been written about this (Bressler, Bahl, *Mayo Clin Proc* 2003;78:1564–1577; see also the editorial and the multiple references in the *Archives of Internal Medicine. Polypharmacy: a new paradigm for quality drug therapy in the elderly? Arch Intern Med* 2004;164:1957–1959).

The EMA has issued a special report on medicines in the elderly. See Web Resource 10-17. The conclusions include recommendations to define elderly, frailty, and adequate age cutoff points for drugs, to continue adding a specific section on elderly in the Committee for Medicinal Products for Human Use (CHMP) guidelines and to up-date these where necessary, to emphasize in discussions with companies the need to recruit an adequate number of elderly of various ages in the studies, and to systematically require the appraisal of elderly exposure for drug approval. See also the "Medicines for the Elderly" section at the EMA website (Web Resource 10-18).

Other Special Groups

It is now generally recognized that there is significant biodiversity among humans. There are probably many reasons for this. One major cause relates to drug metabolism pathways. The cytochrome P450 system, which plays a major role in drug metabolism, is well known to exhibit enormous diversity (genetic polymorphism), producing major differences in metabolism of drugs from individual to individual (see Evans, Relling, Pharmacogenomics: translating functional genomics into rational therapeutics. *Science* 1999;286:487–491; Court, A pharmacogenomics primer. *J Clin Pharmacol* 2007;47:1087–1103; and Nakamura, Pharmacogenomics and drug toxicity [editorial]. *N Engl J Med* 2008;359:856–858). Because of the differences in how drugs are absorbed, metabolized, distributed, and excreted by groups and by individuals, a more rational and tailored use of drugs will allow the maximization of effectiveness and the minimization of AEs. See the table of cytochrome P450 drug interactions at Web Resource 10-19.

Two further examples of special groups (women and African Americans) follow. In practice, one can create scores of special groups; this may indeed occur if pharmacogenomics fulfills its potential and allows subgroups (and perhaps even individuals) to be identified in terms of who will be at risk for or safe from particular ADRs. How pharmacology and medicine will evolve and characterize these differences in the upcoming years is a fascinating and unanswered question.

Women

Women have, in general, a smaller proportion of body water and a greater proportion of body fat than men. Men and women may metabolize drugs differently. For example, men have more alcohol dehydrogenase than women and thus metabolize the same amount of alcohol more rapidly (Frezza, di Padova, Pozzato, et al., *N Engl J Med* 1990;322:95–99). Women also handle cardiac drugs differently from men in many instances (Jochmann, Stangl, Garbe, et al., *Eur Heart J* 2005;26:1585–1595). Pregnant women also handle drugs differently. See Chapter 35.

African Americans

It is well known that different groups in the United States have significant differences in their general health. For example, a review by the Centers for Disease Control and Prevention (*MMWR* 2005;54[01]:1–3) noted that "for many health conditions, non-Hispanic blacks bear a disproportionate burden of disease, injury, death, and disability."

Similarly, African Americans may respond less well to certain drugs, such as antihypertensives (Levy, ed., *Ethnic and Racial Differences in Response to Medicines: Preserving Individualized Therapy in Managed Pharmaceutical Programs*, National Pharmaceutical Council, Reston, VA, 1993) or may have more AEs, such as angioedema associated with angiotensin-converting enzyme inhibitors (Kalow, *Trends Pharmacol Sci* 1991;12[3]:102–107). From these and other data, additional studies of the effects of drugs in various ethnic or racial groups are desirable. See an excellent commentary on the need for greater diversity in clinical trials by Professor Kenneth Davis of the University of Cincinnati in "African-American Health. Clinical Trial Diversity: The Need and the Challenge," at Web Resource 10-20.

There are many references on ethnicity and differences in drug metabolism (for example, see Phan, Moore, McLachlan, et al., Ethnic differences in drug metabolism and toxicity from chemotherapy. *Expert Opin Drug Metab Toxicol* 2009;5[3]:243–257).

The collection and analysis of data based on ethnicity is quite tricky, however. The FDA issued a guidance on the collection of ethnicity data in clinical trials in 2005 (Web Resource 10-21). The guidance offers practical guidelines on how to collect race and ethnicity data in clinical trials and how to present the data in INDs, NDAs, and BLAs. But how ethnicity and the data are to be interpreted in people or groups with mixed ethnic backgrounds is unknown. We await pharmacogenomics.

11

Drug Interactions

Analyzing AEs and ascribing the causality to a particular drug can be quite difficult. This difficulty, however, is magnified when the patient also takes additional drugs. This is sometimes known as "polypharmacy." It is generally believed that the more drugs taken, the greater the risk of AEs and the greater the risk of drug–drug interactions.

In such cases, it may not be possible to ascribe the AE to one particular drug. In most situations of regulatory reporting, the reporter or the company is generally required to specify one or more "suspect drugs" and, if present, one or more "concomitant drugs." The former are presumed to have a suspected causative role in the AE and the latter not.

Further complicating matters are drug interactions, a situation that occurs when two (or more) drugs are taken that influence each other directly or indirectly. That is, the pharmacokinetics (e.g., blood levels) or pharmacodynamics (effects in the body) of one or all of the drugs may be altered.

For example, the coadministration of desloratadine (Clarinex) and erythromycin, ketoconazole, azithromycin, or fluoxetine in pharmacology studies produced increased plasma concentrations (Cmax and AUC0-24h) of desloratadine and its major metabolite but did not produce clinically relevant changes in the safety profile (Clarinex Package Insert, February 2007). This is an example of a drug–drug interaction producing changes in pharmacokinetics (the plasma levels) but not in the pharmacodynamics (no clinical safety untoward effects).

A patient may suffer from a pharmacodynamic interaction when taking several products that share the same adverse reaction. For example, when simultaneously taking aspirin and clopidogrel (both reduce the clotting mechanism) plus a nonsteroidal anti-inflammatory drug like piroxicam and, unknowingly, another nonsteroidal anti-inflammatory drug like ibuprofen (both weaken the gastric lining and promote bleeding), the patient is at great risk of gastrointestinal bleeding.

At the other end of the spectrum is a drug like warfarin, which can be lifesaving but which has more than 55 potential drug interactions listed by drug class and more than 150 drugs and dozens of botanicals (some of which have anticoagulant properties) by specific name in the U.S. labeling. In addition, several "disease–drug" interactions are listed whereby these specific diseases may produce increases in the Prothrombin Time/International Normalized Ratio (PT/INR). The interactions may produce elevations or decreases in the PT/INR. In some cases, the same drug with Coumadin may produce an elevation in these levels in one patient and a decrease in another patient (Coumadin Package Insert, January 2010). These changes have the potential to produce significant clinical effects by putting the patient at risk for hemorrhage or clotting.

It is impossible, in the course of testing new drugs, to run drug–drug interaction studies against all drugs or even all classes of drugs. At best, sponsors run selected interaction studies against

- the most commonly used drugs that the exposed patients would be likely to take because of their age, diseases, sex, and so on.
- drugs that might be expected to produce interactions based on pharmacology data (e.g., cytochrome P450 metabolism) or based on historical data from similar drugs in the class.

These studies tend to be done on healthy patients in short-term clinical pharmacology trials. Drugs that are suspected of producing interactions but are significantly toxic by themselves (e.g., cancer drugs) generally cannot be studied in this manner because of ethical considerations. It is hoped that one day pharmacogenetics may provide better means of answering drug–drug interaction questions.

■ Cytochrome P450

Most data on drug–drug interactions are based on study of the Cytochrome P450 (CYP) system. CYP represents a large group of enzymes whose function is primarily to catalyze the oxidation of organic compounds, in particular drugs but also lipids, hormones, and other chemicals. The enzymes are found primarily in mitochondria or endoplasmic reticulum in cells and are found throughout the body. The enzymes we are most concerned about are found mainly in the liver and handle the biotransformation/metabolism of drugs in preparation for excretion.

Various drugs may increase or decrease the activity of one or more CYP enzymes by inducing the synthesis of the enzyme or inhibiting the enzyme's activity. Thus, if a drug inhibits an enzyme, then another drug that is metabolized by this enzyme may accumulate to toxic (ADR-producing) levels. Conversely, synthesis of more enzyme may increase metabolism of the second drug, lowering its levels and thus producing less efficacy (and perhaps fewer AEs). This may be unimportant if a drug has a wide therapeutic window but may be life-threatening if the window is small and critical concentrations of the drug are needed for efficacy.

Action on the CYP system is not limited to drugs but can be caused by herbals, smoking, and some foods. A good example is the herbal Saint John's wort, which is a potent inducer of CYP3A4. If Saint John's wort induces more CYP3A4, drugs metabolized by this enzyme (the drugs are referred to as substrates), such as cyclosporine or innadivir, may be cleared more rapidly and have less efficacy. (See Risk of drug interactions with St John's wort. *JAMA* 2000;283:1679. There are tables of substrates, inhibitors, and inducers published. See Web Resource 11-1, for example. In addition, the labeling of drugs will discuss drug–drug interactions.)

Note the marked complexity of the issue here if patients are taking multiple drugs. The tables and measurements, which are usually based on studies done in normal individuals during phase I, are really qualitative. They do not indicate whether the changes (induction or inhibition) will be large or small. This is usually due to the great variability in individuals that is seen in the clinical trials. Add on multiple drugs, some of which may inhibit, some of which may induce, some of which may do either, depending on the individual, and it becomes clear that the tables of interactions are at best guides and alerts to pay attention to the possibility of drug interactions. It is necessary, particularly in polypharmacy, to monitor the effects of the drugs, adverse events, and any other clinical issues and changes in the patient. In effect, once more than two drugs are being taken by a patient, it is very hard if not impossible to predict what interactions may occur and their intensity.

For further information, see the excellent section in *Stephens' Detection of New Adverse Drug Reactions*, 5th edition, edited by John Talbot and Patrick Waller (Wiley, 2004). Also see the U.S. FDA's consumer information on drug interactions at Web Resource 11-2. Textbooks on drug interactions are also available. The EMA has an excellent and thorough review of interactions (drug, food, and herbals), covering both in vitro and clinical studies, available at Web Resource 11-3.

As noted above with Coumadin, certain patients who are either debilitated or suffer from certain diseases (e.g., autoimmune disorders, cardiovascular disease, gastrointestinal disease, infection, psychiatric disorders, respiratory disorders, seizure disorders, and others) may be at greater risk for drug interactions, and the more severe the underlying disease, the greater the risk. It should also be noted that there are possible drug–food (e.g., grapefruit juice), drug–nutrient, drug–disease, drug–herbal, and drug–alcohol interactions. It is also worth keeping in mind that drug–OTC interactions may be missed if the over-the-counter products a patient is taking are not asked for by the questioner or remembered by the patient. There have been attempts to mine data on large databases, looking for drug interactions. One method uses the disproportionality scores (see Chapters 7 and 19) for the two drugs in question for an ADR suspected of worsening by an interaction. Individual scores are calculated and then an "interaction" score is determined. This method has not been too successful or widely used. Other methods calculate confidence intervals for each drug and compare them to a confidence interval for a combined "virtual drug" of the two drugs combined in an attempt to estimate the drug interaction effect (see Leone, Magro, Moretti, et al., Identifying adverse drug reactions associated with drug-drug interactions: data mining of a spontaneous reporting database in Italy. *Drug Safety* 2010;1;33[8]:667–675; and van Manen, Fram, DuMouchel, Signal detection methodologies to support effective safety management. *Expert Opin Drug Safety* 2007;6[4]:451–464).

■ Frequency

In reality, drug–drug interactions represent a major problem in medicine today that is not well recognized by clinicians. We may consider some of these to be "medication errors" because known drug interactions where there are significant clinical risks of either lack of efficacy or AEs should not occur. These drugs should not be prescribed or taken together. However, the use of bad drug combinations is common.

In a study in Toronto, Canada, 909 elderly patients receiving glyburide were admitted with a diagnosis of hypoglycemia. In the primary analysis, those patients admitted for hypoglycemia were more than six times as likely to have been treated with co-trimoxazole in the previous week. Patients admitted with digoxin toxicity (n = 1051) were about 12 times more likely to have been treated with clarithromycin in the previous week, and patients treated with ACE inhibitors admitted with a diagnosis of hyperkalemia (n = 523) were about 20 times more likely to have been treated with a potassium-sparing diuretic in the previous week. The authors conclude that many hospital admissions of elderly patients for drug toxicity occur after administration of a drug known to cause drug–drug interactions and that many of these in-

teractions could have been avoided (Juurlink, Mamdani, Kopp, Laupacis, Redelmeier, Drug–drug interactions among elderly patients hospitalized for drug toxicity. *JAMA* 2003;289:1652–1658).

In a database study of 1600 elderly patients in six European countries, the subjects used on average 7 drugs per person; 46% had at least one drug combination possibly leading to a drug–drug interaction. On average, there were 0.83 potential drug–drug interactions per person. Almost 10% of the potential interactions were classified "to be avoided" according to the Swedish interaction classification system, but nearly one third of them were to be avoided only for predisposed patients. The risk of a subtherapeutic effect as a result of a potential drug–drug interaction was as common as the risk of adverse reactions. Furthermore, differences in the frequency and type of potential interactions were found among the countries (Bjorkman, Fastbom, Schmidt, Bernsten, Drug–drug interactions in the elderly. *Ann Pharmacother* 2002;36:1675–1681; Bjorkman, Fastbom, Schmidt, et al., *Ann Pharmacother* 2002;36:1675–1681. For an excellent review of drug therapy in the elderly, see Bressler and Bahl, Principles of drug therapy for the elderly patient. *Mayo Clin Proc* 2003;78:1564–1577).

■ Communication

There is a growing recognition that the mechanism for communicating medical information (in this case drug interaction information) is not adequate and is not achieving its goals. FDA and others have embarked on various new mechanisms and procedures (including the use of social media) to better communicate safety information. Interestingly, in the United States, the responsibility and liability for drug interaction issues seem to be falling more on the pharmacist than on the prescribing physician, perhaps for the following reasons:

- Colleges of pharmacy in the United States include courses in their entry-level degree programs designed to instruct students on aspects of drug interactions, including detection, incidence and significance, types of drug interactions, mechanisms by which interactions occur, and the role of the pharmacist in monitoring drug therapy to either avoid or resolve drug interactions.

- Most pharmacies (particularly the large national and regional chains in the United States) and healthcare systems are heavily computerized, allowing pharmacists to screen patient medication profiles for drug–drug interactions when processing new and refill prescriptions. Some software automatically flags this for the pharmacist and patient. With the movement to electronic prescribing from physician to pharmacy, this is likely to become routine.

- The profession of pharmacy, through its professional organizations such as the American Pharmaceutical Association and the Canadian Pharmacists Association, has publicly proclaimed that the role of the pharmacist in "pharmaceutical care as a practice standard" is to maximize patient outcomes and "taking medication histories and maintaining patient drug profiles to assess patients' drug therapy for possible interactions with current medications and health conditions" (Canadian Pharmacists Association, Web Resource 11-4).

- In the United States, OBRA-90 legislation charged pharmacists with the responsibility to minimize adverse reactions, which includes drug–drug interactions. This legislation, dating back to the 1990s, required pharmacies to maintain good patient records, to provide patient counseling, and to do prospective drug utilization review, including drug–disease, drug–drug, and drug–allergy interactions as well as other good pharmacy practice, including search for therapeutic duplications, over- or under-utilization, and abuse and misuse (see Vivian, OBRA '90 at Sweet Sixteen. *US Pharm* 2008;33[3]:59–65). Similar active duties have been put in place for pharmacists in many other countries.

- The Joint Commission requires that hospitalized patients be educated and counseled on potential food–drug interactions by the pharmacist, dietitian, nurse, and physician. The pharmaceutical care component of the Joint Commission standard specifies that pharmacists are responsible for identifying drug–drug interactions as well as drug–food interactions.

- Various studies suggest a lack of knowledge among physicians about drug interactions, specifically drug–food interactions. These studies also report that fifth-year pharmacy students scored significantly higher than family medicine residents (in their fifth or sixth year of training) in 12 of 14 items on a standardized drug interaction questionnaire.

In the world of drug safety, it behooves the healthcare professionals, sponsors, and health agencies to be aware of polypharmacy and to consider a possible drug interaction even if the reporter has not mentioned it as an AE or even as a suspicion. Certain AEs known to occur in the drug interaction setting (e.g., torsades de pointes, hemorrhage in patients on anticoagulants, seizures, ingestion of grapefruit juice) should raise the level of suspicion in the medical reviewers. It is worthwhile to track suspected drug interactions on a potential "signal list" for continued review.

Conversely, the occurrence of an AE when two or more drugs are being taken does not necessarily imply a drug interaction. Ideally, drug blood-level abnormalities (or other markers suggestive of an interaction) should be obtained to add evidence to the suspicion of a drug interaction in a specific patient. In a more general sense, a clinical study or a demonstration of metabolism issues (e.g., use of the same cytochrome P450 pathway) is needed to add weight to the likelihood of a drug interaction. As noted above, it is difficult, expensive, and sometimes not ethical to perform such studies, and indirect evidence or a high level of suspicion must be relied on to determine a drug interaction.

The astute "pharmcovigilante" should always be aware of the possibility of interactions and pay attention to other medications being taken as well as OTCs, herbals, nutraceuticals, foods, alcohol, and the patient's diseases for clues to interactions. Not an easy task at all!

12

AE Volume, Quality, Good Documentation Procedures, and Medical Records

In spite of all the difficulties inherent in the system for collecting and analyzing Adverse Events (AEs), the number of AEs received by companies and health authorities is rising dramatically. This is likely due to several reasons:

- An increased awareness by healthcare practitioners that reporting AEs to the health authorities (and companies) is critical for public health and better communications.

- An increased awareness among patients and consumers of the importance of reporting AEs, at least in the United States, Europe, and Canada, where these reports are encouraged.

- More clinical trials producing more AEs.

- Increasing prescribing of drugs by physicians and the increasing use of drugs by the general population (both prescription and over-the-counter) producing more AEs.

- More toxic (and more efficacious) drugs being produced, treating diseases that, 20 years ago, were

badly treated or untreatable by drugs (e.g., AIDS, certain malignancies, Crohn's disease, rheumatoid arthritis).

- More drug use by the elderly, more polypharmacy, more drug interactions, and AEs.

- Better communications and easier methods of AE reporting (online, e-mail, EDC, automatic "pulling" of AEs from databases, etc.).

- Better training in pharmacy, nursing, and medical schools as well as increased awareness in hospitals and other healthcare facilities of the need to report AEs.

- People are living longer.

- The spread and use of PV systems to health agencies in countries that either did not have such systems in place or did not pay much attention to them.

The quantity of AEs received by the FDA on marketed products has increased from 170,000 in 1996 (Goldman and Kennedy, *Postgrad Med* 1998;103:3) to 580,000 in 2009 (Table 12.1). See FDA's statistics page (Web Resource 12-1).

Table 12.1	AE Cases Received by FDA for Marketed Products			
Year	Direct	15-Day	Periodic Received	Total Received
2000	16,131	94,931	155,804	266,866
2001	19,308	114,693	150,761	284,762
2002	20,438	128,680	173,375	322,493
2003	22,944	144,271	203,628	370,843
2004	21,655	162,007	239,268	422,930
2005	25,312	213,324	225,183	463,819
2006	20,977	219,956	230,461	471,394
2007	23,033	230,919	228,202	482,154
2008	32,889	275,421	218,207	526,527
2009	34,173	330,476	215,266	580,904

In 2009, about 301,000 of the cases were domestic United States cases and about 178,000 were from outside the United States.

It should be kept in mind that non-United States non-serious AEs and non-United States serious-labeled AEs do not have to be reported to the FDA by companies, so the numbers cited above are less than the total AEs captured. These requirements may change in the future.

The FDA expects that manufacturer-submitted MedWatch forms will be complete and of high quality. In its document "Enforcement of the Postmarketing Adverse Drug Experience Reporting Regulations," September 30, 1999 (Web Resource 12-2), the FDA instructs its inspectors as follows:

Verify the completeness and accuracy of the selected reports against other information in the firm's files as follows:

1. Was information on the form available at the time of submission?

2. Was all relevant information included on the form?

3. Was the initial receiving date supplied to the agency (FDA Form 3500A Section G Item 4) the same date as the initial receipt of information by the manufacturer?

4. Was new information obtained by the firm during the follow-up investigation and was this information submitted to the agency?

5. Where feasible, particularly when hospitalization, permanent disability, or death occurred, did the firm obtain important follow-up information to enable complete evaluation of the report?

In addition, the document further instructs the auditor as follows:

Document deviations from the ADE regulations. Clear deviations such as, failure to submit ADE reports, failure to promptly investigate an ADE event, inaccurate information, incomplete disclosure of available information, lack of written procedures or failing to adhere to reporting requirements, should be cited.

These violations are cited in a "483" addressed to the company. More severe violations may produce a "Warning Letter" (see Chapter 48):

The following violations are considered significant to warrant issuance of a Warning Letter:

- Failure to submit ADE reports for serious and unexpected adverse drug experience events (21 CFR 314.80(c)(1) and 310.305(c)).

- 15-day alert reports that are submitted as part of a periodic report and which were not otherwise submitted under separate cover as 15-day alert reports. This applies to foreign and domestic ADE information from scientific literature and postmarketing studies as well as spontaneous reports (21 CFR 314.80(c) (1) and 310.305(c)).

- 15-day alert reports that are inaccurate and/or not complete.

- 15-day alert reports that are not submitted on time.

- The repeated or deliberate failure to maintain or submit periodic reports in accordance with the reporting requirements (21 CFR 314.80(c) (2)).

- Failure to conduct a prompt and adequate follow-up investigation of the outcome of ADEs that are serious and unexpected (21 CFR 314.80(c) (1) and 310.305(c) (3).

- Failure to maintain ADE records for marketed prescription drugs or to have written procedures for investigating ADEs for marketed prescription drugs without approved applications (21 CFR 314.80(i) and 211.198).

- Failure to submit 15-day reports derived from a postmarketing study where there is a reasonable possibility that the drug caused the adverse drug experience.

In other words, the auditors will cite lack of standard operating procedures as well as late, incomplete, inadequately followed-up, or unsent 15-day reports. It thus behooves the company to be sure that quality and compliance procedures are in place to ensure the following:

- All cases are received in the appropriate department in the company. For example, sales representatives and other company personnel, if told about an AE, must report these cases to the drug safety department for the appropriate handling. This must be documented in standard operating procedures, with training provided and documented and violations noted and corrected.

- Cases must be rapidly triaged in the drug safety unit (or elsewhere if appropriate) to ensure that they are handled in the appropriate time frame. This applies most markedly to cases that may be 15-day postmarketing expedited reports (and, of course, those clinical trial cases that may be 7- or 15-day expedited reports). In practice, this means that all serious AEs should reach the drug safety group within 1 to 2 (working) days after receipt anywhere in the company.

- Serious AEs should be promptly entered into the database and medically reviewed, and those cases that are 15-day expedited reports promptly sent to the health agencies. Follow-up should be requested in those cases where there is incomplete information. It is highly unusual for a case to be complete with the initial report, and, in practice, all serious AEs will have follow-up performed.

- Data should be reviewed against the source documents for completeness and accuracy.

- Data should also be reviewed by a physician for medical content.

Audits and inspections performed by the EMA or other European Union health authorities are similar in their fundamental nature but have certain European Union twists that are different from those in the United States (see Chapter 48). In any case, all the points noted above would apply to a European Union audit as well.

Similarly, the European Union, MHRA, and other agencies stress the importance of quality, timeliness, consistency, and the appropriateness of the skill set of the individuals handling particular functions. Volume 9A (Section 2.3.4, "Expedited Adverse Reaction Reporting") notes that the health agencies (competent authorities) are as follows:

- Monitoring adverse reaction reports received from Marketing Authorization Holders against other sources to determine complete failure to report.

- Monitoring the time between receipt by Marketing Authorization Holder and submission to Competent Authorities to detect late reporting.

- Monitoring the quality of reports. Submission of reports judged to be of poor quality may result in the Marketing Authorization Holders' follow-up procedures being scrutinized.

- Checking of Periodic Safety Update Reports (PSURs) to detect underreporting (e.g., of expedited reports).

- Checking interim and final reports of postauthorization safety.

■ Archiving

The drug safety department must maintain an archive of all paper and electronic records for each case whether serious, whether submitted to the health agencies, and whether considered important. These records should be kept in a secure and protected (from intrusion, fire, water, etc.) file room. Access to the file room or electronic storage should be limited, and files that leave the file room physically to be worked on by the staff or examined by someone else should be formally signed out and tracked. The files should be treated the way a library treats rare and expensive books.

Old cases may be archived off-site either on paper, electronically, or both, in a similarly protected environment, but they must be available for an audit within one working day or less. Hence, the filing, indexing, and retrieval system must be clearly worked out and efficient.

Source documents and cases from outside the country, especially those not in English, may be kept at the source (i.e., the company's subsidiaries or affiliates or business partners) but must be available within a day at most for an inspection or other safety review.

All paperwork, including scrap paper, jotted notes, and telephone logs, must be kept in the permanent files of the company. Some companies scan all documents and retain only the electronic files. These documents, where appropriate, should be kept in the paper folders for each individual case safety report and be easily retrievable during an inspection or audit by internal auditors or health authorities. Pencils, erasers, and whiteout should also be banned from the drug safety department. All notes should be in pen. Sticky notes should also be avoided because they may fall off or disappear and may contain important data. Data corrections or changes should be done by putting a single line through the incorrect value (leaving it still readable) with the new value written nearby and dated and initialed or signed.

The best form and format of archiving should be left to professional archivists. Paper retention produces enormous volumes of files, especially if a company or health authority is receiving tens or hundreds of thousands of cases and hence hundreds of thousands to millions of pieces of paper per year. Thus nonpaper archiving is now, in practicality, obligatory. The problem here is the obsolescence of the electronic storage systems. Data stored on 3 1/2- or 5 1/4-inch floppy disks are now useless because the diskettes themselves may no longer be readable if stored badly and because there are few computers that still have disk drives that can read such disks. Other storage methods (e.g., zip drives) have also come and gone. Any decision made in regard to archiving should be discussed with the appropriate experts (archivists, regulatory, legal, IT) in the institution and reviewed periodically to see whether the methods and procedures in use are still appropriate.

Record Retention Times

There are various time limits that have been established, usually by the legal department or by the records retention department of a company, for all documents. Companies have various time frames for keeping records, allowing their destruction after certain dates, such as 25 years, 3 years after the NDA or MA is closed, 2 or 3 years (depending on product life span) after the last product is sold or used in a clinical trial, and so on. The MHRA (United Kingdom) has explicitly stated in its Q&A PV page under "Record Retention" (Web Resource 12-3):

- The current position of the MHRA is that, as a minimum standard, pharmacovigilance records should be kept while a product is marketed and for several years thereafter.
- However, the term *several years* is difficult to quantify, as it depends on the type of the product, expiry date, therapeutic use, reason for withdrawal from the market, and several other factors.
- Because of these constraints, the MHRA would not encourage the disposal of any pharmacovigilance

records. If a company considers there is a strong case that records can be destroyed several years after marketing has ceased, this should be discussed on a case-by-case basis with the inspectorate.

- The preferred position of the MHRA is that pharmacovigilance records should be kept indefinitely.

So, in practice, safety records should be kept forever. One never knows when one might need the records either for health authority issues or litigation. Keep in mind that diethylstilbestrol produced AEs in the offspring (and even in granddaughters) decades after the original patients took diethylstilbestrol (see Chapter 6).

Good Documentation Practices

Finally, some other comments on good documentation practices:

- If it is not written down, it does not exist and did not happen.
- Documents must be detailed, accurate, and timely.
- Documentation should be contemporaneous; that is, it should be written down at the time it occurs and not at a later date.
- Page numbers, dates, and versions must be tracked.
- No documents should ever be backdated.
- Eschew obfuscation (= avoid lack of clarity)!
- Documents should be written in a businesslike manner, with correct tone, grammar, vocabulary, and syntax.
- Documents should be written so that they are understandable to people whose first language is not that of the document.

Such practices have been codified by some agencies mainly under good manufacturing practices. See the European Union's documentation practices at EudraLex, volume 4, Chapter 4, *Good Manufacturing Practice (GMP) Guidelines* (Web Resource 12-4) and FDA's 1999 "Guidance for Industry—Computerized Systems Used in Clinical Trials" (Web Resource 12-5) for further information.

13

Seriousness, Expectedness, and Causality

The drug safety staff involved in individual case evaluation generally have to make several decisions regarding each case. These decisions must be made rapidly on receipt of an individual case safety report because this determines how the case is handled in the drug safety department and whether, how, and when it is reported to health agencies and business partners.

■ Seriousness

The generally accepted definition of seriousness is as follows:

A serious adverse event (experience) or serious adverse reaction is any untoward medical occurrence that at any dose:

- results in death,
- is life-threatening,

(NOTE: The term "life-threatening" in the definition of "serious" refers to an event in which the patient was at risk of death at the time of the event; it does not refer to an event that hypothetically might have caused death if it were more severe.)

- requires inpatient hospitalization or prolongation of existing hospitalization,
- results in persistent or significant disability/incapacity, or
- is a congenital anomaly/birth defect.

Medical and scientific judgment should be exercised in deciding whether expedited reporting is appropriate in other situations, such as important medical events that may not be immediately life-threatening or result in death or hospitalization but may jeopardize the patient or may require intervention to prevent one of the other outcomes listed in the previous definition. These should also usually be considered serious.

"Examples of such events are intensive treatment in an emergency room or at home for allergic bronchospasm; blood dyscrasias or convulsions that do not result in hospitalization; or development of drug dependency or drug abuse" (ICH E2A).

The European Union also notes that any suspected transmission via a medicinal product of an infectious agent is also considered serious (Volume 9A, page 200).

Note that the FDA slightly altered the definition of "serious" effective March 2011 for clinical trials by adding the concept of "disability" directly into the definition, including the phrase: "substantial disruption of the ability to conduct normal life functions".

Over the years, these definitions have been discussed, parsed, and clarified by health agencies, companies, and other interested observers. In general, the most conservative interpretation is the one drug safety groups should use. Some comments follow:

- Death: Although one would believe this binary concept (alive–dead) would be rather straightforward, there have been some discussions relating to the timing of the death and the circumstances around the AE and the death.

- It is fairly clear that if a patient has a myocardial infarction (the SAE) and then over the next several hours or days goes into shock, has severe arrhythmias, and dies, this death is related to the SAE and this is a "fatal myocardial infarction." It gets trickier, however, if the patient has a myocardial infarction and during a cardiac catheterization goes into an intractable ventricular arrhythmia and dies. Is the myocardial infarction to be classified as a fatal one or is the death a sequelum of the catheterization? There is no clear answer, and it may vary from case to case. The most conservative call is often used by drug safety units; that is, the death is a part of (or consequence of) the SAE. However, if a medically defensible call is made that is less conservative, this should be noted somewhere in the case along with the reasoning behind this decision.

Another example would be that of a fall. If a patient trips while walking on a level surface, falls, and scrapes his or her knee, this is most probably a nonserious AE. If, however, he or she falls while standing on a ledge or walking down a staircase and dies as a result of the fall, the case should be reported as a serious and fatal case but how to classify it is tricky. The fall may be nonserious, but the sum of the case is clearly serious and fatal because of the fatality occurring after the fall, not the actual fall. Again, there is no clear answer; many would take the conservative approach and consider this case (if occurring during a clinical trial) as a serious, fatal, unlabeled fall (presuming "fatal fall" is not in the investigator brochure), and unrelated to the study drug (unless it is believed to be related, perhaps due to accompanying dizziness, which should also be coded). Others would argue that the AE was the fall and everything that happened after it was due to the

circumstances of standing near the ledge. Had the fall occurred on the level surface none of the events leading to the death would have occurred.

- In a 1996 report on a survey done at the United States and European Union Drug Information Association meetings in 1993, Dr. Win Castle and Dr. George Phillips reported marked transatlantic differences in the interpretation of seriousness and expectedness. For example, "total blindness for 30 minutes" was believed to be serious by 89% in the European Union survey and 44% in the United States survey compared with "mild anaphylaxis," which was believed to be serious by 37% of the European Union responders and 98% of the United States responders. Whether this is still the case remains to be seen, but the results nonetheless are most interesting and suggest the need for harmonization and training of safety reviewers (Castle, Phillips, Standardizing "expectedness" and "seriousness" for adverse experience case reporting. *Drug Inform J* 1996;30:73–81).

- Life-threatening: This concept also has interpretation issues revolving around whether the SAE would truly kill the patient if untreated. A mild myocardial infarction with no cardiac function compromise or arrhythmias might be considered serious (medically significant if not hospitalized) but not life-threatening, whereas a myocardial infarction that progresses over the next hour or two to pulmonary edema would be considered life-threatening. This definition thus may overlap to a degree with "medically significant." Again, most would take a conservative approach. Note that FDA changed the definition effective March 2011 to include the requirement that the idea of whether an AE is life-threatening should be commented upon by both the investigator and the sponsor and that if either one feels it is, then the AE should be so considered.

- Hospitalization: Much debate occurred over what actually constitutes "hospitalization" or "inpatient hospitalization." Some patients may be kept overnight (even up to 24–36 hours) in the emergency department for observation and treatment but not "formally" admitted to the hospital as an inpatient. Thus, this patient would not qualify as serious based on a stay in the emergency room (see the Food and Drug Administration's 2001 draft guidance on AE reporting, Section IV.A.3. Web Resource 13-1). In the European Union Directive

2001/83/EC and Volume 9A, refer to the definition of serious adverse reaction, including "inpatient" hospitalization.

- Significant or persistent disability/incapacity: A relatively uncommon criterion in practice. Not formally defined. The FDA gives an interesting example in its 2001 draft guidance:

  > Persons incarcerated because of actions allegedly caused by a drug (e.g., psychotropic drugs and rage reactions) have sustained a substantial disruption in their ability to conduct normal life functions. Thus, these adverse experiences would qualify for the significant or persistent disability/incapacity outcome. Note the change referred to earlier in this chapter about FDA's addition of this concept directly into the definition of "serious."

- Congenital anomaly/birth defect: Usually rather straightforward. It would include even mild birth defects. The FDA also notes that this includes those defects "occurring in a fetus," thus covering abnormalities discovered before birth.

- Important medical events (also called "significant medical events"): This criterion has often been difficult to handle for pharmacovigilance departments because the definition relies on medical judgment. The examples given (allergic bronchospasm, blood dyscrasias, or convulsions) do not necessarily help to clarify other less dramatic situations. The FDA also gives the examples of drug dependency or drug abuse as important events.

Often, cases elicit hours of debate in drug safety units on whether to consider them medically important. Is a mild focal seizure medically important? Is a platelet count 10% below the lower level of normal medically important? Other examples abound. Various rules of thumb have developed:

- If it happened to you or a family member, would you consider it important or medically significant?

- If you discuss or debate whether a case is medically important, it is.

- Another method involves using the FDA's "always expedited" list (see Chapter 8) as published in "the Tome" (see Chapter 4) or the equivalent lists from other health authorities.

- If a member of the marketing or sales department or a nonmedical professional believes it is not important, it is important. (This "rule," though somewhat jocular and cynical, has developed to note the real observation that sometimes there are nonmedical pressures put on personnel in the safety department to interpret cases or make decisions based on sales, financial, or other nonmedical criteria. This is an unfortunate fact of life—not just in the pharmaceutical world but in the world of clinical medicine, where many judgments are now made on a cost-effectiveness basis. Always keep in mind that the primary mission of the drug safety department is to protect the public health.)

■ Expectedness

The United States regulations governing expectedness are fairly straightforward:

> For a pre-marketed product: Any adverse drug experience, the specificity or severity of which is not consistent with the current investigator's brochure; or, if an investigator brochure is not required or available, the specificity or severity of which is not consistent with the risk information described in the general investigational plan or elsewhere in the current application, as amended. For example, under this definition, cerebral thromboembolism and cerebral vasculitis would be unexpected (by virtue of greater specificity) if the investigator brochure only listed cerebral vascular accidents (21CFR312.32(a)). FDA added to this definition effective March 2011 by noting in 21CFR312 that "Unexpected, as used in this definition, also refers to adverse events or suspected adverse reactions that are mentioned in the investigator brochure as occurring with a class of drugs or as anticipated from the pharmacological properties of the drug, but are not specifically mentioned as occurring with the particular drug under investigation." That is, an AE in the class labeling section of the brochure without specific mention for the study drug is considered unexpected.

> For marketed products: Any adverse drug experience that is not listed in the current labeling (package insert or summary of product characteristics) for the drug product. This includes events that may be symptomatically and pathophysiologically related to an event listed in the labeling, but differ from the event because of greater

severity or specificity. For example, under this definition, hepatic necrosis would be unexpected (by virtue of greater severity) if the labeling only referred to elevated hepatic enzymes or hepatitis.

AEs that are "class-related" (i.e. allegedly seen with all products in this class of drugs) which are mentioned in the labeling (package insert or summary of product characteristics) or investigator brochure but which are not specifically described as occurring with this product are considered unexpected" (21CFR314.80(a)).

In the European Union, expectedness is addressed in Directive 2001/20/EC, which simply notes that an unexpected reaction is one "the nature or severity of which is not consistent with the applicable product information (e.g. investigator's brochure for an unauthorised investigational product or summary of product characteristics for an authorised product)."

In theory, this concept is rather straightforward, but in practice, it becomes somewhat harder when synonyms and overlapping concepts are considered. In the report cited previously by Castle and Phillips, 72% of the European Union responders believed that if the labeled event is "dizziness," then "vertigo" would also be considered expected (labeled), but only 50% of the United States responders believed vertigo was labeled. Similarly, 18% of the European Union responders and 3% of the United States responders believed that if "hypotension, wheezing, and urticaria" are labeled, then a reported term of *anaphylaxis* would also be expected. Whether these differences persist, many years after the survey, is unclear. However, it does highlight the fact that well-trained experienced medical personnel doing pharmacovigilance can take the same set of facts and come up with differing and even opposing views.

In general, one should decide expectedness without thought to seriousness. That is, just because a case is non-serious and the AE in question is mildly severe and of little medical import (e.g., a maculopapular rash) compared with a serious AE (e.g., severe hepatitis), the decision on expectedness should be made purely on the basis of the wording in the label and not on the seriousness. Give each AE its due.

With clinical trial drugs, especially those not yet marketed, there may be minimal or no human experience (e.g., the first study in humans or the first phase II study after phase I studies that showed no AEs). In this case, there are no labeled events in the investigator brochure, and everything is thus "new" and unexpected.

Anticipated events based on the pharmacologic properties of the drug should not be considered expected until actually reported in a patient and put into the brochure.

In some cases, it is necessary to consider the route of administration's, dosage's, or indication's being studied when assessing the expectedness. This usually depends on how the investigator brochure or marketed labeling is written. Some describe a different set of AEs for different indications, dosages, or routes of administration. Care must be taken to apply the correct label to each case when doing expectedness.

The general advice would be, as with seriousness, to decide on the side of conservatism. Then, if there are questions on whether an AE is expected, consider it unexpected.

■ Relatedness (Causality)

Of the three criteria revolving around the regulatory reportability of an individual case (seriousness, expectedness, and relatedness), this one is often the most difficult to do for the multiple reasons explained next. Causality may be determined initially at the individual case level, after the receipt of an individual case safety report and again after the review of aggregate data in a case series as for signaling, risk management, and various regulatory reports, such as PSURs.

First, some basic "housekeeping" points should be cleared up to ensure that cases are always handled and collected in the same manner. In doing case assessment, one should be sure that cases are coded using the same MedDRA version and codes (some older dictionaries may still be used and some labeling for older drugs may not be in MedDRA), with trained coders who use consistent methodology and synonym lists. For aggregate reports, the search criteria for the case series should be complete and standardized (using searches from the MSSO and/or CIOMS). Where possible, Standardized MedDRA Queries (SMQs) should be used. See Web Resource 13-2. See Chapter 14 on coding. Cases should be followed up (rapidly upon receipt, not at a later date) as appropriate to ensure the maximum amount of high-quality data.

In practice, many companies have two sets of standards and classifications for causality assessment of individual case safety reports. The first is used in clinical trials by the medical research group and the investigator (a separate causality assessment for each case should be done by the investigator and the sponsor as noted by FDA in the updating of the clinical trial regulations effective March 2011). The second is used in the drug safety unit.

As there is no standard system, various categories (usually three to six) are used in case reports in clinical trials as follows:

- Related
- Probably related
- Possibly related
- Weakly related
- Unrelated
- Unassessable

This methodology is useful in later analyzing signals and in creating tables for investigator brochures, product labeling, and monographs to give a feel for the certainty or lack thereof about the causality of AEs by the drug in question. However, for the drug safety group, which has to determine whether a clinical trial case meets the three criteria (seriousness, expectedness, causality) for expedited reporting, the decision is yes or no. That is, the drug safety group must make the choice between unrelated and related. There is no middle ground or gray zone for causality here. Thus, the drug safety group has to make a rapid decision on whether the case is clearly unrelated (absolutely, positively) or everything else (possibly, probably, unlikely, weakly, etc.). Some drug safety groups consider "unlikely related" to be unrelated and other groups consider it in the broad "related" category. Whichever way is decided, it should be made clear in writing in the SOP or working document (or the protocol for clinical trials) to everyone in the company what is done. Many drug safety officers believe that unless a case is clearly and absolutely unrelated, the causality should be, for reporting purposes, "related." To put it another way, the default causality for all cases is "possibly related" until there is evidence that the case is "unrelated." It is realized that this may not ultimately agree with the case analysis in the final clinical research study report, where a more nuanced opinion may be recorded. So, to summarize, in drug safety there are two causality choices for reporting purposes: unrelated (thus making the case not reportable as an expedited case) and everything else.

Effective March 2011, the FDA changed the causality regulations, introducing the concept of "reasonable possibility" (21CFR32): Suspected adverse reaction means any adverse event for which there is a reasonable possibility that the drug caused the adverse event. For the purposes of IND safety reporting, "reasonable possibility" means there is evidence to suggest a causal relationship between the drug and the adverse event. Suspected adverse reaction implies a lesser degree of certainty about causality than adverse reaction, which means any adverse event caused by a drug. This wording changes the older concept of "possible association" to "reasonable possibility." It is not clear that this will make a major difference in practice.

■ Methodology

Because there are no clear standards or classifications for causality, two broad methods have been developed for causality assessment. (Bayesian analysis is a third method, but this has not proved practical yet.)

Global Introspection

The first is known as "global introspection," which is a somewhat jocular description of having one or more smart experienced drug safety experts (usually physicians) read the case details, in particular the narrative, and decide on "introspective" grounds whether the case is caused by the drug. Obviously, all the expected difficulties exist when the decision is left to one or more human beings using subjective criteria: different training, different experience, untested interrater reliability, biases, and pressure from others within the company or institution. A French group in a 2005 publication on causality found that the overall agreement among five senior experienced experts using global introspection was poor and varied according to level of causality (Arimone, Bégaud, Miremont-Salamé, et al., Agreement of expert judgment in causality assessment of adverse drug reactions. *Eur J Clin Pharmacol* 2005;61[3]:169–173). So, in practice, companies try to get solid, smart, ethical individuals with thick skins and a strong desire to protect the public health to do this job to make the causality judgments.

These criteria are used in global introspection:

Reasons to suspect the AE was caused by the drug.

- The AE occurred in the expected time frame (as a function of the drug's pharmacologic or clinical half-life).
- No problems or symptoms before exposure.
- No other medical conditions that could cause this AE.
- No concomitant medications that could cause this AE.
- A positive dechallenge and (better) a positive rechallenge.
- The AE is consistent with the established mechanism of action of product ("biologic plausibility").

- A known class effect.
- Lack of alternative explanation.
- A dose response.
- A "typical" adverse drug reaction (e.g., low background rate), such as a fixed drug reaction that would not generally be seen except when due to a drug.
- A "clean subject" (e.g., a child).
- Consistency of time to onset (e.g., early for immediate hypersensitivity or long term for tumorigenesis).
- Similar findings in toxicity studies.
- Positive in vitro test (e.g., immunoglobulin E antibodies to allergen and elevated serum tryptase in anaphylaxis).
- Positive in vivo test (e.g., intradermal or prick test for immediate hypersensitivity or patch test for delayed hypersensitivity).
- Identified subset at risk or predisposing factor
- Lack of protopathic bias: a drug given to treat early symptoms may appear temporally associated with the subsequent illness, particularly if the drug's efficacy is low.

Source: Adapted from the Report of CIOMS Working Group III, Guidelines for Preparing Core Clinical Safety Information on Drugs 1995 (see Chapter 36).

Algorithms

Algorithms represent the second method and the usual alternative to global introspection. They have in general not succeeded as well as global introspection when used alone, though they can be useful when used in conjunction with global introspection. Algorithms represent a decision tree that is computerizable and allows yes/no answers to preset questions to determine a causality result. Obviously, the algorithm is only as good as the questions asked and the data provided. Because of the inability to make a "one size fits all" algorithm, there is usually a final human review to ensure that the algorithm results are "reasonable" for the situation. More than 30 algorithms have been developed for both manual and computerized causality assessment of individual cases in pharmacovigilance. One of the earlier used algorithms was developed by Professor J. Venulet in 1980 and updated in 1986 (Venulet, Ciucci, Berneker, *Int J Clin Pharmacol Ther Toxicol* 1986;24:559).

In a study to evaluate agreement between various algorithms and those obtained from an expert panel using the World Health Organization method, 200 reports were studied. The rates of concordance between assessments made using the algorithms and those of the expert panel were 45% for "certain," 61% for "probable," 46% for "possible," and 17% for drug-unrelated terms. Correcting for confounding variables did not significantly improve the results. The authors concluded that full agreement with global introspection was not found for any level of causality assessment (Macedo, Marques, Ribeiro, et al., *J Clin Pharm Ther* 2003;28:137).

■ Comment

Finally, there is another general rule: If there is disagreement between two or more evaluators (e.g., the clinical research team, the investigator, and the drug safety department), the most conservative judgment must be used; that is, if one believes the case is not related and the other believes it is possibly related, the case is considered to be related. The European Union Directive 2001/20/#C article 2(n) notes that if the investigator and sponsor disagree, the sponsor cannot downgrade the investigator's causality, and the more conservative causality is used for reporting purposes. Both opinions should be provided in the narrative of the case when submitted. FDA also wants the investigator and the sponsor to make a judgment and the more conservative wins. Although this has been clarified for situations in which the investigator disagrees with the company, it probably should also apply within the company when there is disagreement. Conservatism and overreporting is preferable to underreporting of SAEs.

For a short and useful summary on how a health authority expert on pharmacovigilance approaches causality from a clinical, pharmacologic, and epidemiologic perspective, see the 2005 article by Diemont (*Netherlands J Med.* 200;63:7, Web Resource 13-3).

■ Health Authority Guidance and Requirements

There is no international standard for causality assessment or classification. The United States and European Union recommendations are summarized below.

■ United States FDA

Current United States regulations require a causality assessment for IND expedited 7- and 15-day reports. These regulations require an IND safety report (21CFR312):

> The sponsor must notify FDA and all participating investigators (i.e., all investigators to whom the sponsor is providing drug under its INDs or under any investigator's IND) in an IND safety report of potential serious risks, from clinical trials or any other source, as soon as possible, but in no case later than 15 calendar days after the sponsor determines that the information qualifies for reporting.... In each IND safety report, the sponsor must identify all IND safety reports previously submitted to FDA concerning a similar suspected adverse reaction, and must analyze the significance of the suspected adverse reaction in light of previous, similar reports or any other relevant information.

> An unexpected adverse event or unexpected suspected adverse reaction is defined by FDA in the regulations as unexpected if it is not listed in the investigator brochure or is not listed at the specificity or severity that has been observed; or, if an investigator brochure is not required or available, is not consistent with the risk information described in the general investigational plan or elsewhere in the current application, as amended. For example, under this definition, hepatic necrosis would be unexpected (by virtue of greater severity) if the investigator brochure referred only to elevated hepatic enzymes or hepatitis. Similarly, cerebral thromboembolism and cerebral vasculitis would be unexpected (by virtue of greater specificity) if the investigator brochure listed only cerebral vascular accidents. "Unexpected," as used in this definition, also refers to adverse events or suspected adverse reactions that are mentioned in the investigator brochure as occurring with a class of drugs or as anticipated from the pharmacological properties of the drug, but are not specifically mentioned as occurring with the particular drug under investigation (21CFR312.32).

For NDA 15-day expedited reports, there is "implied" causality for spontaneous reports. What this means is that if a healthcare professional or consumer takes the time to report an AE to the manufacturer of the drug or to the FDA, the implication is that the reporter believes that to some degree the drug may have caused the AE. This is not clearly stated in the regulations that require 15-day expedited reports, as follows:

> Postmarketing 15-day "Alert reports." The applicant shall report each adverse drug experience that is both serious and unexpected, whether foreign or domestic, as soon as possible but in no case later than 15 calendar days of initial receipt of the information by the applicant" (21CFR80(1)(i)).

In the draft "Guidance for Industry Postmarketing Safety Reporting for Human Drug and Biological Products Including Vaccines" of March 2001 (Web Resource 13-1), the FDA notes the following:

> For spontaneous reports, the applicant should assume that an adverse experience or fatal outcome was suspected to be due to the suspect drug or biological product (implied causality). For clinical studies, an adverse experience or fatal outcome need not be submitted to the FDA unless the applicant concludes that there is a reasonable possibility that the product caused the adverse experience or fatal outcome (see §§ 310.305(c)(1)(ii), 337314.80(e)(1), and 600.80(e)(1)).

> Causality Assessment—Determination of whether there is a reasonable possibility that the product is etiologically related to the adverse experience. Causality assessment includes, for example, assessment of temporal relationships, dechallenge/rechallenge information, association with (or lack of association with) underlying disease, presence (or absence) of a more likely cause, and physiologic plausibility.

In the draft "Guidance for Industry: Good Pharmacovigilance Practices and Pharmacoepidemiologic Assessment" of March 2005, at Web Resource 13-4, the FDA notes the following:

> For any individual case report, it is rarely possible to know with a high level of certainty whether the event was caused by the product. To date, there are no internationally agreed upon standards or criteria for assessing causality in individual

cases, especially for events that often occur spontaneously (e.g., stroke, pulmonary embolism). Rigorous pharmacoepidemiologic studies, such as case-control studies and cohort studies with appropriate follow-up, are usually employed to further examine the potential association between a product and an adverse event.

The FDA does not recommend any specific categorization of causality, but the categories probable, possible, or unlikely have been used. The WHO uses the following categories: certain, probably/likely, possible, unlikely, conditional/unclassified, and unassessable/unclassifiable. Although the FDA does not advocate a particular categorization system, if a causality assessment is undertaken, the FDA suggests that the causal categories are specified.

In contrast to causality assessment at the individual case level, it may be possible to assess the degree of causality between use of a product and an AE when a sponsor or health authority gathers and evaluates all available safety data in aggregate, including the following:

1. Spontaneously reported and published case reports
2. Relative risks or odds ratios derived from pharmacoepidemiologic safety studies
3. Biologic effects observed in preclinical studies and pharmacokinetic or pharmacodynamic effects
4. Safety findings from controlled clinical trials
5. General marketing experience with similar products in the class

FDA concludes: "After the available safety information is presented and interpreted, it may be possible to assess the degree of causality between use of a product and an adverse event."

European Union

The European Union position on causality is explained in ENTR/CT3, "Detailed Guidance on the Collection, Verification and Presentation of Adverse Reaction Reports Arising from Clinical Trials on Medicinal Products for Human Use" (April 2006). (Web Resource 13-5.)

> All adverse events judged by either the investigator or the sponsor as having a reasonable suspected causal relationship to an investigational medicinal product qualify as adverse reactions. The causality assessment given by the investigator should not be downgraded by the sponsor. If the sponsor disagrees with the investigator's

causality assessment, both the opinion of the investigator and the sponsor should be provided with the report.

The MHRA (United Kingdom) comments extensively on this situation (consistent with the general European Union position) in its publication *Good Pharmacovigilance Practice Guide* (Pharmaceutical Press, London 2009, page 133):

> If the investigator states that the event is not related, it is recommended that the SAE form should prompt the investigator to provide details.... If the investigator assigns the causality as "not assessable," the sponsor should adopt a conservative approach in which the event is deemed a suspected adverse reaction until follow-up information is received from the investigator. This scenario also applies should the investigator not supply a causality assessment... the event should be considered as causally related.... The sponsor is also required to make an assessment of causality, as he or she will have greater knowledge of the product upon which to base the causality assessment.

For many years, the French government has used an *imputabilité* decision table based on a combination of a "bibliographic" score (from never reported to well known), chronological criteria (timing, dechallenge, rechallenge), and clinical criteria (specific laboratory findings, suggestive clinical picture, other explanations likely), leading to a five-degree global score (0, unrelated; 1, doubtful; 2, possible; 3, probable; 4, definite) (Begaud, *Drug Inform J* 1984;18:275). It is not used outside of France.

CIOMS I Assessment of Causality

It should be emphasized that manufacturers should not separate out those spontaneous reports they receive into those that seem to themselves to be causally related to drug exposure and those they consider not causally related. A physician in making a spontaneous report to a manufacturer is indicating that the observed event may be due to the drug, i.e. the physician suspects that the event is a reaction. In such a case, it would be inappropriate for a manufacturer to impute to the reporting physician an assessment of causality. Thus all spontaneous reports of serious unlabelled reactions made by medical professionals should be considered as CIOMS reports. However, submission of such a report does not necessarily constitute an acceptance of causality by a manufacturer.

■ Uppsala Monitoring Centre (WHO)

The Uppsala Monitoring Centre uses six categories: (1) certain, (2) probably/likely, (3) possible, (4) unlikely, (5) conditional/unclassified, and (6) unassessable/unclassifiable. They note that these categories are the most widely used, although not everyone uses all of them. See Web Resource 13-6.

Judgment of Cases When Received Versus at the Time of Periodic Reporting and Signaling

Most of this chapter dealt with judging cases at the time of receipt. For causality, this is primarily for clinical trial cases. Judgment of seriousness, expectedness, and causality in the acute phase upon receipt is often done with incomplete information and in a vacuum. At the time of signaling or PSUR preparation, the reviewers now have the benefit of complete (or at least more complete) information on each case, a case series, perhaps a review of animal and other preclinical data, a literature review, and so on. This allows a more nuanced and reasoned judgment. It is not uncommon for causality and the view of the case to change entirely as more data and more cases come in. For example, in the early first in humans clinical trials, every AE is unexpected and new. It is very hard to judge causality. With hindsight, later on and with more data, the judgment may be easier. It is highly unlikely that the first case of valvular heart disease seen with Fen-Phen was felt to be due to the drugs. Only when several occurred did this SAE appear to be linked causally to the drug (see Chapter 53). For cases where there is a high background incidence, assessment of causality may take years and major epidemiological studies to make a valid judgment.

■ Comment

The system for determining seriousness, expectedness, and causality is, to say the least, messy and complicated. One thing that seems to have become clear over the years is that judging causality, particularly for a new drug or for an AE with any drug for which there is a high background rate of that AE, is exceedingly difficult on a case-by-case basis. Some drugs in this category take years, millions of patients exposed, and multiple trials (e.g., Avandia) before an understanding of whether the drug produced a particular AE or group of AEs (e.g., cardiovascular events). The author's view is that a simpler system, which separates reporting to health authorities from causality judgment, should be adopted.

In this setting, all SAEs or the subgroup of unexpected SAES should be reported rapidly (say, within 21 days), all deaths and life-threatening SAEs in 7 days and all nonserious AEs every (say) 90 days. Should electronic medical records come into full and effective use, then all SAEs and AEs could (theoretically) be reported immediately in real time. Then, at various points in time, causality judgments, and relationships to the drug or drug combinations would be made by the companies, health agencies, and perhaps outside experts. This would remove "political" judgments from reporting requirements. Maybe someday.

14

Coding of AEs and Drug Names

As pharmacovigilance becomes more mechanized and computerized, the need for standard terminologies, formats, dictionaries, narratives, and abbreviations grows. The first two major areas that have been standardized are the medical coding of adverse events (AEs) and medical history and the coding of drug names. Medical coding has become standardized in the world of pharmacovigilance with the use of the Medical Dictionary for Regulatory Activities (MedDRA). Several other coding systems have been used. Two prominent ones are COSTART, which the U.S. Food and Drug Administration (FDA) used for AE coding until moving to MedDRA, and WHO-ART, from the Uppsala Monitoring Centre. See Web Resource 14-1 for further information on WHO-ART. Some still use WHO-ART, although MedDRA is now becoming the accepted standard from the International Conference on

Harmonization (ICH). Some older drug labels in the United States and elsewhere still have non-MedDRA terms (e.g., COSTART) but newer labeling had been "MedDRA-ized."

Coding is done so that companies, regulators, and others are able to communicate with each other using the same medical language. AEs are coded so that similar cases are described (coded) in the same consistent way and so that they can easily be retrieved, analyzed, and compared. It is invaluable for signal detection and analysis.

■ AE Coding

MedDRA

MedDRA was developed by the ICH based on earlier work by the United Kingdom health authority. It is owned by the International Federation of Pharmaceutical Manufacturers and Associations, acting as trustee for the ICH Steering Committee. A service organization known as the Maintenance and Support Services Organization (MSSO) serves as the repository, maintainer, and distributor of MedDRA as well as the source for information on MedDRA. Detailed information is available from the MedDRA website (Web Resource 14-2).

MedDRA is a terminology developed for drugs and devices used for standardized coding of medical issues, including AEs and medical history. It is hierarchical, which means that it has multiple levels (five), ranging from the most general to very specific. It is available in English, with some or all of it also available in Czech, Dutch, French, German, Italian, Portuguese, Spanish, and Japanese. A Chinese translation has just been released.

Regulatory Status

European Union: MedDRA use is obligatory in the European Union. All serious adverse event (SAE) reports must be submitted electronically using MedDRA codes. MedDRA is to be used for the reporting of suspected, unexpected, serious adverse events (SUSARs) to the EudraVigilance clinical trial and postmarketing modules. Periodic Safety Update Report (PSURs) must have the AE terms in MedDRA. Product labeling, the Summary of Product Characteristics (SmPC), and Risk Management Plans should also use MedDRA. Volume 9A also recommends using "Standardized MedDRA Queries" for case retrieval when signaling.

United States: It has "more or less" been mandated by the FDA for use in AE reporting. The FDA published a rule mandating its use in 2002, and its use is required in the proposed regulations of March 2003. In 2009, the FDA issued proposed rules requiring AE submission electronically (E2B) using MedDRA. However, these rules have not been put into final regulations and are not in force. Interestingly, in the update of the clinical trial regulations (21CFR312) the FDA explicitly stated that they are not requiring MedDRA for IND safety reporting, though they did not state explicitly why. Nonetheless, MedDRA is used in most AE reporting to FDA. In practice, as MedDRA is obligatory for the European Union, Japan, and elsewhere and has no widely used "competitors," it is wise to use MedDRA consistently for AE reporting.

Japan: Adverse event reports should be submitted in the Japanese version of MedDRA. MedDRA/J is to be used in Periodic Infection Reports and PSURs as well as for reporting infection terms for medical devices with biologic components.

Canada: MedDRA is recommended for coding adverse reaction reports and for the Product Monograph (product labeling).

See the MSSO regulatory website for updates and further regulatory information (Web Resource 14-3).

MedDRA is updated twice yearly (April and October), and, in general, users update their own computer systems within 30 to 60 days of receipt of the upgrade. This too is not fully mandated everywhere but is the common practice. Users may request the addition of new codes to future versions of MedDRA by applying to the MSSO, which then reviews each request. Codes also may be moved, deleted, changed, demoted, and promoted by the MSSO in the updates. The version number "bumps up" each year.

MedDRA terms cover diseases, diagnoses, signs and symptoms, therapeutic indications, medical and surgical procedures, and medical, social, and family histories. MedDRA does not cover drug and device names, study design, patient demographic terms, device failure, population qualifiers (e.g., rare, frequent), and descriptions of severity or numbers. It does not give definitions of AEs.

Originally, MedDRA was developed for postmarketing AEs, but it is now used widely for clinical trial AEs. This has produced complex issues with regard to long trials that might run a year or more and go through one or more MedDRA upgrades. When and how to update the codes in an ongoing trial is complex and has multiple solutions.

MedDRA Version 13.0 now has more than 80,000 terms arranged into five hierarchical categories:

> System organ classes (SOCs): 26
> Higher-level group terms (HLGTs): 335
> Higher-level terms (HLTs): 1709
> Preferred terms (PTs): 18,786
> Lowest-level terms (LLTs): 68,258

An example of coding:

- SOC: Cardiac disorders
- HLGT: Cardiac arrhythmias
- HLT: Supraventricular arrhythmias
- PT: Sinus bradycardia
- LLT: Bradycardia sinus, sinus bradycardia
- Verbatims: Slow heart rate, sinus bradycardia, slow pulse, and so forth

Verbatim terms are not MedDRA terms but rather the terms used by reporters, patients, and investigators. They may be medical, lay, or slang terms. Many companies create verbatim dictionaries in which they map the verbatim terms to MedDRA LLT- or PT-level terms. Note that in this example "sinus bradycardia" is a verbatim, LLT, and PT at the same time. Note also that all PTTs are LLTs (but not vice versa).

Browsers: Because there are so many terms, it is necessary to search for a needed term by computer rather than reading through a printed version of the terminology. For this, the MSSO and other companies have developed software, called "browsers," to allow a user to find the terms he or she needs. The MSSO makes available a downloadable browser to all subscribers (Web Resource 14-4).

Commercial browsers are also available. With the browser, one or more words (e.g., pain in the leg) are typed in, and the browser software determines whether there is a direct word-for-word match at one or more of the hierarchical levels. If so, it gives the direct "hit" along with the hierarchical tree; that is, if the direct hit is an LLT, it will display the PT, HLT, HLGT, and SOC (both primary and secondary if more than one exists). If not, most browsers suggest choices for the user to pick from. Some browsers do autoencoding where one may type in a narrative (prose paragraphs), and the browser will extract and code all medical-sounding terms for the user to examine and accept or reject.

The actual coding of AEs is a very complex subject and cannot be fully covered here, but some general thoughts and issues on coding are addressed. The goal of coding is to create one or more AE codes that capture the essence of the problems that the patient experienced. There should not be too many or too few terms but just enough. That is, we should follow the "Goldilocks Principle" and use codes that are "just right," or as Albert Einstein put it: "Everything should be made as simple as possible, but not simpler." Defining "just enough," however, is difficult. There are many complexities that one encounters when coding:

- Should one be "a lumper or a splitter"? That is, should one code "flu-like syndrome" (the lumper) or "fever," "malaise," "fatigue," "muscle aches," "headache," "chills," and "runny nose" (the splitter)? This may be evident to the reader for a term such as "flu-like syndrome" but less clear for the "Hermansky-Pudlak syndrome" (albinism, visual problems, platelet defects with bleeding, lung disease, and often kidney and gastrointestinal disease).
- Should one code "cascade effects" or "secondary effects"? For example, if a patient becomes dizzy and falls, breaking his or her shoulder and abrading his or her skin, the primary event is dizziness (and should be coded) but should the other terms—the fall, shoulder fracture, skin abrasions—also be coded and thus considered as AEs associated with the drug in question in the database and future labeling?

- Should signs (hepatomegaly) and symptoms (abdominal pain) be coded, or only diseases and diagnoses?
- Should provisional or "rule out" diagnoses be coded?
- How specific should one be? Should one code "skin rash on face and neck" or just "rash"?
- Should one code "low blood glucose" or "hypoglycemia"? This actually represents the question about whether one should code laboratory abnormalities as AEs. In practice, this is done in an arbitrary and inconsistent manner and can be a problem in clinical trial reports or dossiers for Market Authorization (MA) approval when the number of AEs of hypertension do not equal the number of patients whose recorded blood pressure on physical exams went up, clearly demonstrating that not all elevations in blood pressure were considered to be reportable or codable by the investigator or company as AEs.
- Coding may be done at a less specific level, coding "edema" instead of "facial edema" or "lung disease NOS (not otherwise specified)" instead of a more specific diagnosis (e.g., pneumococcal pneumonia). This type of "lumping" can mask or hide certain AEs or problems.
- Coding consistency and variability is often a problem, especially when there are multiple coders or coding is done over time (e.g., in a long clinical trial). One might see "elevated liver enzymes," "abnormal liver enzymes," "elevated ALT," or "elevated AST," all of which are capturing the same condition in different patients at different times. This poses problems when one is attempting to retrieve all the cases of liver problems to do safety signaling (see "Standardized MedDRA Queries" section below) or aggregate AE tables.
- Having too many codes for a particular case makes it hard to understand what the primary or major issues were. In practice, many users try to limit the number of codes in each case to six or eight at most.
- Cultural differences may affect coding across countries or regions. In addition, language issues may alter coding, especially if people are coding in a language (English) that is not their primary language.

There is, in many cases, no single correct answer to a coding question. Rather it is necessary that coders agree on certain standards, or "conventions," that define (sometimes arbitrarily) how to code. The MSSO has published several versions of its coding suggestions entitled "MedDRA® Term Selection: Points to Consider, ICH-Endorsed Guide for MedDRA Users. Application to Adverse Drug Reactions /Adverse Events & Medical and Social History & Indications." See Web Resource 14-5.

The FDA, in its "Guidance for Industry Premarketing Risk Assessment" of March 2005 (Web Resource 14-6), has commented on coding:

> Sponsors should explore the accuracy of the coding process with respect to both investigators and the persons who code adverse events.

- Investigators may sometimes choose verbatim terms that do not accurately communicate the adverse event that occurred.

- The severity or magnitude of an event may be inappropriately exaggerated (e.g., if an investigator terms a case of isolated elevated transaminases acute liver failure despite the absence of evidence of associated hyperbilirubinemia, coagulopathy, or encephalopathy, which are components of the standard definition of acute liver failure).

- Conversely, the significance or existence of an event may be masked (e.g., if an investigator uses a term that is nonspecific and possibly unimportant to describe a subject's discontinuation from a study when the discontinuation is due to a serious adverse event).

- Sponsors should strive to identify obvious coding mistakes as well as any instances when a potentially serious verbatim term may have been inappropriately mapped to a more benign coding term, thus minimizing the potential severity of an adverse event. One example is coding the verbatim term facial edema (suggesting an allergic reaction) as the nonspecific term edema; another is coding the verbatim term suicidal ideation as the more benign term emotional lability.

- Prior to analyzing a product's safety database, sponsors should ensure that adverse events were coded with minimal variability across studies and individual coders.

To limit variability, some companies establish a central coding group that either does all AE coding or checks and verifies that all coding done by others is consistent and correct.

Standardized MedDRA Queries (SMQs)

Standardized MedDRA Queries (SMQs) are groupings of terms from one or more MedDRA SOCs that relate to a defined medical condition or area of interest. They help in retrieving cases to ensure that (hopefully) all the cases that are of interest will be retrieved. This, of course, implies that they were coded correctly on data entry/input of the cases. The included terms may relate to signs, symptoms, diagnoses, syndromes, physical findings, and laboratory and other physiologic test data. Examples of SMQs include cardiac arrhythmias, cardiac failure, cardiomyopathy, hepatic disorders, hostility/aggression, hyperglycemia/new onset diabetes mellitus, malignancies, and nearly 80 more. Others are being developed by the MSSO. See the current list at Web Resource 14-7 and Web Resource 14-8.

Training: Safety departments, regulatory authorities, data entry personnel, and others need to establish detailed coding standards, preferably using accepted (MSSO/ICH) conventions, and to train the staff on their use. Because employees come and go and because MedDRA is updated twice yearly, coding training is usually an ongoing process. The MSSO and many vendors provide basic training courses in MedDRA coding, usually running from 1/2 day to 2 or 3 days.

SNOMED CT

Just when it looked like the AE coding situation was settled, proposals are now under way that are likely to be put in place over the next several years in which MedDRA will be replaced or "augmented" with another system known as SNOMED.

SNOMED CT (Systematized Nomenclature of Medicine—Clinical Terms) is a dictionary of clinical terminology that was created by the combining of terms created by the College of American Pathologists and the United Kingdom National Health Services and is owned, maintained, and distributed by the International Health Terminology Standards Development Organisation (IHTSDO), a nonprofit in Denmark (Web Resource 14-9). IHTSDO acquires, owns, and administers the rights to SNOMED CT. Various countries including the United Kingdom, Spain, Australia, Canada, Sweden, and the Netherlands have joined and are considering implementing SNOMED in their countries.

It is the most comprehensive clinical vocabulary available and has been designated by the U.S. government for electronic exchange of clinical data to include electronic medical records provider order entry, including e-prescribing, laboratory order entry, remote intensive care unit monitoring, lab reporting, emergency room charting, cancer reporting, genetic databases, pharmaceutical use, and more. It will be or is being used by certain U.S. federal agencies for exchanging clinical information for lab result contents, nonlab interventions and procedures, anatomy, diagnoses and problems, and nursing terms. Other governments, particularly in the European Union, are also likely to adopt it. This may replace MedDRA at some point in the future.

■ AE Severity Coding

A common problem for coders is judging the severity (mild, moderate, severe) of an AE. This is, of course, different from the regulatory definitions of "serious" and "nonserious," which may be inconsistent in a sense with severity. For example, mild chest pain that is perceived by the patient as mild but which is due to a myocardial infarction and results in hospitalization may be classified as mild or moderate pain. But in fact the AE was serious because of hospitalization (and "medical importance").

Most reviewers will make a subjective clinical judgment on severity based on the data supplied and their subjective conclusion about the AE or cases. There exists one objective classification system developed by the U.S. National Cancer Institute for use in its protocols. It is to some degree oncology related but can be useful for other indications and trials. It is called the "Common

Terminology Criteria for Adverse Events (CTCAE) v4.0." This version was released in June 2010 and is periodically updated. The document classifies about 800 AEs (including some laboratory values from the Investigations SOC) based on MedDRA 12.0 terms (not the latest MedDRA version, but this is not a problem). The grading scale is 1 (mildest) to 5 (most severe). Information is available free and in the public domain at NCI's site (Web Resource 14-10), and the actual files, in several formats with background information, are at Web Resource 14-11.

See Figure 14.1 for an example.

■ Drug Names and Drug Dictionaries

Another requirement in the pharmacovigilance world is a consistent and up-to-date drug dictionary. Ideally, such a dictionary would have all the names of all the drugs sold throughout the world. Unfortunately, this is not a simple task. It is far harder than developing an AE dictionary:

- Each drug may have multiple names (see below).
- Drug names change.
- Drug formulations change: the excipients, the active ingredient, or both.
- A drug with the same trade name may have different formulations in different countries.
- Spelling varies, and some languages do not use our alphabet.
- Combination drugs have multiple names.

Figure 14.1	**Cardiac Disorders**					
	Grade					
Adverse Event	1	2	3	4	5
Acute coronary syndrome	-	Symptomatic, Progressive angina; cardiac enzymes normal; hemodynamically stable	Symptomatic, unstable angina and/or acute myocardial infarction, cardiac enzymes abnormal, hemodynamically stable	Sympotmatic, unstable angina and/or acute myocardial infarction, cardiac enzymes abnormal, hemodynamically unstable	Death
Definition: A disorder characterized by signs and symptoms related to acute ischemia of the myocardium secondary to coronary artery disease. The clinical presentation covers a spectrum of heart diseases from unstable angina to myocardial infarction.						
Aortic valve disease	Aspympromatic valvular thickening with or without mild valvular regurgitation or stenosis by imaging	Asymptomatic; moderate regurgitation or stenosis by imaging	Symptomatic; severe regurgitation or stenosis by imaging; symptoms controlled with medical intervention	Life-threatening consequences; urgent intervention indicated (e.g., valve replacement, valvuloplasty)	Death
Definition: A disorder characterized by a defect in aortic valve function or structure						
Asystole	Periods of asystole; non-urgent medical management indicated	-	-	Life-threatening consequences; urgent intervention indicated	Death
Definition: A disorder characterized by a dysrhythmia without cardiac electrical activity. Typically, this is accompanied by cessation of the pumping function of the heart.						

Source: Information is available free and in the public domain at NCI's site (http://ctep.cancer.gov/protocolDevelopment/electronic_applications/ctc.htm#ctc_40).

■ Drugs may be very similar, varying only in the salt. They may have the same names or totally different names.

■ Multiple Names and Name Changes

In January 2006, the FDA issued a warning to consumers against filling U.S. prescriptions abroad because drugs with same or similar names may contain different active ingredients from those sold in the United States and may thus pose health risks. See Web Resource 14-12. They gave two examples:

> For example, in the United States, "Flomax" is a brand name for tamsulosin, a treatment for an enlarged prostate, while in Italy, the active ingredient in the product called "Flomax" is morniflumate, an anti-inflammatory drug. In the United States, "Norpramin" is the brand name for an anti-depression drug containing desipramine but, in Spain, the same brand name, "Norpramin," is used for a drug that contains omeprazole, a treatment for stomach ulcers.

A drug, even a "simple" drug, usually has multiple names. For example, here is a list of some of the names for the drug cimetidine that are used around the world: Eureceptor, Gastromet, SKF 92334, Tagamet, Tametin, Tratul, Ulcedine, Ulcimet, Ulcomet, Acibilin, Acinil, Cimal, Cimetag, Cimetum, Dyspamet, Edalene, Peptol, Ulcedin, Ulcerfen, Ulcofalk, Ulcomedina, Ulhys, N-cyano-N′-methyl-N″-((E)-2-([[(5-methyl-1H-imidazol-4-yl) methyl]sulfanyl)ethyl)guanidine,1-cyano-2-methyl-3-(2-(((5-methyl-4-imidazolyl)methyl)thio)ethyl)guanidine, 2-cyano-1-methyl-3-(2-(((5-methylimidazol-4-yl) methyl)thio)ethyl)guanidine, Acibilin, Acinil, Cimetag, Cimetum, Dyspamet, Edalene, Eureceptor, Gastromet, Metracin, and Brumetidina.

As noted above, names may change. Omeprazole was originally sold in the United States as Losec, but the name was changed to Prilosec at the request of the FDA because of possible confusion with Lasix.

In the United States, the U.S. Adopted Names Council (USAN) (Web Resource 14-13), which is officially sponsored by the American Medical Association, the U.S. Pharmacopeial Convention, and the American Pharmacists Association, assigns generic names that are unique and nonproprietary. The USAN works closely with the International Nonproprietary Name (INN) Program of the World Health Organization (WHO) (Web Resource 14-14), which assigns international "generic" names. Different countries or regions may also use different generic names: "acetaminophen" is used in the United States and "paracetamol" in the United Kingdom and elsewhere.

Much attention has been paid in the last several years to medication errors that are felt to be "low-hanging fruit" in the world of drug safety, as errors in naming, prescribing, and handwriting should be more easily rectified than finding the rare SAE. In the FDA, the review of proposed proprietary names is conducted by the Division of Medication Error Prevention and Analysis (DMEPA) in CDER's Office of Surveillance and Epidemiology (OSE). DMEPA, in consultation with the Division of Drug Marketing, Advertising, and Communications (DDMAC) reviews proposed names before approval of an IND, NDA, BLA, and ANDA. FDA does not review proprietary names of products marketed under an over-the-counter (OTC) monograph or those of a distributor or repacker. Similar systems exist in most other countries. See, for example, Health Canada's Guidance for Industry: Drug Name Review: Look-alike Sound-alike (LA/SA) Health Product Names (Web Resource 14-15), the United Kingdom MHRA Guideline on Naming Medicines (Web Resource 14-16), and the European Union's guideline on naming (Web Resource 14-17).

This is obviously a very complex situation. So, in the example above, cimetidine is the "generic" (and the INN and USAN, see below) name of the compound that has a chemical name of N″-cyano-N-methyl-N′-[2-[[(5-methyl-1H-imidazol-4-yl) methyl]thio]ethyl]guanidine, which has the trade names of Tagamet, Peptol, Nu-Cimet, Apo-Cimetidine, Novo-Cimetidine, and others.

See the website of the Institute for Safe Medication Practices (Web Resource 14-18) for an excellent discussion of all aspects of medication prescribing and medication errors, including name issues. They publish a list of Confused Drug Names (Web Resource 14-19).

In the drug safety world, during the preparation of individual case safety reports and aggregate reports (PSURs, NDA Periodic Reports, etc.), comedications are frequently encountered that have not been seen before. Because comedications can play a major role in safety reports, it is critical to know what medications (both prescription, over-the-counter, nutraceuticals, etc.) a patient has taken. Often, however, a strange name is encountered and much time is spent tracking it down to understand what it is chemically. It is far more practical to maintain a drug dictionary with all drug names and formulations that one can refer to as needed.

As with an AE dictionary, it is critical to enter data in a correct and consistent fashion to retrieve it properly. Inconsistent coding produces incomplete searches during signaling or preparing safety reports. Creating and maintaining a drug dictionary, unlike an AE dictionary, is far harder and more complex. With an AE dictionary, the vocabulary is controlled and relatively finite. Few "new" medical terms or diseases occur. Many of the changes to MedDRA represent refinements to the current terms. MedDRA is reaching, to a degree, steady state, with changes each year in the hundreds rather than in the thousands when MedDRA was first released.

Drug dictionaries are quite different. New drugs are developed almost weekly. New drugs, line extensions, "rebranding," new formulations, and new trade names are developed, approved, and launched somewhere in the world every day, and old drugs are withdrawn. To track the names, formulations, and formulas of all these products in more than 150 countries is an impossible task. Whereas MedDRA is updated twice yearly, a drug dictionary, if it is meant to be complete, would need to be updated daily to weekly to remain current. For this and other reasons, ICH has avoided moving into the field of drug dictionaries. When a drug name is encountered that is not found in the drug dictionary normally used, or if it is reported from a country or source that is not usually seen, it is worth doing an internet search to verify what the drug is or contains. Similarly, drugs that are not written in the English (Latin) alphabet should be carefully checked.

■ WHO Drug Dictionary Enhanced

The most useful drug dictionary available is the WHO Drug Dictionary Enhanced, which is a product of the Uppsala Monitoring Centre (UMC). It covers 66 countries and claims to cover nearly 100% of the OTC and prescription products used in these countries. Biotech and blood products, diagnostic substances, and contrast media are also entered when reported. See the website (Web Resource 14-20) for further information.

This dictionary, maintained by the UMC in collaboration with IMS Health, contains 203,199 unique names and 1,568,921 different medicinal products as of June 2010. It is updated quarterly. It contains products registered by the FDA and the European Medicines Agency (EMA) and member states. The dictionary is hierarchical, using system organ classes and the chemical, pharmacologic, and therapeutic properties of each drug. A numerical code is also assigned to each drug. See in particular the monograph and samples at Web Resource 14-21.

The "Anatomic, Therapeutic, Chemical Classification" (ATC) is used in this dictionary. In this classification system, drugs are divided into five different groups:

- First level, anatomical main group: A—alimentary tract and metabolism
- Second level, therapeutic subgroup: A10—drugs used in diabetes
- Third level, pharmacological subgroup: A10B—oral blood glucose-lowering drugs
- Fourth level, chemical subgroup: A10BA—biguanides
- Fifth level, chemical substance: A10BA02—metformin

The coding system is complex. Basically, each product has a unique identifier characterized by

- Medicinal Product Name
- Name Specifier
- Drug Code
- Market Authorisation Holder
- Country
- Pharmaceutical form
- Strength available, quantity, and unit of active ingredient

See the website noted above for details on the specifics of the system.

Companies and other users have handled the dictionary in various ways. Some simply subscribe to the dictionary and use the UMC-issued updates as is. Other companies use the WHO Drug Dictionary as a base and add on to it as new drugs are encountered during their regular handling of individual case safety reports each day. This dictionary may then "grow" separately from the WHO Drug Dictionary into a proprietary company dictionary. This would pose reconciliation problems when the new update of the WHO dictionary is issued, and thus some companies may choose not to use the WHO upgrades but rather maintain their own home-grown version. The logic behind this is reasonable in that companies often sell limited lines of drugs and may only rarely encounter other drugs or classes of drugs. A company that makes primarily diabetic drugs needs to have the latest information on all diabetic comedications arriving on the market but may be less concerned about oncology and asthma drugs, for example. They thus have their dictionary group focus on the drugs they encounter more frequently. The downside is that each company has a different drug dictionary and cannot easily communicate with other companies and with health authorities, especially during electronic transmissions, as they have different dictionaries. From the safety officer's point of view, it is necessary to know what drug dictionary is being used and how coding is done, especially in complicated situations and foreign cases.

■ EudraVigilance Medicinal Product Dictionary (EVMPD)

This is a product dictionary developed by the EMA for the European Economic Area for authorized and investigational products. It has standardized terminology for active ingredients, excipients, pharmaceutical forms, routes of administrations, concentration ranges and units, country codes, MAH, and Sponsor data. It is hierarchical and multiaxial in structure and uses a standardized XML schema. Volume 9A and Volume 10 require all MA holders to enter into the dictionary each medicinal product authorized in the European Union or used in clinical trials. Unlike the WHO dictionary, the EVMPD uses a "multilingual approach" to accommodate the many European languages used. Each MAH must populate the dictionary with its approved and investigational medical products. It is thus an European Union-centric dictionary and is used primarily by the European Union health agencies for signaling, drug identification, and so forth. See Web Resource 14-22.

■ The Future

ICH issued a document, M5, entitled *Data Elements and Standards for Drug Dictionaries* in 2005. There are now efforts underway to create a new global drug dictionary similar to the way MedDRA was created for AE terms. Watch this space.

15

Expedited and Aggregate Reporting in Clinical Trials

There are multiple different safety reports that pharmaceutical companies and other sponsors must submit to health authorities. This chapter reviews the key reports that are required now by most health authorities.

■ Expedited Reporting

Certain serious adverse events (SAEs) must be reported to health authorities within 7 or 15 calendar days. Most countries use "calendar days" rather than "business or working days," as holidays and working days are not the same everywhere. Some countries still retain different rules for local cases, but by and large, thanks to ICH, CIOMS, and common sense, most countries have standardized on the same timing, format, and content of expedited (also called "alert") reports.

■ Clinical Trial Reporting

Another way to express "clinical trial reporting" is reporting for drugs that are not yet marketed (no Marketing Authorization or New Drug Approval (NDA) yet or for the indication in question). Although this refers primarily to clinical trials, it may also refer to SAEs found in named patient use, compassionate use, solicited SAEs, epidemiologic trials, and other "nonclassic" trials and studies.

Most countries require that SAEs, which are unexpected (not labeled), that is, do not appear in the product labeling that is usually the Investigator Brochure, and that have some possibility (even if small) of being caused by the study drug in question, be reported in 15 calendar days from the first notification of anyone in the company (or organization), including its agents, business partners, contractors, distributors, and vendors. This is called a "15-day report," "an expedited report," or "an alert report." Note the triple requirement: serious, unlabeled, and possibly related.

A subcategory of this is the "7-day report." In a 7-day report, the patient in question has died or had a life-threatening SAE, which is also unexpected and possibly related (same as above). This report must be sent to the health authorities within 7 calendar days. Note that all 7-day reports are also 15-day reports. Thus, if a report is communicated as a 7-day report, it must also be followed up as a 15-day report. The 7-day report may be communicated as a phone call, fax, or some other less formal communication compared with the more formal 15-day report (a CIOMS I, MedWatch form, E2B transmission). If the 7-day report is "informal," then it must be followed up with the usual 15-day "formal" report. If the 7-day report is the CIOMS I, MedWatch form, or E2B, it will cover both requirements. Thus, the 7-day report becomes a 15-day report with the same requirements for follow-up and further reporting (see below).

■ United States Requirements for Expedited IND Reports

The Investigator's New Drug Application (IND) obligations are found in 21CFR312. An IND is usually opened and held by a pharmaceutical company, but academics, universities, and individuals may also do so. The term that the FDA uses for the IND holder is generally "the sponsor." The sponsor is obliged to "review and evaluate the evidence relating to the safety and effectiveness of the drug as it is obtained from the investigator" (21CFR312.56(c)). This includes 7- and 15-day expedited reports (21CFR312.32) and annual reports (21CFR312.33). In March 2011, updates to these regulations went into effect.

■ Expedited IND Reports (Alert Reports, 7- and 15-Day IND Reports)

Serious, unexpected (unlabeled), adverse events from clinical trials for which there is a reasonable possibility that the drug caused the event must be reported. Each report identifies all similar reports sent to the FDA, and the sponsor analyzes their significance.

Specifically the FDA regulations state 21CFR312(c)(1): "The sponsor must notify FDA and all participating investigators (i.e., all investigators to whom the sponsor is providing drug under its INDs or under any investigator's IND) in an IND safety report of potential serious risks, from clinical trials or any other source, as soon as possible, but in no case later than 15 calendar days after the sponsor determines that the information qualifies for reporting." In each IND safety report, the sponsor must identify all IND safety reports previously submitted to FDA concerning a similar suspected adverse reaction, and must analyze the significance of the suspected adverse reaction in light of previous, similar reports or any other relevant information.

In each expedited report, all previously submitted expedited reports of similar suspected adverse reactions must be noted and analyzed in light of previous, similar reports or any other relevant information. This analysis may be included in the narrative.

Note that only previously submitted expedited reports need be included in the analysis. However, many companies look at all similar non-expedited SAEs and NSAEs if appropriate. Although not required, this is a wise practice.

Expedited reporting must be done for findings from animal studies, epidemiological studies, pooled analysis of multiple studies, or clinical studies, whether or not conducted under an IND and whether or not conducted by the sponsor, that suggest a significant risk in humans exposed to the drug (312.32(c)(1)(ii)). Data from in vitro studies (e.g., microsusceptibility, drug interaction, or genotoxicity) are to be sent as 15-day IND reports if a significant risk in humans is determined (312.32(c)(1)(iii)).

Any clinically important increase in the rate compared to that in the IB or protocol of a serious suspected adverse reaction must be submitted as a 15-day expedited report. FDA realizes this may not always be available. When it is available, a judgment of "clinical importance" should be based on the study population, nature and seriousness of the AE, magnitude of the increase, and other appropriate factors.

■ The report must be made no later than 15 calendar days after the sponsor's initial receipt of the information (which is day zero and is considered the "clock start date"). Under older regulations the clock start began when there was sufficient information that the three criteria were met (serious, unexpected, associated) for an expedited report and that the report had the four criteria (reporter, patient, AE, drug) to be valid. FDA has changed these rules:

■ Because the four elements of the minimum data set are generally readily available in the clinical trial setting, the agency has determined that the definition and the requirement for the minimum data set are unnecessary and has decided not to require a minimum data set for IND safety reports.

■ The reporting time clock starts (i.e., day zero) as soon as the sponsor determines that the information qualifies for reporting. For a serious and unexpected suspected adverse reaction from a clinical trial, this would be the day the sponsor receives information from the clinical investigator.

- If any information necessary to evaluate and report the suspected adverse reaction is missing or unknown, the sponsor should actively seek such information.

Thus when a study site reports any SAE information, the clock starts–even if the information is incomplete or does not meet the minimum requirements. The sponsor must then rapidly obtain the rest of the (minimum) information needed for the expedited report.

If the case has a serious outcome of fatal or life-threatening (i.e., serious, unexpected, associated, and fatal or life-threatening), the case is to be reported as a telephone or fax report within 7 calendar days of the first receipt. All 7-day reports are automatically 15-day reports and must then be processed and submitted as expedited reports by day 15 unless the 7-day report was a MedWatch or E2B expedited report. Follow-up reports (also expedited reports) are submitted if new information arrives.

For expedited reporting there must be sufficient evidence to suggest a causal relationship between the drug and the SAE, thus creating a "Suspected Adverse Reaction (312.32(c)(1)(i)). FDA does not want to receive as expedited reports those cases that are not likely to be related to the drug.

The FDA has clarified that it requires the investigator to report serious AEs rapidly to the sponsor along with a determination of seriousness/life-threatening as well as a determination of causality ("reasonable possibility"). The sponsor only determines expectedness. The most conservative viewpoint prevails. That is, in terms of seriousness and causality, if either the investigator or sponsor feels a case is serious and that there is a "reasonable possibility" the SAE was due to the drug, it should be expedited.

Determination	Sponsor	Investigator
Serious/Life-Threatening	Yes	Yes
Causality (Responsible Possibility)	Yes	Yes
Expectedness (Labeled/Unlabeled)	Yes	No

The events should be submitted on a MedWatch 3500A form or, if already arranged with the FDA, as E2B transmissions, though the FDA has not officially started accepting IND reports electronically at this writing. Animal reports and other nonindividual case reports (e.g., epidemiologic studies) are usually submitted as narratives rather than on MedWatch forms. Most companies do not want to put animal data into their clinical safety database. Non-U.S. cases may be submitted on MedWatch or CIOMS I forms.

All SAEs from bioavailability and bioequivalence studies must be reported as expedited reports whether labeled (in the investigator brochure or not) or related to the drug (causality).

The sponsor must also notify all participating investigators of these reports. The investigators in turn notify the investigational review boards (21CFR312.32(c)(i and ii)). The notification procedure has become a bit more complex recently, as not every single individual report goes to the investigators and IRBs. Rather important reports or those that alter benefit/risk should be reported. FDA has issued a guidance on this: "Guidance for Clinical Investigators, Sponsors, and IRBs: Adverse Event Reporting—Improving Human Subject Protection" (http://www.fda.gov/downloads/RegulatoryInformation/Guidances/UCM126572.pdf). The sponsor is also required to report information to the FDA from any source, foreign or domestic; clinical, animal, or epidemiologic investigations; commercial marketing experience; literature reports; unpublished papers; and foreign regulatory authorities (21CFR312.32(b)). The FDA retains the right to change the format and frequency of the reports. For marketed drugs, reporting to the IND is not required unless that case is from an IND clinical trial.

Follow-up is required on all safety information received by the sponsor and submitted as a follow-up to the original (initial) 15-day report. Follow-up information is handled with the same 15-calendar-day clock. If a case is received and does not meet the criteria of a 15-day report (e.g., reported as a nonserious case initially) and only later does the receipt of follow-up information show the case to meet the reportability criteria, the clock starts when the follow-up information is received. If a case becomes nonexpedited on receipt of follow-up information, the sponsor should submit this new information as a follow-up 15-day report and indicate that the case no longer meets the criteria for expediting.

Other information the sponsor receives that does not quite fall into these categories but which the sponsor wishes to report should be reported as an information amendment or in the annual report. The FDA notes that reporting of a case by the sponsor does not mean that the FDA or the sponsor believes that the report was necessarily due to the drug. This point may prove to be important in any potential litigation in which the sponsor might become involved (21CFR312.32(c)(3, 4)). Postmarketing trials should be submitted to the IND (whether conducted under an IND or not) only if the case meets the three criteria (serious, unexpected, possibly related) as determined by the sponsor.

The FDA also notes that in some trials, the sponsor and FDA may reach an agreement to be noted in the protocol whereby certain study endpoints (e.g., a particular SAE such as a myocardial infarction or death) which would normally be expedited cases will not be reported as 7- or 15-day reports but rather periodically or at the end of the trial. This must be customized for each situation and FDA must agree to it. Expedited reports should be unblinded and placebo cases should not be reported.

In summary, the sponsor (whether an individual, institution, or company) must submit to the FDA as a 15-day expedited report all clinical trial AEs that are serious, unexpected (not in the Investigator Brochure or Package Insert, depending on which one is used: Investigator Brochure for nonmarketed drugs or new indications of marketed drugs and the package insert—usually—for marketed drugs and postmarketing studies), and reasonably associated with the study drug. As noted above, epidemiologic, animal, and other studies may also generate expedited reporting. If the case is a death or is life-threatening, a 7-day report (phone or fax) must also be made in addition to the 15-day report.

■ IND Annual Reports

In addition to the 7- and 15-day safety reports, the IND holder must also submit annual reports (21CFR312.33). Although the FDA will ultimately change to the Developmental Summary Update Report (DSUR) that ICH has developed, this is not in force yet. Within 60 days of the anniversary date of the IND, a brief report of the progress of the investigation must be submitted that includes the following:

- Individual study information: A brief summary of the status of each study in progress and each study completed during the previous year:
  - The title and number of the study, its purpose, a brief statement identifying the patient population, and a statement as to whether the study is completed.
  - The total number of subjects initially planned for inclusion in the study; the number entered into the study to date, tabulated by age group, gender, and race; the number whose participation in the study was completed as planned; and the number who dropped out of the study for any reason.
  - If the study has been completed, or if interim

results are known, provide a brief description of any available study results.

- Summary information obtained during the previous year's clinical and nonclinical investigations:
  - A narrative or tabular summary showing the most frequent and most serious adverse experiences by body system
  - A summary of all IND 15-day safety reports submitted during the past year
  - A list of subjects who died during the investigation, with the cause of death for each subject
  - A list of subjects who dropped out during the investigation in association with any adverse experience, whether or not it is thought to be drug related
  - A brief description of what, if anything, was obtained that is pertinent for understanding the drug's actions, including, for example, information about dose response, information from controlled trials, and information about bioavailability
  - A list of the preclinical studies (including animal studies) completed or in progress during the past year and a summary of the major preclinical findings
  - A summary of any significant manufacturing or microbiologic changes made during the past year
  - A description of the general investigational plan for the coming year to replace that submitted one year earlier
  - If the Investigator Brochure has been revised, a description of the revision and a copy of the new brochure
  - A description of any significant phase I protocol modifications made during the previous year and not previously reported to the IND in a protocol amendment
  - A brief summary of significant foreign marketing developments with the drug during the past year, such as approval of marketing in any country or withdrawal or suspension from marketing in any country

If the sponsor wishes, it may transfer some or all duties for clinical trials (including safety) to a third party, such as another company or a clinical research organization. In that case, the transfer of obligations must be described in detail and in writing to the FDA (21CFR312.52(a)).

■ Other Clinical Trial (IND) Reporting Issues

Reporting the same 15-day alert case to the IND and the New Drug Application (NDA):

> This issue arises when there is an open IND and an approved NDA for the same drug. Normally in simple situations, before NDA approval and while the IND is open, all 15-day reports are sent to the IND. After the NDA is approved, reporting should now, in general, be to the NDA. There is one situation where there must be reporting to both the IND and the NDA.

> Double reporting is required if the serious AE meets the three IND reporting criteria (serious, unexpected, possibly related) and is from an IND study. In this case the 15-day report must be sent to both the IND and the NDA. If the serious AE report is from a non-IND study, then it is reported to the NDA only.

Reporting serious AEs to comparator drugs and placebos:

> Some countries have been requiring the reporting of placebo and comparator serious AEs. In the United States, FDA has made it clear that placebo cases usually do not meet the four-element criteria (patient, reporter, drug, AE) because there is no "drug" and so are not reported. The European Union also in general does not want placebo cases submitted as expedited reports. However, placebos usually do have excipients and often "benign" products such as lactose that can produce AEs. In addition, in any placebo-controlled trial, there are usually large numbers of AEs seen with placebos. These are reported at the end of the study in the final study report.

> The sponsor of the trial, especially if the trial is a multinational trial, must ensure that all regulatory reporting requirements in each country where there is a clinical trial site are met. These requirements are often different from United States/European Union/ICH requirements and may also require local language reporting for certain serious AEs.

Blinding and unblinding 7- and 15-day alert reports:

> FDA clarified the issue of unblinding in its rewrite of the clinical trial reporting. It wants all expedited reports submitted to them to be unblinded.

They have stated (Federal Register/Vol. 75, No. 188/Wednesday, September 29, 2010/Rules and Regulations. 59947):

"The agency does not believe that unblinding single or small numbers of informative cases will compromise the integrity of the study. However, if patient safety can be assured without breaking the blind, the agency encourages the sponsor to discuss alternative reporting arrangements with the appropriate FDA review division. Any anticipated alternative arrangements to maintain the blind would need to be described in the protocol, including identification of the serious adverse events that will not be reported on an individual basis and the plan for monitoring and reporting results to FDA."

The European Union and the member states generally require that cases be unblinded before submission. See below.

E2A, which the FDA also references and wishes to follow, notes that when possible and appropriate, the blind should be maintained for those persons, such as biometrics (statistics) personnel. In large companies, this often turns out to be difficult to do in practice. Although statisticians may be blinded, in most instances when the blind is broken, a MedWatch/CIOMS I form/E2B file is created, in which case it is noted to be the study drug or control. Usually, serious AE reports are routinely widely dispersed: to the clinical trial physicians, monitors, others in the company, the investigators and the investigational review boards, subsidiaries, clinical research organizations, and data safety monitoring boards. "Leaks" occur and the code is inadvertently revealed to those who are attempting to remain blinded. Thus maintaining a "partial" unblinding is difficult.

Note: Some companies, especially those making ophthalmology products, do not like to use the word "blinded" and prefer to use the word "masked."

Serious AE reporting after the end of the trial:

> There are no clear rules in the United States for the duration of time that serious AEs should be collected and reported in the study report and to the FDA as expedited reports after a trial ends. Many use an arbitrary 30-day period after the patient's last dose. This may come from the long-standing clinical medicine tradition of ascribing postoperative deaths to the surgery if the death occurred

within 30 days of the operation. Clearly, if a drug has a very short or very long terminal half-life (e.g., depot formulations), one may use a different time period.

Survival studies (where all patients are followed until death, such as in cancer trials) present different issues. Here again, many use a 30-day limit after the last dose for collection of serious AEs. All deaths, however, should be collected by the sponsor and, if believed to meet the criteria for a 7- or 15-day report, reported. The issue in survival studies is that periodic follow-up to see whether the patients are still alive, one often has serious AEs reported "in passing." What to do with these is the issue. There is no consensus on this. Some companies collect and report them. Others do not.

■ When to Start Collecting Serious AEs in Trials

Safety data collection starts as soon as the informed consent is signed, and includes the waiting period or washout period (if there is one) when no study drug is administered. This concept was particularly noteworthy in France, where any safety issue that occurred during the "biomedical research" was reportable. This included placebo AEs, complications of medical procedures, auto accidents on the way to the hospital, and so forth. The idea is that the AEs occurred in regard to the study and not just the study drug.

In regard to FDA reporting, a serious AE that occurred before the drug was administered is generally not related to the study drug and thus does not qualify for a 15-day report. There is at least one situation, however, where this might not always be the case. Anticipatory nausea and vomiting before cancer chemotherapy in patients who have already had therapy is rather common, with an approximate 29% and 11% incidence, respectively. See the National Cancer Institute review of this phenomenon at its website (Web Resource 15-2). Thus one may consider that these serious AEs, which may be due to classic Pavlovian conditioning, are possibly related to the study or treatment drug even though it has not yet been taken.

■ European Union Requirements
Expedited Reporting in Clinical Trials

The expedited reporting in clinical trials is covered in the clinical trial directive and Volume 10 Chapter II in three sections (Web Resource 15-3). Specifically, the "Detailed guidance on the collection, verification and presentation of adverse reaction reports arising from clinical trials on medicinal products for human use" (Web Resource 15-4) covers the subject in great detail. Unlike the situation in the European Union for expedited reporting of post-marketing SAEs, which is largely harmonized, clinical trial reporting may still vary somewhat from country to country in the European Union/EEA.

Key points from the above guidance include:

- Reportable cases are SUSARs (suspected, unexpected, serious adverse reactions).
- The sponsor and investigator should both make an independent judgment of causality: "Having a reasonable suspected causal relationship to an investigational medicinal product."
- Expectedness should be determined using the Investigator Brochure for nonauthorized (non-MA) products, and the SmPC for authorized ones.
- In the concerned trial, SUSARs should be reported for the investigational product and comparators. For SUSARs in other trials, refer to the guidance, as the rules are rather complex and depend on whether there is an Marketing Authorization (MA) in a member state.
- For comparators, the case should be transmitted to the MA holder of the comparator.
- Placebo cases normally do not meet the criteria for expedited reporting unless it is possible the reaction is due to an excipient.
- The ethics committee in some countries may only receive ICSRs for SUSARs in the concerned trial in that member state. If so, it is recommended that SUSARs from other member states and third countries be reported to the ethics committee (and health authority) at least every 6 months as a line listing and a summary of the main points. Changes in patient risk and new safety issues as well as changes in the conduct of the trial should be reported in 15 days to the committee.

■ Codes should be broken by the sponsor in blinded trials before reporting to the ethics committee and the health authorities. If the blind break shows the product administered was the test drug, then it should be an expedited report; if a comparator, it should be assessed for expectedness against the SmPC and if unexpected, it should be reported; if placebo, such events normally don't satisfy the requirements for expedited reporting, but "where after unblinding SUSARs are associated with placebo, it is the sponsor's responsibility to report such cases."

■ In trials with high morbidity/mortality with many potential expedited reports, the sponsor may reach an agreement in advance with the concerned health agencies concerning SAEs that are treated as disease-related and not handled as expedited reports. The agreed-on system should be noted in the protocol, and it is recommended that a Data Safety Monitoring Committee be used.

Annual Safety Reports (ASR)

In the European Union, sponsors must submit a safety report once a year while a clinical trial is under way. The report should concisely describe the safety information for one or more trials. See the guidance noted above under European Union expedited reporting for full details. The ASR has three parts:

1. Analysis of the subjects' safety in the concerned clinical trial.

   ■ It should describe all new and relevant safety findings and should consider reversibility; previously unidentified or increased frequency of known toxicity; overdose; interactions; special populations, such as the elderly, children, or any other at-risk groups; pregnancy or lactation; abuse; risks with the investigation or diagnostic procedures; and so forth.

   ■ It should also contain an analysis of measures previously or currently proposed to minimize the risks found and a detailed rationale for whether it is necessary to amend the protocol or to change or update the consent form, patient information leaflet, and the Investigator Brochure.

2. A line listing of all suspected serious adverse reactions (including all SUSARs) that occurred in the concerned trial, including also serious adverse reactions from third countries, tabulated by body system for each trial.

3. An aggregate summary tabulation of suspected serious adverse reactions that occurred in the concerned trial for each body system, for each AE term and for each treatment arm.

The report should be submitted on the anniversary of the first authorization in any member state and within 60 days of the data lockpoint. If there is also an MA for the product, the Periodic Safety Update Report (PSUR) and ASR dates may be harmonized.

Investigators should be informed in writing with a line listing of SUSARs and a summary of any safety issues that could adversely affect the study subjects.

Each member state in the European Union may add more requirements in terms of aggregate reporting.

■ Canadian Requirements

Expedited reporting in Canada follows the 7- and 15-day requirements for expedited reporting whether the case occurred inside or outside Canada. See Web Resource 15-5.

Currently there is no specific timing in the regulations for the ethics committee (called a Research Ethics Board) in Canada to receive periodic reports. Requirements are thus usually set out by the individual board in its charter or Standard Operating Procedures (SOPs). This is undergoing much discussion in Canada.

Health Canada also does not require an annual safety review. Although in the past there was an Annual Clinical Trial Report for IND products, this is now functionally replaced by a yearly submission of the updated Investigator Brochure, which is submitted to the dossier. This allows Health Canada to get an overview of the drug and trial. There is discussion in Canada about whether an annual safety report/Development Safety Update Report and PSURs for marketed products will be required. It is expected that they will be at some point. See Web Resource 15-6.

■ Elsewhere

The requirements for expedited and periodic reporting vary significantly from country to country, even within the European Union, and companies should check locally and frequently about reporting requirements, particularly if there is a study site in that country. Requirements and submissions may not always be in written in English. This differs somewhat from the existing situation for postmarketing reporting, which is largely harmonized.

16

Postmarketing Spontaneous ICSR/SAE Reporting

Postmarketing spontaneous reporting of Individual Case Safety Reports (ICSRs) is the mainstay of drug safety at this time.

■ General Principles

The requirements for reporting revolve around ICSRs of various subsets of serious adverse events (SAEs) and then the periodic aggregate reporting of the remaining cases (and some SAEs already reported) with some degree of medical analysis. This system, on its face, is quite extraordinary as it relies on the good will and beneficence of

- healthcare professionals, to voluntarily report bad reactions to drugs that they have prescribed or administered, and who are not compensated for their efforts
- patients and consumers

This situation is likely to change over the years for many reasons, including cost and better technology. But for now, this is the system that we use to elucidate the safety profile of marketed drugs.

The regulations governing postmarketing reporting are complex, scattered, and only partially harmonized. Various updates and guidances are published irregularly, often changing the rules significantly. There is no single source tracking all changes, and the changes are often but not always published in English. (Why countries with their own national languages should publish their internal rules in English is another discussion entirely.)

■ Postmarketing ICSRs Versus Clinical Trial ICSRs

Although postmarketing New Drug Application (NDA) or Marketing Authorization (MA) reporting of SAE reports are conceptually quite similar to premarketing clinical investigation (IND) SAE reports, there are significant differences. The sources and reporters of the events are varied (not just from clinical trial investigators). The handling and reporting to health agencies are also somewhat different. These are explained later.

As with clinical trial reporting, there is an obligation for safety reporting after approval of the NDA or MA. Postmarketing reporting is usually obligatory after approval whether or not the drug is actually marketed (some companies delay marketing for operational or seasonal reasons). In clinical trials, AEs are reported by investigators who are health professionals and usually have a relationship with the company (e.g., sponsored trials). Thus, cooperation and complete medical reports from a healthcare professional are usually ensured. Under governmental regulations, reporting is obligatory for the investigator and the sponsor.

The postmarketing period, however, is quite different. Reports may come from many sources, including patients, families of patients, healthcare professionals, sales representatives, literature reports, news reports, health authorities, the internet, blogs, social media, poison control centers, other pharmaceutical companies, lawyers, and more. Reporting is purely voluntary for everyone except pharmaceutical companies and rests on the goodwill of the reporters. However, sometimes patients that report the AE are upset that the AE happened at all. They may assume that drugs are safe and this AE should not have happened. At least in the United States, they often want their money back and, in fact, may have called the company not to report the AE but rather to get a refund.

Healthcare professionals often contact the health agency or the pharmaceutical company to report an AE and are not quite aware that the company, obliged to follow up and report the case to the authorities, will do extensive follow-up and request copies of reports from the physician's office, the hospital, the laboratory, and even the ambulance service. Busy pharmacists, nurses, or physicians often do not realize what they are getting into when they simply called to do their duty by making a "quick" report of an AE. They did not want to get burdened down with pulling records from perhaps multiple sources and sending them to the company.

Report quality is also an issue compared with clinical trial reports, as the quality of the postmarketing reports is quite variable, especially when reported by nonmedical people. Consumer reports should have follow-up attempted with the treating physician where possible. The problem is more difficult if the patient used an over-the-counter (OTC) product and self-prescribed; there may be no physician or pharmacist involved at all.

The four elements or criteria for a valid 15-day safety report (sometimes called the minimal data set for reportability) are

1. An identifiable patient
2. An identifiable reporter
3. A suspect drug(s)

4. An AE (or fatal outcome if no AE is reported other than "found dead")

If these four elements are present, then the case is considered reportable to the U.S. Food and Drug Administration (FDA). If they are not, the company should make due diligent efforts to obtain the missing data. The data should be stored in an electronic database.

An identifiable patient usually means one or more identifiers are present: age, sex, initials, name, and so on. Vague reports such as "I heard there was a patient or two upstate who took drug X and had a stroke" or "a few people had strokes" are not specific enough to meet the criteria for identifiable patient. "A man" or "a young girl" or "six men had strokes" are sufficient to be considered identifiable.

An identifiable reporter is usually clearer. It may be the patient or a family member. As a rule of thumb, an identifiable reporter should be one who can be contacted. Thus, an e-mail AE report where there is no information on the sender other than the e-mail address would be a valid reporter because one can respond to the e-mail and get follow-up.

The suspect drug is also usually not a problem. However, issues do occur:

- Occasionally, someone will send in an AE report and make the comment, "I don't think this is due to your drug but thought I should report it anyway, just in case." This should still be considered the suspect drug (unless another one is noted) and the reporter's comment noted in the narrative.
- If it is clear that the drug is the product of another company (e.g., same chemical entity but different manufacturer, whether branded or generic), the case should be sent within 5 days to that manufacturer or company if it is located in the United States; elsewhere rules vary, but in general, the case should go to the manufacturer/MA holder. If, however, it is unclear whether it is the company's product or another manufacturer's product, then the company must process it as if it were clearly its own product. The lack of clear "ownership" and product identification should be noted in the report.
- Different formulations of the same active moiety must be entered into the database and reported, if appropriate, unless the product is clearly found to be from another company. Thus, a topical version of a company's product made by another company (but unclear which one) needs to be reported.

■ Combination products that contain the active moiety should also be reported.

The identifiable AE is also usually clear and relates to any "bad thing." The AE could include signs, laboratory abnormalities, symptoms, or diseases. More general terms like "experienced unspecified injury" or "irreparable damages" should be excluded. Fatal outcome with no AE should be considered reportable ("found dead in bed"). This is the only instance in which an outcome is considered an AE. Death is an outcome and not an AE unless there is no other AE reported.

One should also be sure to distinguish medication errors and product quality issues. Sometimes two or more things may occur in the same report ("The tablet was blue instead of green and smelled funny; I took two instead of one and then had a bad headache. And I want my money back and I have a question."). The product quality, medication error, AE, question, and refund issues should each be handled by the appropriate personnel in the company.

In most countries, the company ("applicant," "sponsor," or MAH) must report each AE that is serious and unexpected (not in the approved labeling = Package Insert for the United States, the SmPC for the European Union, the product monograph in other countries, etc.), whether domestic or abroad, within 15 calendar days of initial receipt of the information. Note that this is different from the criteria used for clinical trial reporting, which, in most countries, requires three criteria (serious, unexpected, possibly related to the drug). Postmarketing reporting only requires two (serious, unexpected) because it is believed that spontaneous reports have "implied" causality or suspicion. The reporter would not have contacted the health agency or the company to report the case if he or she did not believe there was some level of causal relationship between the drug and the AE.

The company must promptly investigate all serious AEs that produced 15-day alert reports and must submit follow-up reports within 15 calendar days of receipt of new information or as requested by the health agency. If additional information is not obtainable, records of the unsuccessful steps taken to seek additional information should be maintained.

The company selling or making the drug is not the only one obliged to report serious AEs. This requirement also applies to any person or entity whose name appears on the label of an approved drug product as a manufacturer, packer, or distributor. By extension, this applies also to any agent, comarketer, and distributor, that is, anyone or any company or entity that may receive an AE and with which the company has a relationship.

Solicited safety information (e.g., from patient outreach or support programs) should be handled as if this were a postmarketing trial and the three clinical trial reporting criteria are applied: serious, unexpected, and a reasonable possibility that the SAE is related to the drug. That is, the criteria are not those of the postmarketing situation (serious, unexpected) but of the clinical trial situation. There are no 7-day reports in the postmarketing setting.

■ Sources of AEs

Postmarketing AEs may come from many sources: sales representatives; the regulatory, quality, compliance, or telephone operator departments and other company employees (such as the chief executive officer's secretary/administrative assistant); lawyers and lawsuits; individual patients, consumers, and family; pharmacists; nurses; physicians and other healthcare professionals; health agencies; company subsidiaries; associated business partners (not part of the company); websites; e-mail; social media; newspapers; the medical literature; poison control centers, TV, and radio. The company must set up the appropriate internal procedures (standard operating procedures) to ensure that AEs arriving anywhere in the company reach the drug safety group in a timely manner (usually no more than one or two working days).

Unlike clinical trial reports, where the reporters are usually clinical investigators or their staff, many postmarketing reports arrive by telephone from unhappy patients or harried medical professionals. The company needs to establish a careful triage of calls to identify those that are product-related and ensure they are sent to a medical professional quickly after the operator answers so that AEs and other product issues are not missed. It is not wise to bounce the call to multiple departments until the right one is found. Voice response systems may fail to elicit the problem ("Press one to get your money back. Press two to report an AE...").

A rather special skill set on the part of the staff (whether medical professionals or not) in the company who field these calls is required. The caller, especially a patient, usually wants something (money or replacement drug) and may be angry and hostile. The call center responder must be cool and calm and obtain the needed medical and demographic information while maintaining empathy and sympathy. Often the caller has contacted the company with a question ("Can drug X cause heart attacks?"), not realizing that the company will explore to see whether there is an AE there. Thus, the call is transformed from a request for information to supplying information that may anger the caller. The call center responder should write down (on paper or directly into a database) the caller's information, using direct quotes where possible without admitting that the drug necessarily caused any AEs or produced problems. When the call is from a consumer, an attempt should always be made to obtain the contact information of the patient's physician or other healthcare provider to "medically validate" the report. If follow-up is needed with the caller (e.g., after obtaining medical records), another contact should be arranged.

■ Literature and Publications

Formal and frequent searches of the published literature using a computerized system (commercial services) that searches large numbers of publications and databases for publications on the company's products (both by trade name and generic name) is required. If the search reveals a citation, article, or abstract that contains a case report or clinical trial with information that meets the four criteria, a 15-day postmarketing alert report must be sent to the health agency along with a copy of the article (in English usually) in most countries. This is handled like any other 15-day report, with follow-up sought. If an article describes multiple cases, then a separate report should be filed for each (for the United States, see 21CFR31.480(d)(1,2)). Note that such literature searches are required *weekly* for drugs marketed in the European Union and are included in PSURs. The European Union requirements for reporting literature are very specific in terms of style ("the Vancouver Style"). Member states may request translation of the article into their national language, though English may be used in the ICSR submitted as an expedited report. See Volume 9A Chapter I.4, Section 3.2 and Part III 7 for further detail.

The issue of translation arises periodically. If a publication title suggests that the article contains reportable safety information and if the article and the abstract are in a language that no one on staff is able to read (or even minimally decipher), then the article should be translated to determine whether there is a case. This may be very costly for certain languages. Fortunately, most cases are published in English or one of the other major medical languages. There are free internet tools that will do rough (usually very rough) computer translations of text that may give an idea of whether the article contains safety information and a possibly reportable case. It is not clear yet whether this would suffice for translation. This could avoid delays and costs but at the expense of a possibly faulty translation. The regulatory reporting clock starts when the four elements of a valid case are identifiable. This may mean the clock starts only when the translation is received, if the abstract did not supply the four elements. Companies are expected to search local journals not tracked in the major computer literature databases (e.g., Embase, PubMed) if the company sells in that language market.

For multinational companies with offices around the world, who searches which journals should be addressed early on and up front to avoid duplication of efforts. The international offices are usually useful for obtaining follow-up from faraway reporters and non-English-speakers. However, it is usually not productive to have each international office search its country's journals for AEs unless they are not tracked in the major computerized literature database. This is best done through the central database search.

■ Other Sources of Reports

Periodically, certain large organizations (such as poison control centers and teratology centers) publish summary or review articles detailing dozens to thousands of reports of AEs with drug names associated. Often there is insufficient information to create individual cases, but occasionally there is a minimal data set (patient identifier, poison control center as reporter, a drug, and an AE). This may pose a problem in regard to reporting. Usually, follow-up is impossible or impractical. In such cases, it is worth communicating with the health authority(ies) on the best way to proceed. No agency wants to receive 5000 ICSRs each with minimal data any more than the company wants to generate them. A summary letter or a single report covering multiple patients may be acceptable.

■ Follow-Up

Follow-up on all serious AEs should be done. There are no absolute rules on what is sufficient in terms of due diligence, but a common rule of thumb in the industry is two or three follow-up requests (registered letters, voice mail messages, or contacts with physician's staff, etc.) for "routine" serious AEs are sufficient. New, dramatic, unexpected, fatal, or life-threatening serious AEs may require many more attempts to obtain adequate data to make sense of the case (the true goal of all these efforts). Many in the industry have "war stories" of flying to far-off sites or doing various maneuvers to try to obtain follow-up information on critical cases.

Follow-up on nonserious expected cases is often not done or expected by regulatory agencies, especially if the AE is already in the labeling. Follow-up on nonserious unexpected cases is, however, generally a good idea and is obligatory in some countries. Efforts are usually limited to one or two follow-up e-mails or calls.

■ Notes on United States Requirements for Postmarketing NDA Reporting of SAEs

The U.S. regulations are found in 21CFR314.80 and basically state that the NDA holder has an obligation to promptly review all adverse drug experience information received from any source, "foreign or domestic including information derived from commercial marketing experience, post marketing clinical investigations, post marketing epidemiological/surveillance studies, reports in the scientific literature, and unpublished scientific papers" (21CFR314.80(b)). Companies do not have to resubmit to the FDA reports received from the FDA.

There are multiple, scattered guidances, draft guidances, and other documents that cover reporting requirements. They are, unfortunately, incomplete, vague, and in many cases nonspecific. The FDA has various Web pages available on its site with instructions for industry, including the following:

- Postmarket Drug Safety Information for Patients and Providers
  - Web Resource 16-1
- Guidances, Information Sheets, and Notices
  - Web Resource 16-2
- Regulations and Policies and Procedures for Postmarketing Surveillance Programs
  - Web Resource 16-3
- Guidances (Drugs)
  - Web Resource 16-4
- Guidance, Compliance & Regulatory Information (Biologics)
  - Web Resource 16-5
- Industry (Biologics)
  - Web Resource 16-6
- Staff Manual Guide: Chapter 53; Postmarketing Surveillance and Epidemiology: Human Drugs
  - Web Resource 16-7
- Potential Signals of Serious Risks/New Safety Information Identified from the Adverse Event

Reporting System (AERS)
  - Web Resource 16-8
- MedWatch
  - Web Resource 16-9
- Adverse Event Reporting System (AERS)
  - Web Resource 16-10
- Over-the-Counter (OTC) Related Federal Register Notices, Ingredient References, and other Regulatory Information
  - Web Resource 16-11
- If it is a foreign-originated report with the same active ingredient (moiety), then the case should be entered into the database and reported if the reporting criteria are met:
  - The FDA's 2001 postmarketing AE draft guidance states the following for foreign literature: "Reports of serious, unexpected adverse experiences described in the scientific literature should be submitted for products that have the same active moiety as a product marketed in the United States. This is true even if the excipient, dosage forms, strengths, routes of administration, and indications vary."
  - In regard to the definition of an active moiety, "An active moiety means the molecule or ion, excluding those appended portions of the molecule that cause the drug to be an ester, salt (including a salt with hydrogen or coordination bonds), or other noncovalent derivative (such as a complex, chelate, or clathrate) of the molecule, responsible for the physiological or pharmacological action of the drug substance." From the FDA's "Frequently Asked Questions for New Drug Product Exclusivity." See Web Resource 16-12.

If a company holds more than one NDA for the same chemical entity, the 15-day report should be addressed to the oldest (original) approved NDA if the actual product or formulation is not known or specified. If a company has more than one of its products listed in the report, the case should be sent to the NDA for the first listed product on the report, which is usually the "more" or "most" suspect drug.

■ MedWatch to Manufacturer Program

The FDA established the MedWatch to Manufacturer Program, in which serious spontaneous AEs reported directly to the FDA are sent to the manufacturer as

MedWatch forms. See the FDA website (Web Resource 16-13). The reports contain the reporter's name and address, permitting the manufacturer to do follow-up. The reporter must consent to this. The original MedWatch received from the FDA should not be re-sent to the FDA (see 21CFR3.14.80(b)), but any follow-up information should be. Other reports may be received from the FDA under the Drug Quality Reporting System that the FDA established for reporting and receiving quality issues on products analogous to the MedWatch Program (Web Resource 16-14).

Reports from the FDA via the Freedom of Information Act

This is a system that allows anyone to obtain information from the U.S. government that is not classified or proprietary (commercial secrets). For a nominal fee, it is possible to obtain from the FDA MedWatch reports on any drug (one's own or competitors'). It is a one- or two-step process. The initial request produces a standardized printout or CD/DVD with a line listing of AEs. Any specific case (the MedWatch form) may be obtained by then requesting it using its identification number (accession number). The cases received are anonymous in regard to the patient and reporter, thus preventing follow-up. Unfortunately, some follow-up reports are not tied or referenced to the initial reports. If one goes through FOI for information, the request itself is public information and can be found out (by a company's competitors, for example). Thus, there are commercial ventures that perform the search for a company and make the search anonymous. One such company is FOI Services. Their website is listed in Web Resource 16-15.

There are reasons both for and against obtaining cases on one's own drugs:

- Pros
  - The company will know what the FDA knows and will have as complete a data set as possible. There should be no "surprises," such as communications from FDA about safety matters the company does not know about.
  - The company will be better able to look for signals and perform signal analysis (including data mining) with a complete database.
- Cons
  - No follow-up is possible on a case. What you have is what you have.

- It may not always be possible to determine whether a case is a duplicate (e.g., it was reported to the FDA in addition to the company, perhaps by a different reporter). As the reporter and patient identifiers are removed, it may be hard to ascertain whether the case is a duplicate.
- Coding and case handling (e.g., narrative style and content) may be different. At this point, a decision on whether to recode must be made.

Most people nowadays feel that it is wise and ethically appropriate to obtain the FDA reports and any other safety reports available from other health agencies (e.g., Data Analysis Prints from the United Kingdom MHRA or periodic searches online of Health Canada's safety database). The large majority of cases in the FDA database come through the company, so, in theory, there should be few cases received directly by FDA. Some companies obtain competitor safety information in this way. Such data, however, are not permitted to be used in marketing or sales. Similar FOI systems exist already or are being developed in other countries. Again, issues arise such as duplication, consistency, language, and follow-up when obtaining case reports. Many multinational companies have their local offices obtain these cases where possible. The Uppsala Monitoring Centre in Sweden maintains the largest worldwide safety database, with cases obtained from national health agencies. However, the data are usually only line listings and may be difficult to use to identify new or important cases.

Instructions on Filling Out the MedWatch Form

There are very detailed instructions on the FDA's MedWatch website (Web Resource 16-16) on how to fill out the MedWatch form (3500A form for manufacturers), and for healthcare professionals (3500 form for all others) at Web Resource 16-17. Companies should review the instructions and put them into place. For electronic submission (E2B) of ICSRs with and without attachments, detailed information is available at Web Resource 16-18.

European Union Regulations

The European Union regulations and requirements for medicinal products (defined broadly to include drugs, biologics, herbals, etc.) are all found in one document:

Volume 9A (Web Resource 16-19). It was last updated in September 2008 and runs over 220 pages. It is thorough, clear, complete, well written, and available in a searchable PDF format. It is essentially "one-stop shopping" and is a must-read for anyone doing pharmacovigilance, even those not doing European Union drug safety.

Its sections include:

- The legal framework for pharmacovigilance
- Guidelines for MA holders, including requirements for

  - Systems monitoring of compliance and PV inspections, the QPPV, risk management
  - Expedited reporting of ICSRs
  - Special situations (e.g., pregnancy, compassionate use, overdose, misuse, medication errors, lack of efficacy)
  - PSURs
  - Company-sponsored postauthorization studies (PASS)

- Guidelines for the Member States Competent Authorities and the EMA
- Electronic exchange of information
- PV communications
- Annexes on terminology, abbreviations, ICH guidelines, templates (including RMPs, PSURs, direct healthcare professional communications), and distribution requirements for ICSRs and other reports to the member states.

Summarizing all of these requirements and details is beyond the scope of this book. However, an excellent resource for a summary of these requirements, as seen through British eyes, is available in the book published by the MHRA entitled *Good Pharmacovigilance Practices*, Pharmaceutical Press, London, 2009. See their website for information (Web Resource 16-20).

■ Canadian Regulations

Canada's core document on drug safety is Guidance Document for Industry—Reporting Adverse Reactions to Marketed Health Products, found at Web Resource 16-21.

■ Australian Regulations

Australian guidelines for pharmacovigilance responsibilities of sponsors of registered medicines regulated by Drug Safety and Evaluation Branch are found at Web Resource 16-22.

Each country's requirements can usually be found on the national website of the drug agency or ministry of health. In many cases, however, the requirements are not available in English.

■ Frequently Asked Questions

Q: This is rather messy, it seems. Would this not be an ideal situation for full harmonization, since the rules are fairly similar already?

A: Yes, indeed. However, the devil is always in the details. It is likely we will get there as data standards for format, contents, and transmission develop. Of course, there will likely be multiple standards, and then we will have to standardize the standards. The issue of language will not be resolved until adequate computer translation abilities are developed. The logical (albeit utopian) outcome of all of this is the reporting of each AE in the reporter's native language to a single global repository from which anyone can obtain complete information. Perhaps this will go even one step further if electronic medical records become a practical reality. In this setting, it would be possible to "pull" the AEs and the complete medical records from this megadatabase (or linked databases/warehouses) without requiring active submission by reporters.

17

Periodic Adverse Drug Experience Reports (PADERs): NDA Periodic Reports and Periodic Safety Update Reports (PSURs)

Most countries now accept and usually require the submission of Periodic Safety Reports for aggregate postmarketing safety reporting. The U.S. Food and Drug Administration (FDA) accepts PSURs, though this must be agreed on with the agency in writing beforehand. The older format, NDA Periodic Reports, also called Periodic Adverse Drug Experience Reports (PADERs), are still required according to the regulations (unless there is the PSUR waiver), though FDA will likely require PSURs in the near future.

In addition to the 15-day alert reports, the FDA requires the submission of New Drug Application (NDA), Abbreviated NDA, and Biologic License Application (BLA) periodic reports. The regulations covering this are found in 21CFR314.80(c)(2)(I,II).

■ NDA Periodic Reports

As with Investigational New Drug application (IND) regulations, there are updates scattered in various other FDA documents. Some are arguably specific to premarketing settings (e.g., drug-induced liver injury) but should be kept in mind with postmarketing aggregate reporting too:

- Postmarketing Reporting of Adverse Drug Experiences (March 1992)
- Guideline for Adverse Experience Reporting for Licensed Biological Products (October 1993)
- Postmarketing Adverse Experience Reporting for Human Drug and Licensed Biological Products: Clarification of What to Report (August 27, 1997)
- Post-marketing Safety Reporting for Human Drugs and Biological Products Including Vaccines (March 2001)
- Conducting a Clinical Safety Review of a New Product Application and Preparing a Report on the Review (February 2005)
- Drug-Induced Liver Injury: Premarketing Clinical Evaluation (July 2009)
- Drug Safety Information—FDA's Communication to the Public (March 2007)
- Format and Content of Proposed Risk Evaluation and Mitigation Strategies (REMS), REMS Assessments, and Proposed REMS Modifications (March 2009)

- Postmarketing Studies and Clinical Trials—Implementation of Section 505(o) of the Federal Food, Drug, and Cosmetic Act (July 2009)
- Enforcement of the Postmarketing Adverse Drug Reporting Regulation. Staff Manual Guide: Chapter 53; Postmarketing Surveillance and Epidemiology: Human Drugs. Adverse Drug Effects

See FDA's guidance pages (Web Resource 17-1).

The basic regulations state the following (21CFR314.80(c)(2)(I,II)):

All "adverse drug experiences" not submitted as 15-day alert reports must be submitted in the periodic report. A periodic report for each NDA must be submitted quarterly (every 3 months) for the first 3 years after the approval of the NDA. After the 3-year period is over, the reporting frequency is then yearly unless the FDA requests otherwise.

Each report must be submitted 30 days after the close of the quarter for quarterly reports and 60 days after the close of the anniversary date for yearly reports. Thus, the company has 30 or 60 days to prepare the report. The FDA may alter this schedule if they wish to continue quarterly reporting after the 3-year period is over.

Each periodic report is required to contain the following:

- A narrative summary and analysis of the information in the report and an analysis of the 15-day alert reports submitted during the reporting interval (all 15-day alert reports must appropriately reference the applicant's patient identification number, adverse reaction term(s), and date of submission to the FDA).
- A MedWatch form (3500A) for each adverse drug experience not reported as a 15-day expedited report (with an index consisting of a line listing of the applicant's patient identification number and adverse reaction term(s)).
- A history of actions taken since the last report because of adverse drug experiences (e.g., labeling changes or studies initiated).
- Periodic reporting, except for information regarding 15-day alert reports, does not apply to adverse drug experience information obtained from postmarketing studies (whether or not they were conducted under an investigational New Drug Application), from reports in the scientific literature, or from foreign marketing experience.
- Follow-up information to adverse drug experiences submitted in a periodic report may be submitted in the next periodic report.

In August 1997, the FDA published a guidance encouraging NDA holders to submit requests to waive the requirements to submit MedWatch forms for nonserious labeled AEs (Web Resource 17-2).

The March 2001 Guidance at Web Resource 17-3 explains the requirements for a periodic report and is officially in effect even though it remains a draft a decade after being published. It is summarized below.

■ PSURs to the FDA

The March 2001 Guidance describes the mechanism to obtain a waiver to submit PSURs using the ICH E2C requirements (see Chapter 37) instead of NDA Periodic Reports:

- If all dosage forms and formulations for the active substance, as well as indications, are combined in one PSUR, this information should be separated into specific sections of the report when such separation is appropriate to portray accurately the safety profile of the specific dosage forms. For example, one should not combine information from ophthalmic drop dosage forms and solid oral dosage forms.
- Copies of the FDA Form 3500A or VAERS form that are required by the regulations must be included. These forms should be included with the PSUR as an appendix. You can request a waiver for submitting certain nonserious, expected adverse experiences on an FDA Form 3500A.
- A summary tabulation should be included as an appendix listing all spontaneously reported U.S. individual case safety reports from consumers if such cases are not already included in the PSUR. Summary tabulations should be presented by body system of all adverse experience terms and counts of occurrences and should be segregated by type (i.e., serious/unexpected; serious/expected; nonserious/unexpected; and nonserious/expected).
- A narrative should be included as an appendix that references the changes, if any, to the approved U.S. labeling for the dosage forms covered by the PSUR based on new information in the PSUR. A copy of the most recently approved U.S. labeling for the product(s) covered by the PSUR should be included.
- Submission Date and Frequency for PSUR Reports. Applicants can request a waiver to submit PSURs to the FDA based on the month and day of the international birth date of the product instead of the

month and day of the anniversary date of U.S. approval of the product. The waiver request should specify that these PSURs would be submitted to the FDA within 60 calendar days of the data lock point (i.e., month and day of the international birth date of the product or any other day agreed on by the applicant and the FDA). Applicants can also request a waiver to submit PSURs to the FDA at a frequency other than those required by regulation.

Postmarketing Periodic Reports

The information contained within a classic NDA Periodic Report should be divided into four sections in the order described below and should be clearly separated by an identifying tab. If information for one of these sections is not included, the applicant should explain why the information is not provided.

Section 1: Narrative Summary and Analysis

A narrative summary and analysis of the information in the postmarketing periodic report and an analysis of the 15-day reports (i.e., serious, unexpected, adverse experiences) submitted during the reporting period must be provided and should include the following:

- The number of non-15-day initial adverse experience reports and the number of non-15-day follow-up reports contained in this periodic report and the time period covered by the periodic report.

- A line listing of the 15-day reports submitted during the reporting period. This line listing should include the manufacturer report number, adverse experience term(s), and the date the 15-day report was sent to the FDA.

- A summary tabulation by body system (e.g., cardiovascular, central nervous system, endocrine, renal) of all adverse experience terms and counts of occurrences submitted during the reporting period. The information should be taken from

  - 15-day reports submitted to the FDA

  - Non-15-day reports submitted in the periodic report

  - Reports forwarded to the applicant by the FDA

  - Any nonserious, expected, adverse experiences not submitted to the FDA but maintained on file by the applicant

For the adverse experience term "product interaction," the interacting products should be identified in the tabulation.

- A summary listing of the adverse experience reports in which the drug or biologic product was listed as one of the suspect products but the report was filed to another NDA, Abbreviated NDA, or BLA held by the applicant.

- A narrative discussion of the clinical significance of the 15-day reports submitted during the reporting period and of any increased reporting frequency of serious, expected, adverse experiences when, in the judgment of the applicant, it is believed the data reflect a clinically meaningful change in adverse experience occurrence.

This narrative should assess clinical significance by type of adverse experience, body system, and overall product safety, relating the new information received during this reporting period to what was already known about the product.

The narrative should also state what further actions, if any, the applicant plans to undertake based on the information gained during the reporting period and include the time period for completing the actions (i.e., when the applicant plans to start and finish the action and submit the information to the agency).

- The narrative discussion should indicate, based on the information learned during the reporting period, whether the applicant believes either that (1) no change in the product's current approved labeling is warranted or (2) there are safety-related issues that need to be addressed in the approved product labeling. If the FDA is considering changes in the approved product labeling, the applicant should state in the narrative the date and number of the supplemental application submitted to address the labeling changes.

Section 2: Narrative Discussion of Actions Taken

A narrative discussion of actions taken must be provided, including any labeling changes and studies initiated since the last periodic report. This section should include:

- A copy of current U.S. product labeling
- A list of any labeling changes made during the reporting period
- A list of studies initiated

- A summary of important foreign regulatory actions (e.g., new warnings, limitations in the indications, and use of the product)
- Any communication of new safety information (e.g., a Dear Doctor letter)

Section 3: Index Line Listing

An index line listing of FDA Form 3500As or Vaccine Adverse Event Reporting System (VAERS) forms included in section 4 of the periodic report must be provided. The line listing for each FDA Form 3500A or VAERS form submitted should include:

- Manufacturer report number
- Adverse experience term(s)
- Page number of FDA Form 3500A or VAERS form as located in the periodic report
- Identification of interacting products for any product interaction listed as an adverse experience

Section 4: FDA Form 3500As or VAERS Forms

FDA Form 3500As or VAERS forms must be provided for the following spontaneously reported adverse experiences that occurred in the United States during the reporting period:

- Serious and expected
- Nonserious and unexpected
- Nonserious and expected

Applicants are encouraged to request a waiver of the requirement to submit individual case safety reports of nonserious, expected, adverse experiences for drugs and certain biologic products as described below. Adverse experiences due to a failure to produce the expected pharmacologic action (i.e., lack of effect) should be included in this section.

For individual case safety reports of serious, expected, adverse experiences, the FDA encourages applicants to include relevant hospital discharge summaries and autopsy reports/death certificates as well as lists of other relevant documents as described for 15-day reports of serious, unexpected, adverse experiences.

Initial non-15-day reports should be included in the periodic report in a separate section from non-15-day follow-up reports. All initial and follow-up information obtained for an adverse experience with a given periodic reporting period should be combined and submitted in the periodic report as one initial non-15-day report (i.e.,

an initial non-15-day report and a non-15-day follow-up report describing the same adverse experience should not be submitted in the same periodic report). An FDA Form 3500A or VAERS form for a serious, unexpected, adverse experience should not be included in a periodic report because this adverse experience should have been previously submitted to the FDA as a 15-day report.

If no adverse experiences were identified for the human drug or biologic product for the time period involved and no regulatory actions concerning safety were taken anywhere in the world where the product is marketed, the periodic report should simply state this and be submitted to the FDA along with a copy of the current U.S. labeling. The FDA has encouraged the use of Periodic Safety Update Reports in place of periodic reports.

■ Other Reports

The FDA requires other reports for "NDA maintenance":

- Distribution reports (21CFR600.810): This is a 6-month report requiring the submission of all information about the quantity of product distributed under licensing agreements. It does not touch drug safety.
- Annual reports (21CFR314.81(b)(2)): This is a yearly report requiring the submission of information from the previous year that might affect safety, efficacy, or labeling as well as information on labeling changes, distribution, chemistry, manufacturing and controls changes, nonclinical laboratory studies, clinical trial data, and pediatric data.

■ PSURs

The PSUR in one form or another is now the basic postmarketing aggregate report submitted around the world. As noted, it was "created" in ICH E2C and addenda. See Chapter 37. In the European Union, Volume 9A Part I, Section 6 covers PSURs. This section is extensive and runs some 26 pages. The UK Medicines and Healthcare Products Regulatory Agency (MHRA) also summarizes information on PSURs in its Good Pharmacovigilance Guide. Those who prepare PSURs should refer to these documents as well as any local requirements in other countries.

PSUR (like the NDA Periodic Report) is the major document for aggregate safety analyses by the authorities. Lateness, poor quality, incompleteness, and errors will be noted and will precipitate inspections and punishment ranging from chastisement to more severe sanctions. In the European Union, the Qualified Person for PV has personal responsibility and liability for the report and its contents.

The PSUR serves multiple purposes, including the maintenance and requirements for the authorization, product use, the benefit–risk analyses, the Marketing Authorization's (MA) views on the product, and the safety issues for the reporting period and, for some safety issues, for the whole history of the drug. The PSUR is used for signaling but should not be the sole mechanism used for signaling.

The periodicity in the European Union and certain other countries is every 6 months for 2 years after authorization (even if marketing has not begun anywhere), then every year for 2 years and then every 3 years. In some situations, the authorities may request that the every-6-month or every-1-year schedule be maintained after the time for every-3-year-reports has arrived. A PSUR is usually required at the renewal of the MA (every 5 years) in the European Union. Most countries allow harmonization with the first approval anywhere (International Birth Date, or IBD), and the report is due no later than 60 days after the end of the reporting period. The U.S. periodicity is that of the NDA Periodic Report (every 6 months for 3 years, then yearly).

For drugs with significant sales, the document can be very large and time-consuming to prepare. It is usually a multidisciplinary effort (Drug Safety, Regulatory, Clinical, Epidemiology, Signaling, Quality, etc.). A written Standard Operating Procedure (SOP) or guideline or manual should exist on PSUR preparation. The previous PSURs and regulatory responses to them for the product should always be consulted before preparing the current PSUR as there are commitments, requests, special analyses, and so forth, that may be required on a continuing basis and should not be omitted until the commitment is completed or the health agencies agree. The appropriate labeling should be used. It is usually the Company Core Safety Information (CCSI), but it may be the Summary of Product Characteristics (SmPC) if no CCSI exists.

The contents, in brief, include:

- Executive Summary: Brief overview of the key information
- Introduction with product characteristics, period covered, and PSUR number (e.g., 3rd)
- Marketing Authorizations in a table with countries and dates, including disapprovals and withdrawals

- Update on health agency actions taken for safety reasons
- Patient exposure
- Presentation of Individual Case Histories (by MedDRA SOC)
  - Brief description of criteria used for cases shown
  - Description and analysis of selected cases
    - Including fatal cases
    - New and relevant safety information
- Line Listing of ICSRs
- Serious ADRs and nonserious unlisted ADRs from spontaneous sources
- Serious ADRs available from postapproval commitments and studies and named patient and compassionate use
- Serious ADRs from Regulatory Authorities
- Serious ADRs and nonserious unlisted ADRs from the medical literature
- Other listings as specially required (e.g., consumer reports not validated)
- Studies and Trials
  - Studies completed during the PSUR reporting period that provide relevant safety information, including epidemiology studies
- Other important information
  - Any information provided after the data lock point for the PSUR
  - Risk Management Plans and changes to them
- Overall safety evaluation
  - Key new information on serious and nonserious ADRs
  - Drug interactions, overdose, pregnancy issues, etc.
  - Epidemiology, signal and trends, white papers, class effects, etc.
- Conclusion
  - Overall risk–benefit analysis
  - Differences with the current reference labeling document (CCSI or SmPC)
  - Actions to be taken or initiated
    - Changes to reference labeling documents
  - Risk Management activities
- Appendices

Note that individual countries may require additional information and reports or summaries in the local language. Canada, for example, does not require that PSURs be submitted obligatorily but that they be available on rapid notice if requested. The United States requires certain additional sections (see below). Some countries may require additional sections in the local language.

PSURs to the FDA

The March 2001 Guidance describes the mechanism to obtain a waiver to submit PSURs using the ICH E2C requirements instead of NDA Periodic Reports:

- If all dosage forms and formulations for the active substance, as well as indications, are combined in one PSUR, this information should be separated into specific sections of the report when such separation is appropriate to accurately portray the safety profile of the specific dosage forms. For example, one should not combine information from ophthalmic drop dosage forms and solid oral dosage forms.

- Copies of the FDA Form 3500A or VAERS form required by the regulations must be included. These forms should be included with the PSUR as an appendix. You can request a waiver for submission of certain nonserious, expected adverse experiences on an FDA Form 3500A.

- A summary tabulation should be included as an appendix listing all spontaneously reported U.S. individual case safety reports from consumers if such cases are not already included in the PSUR. Summary tabulations should be presented by body system of all adverse experience terms and counts of occurrences and be segregated by type (i.e., serious/unexpected; serious/expected; nonserious/unexpected; and nonserious/expected).

- A narrative should be included as an appendix that references the changes, if any, to the approved U.S. labeling for the dosage forms covered by the PSUR based on new information in the PSUR. A copy of the most recently approved U.S. labeling for the product(s) covered by the PSUR should be included.

- Submission Date and Frequency for PSUR Reports. Applicants can request a waiver to submit PSURs to the FDA based on the month and day of the international birth date of the product instead of the month and day of the anniversary date of U.S. approval of the product. The waiver request should specify that these PSURs would be submitted to the FDA within 60 calendar days of the data lockpoint (i.e., month and day of the international birth date of the product or any other day agreed on by the applicant and the FDA). Applicants can also request a waiver to submit PSURs to the FDA at a frequency other than those required by regulation.

Note that the FDA, the European Union, and other jurisdictions have mechanisms in place to harmonize the submission dates. An international birth date (usually the first approval anywhere in the world) can be established with the health agencies, allowing the company to prepare and submit all reports based on this date. Harmonization of periodicity is not possible using addenda reports to get all the PSURs into synchronization. Thus reports may need to go into some agencies every 6 months, yearly, three-yearly, etc., but at least they are all prepared on the same anniversary date each year (e.g., if February 1st is established as the international birth date, then reports would go in with a data lockpoint of February 1st for yearly or multiyear reports and February 1st and August 1st for 6-month reports).

The European Union and other groups are now proposing to make the PSUR into a much broader benefit-risk document with major changes in the format and contents. How this will play out in the European Union and then whether it will be agreed upon by the U.S., Japan, and other countries remains to be seen.

Frequently Asked Questions

Q: So should we start to do PSURs for the FDA now?

A: Yes that would be a good idea. FDA will require PSURs at some point in time, probably sooner rather than later, and with perhaps no more than six months' notice before the requirement goes into effect. If the company is already preparing PSURs for other health authorities, the move to U.S. PSURs should be relatively doable. If the company has no experience in doing PSURs at all, indeed now is the time to learn and to start.

Epidemiology and Pharmacoepidemiology: What Are They? What Are Their Limitations and Advantages?

This chapter is not meant to be an introduction to epidemiology or pharmacoepidemiology. There are many excellent textbooks and references in those fields. Rather, this chapter attempts, briefly, to place epidemiology and pharmacoepidemiology in the context of their use in the practical world of drug safety. An excellent website to visit is that of the International Society of Pharmacoepidemiology (Web Resource 18-1).

What is epidemiology? There are several similar definitions:

■ The study of the distribution and determinants of diseases in populations. Epidemiological studies can be divided into two main types:
   ■ Descriptive epidemiology describes disease and/or exposure and may consist of calculating rates, for example, incidence and prevalence. Such descriptive studies do not use control groups and can only generate hypotheses, not test them. Studies of drug utilization would generally fall under descriptive studies.

■ Analytic epidemiology includes two types of studies: (1) observational studies, such as case-control and cohort studies, and (2) experimental studies, which would include clinical trials, such as randomized clinical trials. The analytic studies compare an exposed group with a control group and are usually designed as hypothesis-testing studies. (From the International Society of Pharmacoepidemiology, Web Resource 18-2.)

■ The study of the distribution and determinants of health-related states or events in specified populations, and the application of this study to the control of health problems. (From the Centers for Disease Control and Prevention, Web Resource 18-2.)

■ The study of the frequency, distribution, and behavior of a disease within a population (Web Resource 18-3).

■ The study of the incidence, distribution, and control of disease in a population (Web Resource 18-4).

■ The study of a disease that deals with how many people have it, where they are, how many new cases develop, and how to control the disease (Web Resource 18-5).

- Study of disease incidence, distribution, and behavior in populations, as well as the relationship between environment and disease.

- The branch of medicine that deals with the study of the causes, distribution, and control of disease in populations (Web Resource 18-3, the American Heritage Dictionary).

- The study of the incidence, distribution, and determinants of an infection, disease, or other health-related events in a population. Epidemiology can be thought of in terms of who, where, when, what, and why. That is, who has the infection/disease, where are they located geographically and in relation to each other, when is the infection/disease occurring, what is the cause, and why did it occur (Web Resource 18-4).

What is pharmacoepidemiology?

- The study of the utilization and effects of drugs in large numbers of people. To accomplish this study, pharmacoepidemiology borrows from both pharmacology and epidemiology. Thus, pharmacoepidemiology can be called a bridge science spanning both pharmacology and epidemiology. (From the International Society of Pharmacoepidemiology, Web Resource 18-2.)

- The study of the utilization of drugs, good and bad, by populations, and the effect of these drugs on those populations, for better or for worse.

For the purposes of this chapter, the terms *epidemiology* and *pharmacoepidemiology* will be used interchangeably even though purists will object to this since the two are not entirely the same.

Of necessity, pharmacoepidemiology uses numbers and statistical analyses. It is the study of populations as opposed to the study of individuals. Thus, it is used to answer questions about groups of people rather than about individual patients. It is also used to extrapolate and generalize from individuals to groups and populations. Thus, it would answer questions like "Are the women who live on Long Island, New York, at greater risk for breast cancer than those who live elsewhere?" or "Is the use of drug X associated with a higher incidence of atrial fibrillation in elderly men?" as opposed to questions like "Does Ms. Jones have breast cancer because she lives on Long Island?" or "Did drug X produce atrial fibrillation in 79-year-old Mr. Jones?"

In the world of drug safety, epidemiology is used to answer questions about adverse events (AEs), and in particular serious adverse events (SAEs), in populations after (usually) a signal has been generated based on one or more individual case reports. The purpose is to confirm and quantify the signal or to rule it out. Such studies can rarely answer questions about causality but rather give information on risks and associations.

In this chapter, we give a very high-level view of the handful of concepts that continually appear in the drug safety and pharmacovigilance literature and for which a passing knowledge (at least) is useful. Pharmacoepidemiology is now an area of much research and interest and it will play a greater role in drug safety as risk-based pharmacovigilance becomes the mainstay of drug safety and better and bigger databases and data warehouses are developed and populated.

■ Case Report or Individual Case Safety Report (ICSR)

A case report, also called an "individual case safety report" (ICSR), is a clinical observation of a patient who received a drug and experienced one or more AEs. The most common paper formats for presentation of a case report are the MedWatch form and the CIOMS I form. The electronic equivalent is the E2B report, which is an electronic file transmitted to a health authority or company or elsewhere with all the elements of the ICSR. Sometimes cases are published as short reports in medical journals, some of which have been previously reported to health authorities and some not. These cases are picked up in the periodic review of the medical literature done by companies.

■ Aggregate Reports

Aggregate reports are descriptions, or compilations and analyses, of a group of patients exposed to a drug (or sometimes more than one drug, e.g., combination products) and the AEs and other safety issues such as medication errors or quality problems. There are multiple standard formats, of which the Periodic Safety Update Reports (PSUR) is the main one. The U.S. aggregate reports are called, sometimes confusingly, NDA Periodic Reports, Periodic Reports, and PADERs (Periodic Adverse Drug Experience Reports). To worsen the situation, PADERs is also occasionally used to refer to PSURs. And the FDA also accepts PSURs. Whatever they are called, companies are obliged to prepare them in a serious and careful manner and to submit them on time to concerned health authorities.

■ Randomized Clinical Trial (RCT)

This is the type of study that most people are familiar with. It is an experimental study, not an observational study, because a protocol, used by the investigators, determines who receives what drug treatment; the protocol may differ from the normal practice of medicine. In an observational trial, one merely observes and records what happens in the normal course of medical practice and treatment. An observational trial may have a protocol, but it does not dictate treatment, which is left up to the treating physician/investigator.

A randomized clinical trial is prospective. It involves two or more groups of patients with a disease receiving different treatments. For example, one group may get drug A and the other group may get drug B or placebo. It may be single blinded (the patient does not know what the treatment is) or double blinded (neither the patient nor the investigator knows what the treatment is). The study may also be randomized to minimize known and unknown biases (factors other than the drugs tested that may alter or explain the results). These studies are often long and costly. They represent the gold standard of research: the double-blind, randomized, controlled trial. These studies are usually done during phases I, II, and III of drug development, and for many reasons (ethical, availability of patients, etc.), may not be feasible after the drug is marketed. The results are usually clear and easily understandable with the calculation of a risk difference between groups. For example, the group receiving drug A had a 4.1% incidence of AEs and the placebo group a 2% incidence of AEs, a difference of 2.1%. These trials, especially before approval for marketing, are usually prepared primarily to examine efficacy. The patient numbers and design are done to maximize the likelihood of finding a meaningful clinical and statistical result with the primary efficacy endpoints. The studies are usually "powered" to show this one way or the other. (Statistical power refers to the likelihood that the trial and statistical test will reject a false *null hypothesis*, or, to put it another way, power is the probability that one will observe a treatment effect in the trial when such effect really occurs.) The safety data from the trials are rarely sufficient to draw conclusions because rare adverse drug reaction (ADRs) will not be picked up with only a few to several thousand patients studied. The studies are not powered to pick up safety

information and one might falsely conclude that a drug is "safe" or, more precisely, that doses do not differ from the comparator drug in terms of safety. Thus, the safety information is just presented as tables or listings without statistical tests. This is sometimes known as "descriptive statistics."

A newish methodology in clinical trials is being used more frequently and is called "adaptive clinical trials." They have been used for some years in phase I in sequential dose tolerance studies in which three or four patients are treated with a fixed dose. If well tolerated, another three patients are then treated with a higher dose, and so on until a toxicity occurs that precludes further dose elevations. Many different methodologies have been developed, all of which have in common the use of the early data to determine what changes to make (to adapt) in the next patients being treated in that trial. Bayesian techniques are used to determine how the trial will be adapted. The goals of these trials are to obtain efficacy information and minimize toxicity by eliminating cohorts or treatments that do not work or are toxic. When successful, efficacy information can be obtained more rapidly and with fewer patients or cohorts. In terms of safety, however, fewer patients will be exposed to different treatments (as the unsuccessful ones are rapidly abandoned). If this means that efficacy is determined with fewer patients treated, a clear upside, the number of patients examined for adverse events will drop and the infrequent AEs will be less likely to be found, a clear downside. How this methodology, which the health agencies support in general, plays out in terms of safety remains to be seen.

■ Case-Control Study

This concept is sometimes hard to grasp intuitively. This type of study determines the chance ("odds" or "probability") of having taken the suspect drug in a group of patients already suffering from an AE and compares that with the chance of having taken the drug in a group of patients who did not have the AE. To put it more simply, take a group of patients who had the AE and another group who did not have the AE and see how many in each group took the drug in question.

Using a large database (e.g., a claims database, a hospital database), patients with the AE (cases) are selected who have experienced the AE in question. Another group that did not experience the AE (control subjects) is also selected. Usually, the investigator attempts to match the two groups as closely as possible (ideally they should be identical) based on demographic characteristics (e.g., age, sex, race, indication treated, concomitant diseases, and medications) so that the groups are comparable. Both groups should have the same medical profile and opportunity to receive the drug. For example, if a hospital database is used, the drug should be on the pharmacy formulary for the entire time period examined in the study. This is a retrospective study because the AE has occurred and the investigator is looking back in time into the medical history of the patient, to before the AE occurred.

The patients' medical histories are then examined to see which patients in each group used the drug in question. The data are then filled in a 2 × 2 table as follows:

Took the Drug

	Yes	No		
	a	b	Yes	Experienced the AE
	c	d	No	

$$\text{Odds ratio} = \frac{a/(a + c)/c(a+ c)}{b(b + d)/d(b + d)} = ad/bc$$

After the data are filled in, the odds ratio is calculated.

For example, the data might show the following:

- 120 patients experienced the AE
  - 90 took the drug and
  - 30 did not
- 120 control patients did not experience the AE
  - 50 took the drug and
  - 70 did not

The table would look like the following:

Took the Drug

	Yes	No		
	90	30	Yes	Experienced the AE
	50	70	No	Did not experience the AE

The odds ratio is calculated by dividing the odds of having the AE in the group that took the drug (90 of 140 patients or 90:50 = 1.8) by the odds in the group that had the AE but did not take the drug (30 of 100 patients or 30:70 = 0.43). The division is 1.8/4.3 = 4.2. Using the formula above

$$\text{Odds ratio} =$$
$$\frac{90/(90 + 50)/50/(90 + 50)}{30/(30 + 70)/70/(30 + 70)} = (90 \times 70)/(50 \times 30) = 4.2$$

A value greater than 1.0 is suggestive of an association between the drug and the AE. As a rule of thumb, anything greater than 2.0 is believed to be fairly strong and quite suggestive of an association. In our example, this is a high value (4.2) and suggests that there is an association between taking the drug and having the AE.

Advantages of case-control studies are that they are useful for studying very rare AEs because the investigator seeks out a database where this AE is found in a large enough number of patients. Obviously, the patients also had to have the opportunity to take the drug if this database is to be used. These studies are fast and relatively inexpensive. However, they are liable to significant bias both in the selection of the patients for the two groups and in the amount and quality of the drug exposure and medical history data.

■ Cohort Study

A cohort study is the other basic type of epidemiologic study used in pharmacovigilance. This type of study is easier to grasp intuitively. Two groups of patients are chosen from a database. The first group is those who took the drug in question for a certain amount of time, and the second group (the "cohort") is those that did not take the drug. The investigator attempts to choose ("match") a cohort that is as close demographically to the drug group as possible.

The patients' medical records are reviewed and the incidence of the AE in question is calculated for each group. These studies are prospective, as the investigator picks a point in time and studies the two groups as they move forward in time to see whether they develop the AE. This study may be done on data that have already been collected and stored in a database or it may be done on data that are being collected now and moving forward. The advantage of the cohort over the case-control study is the ability to calculate the excess risk, the absolute risk difference. The excess risk is useful in determining the number needed to harm, that is, the number of patients who need be exposed to a drug to produce a specified AE.

Took the Drug

	Yes	No	
	a	b	Experienced the AE
	c	d	

Relative risk = $[a/(a + c)] \div [b/(b + d)]$ or the rate in exposed divided by the rate in the unexposed.

Absolute risk = $[a/(a + c)]–b/(b + d)]$ or rate in exposed minus rate in unexposed.

After the data are filled in, the absolute and relative risks are calculated. Using the same example as above:

Took the Drug

Yes	No	
90	30	Experienced the AE
50	70	

Relative risk = [90/(90 + 50)]/30/(30 + 70)] = 0.643/0.300 = 2.14 times more cases of AE, whereas absolute risk = 0.643 − 0.3 = 0.343.

This tells us that the drug group is more than two times at risk for this AE compared with the cohort group. If the relative risk were 1, the likelihood of getting the AE is the same in the drug and cohort group. If the relative risk is less than 1 (but greater than zero—the value in this calculation is always greater than zero), then the risk of getting the AE in the drug group is less than that in the cohort group.

The absolute risk tells us there were 343 additional cases of AE per 1000 patients exposed to the drug. Therefore, the number needed to harm is about 3; that is, every third patient on the average will develop the AE (something the clinician should keep in mind).

For an excellent discussion of risk ratios and odds ratios, their differences, when they are close to being the same (i.e., when the AEs are very rare), and other complex issues, please see the article by Jon Deeks of The Centre for Statistics in Medicine Oxford, at Web Resource 18-5. The entire Bandolier site (Web Resource 18-6) is worth looking at for, as they put it, "evidence based thinking about health care."

■ Nested Case-Control Study

This type of case-control study is inside, or nested in, a cohort study. The nested case-control design uses estimates from a sample of the cohort rather than the whole cohort. It permits the collection of less data than in a full cohort study with an acceptable statistical analysis and saves time and money.

■ Confidence Intervals

Most studies are based on samples, not entire populations. The confidence interval reflects the resulting uncertainty.

Based on the sample of the population, a particular result is obtained (e.g., 15% of the users of drug A had serious AEs). Because we did not study the whole population, we cannot be totally sure that the 15% figure represents the true value for the whole population rather than just for the smaller sample studied. The confidence interval represents the range of the correct or true value for the whole population. One can calculate various levels of "assurance," 90%, 95%, 99%, 99.9%, and so on, for the confidence interval. Usually, the 95% level is used. The narrower or smaller the distance between the upper and lower values of the confidence interval (called the "confidence limits"), the better. In general, the more patients in the study, the narrower (better) the confidence interval. To put it another way, if the 95% confidence interval for a study group is [43–79 units], then we can be 95% sure that the true value for the entire population is between 43 and 79. If the 95% confidence interval is narrower [59–66] because more patients were studied or for various other reasons, we have a more precise sense that the true population value is closer to the value found in the sample studied.

With the arrival of risk management as an integral part of the development and life span of all drugs, the fields of pharmacoepidemiology and drug safety are now more tightly linked than ever. Health authorities require epidemiologic safety studies, particularly as postmarketing commitments. Large databases and practitioners who know how to do these studies become more and more available and the methodology becomes more refined and automated. Most pharmaceutical companies now have risk management/pharmacoepidemiology departments to handle these studies.

■ Frequently Asked Questions

Q: I never was particularly gifted with math and numbers. Do I really have to learn this stuff? Do I really need it in drug safety?

A: Yes, you really need it. As electronic medical records become more widespread and large databases are used for epidemiology and non-interventional studies, data mining, Bayesian analysis, and other statistical techniques, numerical literacy—as it is called—will be very useful and probably obligatory at some point. Sorry.

19

Signals and Signaling in the Context of Risk Management

E normous efforts are made, in terms of people, time, cost, and technology, to collect AE data in companies, governments, and elsewhere. The collection of vast amounts of data is meaningless in and of itself. It is only when these data are organized and analyzed for new safety issues (which are then acted on in the context of risk management) that the true value of this effort becomes apparent. The hunt for meaning is known as "signaling."

■ The Signal

The Uppsala Monitoring Centre defines a signal as follows:

> Reported information on a possible causal relationship between an adverse event and a drug, the relationship being unknown or incompletely documented previously. Usually more than a single report is required to generate a signal, depending upon the seriousness of the event and the quality of the information (Web Resource 19-1).

They comment further:

> This describes the first alert of a problem with a drug. By its nature a signal cannot be regarded as definitive but indicates the need for further enquiry or action. On the other hand it is prudent to avoid a multiplicity of signals based on single case reports since follow up of all such would be impractical and time consuming. The definition allows for some flexibility in approach to a signal based on the characteristics of individual problems. Some would like a "signal" to include new information on positive drug effects, but this is outside the scope of a drug safety Programme (Delamothe, *Br Med J* 1992;304:465).

A newer definition has been proposed:

> Information that arises from one or multiple sources (including observations and experiments), which suggests a new potentially causal association, or a new aspect of a known association, between an intervention and an event or set of related events, either adverse or beneficial, which would command regulatory, societal or clinical attention, and is judged to be of sufficient likelihood to justify verificatory and, when

necessary, remedial actions (Hauben, Aronson. Defining "signal" and its subtypes. *Drug Safety* 2009;32[2]:99–100).

Not everyone agrees that all signals based on single cases should not be pursued. Sometimes, however, rare events are picked up after a single case, and certain AEs are almost always due to drugs (e.g., Stevens-Johnson Syndrome, fixed drug reactions). Thus, a single case can be a signal. More common problems (e.g., myocardial infarctions) might not be worth pursuing as a signal if there is only a single case in a middle-aged diabetic smoker. But in a 12-year-old it is worth pursuing.

Signals may be "qualitative" (based on spontaneously reported data) or "quantitative" (based on data mining, epidemiologic data, or trial data). The signal may be a new issue never before seen with this product, or it may be the worsening or changing of a known AE or problem (e.g., a previously unaffected patient group is experiencing this problem, or the incidence has increased, or it is now fatal in those it attacks, whereas before it was not). As noted above, qualitative signals may be based on one single striking case or on a collection of cases. In addition, qualitative signals may also be based on preclinical findings; experience with other similar products in the class ("class signals"); new drug or food interactions; confusion with a product's name, packaging, or use; counterfeiting issues; quality problems; and more. Thus, the word "signal" is being expanded.

"Signal" is primarily used to refer to marketed products, although the term is occasionally used for new issues in clinical trials. Some people use the term "potential signal" to indicate an issue with minimal data (e.g., only one case report), whereas others use the term "weak signal."

Some signals are very difficult if not impossible to pick up. Signals with very long latencies (onset well after the drug use has ended) or which skip a generation (DES and vaginal cancer; see Chapter 6) require exceedingly astute observers or great luck to be found.

Identifying signals, however, is not enough. The signal must be further investigated by doing what is variously called a "signal workup," a "signal inquiry," or a "pharmacovigilance investigation." The ultimate goal and true raison d'être of signal discovery and investigation is to determine whether the newly identified problem is indeed due to the drug, and is of sufficient severity and frequency in relation to the benefit, to require alerting physicians, nurses, pharmacists, and patients via a change in the product labeling, television, internet, social media, and other announcements or, in more severe cases, recalling of the product or stopping a clinical trial.

Signaling is not passive. It is proactive. No longer does one wait for AEs or SUSARs before acting. Rather an active signaling effort must be done throughout a product's life cycle. The goal is to anticipate, evaluate, and minimize problems, not to react to them after the fact.

■ Signal Sources and Generation

Signals are looked for in multiple ways. The oldest method is essentially passive and relies on the collection by pharmaceutical companies, government health authorities, or third-party organizations (academic centers, medical registries) of spontaneous AE reports and aggregate analyses of these reports plus any others picked up from other sources, such as solicited cases, compassionate use, surveys, etc. They are then reviewed individually and in aggregate, looking for "striking," "unusual," or "unexpected" AEs. Medically qualified people (physicians, nurses, pharmacists) examine large quantities of data, attempting to find the proverbial needle in the haystack, and either discuss within the organization the "potential signals" found or post them publically (see FDA's potential signal website in Chapter 21). This technique is elegantly known as "global introspection." It is quite time-consuming and laborious, but in the hands of astute and clever clinicians does indeed pick up major problems and still remains, in many respects, the cornerstone of signal generation and identification around the world. It obviously relies on the good will and perspicacity of the reporting physicians, nurses, pharmacists, and patients to send AE reports into the companies or health authorities (without remuneration) and on the goodwill and competence of the data analysts.

It is most sensitive when

- The signal is very unusual and rarely seen in general (e.g., aplastic anemia).
- The signal is rarely seen with that drug class (pulmonary fibrosis with beta-blockers, e.g., practolol).
- The signal is rarely seen in that cohort of patients (e.g., cataracts in young nondiabetic patients).
- The signal is fatal, particularly in patient groups who classically do not have high mortality rates (e.g., deaths in 20-year-olds).
- The signal is expected to be seen because it has been reported in other drugs in the same class (e.g., rhabdomyolysis with a new statin).
- The signal is expected because it is due to an exaggeration of the drug's pharmacologic effect (e.g., syncope in patients taking an antihypertensive).

- The AE in question is seen almost exclusively with drugs (e.g., fixed drug reaction).
- The causality is crystal clear (e.g., the tablet is large and sticky and gets stuck in the oral pharynx, producing obstruction; or when immediate swelling and itching is seen at the site of a drug being injected).
- No other drugs, OTC products, neutraceuticals are being taken by the patient(s) in question.
- The drug is being taken for a short time, and there are no or few confounders.
- The patients are otherwise healthy and have no other medical problems beyond the one being treated with the drug in question.
- There is a positive rechallenge (reaction reappears upon drug reintroduction after a positive dechallenge).
- The AE is different from the signs, symptoms, and problems seen with the disease being treated and would not be confused with the disease itself.

It is less sensitive when

- The signal has a high background incidence in the general population (e.g., headaches, fatigue).
- The signal has a high background incidence in the population being treated (e.g., myocardial infarctions in middle-aged hypertensive smokers).
- The signal represents a worsening of the problem being treated (e.g., fialuridine's, producing worsening and fatal hepatitis in patients being treated for hepatitis; see Chapter 52).
- The patients are taking multiple drugs (polypharmacy, intensive care unit).
- The patients have major underlying medical problems producing disease, signs, and symptoms (e.g., oncology patients).
- The drug is taken chronically, and many intercurrent illnesses and problems occur over time (confounders).
- There is a negative dechallenge (reaction continues even after stopping drug), or the drug in question is not stopped in the patient and the AE disappears by itself anyway.

Increased Frequency

This is a technique that has been on-again, off-again. It has been in favor and out of favor. It basically relies on a statistical calculation of reporting frequency in the current period versus a previous period (e.g., 1Q2011 vs. 1Q2010) to see if there is an increase in reporting of a particular AE. The technique is easy to do, and can be computerized and run for all reported AEs for a drug. It has, in practice, turned out to be not very useful. Although signals are, by definition, generated by this process (some AEs go up [i.e., are more frequent and thus a signal], some go down, and some remain the same), they have, in general, turned out to be false alarms or meaningless, or were easily picked up by other means.

Nonetheless, it is recommended that frequency analyses be done in PSURs. See Volume 9A Section 6.3.10, "An increased reporting frequency of listed adverse reactions, including comments on whether it is believed the data reflect a meaningful change in adverse reactions occurrence." The U.S. Food and Drug Administration (FDA) also required frequency analysis until 1997 in its NDA periodic reports, but ended that because it was found to be of little practical use. The FDA has, however, in the proposed regulations published in 2003 ("The Tome"), proposed reinstating its use. Nonetheless, some organizations still do this on a routine basis. The FDA has also recently asked that frequency analyses be done in clinical trials to see whether an SAE's occurrence (incidence) is rising.

Data Mining

This term is used, sometimes somewhat pejoratively, to describe various automated or semiautomated techniques that generate signals from existing databases. These techniques use raw case report data and arrays of drug-AE combinations to calculate "expected" versus "observed" numbers or reporting rates, and use observations of excess reporting as signals. Various techniques exist, including proportional reporting rate (PRR), gamma poisson shrinker (GPS), urn-model algorithm, reporting odds ratio (ROR), Bayesian confidence propagation neural network—information component (BCPNN-IC), adjusted residual score (ARS), and others. These techniques attempt to extract signals that are not obvious using global introspection. Some feel that this is a largely futile exercise since spontaneous reports are "dirty" data with unknown and unknowable numerators and denominators and you cannot "make a silk purse out of a sow's ear."

However, much work is being done on making better use of "dirty" data. One example of a success is called fractional or proportional reporting rates (PRR), also know as "disproportion" reporting rates or "signals of disproportionate reporting (SDRs)":

For each AE, the calculation of the proportion of that AE as a function of all AEs reported for a drug is calculated and compared with the proportion of that AE for all other drugs in the database.

For example, liver failure for drug X was reported 95 times out of the 1418 total AEs for drug X. For the entire AE database of all drugs (except drug X), the score of liver failure was, for example, found to be 2,243/41,540 = 0.054.

	Drug X	All Other Drugs
Liver Failure	95	2,243
All Other AEs	1,418	41,540

Calculation

(95/1418) / (2243/41540) = 1.24

0.067/0.054 = 1.24

So liver failure with drug X is seen with a proportion (or "score," "statistic," "disproportion," or PRR) of 1.24 (that is, 24% more liver failure with drug X compared to the rest of the drugs in the database).

Is this a signal? In theory it is, since the proportion is higher than for other drugs. But at only 24%, this is somewhat small if other AEs show a proportion of 200% or 400%. If the proportion of the AE for the drug in question was the same as the proportion for the whole database, the number would be 1.00. This means that the same reporting rate for liver failure is seen with drug X and the rest of the drugs in the database. If there were proportionally fewer liver cases with drug X, the score would be <1.00. Does this mean that drug X actually protects against this AE? In theory, this is the logical extension of this line of reasoning, but it would take much more than this to think there is a therapeutic effect (of sorts) to prevent this AE.

The level at which one considers a signal to be generated could be chosen as anything >1.00, although this will probably produce many false positives. In practice, one might take a high score above, say, 2.0 or more before one starts considering these to be signals. If one does this for all 80,000 or so MedDRA terms, then one might expect about 40,000 signals (values >1.0) if the distribution were random. This is obviously not practical. Alternatively, one might look at the top 10 or 20 scores. Another technique would be to use more complicated filters such as a PRR>3 and a chi-squared test >5 and more than three cases with the drug in question.

It is also useful to look at the scores periodically to see whether a particular AE is increasing. That is, it is becoming more disproportional over time and thus may be a stronger signal.

To be useful, the database must be reasonably large (though it is hard to say how large). If additional cases are needed to expand the database, it is possible to download cases from the FDA AERS database from the FDA website, from the Health Canada safety database, the MHRA DAP reports, the EMA Eudravigilance database, or the UMC's Vigibase (see Chapter 8). There may be significant logistical issues in uploading or manually entering cases from these databases into another database. There are many other issues than can make this technique less useful. The other drugs, patients, diseases, and characteristics of the rest of the database should be similar to that of the drug in question. An extreme example would be studying injection site reactions for drug X compared to the rest of the drugs in the database, none of which is given by injection. There would be no injection site reactions for tablets. Or more subtly, if the drug in question is given mainly to elderly diabetics, comparing it to the AE pattern of other drugs given to children would similarly not be very meaningful.

For further details, see Evans, Waller, Davis, Use of proportional reporting ratios for signal generation from spontaneous adverse drug reaction reports (*Pharmacoepidemiol Drug Safety*. 2001;10:483–486). A comparison of different techniques and thresholds is found in Hochberg, Hauben M, Pearson RK, et al., An evaluation of three signal-detection algorithms using a highly inclusive reference event database, *Drug Safety* 2009;32(6):509–525; and Deshpande, Gogolak, Weiss Smith, Data mining in drug safety: review of published threshold criteria for defining signals of disproportionate reporting (*Pharm Med* 2010;24(1):37–43). Various data mining techniques are also described in FDA's 2005 Guidance on Good PV Practices (see below). Whether these or other methods will ultimately prove useful remains to be seen.

■ Other Sources of Signal Data

Information should be obtained, as appropriate, from sources other than spontaneous reports. Other sources include nonclinical study data, such as toxicology and pharmacology data, including animal data, the medical and scientific literature, clinical trial data (not all of which may be found in the drug safety data base—nonserious trial AEs may not be kept in drug safety's database), external databases (FDA, UMC, etc.), product quality complaints and manufacturing deviations, regulatory authority comments in PSURs or direct communications to the company, and so on. If a Risk Management Plan (RMP) or REMS is in place, signaling should be done with this in mind.

■ Putting It All Together

After data have been found from all of the sources noted above (ICSRs, aggregate data, data mining, solicited cases, etc.), the results should be tabulated, reviewed, and "triaged" to determine which findings deserve further consideration now and which go into a "holding box" waiting for more data. There is no precise formula to determine which signals should be investigated rapidly and aggressively and which can sit. Some factors to consider include whether the drug is widely used, whether the signal in question is serious/severe or not, whether the patients are seriously ill, whether the problem is reversible, whether the investigation is easily done, whether the outcome of the investigation can be known in a shortish time rather than years, whether there is health authority or other external pressure (e.g., publicity, internet activity), and (probably unfortunately) monetary cost.

Organizational Team

Each organization, whether a drug company or a health authority, needs to have a team (formal usually but may be ad hoc if appropriate) to evaluate the signals. This is usually a multidisciplinary team that reviews, analyzes, and may also make recommendations on signals. It may be empowered to make decisions or it may function to deliver data and multiple action choices to more senior management personnel. Members include physicians and healthcare personnel from drug safety, epidemiology, clinical research/development, regulatory affairs, biostatistics, quality, risk management, legal (sometimes), pharmacology/toxicology (sometimes), manufacturing (sometimes), and others as needed, including external subject-matter experts. Marketers and sales personnel should not be on the team.

Signal Workup

Once the signal list has been prepared, the list needs to be prioritized for workup according to the criticality of the signals and the resources available. Of course, lack of resources is never an acceptable excuse for not working up a signal that is important to the public health. This will be an unacceptable reason with the HA (or in court!) for incomplete, inadequate, or slow signal workup, which jeopardizes public health. But realistically speaking, resources will play a role in prioritizing.

Prioritize

There are many ways to prioritize signals. Red, yellow, green is one way, or numerical priorities on a 1 to 5 scale are used. Whatever method is chosen, though, it should be documented and consistently used. Exceptions will not be well looked-upon by inspectors.

Do an initial priority assessment. Highest priority should go to drugs that are new, where the AEs are serious or severe, where there are tampering or counterfeiting issues, where the patient population is ill or apparently at high risk, where the drug is known to be toxic, where many people use the drug, and to black triange drugs (the designation in United Kingdom labeling of a new and/or dangerous drug), etc. For better or worse, other issues also enter into prioritization, ones that are less related to public health, such as politics, sales volume, need to "protect" the drug, adverse publicity, showing due diligence in tracking, and working up safety issues (e.g., FDA's Potential Signal website, Web Resource 19-2). Conversely, drugs whose AE profile is mild and where few adverse consequences on the public health are seen or expected would have lower priority. Minor AEs of toxic drugs would probably fall somewhere in the middle of prioritization.

Although difficult to do, efficacy should also be taken into some account when deciding on initial prioritization. Drugs with minimal efficacy with potential new, severe AEs should have a higher priority. To put it another way, if the drug in question was "placebo" such that no efficacy was expected (forgetting placebo effects for the moment), then no AEs at all should be tolerated, and this drug would get a high priority for signal workup.

The CIOMS VIII Working Group suggests the following points to consider in prioritizing signals: medical significance (serious, irreversible, etc.), increasing PRR scores, an important public health impact, easily retrievable data elements, and temporal clustering. See Practical Aspects of Signal Detection in Pharmacovigilance, Report of CIOMS Working Group VIII, Geneva 2010 (see Chapter 36). This publication is a fine review of the state of the art in signaling as of 2010.

Arrange and Review

Next, the drugs in question should be arranged on a spreadsheet or put into a database. There are various ways to do this. Some suggestions are made here.

One may create an overall summary signaling spreadsheet and then a daughter spreadsheet for each drug/signal combination (e.g., one sheet for Drug X and elevated liver tests or another sheet for Drug Y and atrial arrhythmias). Cases or case series should be arranged on the sheet using a simple or augmented CIOMS II line-listing format, with "augmented" referring to adding additional data to the line listing, such as a brief narrative, clinical course, or causality (see below). Cases may be arranged by date, by seriousness, or by some other factor. Various software programs are available for useful and creative displays of the data (see below).

Next, it is often useful to do causality assessments. In many cases, this should be done again at the time of signal evaluation even if the cases have an earlier causality from the investigator, reporter, company, or patient. Note that many companies do not do causality assessments on spontaneous reports, as they are presumed to be possibly related by convention. Thus causality on these cases should be done now. Hindsight, time, and new data may change the original causality determinations. There is no uniformly accepted international classification. Choose a system and stick to it (e.g., related, possibly related, weakly related, unrelated, insufficient information/unknown).

Causality should be assigned to individual cases and to the group of cases as a whole. In a case series, no single case may be clearly due to the drug, but the weight of the evidence of the sum of the cases may strongly suggest a likely signal.

The signal should be assessed in terms of

- Magnitude and seriousness of the reaction—public health risk
- Demographics—age, gender, ethnic background, weight
- Effect of exposure—duration and dose—changes in risk over time
- Concomitant medications
- Drug interactions
- Comorbid conditions and other confounders
- Biological plausibility
- Alterative treatments and therapies
- Other issues (e.g., HA request for workup, publicity)

Next, each drug/signal combination should be assigned a signal level based on review of the cases and causalities. Be reasonable in terms of what constitutes a signal. Always keep in mind the benefit–risk balance: not all risks can be eliminated. One such classification is

- Strong: a series of well-documented cases with no alternative causes and ideally with at least one positive rechallenge (rechallenge criterion not applicable in, for example, irreversible adverse events, hepatotoxicity, etc.)
- Fairly strong: a series of generally well-documented cases with few alternative causes and ideally at least one positive dechallenge
- Average: a series of cases of variable quality
- Fairly weak: a series of cases that have significant limitations regarding plausible temporal associations or for which there are likely alternative explanations
- Weak: a series of cases that are generally incompletely documented, lack plausible temporal associations, or are generally explainable by alternative causes or similarly

And then assign an action:

- A signal warranting immediate action to protect public health. These actions may be temporary (if the signal is ultimately determined to be unfounded) or permanent.
- Signal warranting intensive follow-up and further investigation in the form of a clinical trial, an epidemiologic trial, outside consultation, and so on.
- Signal warranting further investigation and follow-up of the current cases (e.g., for outcomes); to be reexamined in 60 days.
- Weak signal: continue watching; no further action at this time.
- Not a signal: no further investigation needed.

The Workup

At this stage, the signals that have been chosen for workup should be so designated and the workup begun. Various steps that can be done include the following:

- Search for additional cases using the appropriate MedDRA terms (or SMGs) in the clinical trial database if some cases (e.g., nonserious clinical trial AEs) are not also found in or have been reconciled with the safety database.
- Search for similar or additional cases in external databases (see Chapter 8) such as the UMC database in Uppsala, Health Canada's database, the

MHRA Drug Analysis Printouts (DAPs), FDA's AERS database, and FDA potential signals listing (see Chapter 21).

- Consider other databases that can be used for epidemiologic studies in addition to the spontaneous reporting databases noted in the previous bullet. These include Prescription Event Monitoring Databases (Drug Safety Research Unit in the United Kingdom, Web Resource 19-3), Linked Administrative Databases (U.S. private healthcare databases), United Kingdom General Practice Research Database (GPRD) (Web Resource 19-4), as well as specialized databases, such as teratology databases or disease-specific databases (e.g., cystic fibrosis), and governmental databases (e.g., Canadian provinces). The organization Bridge to Data (Web Resource 19-5) has a compilation of more than 90 worldwide databases with descriptions of their characteristics, allowing the user to find databases that may suit the signal workup.

  It may be useful to engage an expert in pharmacoepidemiology at this point to find the right databases and assist in designing the appropriate study.

- Search out additional literature cases using PubMed, Google Scholar, or other search engines and databases. See if the signal is listed on FDA's potential signal database.

- Consider reviewing the AE profiles and class effects of similar drugs in that class.

- Consider more complex, time-consuming, and expensive procedures to validate, strengthen, or refute a signal, such as epidemiologic (observational) studies in large databases (e.g., claims databases), to detect or find rare AEs and obtain information in large patient populations (e.g., tens of millions of patients), targeted clinical trials, and large simple safety studies (LSSS).

The Conclusions and Next Steps

The reviewers should come to a conclusion or conclusions for recommendation to the decision maker or safety committee (see below). As noted, many classifications are available; pick one and stick to it. The conclusions may be along the lines of

- Red Signal–High Priority: SAE previously unknown or unlabeled or inadequately labeled. Quality issues such as adulteration or contamination. May be accompanied by media attention and public scrutiny

despite the only weak or incompletely documented cases. If confirmed, will lead to a reevaluation of the benefit–risk analysis and likely a change in labeling, product withdrawal, and so on.

- Yellow Signal–Medium Priority: Further evaluation of the signal is required but the criteria of the Red category are not met. If confirmed, these signals are expected to lead to a change in the risk–benefit analysis and may require changes in the labeling/packaging in the AE section and possibly also in the indications, contraindications, warnings, and adverse event sections.

- Green Signal–Low Priority: AEs that are already known or labeled and felt not to be a significant safety problem. Signal investigation at this time may be minimal, deferred, or simply kept on a "watch list" looking for further case reports (if any) before reevaluation. Workup now would not be a good use of resources.

The Safety Committee

Following the prioritization and workup, a mechanism to conclude and act on the signals is needed. This may be a senior safety/risk management committee or it may be an individual (the chief medical officer, for example). Whatever mechanism is used, there must be a formal written procedure to review and adjudicate signals on a regular basis. There should be an empowered decision maker in the form of either a person or a committee.

For emergency signals, the committee should be able to meet within 24 hours (or even sooner). In a pharmaceutical company, this could be a senior safety committee composed of the chief medical officer, chief safety officer (if not the same person), and heads or senior people from drug safety/pharmacovigilance, regulatory affairs, labeling, clinical research, the legal department, preclinical (animal) toxicology/pharmacology, risk management, epidemiology, and other corporate subject matter experts as needed (e.g., formulations). If the product is studied or marketed outside the home country, the needs of these countries must also be represented in the decision and action steps. The marketing and sales and similar departments should not, in general, be represented on this committee, as this must be a medical–public health decision. In occasional instances, outside expert consultants, as neutral as possible, given that they are paid consultants to the company, may be invited to join if appropriate.

In a health authority, the committee structure should be constituted in a similar manner, with senior medical, toxicology, pharmacology, labeling, risk management, epidemiology, and legal subject-matter experts as well as any other members needed, depending on the structure of the health authority. Attention should also be paid to actions of other health authorities around the world.

The safety committee needs to come to conclusions about issues presented to it. It should never routinely request more data at successive meetings for a particular problem or use other bureaucratic mechanisms to delay a decision. Relevant data should be requested and rapidly obtained and decisions made. These decisions should be documented in minutes. The outcomes should consider the public health and risk management/minimization and what action steps, if any, need to be taken:

- Label change, variation, and so forth, for marketed drugs (e.g., new ADR, warning, precaution, contraindication); dear doctor/healthcare professional letter; drug withdrawal and, if so, to what level (consumer, pharmacist, wholesaler); and communication plan to the health authorities, public, and healthcare professionals.

- Further study and consultation regarding this signal.

- If in clinical trials, stop or change studies to enhance patient protection, notification of the data monitoring committee and/or IRB, adjudication committee, changes in the investigator brochure, and informed consent.

- Notification of the applicable health agencies (competent authorities) by phone, e-mail, or letter.

- Other follow-up actions and further review by the committee at a later date.

- Effect on the Risk Management/REMS program in place or, if one is not in place, whether to put one in place rapidly.

- Mechanisms to handle the public announcement and any issues that might arise from that, including legal actions and adverse publicity.

- If a REMS or RMP is in place, the signal should be considered in context with the plan. It may be necessary to revise, change, or update the plan in consultation with the health authority.

- Either inside or separate from the plan, it may be necessary to take further risk minimization actions.

- Recall, withdrawal, etc.

When the committee is in a health agency, depending on legal responsibilities and regulations, the committee needs to decide on label changes, withdrawal, and study cessation in the same manner as noted above for companies.

For an excellent review of signaling, see Practical Aspects of Signal Detection in Pharmacovigilance, Report of CIOMS Working Group VIII, Geneva 2010 (see Chapter 36).

■ Computerized Tools for Signal Detection and Workup

Several companies now produce software or tools that can be used as add-ons to a drug safety or clinical trial database. These programs allow for graphic displays, tables, cross-references, lumping, splitting, and various other ways to look at data. They are useful for large numbers of cases when "eye-balling" the data is infeasible. The programs allow for aggregate charts or displays of data in which hyperlinks allow the reviewer to click on a bar, point, or line and see the cases that lie behind that data point. Thus, one can look at a chart of the most frequent SAEs and then click to see the cases either as a case series or as individual case data. Ad hoc queries and analyses can be done, such as analyses by age, sex, comeds, diagnosis, and so forth. One can focus only on outliers or particular AEs. Comparisons over time, with different drugs and other sorts of comparisons, can be made. Obviously, this is data-dependent. If there is little data, no comparative data, or incomplete data, the tool cannot really help.

These systems vary but functions found in these tools include a drug profile portal to document and track issues and potential signals with built-in workflow and using various statistical methods, including empirical Bayesian geometric means, relative ratios, proportional reporting, logistic regression, Bayesian multi-item gamma poisson shrinker, and Kaplan-Meier plots, drill down into the data to the patient level, "what if" scenarios, and so forth. Most can be used for clinical trial data and safety data from different databases. Imports of FDA AERS and other external database information are also possible in most cases.

Several vendors make useful products. Some include:

Integrated Review and J Review (Web Resource 19-8)

Empirica Signal (Oracle/Phase Forward) (Web Resource 19-6)

TIBCO Spotfire (Web Resource 19-7)

agSignals (Web Resource 19-9)

■ Key Documents on Signaling and Good PV Practices

The FDA Guidance on Good Pharmacovigilance Practices of 3/2005

In March 2005, the FDA (Center for Drug Evaluation and Research and Center for Biologics Evaluation and Research) released a Guidance for Industry entitled, "Good Pharmacovigilance Practices and Pharmacoepidemiologic Assessment." This is an excellent document (though several years old now) and summarizes the FDA's thinking on the topic. It also, to a large degree, reflects current practices in the industry. It references three guidances initially issued in May 2004 and revised and reissued in May 2005. Note that many of the items in this guidance have been changed or superseded by the 2007 PDUFA/FDAAA, such as the change from RiskMAPs to REMS. Nonetheless, this document is still well worth reading, as its concepts remain the same:

1. Premarketing Risk Assessment
2. Development and Use of Risk Minimization Plans (RiskMAP Guidance)
3. Good Pharmacovigilance Practices and Pharmacoepidemiologic Assessment

Key parts of this document concerning signaling are as follows:

- Identifying and describing safety signals: From case report to case series.
- Case reports. The FDA recommends that sponsors make a reasonable attempt to get complete information for case assessment during initial and follow-up contacts. Companies should use trained healthcare practitioners. If the report is from a consumer, it should be followed up with contact with the healthcare practitioner. The most aggressive efforts should be directed at serious AEs, particularly those not previously known to occur with the drug.
- Case series. After an initial postmarketing spontaneous case report is found, additional cases should be sought in the sponsor's database, the FDA Adverse Event Reporting System database, published literature, and other databases. Cases should be evaluated and followed up for additional information where needed and where possible. Of importance are data that would support or reject a causal association with the drug. Although the FDA notes that there is no internationally agreed-on causality classifications, they do note that prob-

able, possible, and unlikely have been used. Cases with confounders should be analyzed too and not routinely excluded.

- After such a review, the cases that support the signal's further investigation should be summarized in a table or other manner to describe the important clinical characteristics.
- The FDA refers to the use of data-mining techniques but notes that their use "is not a required part of a signal identification or evaluation."
- The FDA then gives guidance as to which signals should be further evaluated: new unlabeled serious AEs; an apparent increase in the severity of a labeled event; occurrence of serious AEs that are extremely rare in the general population; new drug–drug, drug–food, or drug–dietary supplement interactions; identification of a previously unrecognized at-risk population; confusion about a product name, label, package, or use; concerns about product usage (e.g., use at higher-than-labeled doses); concerns that the current risk management plan is not adequate; or "other."
- Calculation of reporting rates. In a somewhat controversial section, the FDA recommends that the sponsor calculate the crude AE reporting rates using the number of reported cases of that signal AE in the United States as the numerator and the estimate of U.S. patient exposure (as patients or patient-time) as the denominator. Where feasible, the reporting rates over time or versus similar products or drug classes or versus estimates of the background rate for this even in the general population may be useful. The FDA does warn, however, that these figures are generally used for exploratory purposes or for hypothesis generation. They note that reporting rates are not incidence rates.
  In practice, use of these figures is fraught with danger. The numerator is bad because there is always underreporting of an unknown degree; the denominator is worse because it is hard to know how many patients truly took the drug (as opposed to filling the prescription) and for how long. Thus, the ratio is often meaningless. A high reporting rate may suggest that the signal is real, but a low reporting rate does not exonerate the drug.

■ Investigating a Signal

- Pharmacoepidemiologic studies are cited by the FDA. There are various types of nonrandomized trials that can be done, including cohort (prospective or retrospective), case-control, nested case-control, and others. They can be done at any time (before or after marketing), although they are often done after a signal has been suggested by postmarketing adverse events. The FDA suggests that bias be minimized and that confounding be accounted for. They also suggest that "it is always prudent to conduct more than one study, in more than one environment and even use different designs."

- Registries. The FDA defines a registry as "an organized system for the collection, storage, retrieval, analysis and dissemination of information on individual persons exposed to a specific medical intervention who have either a particular disease, a condition (e.g., a risk factor) that predisposes [them] to the occurrence of a health-related event, or prior exposure to substances (or circumstances) known or suspected to cause adverse health effects." A control or comparison group should be included where possible.

- Surveys. Without clearly defining surveys, the FDA recommends that they be done when information gathering is needed. For pharmacoepidemiologic studies, registries, and surveys, the FDA encourages consultation with the agency before beginning.

Interpreting a Signal

The FDA recommends that the sponsor conduct a case level/case series review, using data mining and calculating reporting rates where feasible. Then the sponsor should consider a further study to establish whether a safety risk exists.

When the sponsor believes a safety risk is possible, a synthesis of all information should be prepared and submitted to the FDA, including the following:

- Cases (spontaneous and literature) with exposure information
- The background rate for the event in general and the specific patient population(s)
- Relative risks, odds ratios, or other pharmacoepidemiology study results
- Biologic effects from animal work and pharmacokinetic and dynamic studies
- Safety data from controlled clinical trials
- General marketing experience with similar products

The sponsor should provide an assessment of the risk-to-benefit balance for the population as a whole and for at-risk groups (if any). The FDA notes that this is an iterative process, and not all actions described in the guidance are done at all times. Proposals on further steps should also be provided along with risk minimization actions. The FDA then makes its own judgment based on the data.

The FDA recommends that sponsors develop and continually reevaluate their risk management plan. In some cases, postmarketing reporting of spontaneous AEs will suffice. In other situations, much more may be needed. The FDA notes it may bring potential safety risks to its Drug Safety and Risk Management Advisory Committee or the specific advisory committee dealing with the product in question.

These actions described above represent a careful, step-by-step, well-planned proposal for investigating a signal that allows a thoughtful and logical response to a signal. In many and probably most situations, especially those for nonserious signals or drugs not in the public eye, this process unfurls as described above. However, for situations that make the public eye (e.g., Vioxx, Fen-Phen), the pressures to act before all the evidence is in are enormous.

Signal review does not occur in a vacuum. Multiple influences play a role:

- Changes in personnel in the company and the FDA may cause loss of continuity in a signal investigation.
- Publicity from consumer groups, the media, and other companies, some of which may be premature or unnecessarily scary and inflammatory.
- Lawsuits.
- Actions by other health agencies outside the United States.
- The time needed to prepare and carry out whatever actions are proposed, such as registries, studies, data mining, and surveys.
- Further spontaneous reports or lack thereof during the investigation ("Oh no, we just got another case!").
- Pressures from various areas to continue marketing or to stop marketing.
- Extreme positions based on little data.
- Sponsor marketing and financial pressures (lost market and money).
- Pressures on the FDA (Congress, companies, consumer groups, media).

- Pressure to do interim analyses or to stop ongoing trials (often for different indications) of the drug in question, which jeopardizes the integrity of the study.

- Privacy and data protection issues.

In addition, the points of view ("agendas") of the protagonists in the drama are clearly different in many regards, although everyone really does want to protect the public health and not hurt people. Here are the points of view using some of the language each group might use to make its case:

- The company wishes to protect its (enormous) investment in a product that took years to develop and to market and that is paying the salary of hundreds or thousands of employees. A "handful" of not clearly proven cases with causality in doubt should not be made public and should not be allowed to "destroy" the drug before the full scientific and medical investigations are completed. The drug is clearly helping the "vast majority" of the patients using it, and the possible occurrence of AEs (even serious ones) should not deprive the rest of the public of the product. Because the drug has a finite life (i.e., patent expiration), the company believes it must protect it as much as possible. The investigation of the signal should be done in private without release of the "debate" to the public. Even if the drug is totally exonerated after the signal investigation, there is usually lost market share and harm to the drug. Within the company, no one wants to be the one to "kill the drug," because this can be a career-ending and a stock price-destroying event. Lawsuits will doubtless follow (often no matter what the result of the signal investigation), and the personal and financial liability can be enormous. When lawsuits occur, employees move into defensive mode, spending more and more time with attorneys. In summary, the company will, of course, do the right thing, but only when the data are in and the science is clear. It will not act prematurely.

- The FDA wishes to protect the public health as its primary goal. It wants to do this as early as possible to minimize the risk to the public. Better to err on the side of patient protection than to allow a toxic product to stay on the market (or remain inadequately labeled) for too long. The agency cannot appear to be too cavalier with the data or to "be in the pocket of the drug companies." It is also far easier to take the position against the "big bad drug companies." In some sense, the drug should be considered guilty until proven innocent. *Primum non nocere* ("Above all do no harm") is an aphorism originally attributed to the ancient Greek physician Galen, but it more likely arose in the seventeenth century. If something bad happens, the Congress, the Secretary of the Department of Health and Human Services, the media, and the consumer groups will attack the companies and the FDA unmercifully.

- With the new Drug Watch regulations, more data (much unconfirmed and incomplete) will be released earlier. This will both help the agency protect itself and get the information before the public, but it will also change the shape of the investigation and diminish the use of the drug, perhaps prematurely.

- Consumers want totally safe and totally effective drugs with no risk. When bad things occur (because the companies may have withheld data or did not do their job or the FDA may have acted too quickly and did not do its job), someone is at fault and someone must pay and be punished. All data should be available, and the entire process should be transparent. In general, better to err on the side of stopping the use of the drug than continuing its sale and use. And drugs are indeed guilty until proven innocent.

- The media are delighted when the spectacle plays out, especially with data dribbling out over time and errors with alleged misdeeds by the company or the FDA surfacing. The more sensational, the more errors or inappropriate or illegal actions, the more individuals hurt, the more the story captivates the public, moving into websites and blogs and selling papers and TV time.

- For competitor pharmaceutical companies, there are mixed feelings. Clearly, what is happening to another company could happen to them at anytime too, with one of their products. However, the competitors are not unhappy if more patients now switch to their drugs rather than using the one undergoing a signal investigation. And finally there is an element of Schadenfreude (from the German meaning "pleasure taken from someone else's misfortune") that is common in human nature.

All of this suggests that rather than thinking of the signal investigation process as a careful, rational, well-planned program done in a timely and deliberate manner, one should rather think of the process, for dramatic or serious issues, as the "fog of war," with multiple pressures (some known and some unknown to each player) acting to force rapid and urgent "action" to protect the public.

The consequences of whatever action is taken may have far-reaching and irreversible effects. Drugs that are withdrawn rarely return to the market even if the signal has subsequently been disproven. Label changes adding a new safety warning, AE, or other are rarely taken out of the label even if disproven. The change in medical practice to the use of different drugs (which may be more or less expensive, available, effective, safe, etc.) is similarly hard to reverse.

European Union Volume 9A on Signal Detection

Section 8.2 Signal Detection and Evaluation:

Signals of possible unexpected adverse reactions or changes in severity, characteristics or frequency of expected adverse reactions may arise from any source including preclinical and clinical data (e.g. spontaneous reports from Healthcare Professionals or Consumers; epidemiological studies; clinical trials), published scientific and lay literature. Standardised MedDRA Queries (SMQs) may be used for signal detection and the use of SMQs is recommended in order to retrieve and review cases of interest where signals are identified from adverse reaction databases. Rarely, even a single report of an unexpected adverse reaction may contain sufficient information to raise a signal on or establish a causal association with the suspected medicinal product and impact on the risk-benefit balance.

Volume 9A also notes various methods and sources of information where signals can be found. These include individual case review, trend analyses of case reports, complex statistical methods (data mining), and others.

MHRA Comments on Signal Detection

In a Q&A, the MHRA comments on its website in regard to signal detection (Web Resource 19-10).

One question was asked regarding the issue that signal detection can be a burden for companies, especially small companies and generic manufacturers, and thus requests more information on signaling. MHRA notes that Volume 9A (as noted above) suggests ways of signaling. The MHRA then notes that the MAH should determine which methodology it will use based on a risk assessment of the product portfolio. The MHRA expects all MAHs to have systems and formal procedures in place and documented in writing (SOPs). The documentation should include definitions of a signal and potential signal so as to determine which signals need further investigation. The personnel and their roles and responsibilities must be specified, as well as escalation procedures after a signal or potential signal is identified. MHRA does not give specific minimum requirements for signal detection but does give guidelines, which include the following:

- The methodology for signaling is appropriate for the data in question. Statistical analyses may not be useful if the data set is small.
- A quality system to ensure proper signaling must be in place.
- Findings from signal data reviews must be rapidly and appropriately assessed, and the QPPV must be kept informed.
- Rapid and appropriate decisions are made after data review.
- All procedures and evaluations must be documented.

MHRA notes specifically that signal detection only at the time of each PSUR is unlikely to be adequate in most cases. For generic products with few AEs on a 6-monthly PSUR cycle, signaling at PSUR time may be appropriate.

In its book *Good Pharmacovigilance Practice Guide*, the MHRA expands on these points.

Practical Comments on Signaling Techniques: How to do it:

- Read the latest and earlier PSURs for signals and regulatory responses to the PSURs.
- Review the signal list your organization keeps (if it doesn't keep one, start one).
- Review all expedited cases for signals.
- Scan either manually or in an automated fashion in the database for "Always Expedited Cases." (FDA's 2003 proposal of cases that are always important and expeditable).
- Scan for cases that are usually or have a high probability of being drug related (Stevens-Johnson, aplastic anemia, injection site reactions, anaphylaxis, etc.).
- Although expedited cases are likely to produce new

signals (since they are serious and by definition unlisted—not in the labeling), this is the first place to look for new signals. Next, look at other serious cases (listed) and nonserious unlisted cases.

■ Review lab data separately if the database allows analysis of data from spontaneous cases.

■ Consider looking for cases using several levels of MedDRA. That is, many will scan AE lists of LLTs. Consider being a "lumper" and looking at PTs, HLTs, and HLGTs. Although granularity is lost as one looks in this manner, signals may turn up.

■ Use MedDRA Standardized MedDRA Queries (SMQs), which can be run automatically in a mechanized way in the database (see Web Resource 19-11 and Chapter 14 on MedDRA).

■ If clinical trials for a marketed drug are under way either as postmarketing studies (e.g., commitments, large safety studies) or new indications, review the AEs from these trials.

■ Look for clinical patterns rather than just isolated AE listings. Relate laboratory or test findings to signs and symptoms. For example, look for AEs of jaundice and lab tests of elevated AST, ALT, bilirubin.

■ If the database is able to generate such tables, look at the drug in question along with concomitant medications to see whether there are patterns of AEs with particular drug combinations.

■ Look at all overdose cases. These are often fruitful areas to pick up signals.

■ Do a literature review.

■ Look for cases in the easily available databases (Health Canada, FDA, MHRA), and use the less easily available databases if necessary or feasible.

■ Consider doing increased frequency analysis (with care).

■ Consider doing routine proportionality calculations as noted above.

■ After doing a signal hunt, make a list of all the signals or possible signals found and try to group them. For example:

　■ Elevated AST, jaundice, weakness, fatigue = drug-induced liver disease

　■ Malaise, fever, weakness = flu-like syndrome

　■ Seizures, fainting, epilepsy, petit mal, grand mal, focal seizures = seizure disorder

■ After doing a preliminary review and grouping, search for additional cases not picked up on the first round. For example:

　■ Seizures are a possible signal. Look at the database for more subtle clues for seizures: loss of consciousness, abnormal EEG, syncope, sudden death, and see whether any of these cases may be added to the case series.

■ Clues to which cases are significant:

　■ All serious AEs are significant.

　■ The case was severe in intensity.

　■ It led to discontinuation of treatment.

　■ It was sustained rather than transient.

　■ It put the patient at risk for developing a clinically significant outcome.

　■ The drug effect was large (e.g., a 20 mmHg increase in diastolic blood pressure).

　■ The outcome of the drug effect was permanent (caused total blindness) or resulted in sequelae (e.g., decreased visual acuity).

　■ The drug effect could not be prevented or minimized (e.g., by reducing the dose).

There is no one-size-fits-all technique for signaling. Some combination of the techniques described here and elsewhere should be customized for each product. Products with few AEs will be handled differently from those with large volumes of AEs. New products, new indications, new patient populations, new formulations, and any other major changes should raise the reviewer's sensitivity level to new signals. Prioritize the signals found and begin the signal evaluation (see Chapter 20).

■ Frequently Asked Questions

Q: Again, why would anyone want to work in drug safety for a living?

A: For many reasons. Signal detection and analysis is usually a fascinating exercise requiring medical, investigative, tactical, logical, and political skills. One really is acting to help the public health. Most signals, perhaps the vast majority, are rather unextraordinary and nonserious and can be worked up in a thoughtful and timely manner. In these instances, it is very satisfying. Similarly, even in the dramatic instances, the right thing usually does end up being done, and that also is quite satisfying. The probability of a horror scenario is less likely, but that is the risk one takes in this business. As with signaling (and most of life), it all boils down to a benefit-to-risk analysis.

Q: Should the companies try to find signals before the health authorities? If the FDA picks up the signal before the company, isn't that a "failure" on the part of the company?

A: This is not a contest in which the fastest pick-up wins. The goal is bettering the public health. Sometimes the company picks up the signal first; sometimes the agencies do. Often, the health agencies see more data than the companies and often the agencies see the safety profile of similar drugs in that class. They may thus have a broader overview and their case series may be more complete than that of the companies. What may be a weak signal to the company may be seen in many or all of the drugs in the class, making it a much stronger signal. Drug safety is tough enough as it is; you don't have to beat yourself up any more than necessary!

Information Technology, Databases, and Computers

Any company that receives more than a handful of AEs, whether for marketed products or for products only in clinical trials, needs a database to collect, assemble, and report on these AEs. As the rest of the chapters in this book indicate, the regulations and reporting requirements are voluminous and follow tight standards in terms of content, format, and timing for reports to HAs. It is thus necessary to have an AE database that allows, at the minimum, either easy data entry manually and by E2B or a customized upload, preparation, and printing of MedWatch and CIOMS I forms and various other aggregate data reports for PSURs, IND annual reports, Development Safety Update Reports (DSURs) (soon), and NDA periodic reports as well as any other customized or national/local reports. Export capabilities are also necessary as E2B files or other customized exports. Many of the databases used for drug safety also allow for complex analysis and data mining of AEs, such as increased frequency and disproportionality calculations (see Chapter 19). Some have Eudravigilance export capabilities.

Many databases also have workflow and quality components built in with e-mail and messaging functionality. Some companies customize their databases, though more and more companies are buying one of the standard packages ("shrink-wrapped software") available from various vendors. As databases get larger and larger and more and more complex, the ease and ability of transferring data from one database to another database becomes more difficult and costly. Thus, once a company commits to one database, it often will use that database "forever." Mergers and acquisitions of the database company can produce significant headaches for the user community if the database is no longer supported or upgraded. This, however, is just the tip of the iceberg. Many more functions are needed for a modern drug safety department, especially if the department has worldwide data input and reporting obligations. This chapter reviews the issues and specialized needs around safety databases.

■ Required Safety Database Functionality

The following list represents a high-level view of the functions that a safety database must have to meet the needs of a multinational drug safety department. For smaller single-country departments, the needs may be somewhat less. There will surely be other requirements needed now or in the future that are not listed here. The ability to change and customize the database as requirements change is critical. Note there is some duplication and overlap among the sections below as some requirements are common to multiple areas.

- Data Entry
    - Upload capabilities from other databases (e.g., phone center and clinical research databases) via E2B or other formats.
    - Case data entry to include all needed fields to produce a completed MedWatch form, CIOMS I form, PSUR, CIOMS line listing, E2B transmission, and so forth.
    - Tabular entry of laboratory data as well as manual entry.
    - Seriousness, expectedness (labeledness), causality at the case, and AE level by the investigator, company, CRO, others. (That is, multiple entries possible for causality in particular.)
    - Multiple narratives for the same case (e.g., short narrative, long narrative, non-English narrative, case comments, blinded narrative). Mechanism to handle follow-up information in the narrative (overwrite vs. append). Size limitations on the field.
    - Ability to handle multiple labels (e.g., Summary of Product Characteristics, U.S. Package Insert) producing different expectedness classification depending on label.
    - Ability to handle one or more reporters for a single case.
    - Versioning ,with multiple versions possible for each case (e.g., by country).
    - Tracking of information in and out (case log).
    - Support of the Medical Dictionary for Regulatory Activities (MedDRA) (multiple versions and languages), WHO-ART (and other) drug dictionaries, as well as dictionaries for other functions (such as abbreviations, laboratory units, SNOMED, etc.).

- Tight link to a MedDRA browser to allow easy coding.
- Tight link to the drug database.
- Ability to handle central and computerized lab data imports (uploads) with multiple normal ranges.
- Handling of devices, drugs, biologics, medication errors, product quality complaints, blood products as needed.
- Duplicate check for cases using multiple fields (e.g., name, postal code, age).
- Ability to add fields as needed (e.g., new business partner case reference numbers).
- Ability to close/complete a case and reopen it as needed.
- Ability to have scanned source documents attached or linked to cases.
- Required fields customizable by users.
- Edit checks (e.g., system will not allow entry of data to show that a 50-year-old patient has a birth date of January 12, 2005, or that a male is pregnant).
- Ability to handle clinical trial, spontaneous, solicited, named patient, literature, and other types of cases.
- Ability to handle multiple doses of each drug (to account for starting, stopping, restarting, dose change, etc.).
- Spell check in multiple languages.
- Automated case narrative.
- Ability to handle combination drugs, drug-devices, OTC, and so forth.

- Work Flow
    - Ability to track and move a case through its processing using customized business rules set up by the users.
    - Communication ability at the user and case level (e.g., a reviewer can electronically ask a question of the person who entered the case data via email, SMS, etc.).
    - Version tracking of each case with multiple different versions existing simultaneously for a case (e.g., U.S. version 2, EMA version 3, Japanese version 4).
    - Metrics to measure status of groups of cases with groups customized by the user (e.g., each work team has its own metrics and management

has aggregate metrics).

- Duplicate checking and ability to duplicate a case or archive a case.
- Ability to handle customized case identification numbering with each case having multiple numbers.
- Multiple clock start dates (e.g., varies by country).
- Follow-up letter generation to reporter or patient.
- Correspondence tracking.
- Returned product request and tracking.
- Ability to use external software tools, bolt-ons, apps.

- Administration
  - Customized access limits at user, country, group, case, drug level (e.g., France cannot read Germany's cases, team handling drug X cannot see drug Y cases).
  - Security and passwords—21CFR11 compliant.
  - Scalability (able to add more users, countries, drugs easily).
  - International use (if needed).
  - Multiple language support.
  - Tickler (reminder) system.
  - Audit trails (full unless there is a clear reason not to have complete audit trails).
  - Validation.
  - HIPAA and European Union 95/46 (data privacy) compliant—ability to anonymize a case.
  - Tracking of submissions for expedited and aggregate reports to multiple HAs.
  - Case cannot be downgraded (serious to nonserious or unexpected to expected) without senior signoff.
  - A Japanese version with the ability to produce the appropriate E2B file ("the J file") in the Japanese language.

- Vendor Support and Information Technology Issues
  - User groups.
  - Support from vendor and internal IT colleagues at home-base and worldwide user sites.
  - Ability to customize when new regulations and requirements are put in place
  - IT support capability in-house.

- Upgrade policy and support for older versions.
- Hardware needs and compatibility with other hardware and software.
- Backup system (e.g., every hour, nightly, weekly) with ability to reconstitute database contents within 24 hours in case of emergency.

- Validation
  - A fully validated system and validation strategy in place going forward.
  - Change control in place.
  - Acceptable to United States, European Union, MHRA, and other inspectors.

- Labeling Functions
  - The database should be able to store the AEs that are labeled/listed for each drug and formulation, and to identify which cases, based on the labeling, seriousness, and causality (for clinical trial cases), are 7- and 15-day reports to HAs in various countries, which go into PSURs, and so forth.
  - Labels for multiple countries should be storable and useable in this manner. Strategy on handling labeling in non-English languages.

- Reporting Functions
  - Draft and final versions of all usual reports: MedWatch, CIOMS I, PSUR tables, listings, NDA periodic, and IND annual tables, Investigator Letters, cover letters to regulatory agencies in English or other languages with the agency address, case number and drug automatically inserted into the letter.
  - Other reports: United Kingdom Yellow Card, French inputability in French, English, and other languages.
  - Export to EudraVigilance for both clinical trial and postmarketing cases.
  - Ability to identify, based on algorithms that are entered into the database, which cases are 7-day and 15-day reports and which cases go into PSURs, NDA periodic reports, including follow-ups.
  - Ability to import E2B files and data from other database and place into templates (e.g., insert case numbers, drug name, and dates into MS Word documents).
  - Ability to query easily (e.g., Query By Example) on all fields to produce queries that can be made into reports without the need of a programmer

to develop an SQL query.

- Batch printing, transmission of MedWatch forms, or line listings of query or report results in PDF files.

- Ability to save queries and reports at the user level.

- Ability to do SQL queries.

- Ability to anonymize reports and queries (e.g., no initials, no reporter names or addresses).

- Eudravigilance reporting.

- Epidemiologic, data-mining, and other reports using internal functions or add-on ("bolt-on") tools.

- Data Export and Import

  - E2B import with strategy on how to triage, flag, or "accept" a case before adding it to the database, especially if an earlier MedDRA version or different drug dictionary was used.

  - E2B export to multiple sources with automated receipt acknowledgment and multiple headers or content changes (e.g., different file for Japan, United States, and European Union for each case).

  - Automated transmission of cases based on business rules to internal and external recipients (e.g., a particular drug's cases go to licensing company externally and recipients internally 10 calendar days after first receipt date).

  - Ability to generate other formats for data export (Excel, PDF, etc.).

- Pharmacovigilance Functions

  - Note that some or all of these functions may be done by external software or databases separate from the PV/drug safety database. The external operations may or may not be tightly linked to the safety database.

  - Ability to produce pharmacovigilance reports and data-mining, both defined in the software and customized by the user.

  - Ability to use add-on statistical, epidemiologic, and other tools and reports

  - Drug usage data stored and used in queries and reports.

  - Ability to use a third party's software.

  - Signal detection and trend analysis.

■ Database Support

With a complex safety database in place, the drug safety group will need dedicated support from the technical services handling computers and information within an organization (be it a health agency or a pharmaceutical company). This will usually require one or more people working full time with the drug safety group. This is critical, as the IT personnel, to better serve, must learn a significant amount about how the safety business runs.

The IT group will serve multiple functions, including administering hardware and software, upgrades, user access and security, ad hoc queries (by the programmers), ongoing maintenance, bug fixes, new reports and projects, audit and inspection support, and validation and change control. In addition, there will be many behind-the-scenes personnel (e.g., database administrators, server maintenance, network personnel) involved in support of the drug safety database. If some or all of these functions are outsourced, an internal IT expert should oversee the operations of the outsourced companies and ensure that all requirements (regulatory, legal, and contractual) are followed.

It is usually good for both the drug safety medical staff and the IT personnel to have "one-stop shopping." That is, requests for IT support or for new projects should go through one person within the drug safety department to one person in the IT department to manage the flow of work and requests, track projects, and clarify needs. The IT person will then coordinate the behind-the-scenes actions in the IT department (e.g., network personnel, database administrators). Thus, the drug safety personnel should be able to go to one IT person for any computer issues and not have to figure whom to go to in IT: the database coordinator, the software support team, or the hardware support team. And the IT personnel do not have to figure out whom to contact in drug safety.

The database must support all privacy and security requirements from around the world. In particular, the European Union has in place very strict privacy regulations (Directive 95/46). The United States has Health Insurance Portability and Accountability Act (HIPAA) requirements in place as well (see Chapter 28). Whatever database is used, it must be able to handle multiple and sometimes conflicting privacy and data protection requirements. This may involve storing personal identifier information (names, addresses, reports, etc.) in separate files in separate servers, sometimes within the European Union. These rules are complex and changing. Many companies now have dedicated privacy officers who can assist in these issues.

Data Entry

Companies must make strategic, organizational, and operational decisions on where data entry should occur, especially if they are multinational companies. Single-country companies are able to have their safety data entered centrally in one or at most two facilities. This streamlines operations and allows for standardization across all data entry personnel and for backup data entry if one site should go out of service (e.g., fire, loss of electrical power). Some companies will outsource some or all of the safety functions.

Multinational companies must deal with issues of multiple languages, the need for follow-up on AE cases by local personnel in the local language, local reporting requirements (again, often in the local language), and the need for consistency and a single message (saying the same thing to all HAs in each AE case or safety issue). Companies respond to these needs in multiple ways:

- Headquarters data entry: For small companies or AEs from only one or two countries, it is sometimes feasible to ship all AEs to the main drug safety department for data entry.

- Geographic data entry by region: One (or sometimes two) regional data entry center each for North America, Europe, South America, and Asia/Africa. Follow-up of cases is done locally in the local language and the data transmitted to the regional data center for entry into the corporate safety database. This requires careful timing and coordination for cases sent from each country to remain in full compliance.

- Country data entry: Some companies have more dispersed data entry than by region. They may designate major affiliates or subsidiaries, particularly those with high volumes of AEs, to do data entry for their country (and possibly other countries nearby), thus having data entry done, for example, in the United States, Canada, Mexico, France, the United Kingdom, Germany (also handling Austria), Spain, Benelux (all done out of one site), Australia, South Africa, Japan, Singapore (covering the rest of Asia outside of Australia and Japan), and so forth.

- Outsourcing for some or all data entry: Companies may hire CROs to do data entry for them, shipping completed cases for review back to the company.

This could occur for all cases or only for those cases in a country where the company chooses not to set up a data entry function.

- Some countries handle clinical trial data entry separately from postmarketing data entry even if the data goes into the same safety database.

The critical issues, whichever mechanism is chosen, are as follows:

- Maintaining standards and consistency across multiple and diverse data entry sites, often speaking different languages and working under different conditions and time zones, is always challenging.

- Organizational reporting may also present issues if the safety personnel abroad report only locally and not "dotted line" or directly to the head safety office.

- Training is harder over greater distances even with online and other high-technology training tools.

- Quality is harder to measure and maintain.

- IT issues occur in terms of storage, networks, security, data transmission speed, and support.

- Data privacy issues may arise if data is shipped from a region with tight data privacy and security rules to areas of less stringent data protection rules (e.g., the United States, in the eyes of the European Union).

- Time zones interfere with workflow. It is almost impossible to arrange a simultaneous teleconference among Asia, the United States/Canada, and Europe due to time differences without pulling somebody out of bed. The International Date Line also presents some dating problems ("This report came into the United States today from Japan, where it was received tomorrow"). In addition, business hours don't overlap: the day crew working in North America will have to interact with the night crew working in Asia.

Data Transmission (E2B)

See Chapter 37 regarding the E2B documents issued from ICH. In this section, the practicalities of setting up E2B for data import and export are discussed.

E2B export of individual case safety reports is now obligatory for manufacturers to HAs in Japan and the European Union and certain other countries. In the United States, the FDA has encouraged the use of E2B by manufacturers for postmarketing expedited and nonexpedited reports but has not yet made it obligatory. It is expected that the FDA will do so soon.

There are several issues in E2B export:

- The E2B file differs somewhat in each of the three major regions. In particular, a separate file ("the J file") for each case must be prepared for Japanese reporting, as it is required by the Japanese HA in addition to the standardized E2B file. The European Union and the United States also have some differences in requirements that are forcing some companies to prepare three separate files, one each for the United States, Japan, and the European Union.

- The database structure of some old databases or cases is not fully compatible with E2B transmissions. For example, laboratory data may be entered into structured fields or as free text. Some companies have dozens of years of laboratory data stored as free text in their database. It is usually not necessary or worth the effort to reenter the data into structured tables. However, decisions must be made on how these data will be entered moving forward. Electronic data entry or downloading of laboratory data may alleviate much of this problem.

- Technical issues exist on gateways, drug dictionaries, and MedDRA versions.

- A process must be set up within a company to verify that all appropriate reports have been sent to the appropriate HAs (and/or business partners) on a timely basis and that they were received and successfully uploaded into the receivers' database(s).

Most of the modern commercially available drug safety databases handle these issues fairly well and companies are now expected by the regulatory agencies to handle these technical differences and submit cases correctly and on time. Outsourcing companies (CROs) are able to do E2B and EudraVigilance transmissions for companies that have not set up the system and processes needed for direct E2B transmission themselves.

There are corresponding issues in regard to E2B (or database-to-database) import of files from business partners and other companies. In addition, there are other issues:

- How to screen and triage a report coming in. Should it be uploaded automatically into the receiver's database or should it be kept in a "holding area" until drug safety personnel are able to review the file for content and format to ensure that it meets the appropriate criteria for entry into the database?

- How is the file actually reviewed by the staff? Online? Printed out?

- Screening for duplicates may be done in the triage area or after uploading. Duplicates are defined as receipt of the same case containing no new information whatsoever.

- A strategy must be found for identifying, handling, and versioning follow-up reports for cases already in the database.

- Dictionary incompatibility. If the sender has not yet upgraded to the latest version of MedDRA or the drug dictionary and the receiver has, how is the case handled? If different, and possibly incompatible, drug dictionaries are used, how are the data handled?

- How is security handled regarding encryption, viruses, and so on?

The Future of E2B (R3)

Things are changing rapidly. ICH has decided that the future versions of E2B will be created in collaboration with other organizations to widen the use around the world and for use by more than drug safety transmissions by pharmaceutical companies and health agencies. Thus, the International Organisation for Standards (ISO), Health Level 7 (HL7), the Clinical Data Interchange Consortium (CDISC), the International Health Terminology Standards Development Organisation (IHTSDO), European Committee for Standardization (CEN), and others are now are working together to create a single, common ICSR standard. They are developing the ISO/DIS 27953-1 Health informatics—Pharmacovigilance—Individual case safety report—Part 1: The framework for adverse event reporting and ISO/ DIS 27953-2 Health informatics—Pharmacovigilance—Individual case safety report—Part 2: Human pharmaceutical reporting requirements for ICSR. Testing is under way, and over the next several years, electronic transmission standards and requirements will be changing.

Safety Databases

Some companies develop their own customized ("bespoke") databases, but this is becoming less and less common as the commercially available products have become quite sophisticated and widely available to meet the needs of large and small companies. In some cases, both full-scale and "light" versions of the database are available. However, mergers of the software companies that have designed databases have occurred, which may decrease the number of available commercial safety databases.

There are several major safety database products on the market currently:

- ArisG by ArisGlobal. See Web Resource 20-1.
- Argus by Oracle, Inc. See Web Resource 20-2.
- Empirica Trace (formerly called Clintrace) by Phase Forward, Inc. See Web Resource 20-3.
- AERS by Oracle, Inc. See Web Resource 20-4.

Each has its strong and weak points, but all seem acceptable for AE database use. Phase Forward and Relsys (the creator of Argus) have been purchased by Oracle. It is not yet clear which databases will be maintained and for how long. Thus, data migration will likely be needed at some point for users of the non supported databases.

Some small companies with few AEs may still use spreadsheets to capture AEs. This is, in general, not practical and should be replaced by a standard safety database as soon as is feasible. If it is done that way, the data must still be protected and "validated."

■ Database Migration

At some point, most companies will have to migrate their safety data (often called "the legacy data") to a new or upgraded safety database. Many companies will also, at some point, have to import safety data should they acquire an already marketed product. Sometimes companies merge and combine their safety systems.

These situations will require the transfer of data from the originator's database into the acquirer's database. This data transfer is generally a painful exercise requiring the expertise of the drug safety, IT, regulatory, and other groups. It can be difficult and time-consuming if patient numbers are in the hundreds of thousands to millions, with billions (or more) of data points!

The data will have to be examined and mapped into the new database. Some fields will be easily moved (e.g., last name). Others will usually be feasible (e.g., date of birth) but can become tricky if data are incomplete (e.g., the birth date is recorded as January 1961 without specifying a day). Some databases cannot accommodate this and a filler (or fake) day may need to be entered to populate the field. Over time, this maneuver to create

an "acceptable" birth date will likely be forgotten, and it will not be realized by the staff handling the transfer that the birth date is not really correct. This may or may not matter. Sometimes data are imprecise and must be moved to precise fields (e.g., the age is recorded as "teenager" or given as a range "10 to 20 years old" in the originating database but must be exact in the new database). Thus, all sorts of data "cleaning" will be necessary to upload the data. Although much of the data can be automatically transferred using algorithms, some of the data will need to be examined and transferred manually. The transferring team will find inexplicable data and not be able to trace the "cleaning rules" applied when the data were entered or transferred in the past. Multiple moves of data over the years worsen this problem.

The migration process can take months to a year for large and complex databases. An internal team, sometimes with outside consultant assistance, should be assembled for this project, with careful project management, quality control, validation, and full documentation of all processes, changes, and alterations. The company should expect an inspection by the concerned health agencies (FDA, EMA, MHRA in particular) after the migration.

■ Health Level 7 (HL-7)

HL-7 is a nonprofit organization headquartered in the United States with offices or affiliates in more than 40 countries. It is a "standards developing organization dedicated to providing a comprehensive framework and related standards for the exchange, integration, sharing, and retrieval of electronic health information that supports clinical practice and the management, delivery and evaluation of health services" (Web Resource 20-5). The term HL-7 also (confusingly) refers to the standards themselves in addition to referring to the organization.

The organization develops standards (also called "specifications" or "protocols") for various healthcare areas, such as clinical trial data, pharmacy data, medical device information, imaging, and insurance claims forms. They do not develop software, but rather produce specifications so that everyone will create and store and transmit the data in a standard way no matter what computers, software, or databases are used.

Among other things, they have been creating and issuing standards for electronic health records, data transmission of these records, structured product labeling for drugs, and others. It is likely that HL-7 will ultimately encompass E2B reporting.

The FDA plans to use HL-7 standards for all data being submitted to the agency, including adverse events, product complaints, problem reports, drug labeling, and IND and NDA submissions. The FDA is using HL-7 standards for the transmission of some device individual case safety reports (ICSRs). See Web Resource 20-6.

■ CDISC

CDISC is a global, multidisciplinary, nonprofit organization that has established standards to support the acquisition, exchange, submission, and archive of clinical research data and metadata. Their goal is to develop and support global, platform-independent data standards that enable information systems to easily exchange data to improve medical research and healthcare.

CDISC standards are vendor-neutral, platform-independent, and freely available.

See Web Resource 20-7.

One outcome of these efforts will be multiple standardized vocabularies and dictionaries that will include MedDRA, drug dictionaries, and many other standards.

■ Systematized Nomenclature of Medicine Clinical Terms (SNOMED CT)

SNOMED is a hierarchical, clinical terminology or dictionary that covers diseases, clinical data, microorganisms, drugs, procedures, adverse events, and more. It has more than 344,000 "concepts." It will encompass MedDRA and much more. It was created by the College of American Pathologists and the United Kingdom National Health Service in 2002. The U.S. Department of Health and Human Services in 2007 agreed to participate in the development of SNOMED CT for use with electronic health records. It is available free of charge to everyone in the United States. Similar efforts are under way in other countries around the world.

This is a highly complex area that is constantly changing and evolving. Not all efforts are fully harmonized around the world, and it is possible if not likely that multiple standards will develop over time. Although these efforts are just beginning to touch drug safety, it is expected that the systems, procedures, business models, IT, and all other aspects of drug safety will change over the years as these standards are put into practice.

21

The United States Food and Drug Administration (FDA) and MedWatch

The "granddaddy" of drug safety "regulatory agencies" dates back to eighteenth-century Japan, when the eighth shogun, Yoshimune Tokugawa (1716–1745), upon recovering from an illness, awarded 124 medicinal traders in Osaka special privileges to examine medicines throughout the country. However, the safety of the medicines was difficult to guarantee despite these efforts. A shrine in Osaka, called Shinno-san, was created and dedicated to Shinno, the guardian of the pharmaceutical industry and the divine founder of medicine from China. This information was found at the Osaka tourism website (Web Resource 21-1).

Since the time of the shoguns, multiple other government authorities have become involved in drug safety. In the past 20 or so years, the number of organizations devoted to drug safety has increased markedly, in particular outside the United States. This chapter deals with the U.S. Food and Drug Administration (FDA) and focuses on the major players involved in handling drug safety.

The FDA handles safety in several different areas. The two largest areas touching drug safety are the Center for Drug Evaluation and Research (CDER) and MedWatch.

The FDA has undergone and continues to undergo major changes following various controversies, drug withdrawals, investigations, and changes in the law. This chapter will summarize the key divisions and functions that deal with drug safety (CDER, Risk Management, MedWatch, CBER, and CDRH) and will outline some of the initiatives currently under way that will lead to further changes in the next several years.

■ CDER (Center for Drug Evaluation and Research)

This is the prime center in the FDA for handling drugs. CDER handles new drugs from the IND stage (when a product first moves into human study) to the evaluation of the NDA for approval or rejection of the request to market the product in the United States. CDER then evaluates the postmarketing safety of the product. Although simple in theory, the actual practice is complex and has evolved over time. It continues to change and should be viewed as a work in progress.

The organization chart is posted online and is quite useful. It gives names, addresses, and contact information (Web Resource 21-2). There are more than 20 "offices" in CDER covering many areas, including biotechnology, new drug evaluation, counterterrorism, pediatric drug development, generic drugs, compliance, and, of course, drug safety. There are also advisory committees that consist of outside experts who meet periodically to review data and advise the FDA on various issues, including drug approvals and policy issues. See CDER's website (Web Resource 21-3). There are advisory committees made up of external members that give expert consultation to the FDA (Web Resource 21-4). There is an advisory committee on Drug Safety and Risk Management that looks at safety issues.

The FDA reorganizes periodically. The current structure is as follows: the Office of the CDER Center Director has under it approximately 13 offices, including the Office of Surveillance and Epidemiology. This office has under it five divisions:

- Division of Pharmacovigilance I & II (2 divisions): The staff includes safety evaluators whose primary role is to detect and assess safety signals for all marketed drug products. They work closely with medical reviewers in the Office of New Drugs so that potential safety signals are placed in the context of existing preclinical, clinical, or pharmacologic knowledge of the drugs in question.

- Division of Epidemiology: The staff reviews epidemiologic study protocols increasingly required of manufacturers as postmarketing commitments. They evaluate various postmarketing surveillance tools that may be incorporated into risk management strategies, such as patient registries and restricted distribution systems. They estimate the public health impact of safety signals by evaluating computerized databases and the published literature.

- Division of Medication Error Prevention and Analysis: The staff provides premarketing reviews of all proprietary names, labels, and labeling in CDER to reduce the medication error potential of a proposed product. The division also provides postmarketing review and analysis of all medication errors received.

- Division of Risk Management: The staff handles data resources, risk communication, and outcomes and effectiveness research components of drug safety risk management programs (REMS). This division oversees MedWatch, risk communication

research, and activities such as Medications Guides, Patient Packet Inserts, and pharmacy information surveys, and international regulatory liaison activities (such as videoconferencing) for all drug and biologic postmarketing safety issues.

In 2005, the FDA created the new Drug Safety Oversight Board (DSB), which advises the CDER Center Director on handling and communicating important and emerging drug safety issues. The board meets monthly and is composed of representatives from three FDA Centers and six other federal government agencies: the Agency for Healthcare Research and Quality (AHRQ), Centers for Disease Control and Prevention (CDC), Department of Defense (DOD), Indian Health Service (IHS), National Institutes of Health (NIH), and Department of Veterans Affairs (VA). See Web Resource 21-5. The DSB provides scientific and regulatory recommendations on drug safety and communication issues and policies to the senior FDA management on

- Potentially significant drug risks and safety issues
- Effective communication of drug safety information to healthcare professionals, patients, and the general public
- Establishment of general policies regarding drug safety issues and approaches to resolving internal FDA policy differences and disagreements
- Disputes between a sponsor and CDER concerning a Risk Evaluation and Mitigation Strategy (REMS) that occurs after approval of a prescription product if the sponsor requests DSB review

FDA's SOP for the board is available at Web Resource 21-6.

The FDA has an extensive, useful website, although the information tends to be scattered and difficult to find. There is a search engine that is somewhat useful. The website has extensive information on how the FDA works, its history, drug availability, counterfeits, internet purchases of drugs, labeling and medication guides for drugs on the market, signals, REMS, guidances, laws and regulations covering pharmaceuticals (as well as devices, biologics, radiologics, OTC products, nutraceuticals and more). The main CDER website (Web Resource 21-3) lists late news and provides a jumping off point to other CDER information, including:

- "FDA Basics": Fundamental information on the various divisions, functions, and leaders at FDA (Web Resource 21-7).
- "Drug Specific Information": This is an alphabetical

list of drugs that have an information sheet, Early Communication about an Ongoing Safety Review, or other important information (Web Resource 21-8).

- "Development & Approval Process for Drugs": Information on how drugs are developed and approved (Web Resource 21-9).
- "Guidance, Compliance, and Regulatory Information": For industry. This key page for pharmacovigilance (PV) professionals has links to information on laws, acts, rules, good review practices, enforcement activities, surveillance, postmarketing commitments requirements, warning letters, enforcement actions, new guidance documents, cyber letters, and the CDER manual of policies and procedures (Web Resource 21-10).
- "Information for Industry": A page for the pharmaceutical industry with links to guidances, postmarketing information, the Prescription Drug User Fee Act (PDUFA), warning letters, electronic submissions, the Orange Book (approved drug products with therapeutic equivalence evaluations), abbreviations, and types of applications (Web Resource 21-11).
- "MedWatch": See below for more detailed information (Web Resource 21-12).
- "Drugs at FDA": A link to the page that has an alphabetical list and search engine to find approved drugs by name, active ingredient, or application number (Web Resource 21-13).
- "Recalls, Market Withdrawals & Safety Alerts" (Web Resource 21-14).

■ The Safety Portal

FDA has launched a "one-stop shopping" safety portal in which safety reports for nearly all products regulated by FDA (and NIH) can be reported. Food (human or animal), drugs, biologics, blood products, gene-transfer research issues, and more can be reported by manufacturers, healthcare professionals, researchers, public health officials, and "concerned citizens." This portal is being developed and changes will be made as experience is gained. It allows for initial and follow-up reports. One can enter a case as a "guest" or one can establish an account and use it repeatedly. See Web Resource 21-15. It is not meant for emergency reporting. See also their FAQ page (Web Resource 21-16).

Other pages of interest include:

- "Potential Signals of Serious Risks/New Safety Information Identified from the Adverse Event Reporting System (AERS)": This page contains information about ongoing signals (Web Resource 21-17).
- "Postmarket Drug Safety Information for Patients and Providers": This site contains information on postmarket study requirements and commitments, a link to the clinical trials registry, and other safety-related information.
- "Approved Risk Evaluation and Mitigation Strategies": This site contains information and links to REMS that are in place (Web Resource 21-18).
- "Guidances": This site contains FDA's new, current, revised, and withdrawn guidance on all areas, including Drug Safety, ICH, OTCs, Good Review Practices, and the FDAAA Food and Drug Administration Amendments Act (Web Resource 21-19).
- "Postmarket Drug Safety Information for Patients and Providers: Selected Safety Regulations": This page has links to the relevant sections of the Code of Federal Regulations covering safety matters for drugs and biologics, as well as INDs, NDAs, and labeling (Web Resource 21-20).
- "Warning Letters": A site with many years of warning letters for all matters, not just safety, that are browsable and searchable by company, issuing office, and so forth (Web Resource 21-21).
- "Pregnancy & Lactation Labeling" (Web Resource 21-22).
- "Prescription Drug User Fee Act (PDUFA)": The main web page for information on PDUFA, with several links (Web Resource 21-23).
- "Office of Surveillance and Epidemiology (OSE)" (Web Resource 21-24).
- "Guidance, Compliance, & Regulatory Information": This page has links to the various laws, acts, guidances, and so forth.
- "Surveillance: Post Drug-Approval Activities": Links to the staff guide, regulations and policies, advertising, and promotional information.
- "Adverse Event Reporting System (AERS)": This site has the description of the FDA drug safety database, with data files and statistics (Web Resource 21-25).
- "MedWatch to Manufacturer Program": The system whereby FDA informs manufacturers of SAEs

that are received directly by FDA (see "MedWatch" below) (Web Resource 21-26). Note the MHRA in the United Kingdom has a similar program (Web Resource 21-27).

- "DailyMed": This is actually an NIH website that provides "high quality information about marketed drugs." It is not a complete listing but does have information on more than 7000 drugs. See the Drugs@FDA site (Web Resource 21-28).
- "Medication Guides" (Web Resource 21-29).
- "Medication Errors" (Web Resource 21-30).
- "Safe Use Initiative": FDA's program to reduce preventable harm from medications (Web Resource 21-31).

The FDA website is extensive, and almost everything that one wants to find relating to the FDA, drugs, and drug safety are present, though often not easy to find. In addition, FDA changes its websites frequently, and pages may jump or move, or URLs may be dead links. It may be necessary to search for the new URL using the FDA search engine on the home page. Note that most of the drug safety information is in the CDER section of the website.

■ Risk Management

On the FDA website there is extensive information on risk management initiatives, which are covered in Chapters 30 and 31. Other FDA activities are covered in this chapter and in other chapters in this book.

In 1997, the federal government put forth a global framework for federal risk management of drug products (Web Resource 21-32). The fundamental concepts include the following:

- *Risk assessment* is the estimation and evaluation of a risk in the pre- and postmarketing areas.
- *Risk confrontation* determines the acceptable level of risk in the large context, including social and community values as well as the technical judgments of professionals. This includes the use of advisory committees, which get input from various concerned stakeholders. In addition, the FDA has relationships with various groups of health professionals, consumer and patient advocacy groups, industry organizations, and other governmental agencies to gather information and advice.
- *Risk intervention* is the evaluation of alternative risk control actions, selection among them, and their implementation. After the risks are identified and assessed, they must be managed or minimized. The

FDA can refuse to allow the product to be marketed if the product's risk outweighs its benefits. If the product is permitted on the market, the FDA minimizes risk by various mechanisms, including the review and approval of the original labeling and any subsequent changes. FDA also regulates the advertising and promotion of marketed products. Promotional materials must not be false (i.e., they must conform to the label and be substantiated), and they must not be misleading (i.e., they must be balanced and include the material facts). FDA also tracks medication errors and can act on issues there. FDA also can require other risk minimization measures, including mandating education for product users, limiting product distribution (e.g., to specific hospitals or specialists), requiring prescriber qualifications, training, or informed consent, etc. The FDA may also require postapproval clinical or epidemiologic studies after marketing. In severe or urgent situations, there are various mechanisms to remove products from the market.

- *Risk communication* is aimed at conveying the needed information to the public. There are ongoing and rapidly changing mechanisms of risk communication using traditional as well as new social media mechanisms to convey information to consumers and healthcare practitioners. The internet and various new means of wireless communication challenge all parties to get the correct message out in the large sea of information. The product labeling (Package Insert) has been the classic mechanism of communication. The FDA has redone and revised how labels are made and communicated both to patients and practitioners. This is a controversial area as some feel the changes make labeling more complete but less useful and more ponderous. Medication guides for patients are also used in risk programs. Whether these changes lead to lowering risks for particular products remains to be seen. Another controversial area is Direct-To-Consumer advertising and promotion, which is allowed in the United States but not in many other developed countries. Whether this promotes product use that is safer or more dangerous is a much-debated topic, with no clear answer.

■ MedWatch

The MedWatch program is the FDA's national pharmacovigilance program. It provides clinical information about safety issues involving prescription and over-the-counter drugs, biologics, medical and radiation-emitting devices, and special nutritional products (e.g., medical foods, dietary supplements, and infant formulas). See the MedWatch site (Web Resource 21-12).

The website provides "one-stop shopping" for information or links to information on medical product safety alerts, recalls, withdrawals, current new and hot topics, educational materials and a glossary, the NIH Daily Med site (Web Resource 21-33), from the National Library of Medicine, containing up-to-date drug labeling information, Medication Guides, drug-specific information (more labeling), drug shortages, and more.

There is also a set of links to receive periodic e-mail notifications and RSS feeds (which you can have automatically sent to your internet home page if it accepts such feeds).

Another little-known MedWatch function is the MedWatch to Manufacturer Program (Web Resource 21-26), which allows drug and biologics manufacturers to receive certain SAEs submitted directly to FDA that would not otherwise be known to the manufacturer. One can subscribe at anytime after approval for a period of 3 to 4 years.

The other key part of the MedWatch site is information on reporting serious AEs to the FDA using the MedWatch form, which comes in two very similar varieties—the 3500 form for the public to voluntarily submit AEs and the 3500A form for mandatory reporting by manufacturers.

An information page for health professionals describes the systems used for drug and device reporting (Web Resource 21-34), which then has links to the other pages giving further information. There is a link to a downloadable PDF version of the MedWatch voluntary form for the public and the mandatory form (3500A) for manufacturers. There is also a link to an online reporting form for the public (Web Resource 21-35).

There is a page (Web Resource 21-36) with information for industry on the three key SAE reporting areas. Information and links to the appropriate regulations and forms are included:

- OTC Products and Dietary Supplements (Web Resource 21-37)
- Drug/Biologic/Human Cell, Tissues and Cellular and Tissue-Based Product Manufacturers, Distributors, and Packers (Web Resource 21-38)
- Human Cell & Tissue Products (HCT/P) Adverse Reaction Reporting (Web Resource 21-39)

For newly approved new chemical entities, FDA has a MedWatch to Manufacturer Program, whereby certain serious cases sent directly to FDA are transferred to the manufacturer (Web Resource 21-26).

■ Safety Databases

The FDA maintains several databases that contain safety information:

- Adverse Event Reporting System (AERS) (Web Resource 21-40). This is a computerized information system for FDA's postmarketing safety surveillance program for drugs and biologics. It is compliant with the ICH E2B guidance. This database is one of the largest of its kind. Quarterly (noncumulative) data files since January 2004 are available for downloading as zipped SGML or ASCII files (Web Resource 21-41). The data are not cumulative and not searchable online, though Freedom of Information (FOI) requests for AERS data, and actual (redacted) MedWatch forms are possible. Data include information on patient demographics, the drug(s) reported, the adverse reaction(s), patient outcome, and the source of the reports.
- Postmarket Requirements and Commitments (Web Resource 21-42). This database contains information on studies and trials that sponsors have committed to carrying out after drug approval.
- Vaccine Adverse Event Reporting System (VAERS) (Web Resource 21-43). VAERS is a cooperative database from the CDC and the FDA. VAERS collects information about AEs that occur after the use of licensed vaccines. See below under CBER.
- Manufacturer and User Facility Device Experience Database (MAUDE) (Web Resource 21-44). This database contains device information on reports since 1991. See below under CDRH.
- Clinical Trials Database (Web Resource 21-45). This is not a safety database but has information about governmental and private clinical trials under way in the United States and globally. There are tens of thousands of trials in more than 170 countries on file. Some contain safety information. The new PDUFA/FDAAA laws require safety information to be put online, though this will not become operational for several more years.
- Other databases include a poisonous plant database (Web Resource 21-46).

Other Useful FDA Web Pages

- Postmarket Drug Safety Information for Patients and Providers: A one-stop shopping page for just about everything you want to know about safety (Web Resource 21-47).
- FDA guidances for FDA-regulated products (Web Resource 21-48).
- Office of Non-Prescription Drugs (OTCs) (Web Resource 21-49).
- Potential Signals of Serious Risks New Safety Information Identified from the Adverse Event Reporting System (AERS) (Web Resource 21-17).
- Prescription Drug User Fee Act (PDUFA) (Web Resource 21-23).
- Food and Drug Administration Amendments Act (FDAAA) of 2007 (Web Resource 21-50).
- Warning Letters (Web Resource 21-51).
- Approved Risk Evaluation & Mitigation Strategies (REMS) (Web Resource 21-18).
- Global Health Agencies (links) (Web Resource 21-52).
- Dietary Supplements (Web Resource 21-53).
- Code of Federal Regulations (Web Resource 21-54).
- Drugs@FDA—the U.S. labeling for most approved drugs (Web Resource 21-13).

Finally, there is an excellent page (Web Resource 21-20) that covers mandatory postmarketing reporting by drug and biologic manufacturers, distributors, and packers. There are hyperlinks to the applicable federal regulations:

- Labeling
  - 201.56 – Requirements on content and format of labeling for human prescription drug and biological product
  - Other labeling regulations
  - 208 – Medication Guides for Prescription Drug Products
  - 310.501 – Patient package inserts for oral contraceptives
  - 310.515 – Patient package inserts for estrogens
- 312 – Investigational New Drug (IND) Application
  - 312.32 – IND safety reports
  - 312.33 – Annual reports

- 312.88 – Safeguards for patient safety
- 314 – Applications for FDA Approval to market a New Drug (NDAs)
  - 314.80 – Postmarketing reporting of adverse drug experiences
  - 314.81 – Other postmarketing reports
  - 314.97 – Supplements and other changes to an approved abbreviated application
  - 314.98 – Postmarketing reports
  - 314.520 – Approval with restrictions to assure safety use
  - 314.540 – Postmarketing safety reporting
  - 314.630 – Postmarketing safety reporting
- 601 – Biological Licenses
  - 601.12 - Changes to an approved application
  - 601.32 – General factors relevant to safety and effectiveness
  - 601.35 – Evaluation of safety
  - 601.93 – Postmarketing safety reporting
- 610 – General Biological Products Standards
  - 610.11 – General safety

In addition, other key documents such as FDA instructions for field staff, E2B AE submission information, ICH documents, and others are available.

CBER (Center for Biologics Evaluation and Research)

The CBER website contains less information regarding product safety than the CDER site because the regulatory responsibility for approval and postmarketing evaluation of many CBER products was transferred to CDER in 2003. The products remaining in CBER include cellular products (e.g., pancreatic islet cells for transplantation, whole cells, cell fragments, or other components intended for use as preventative or therapeutic vaccines); allergenic extracts used for diagnosing and treating allergic diseases and allergen patch tests; antitoxins; antivenins; venoms; blood; blood components; plasma-derived products (e.g., albumin, immunoglobulins, clotting factors, fibrin sealants, proteinase inhibitors), including recombinant and transgenic versions of plasma derivatives (e.g., clotting factors); blood substitutes; plasma volume expanders; human or animal polyclonal antibody preparations, including radiolabeled or conjugated forms; certain fibrinolytics such as plasma-derived plasmin; and red cell reagents.

More extensive information on this subject can be found at the CBER website (Web Resources 21-55 and 21-56).

In regard to safety, there is information covering recalls, shortages, biological product deviation reporting (i.e., errors and accidents in manufacturing), AE reporting, and specific information about safety issues on various products such as flu vaccines, HIV test kits, tissue products, and blood products. As noted, most AEs are reported via MedWatch using the 3500 voluntary reporting form.

One exception is vaccine AEs (Web Resources 21-57 and 21-58). These are reported to the Vaccine Adverse Event Reporting System (VAERS), which is sponsored by the FDA and the CDC. As with drugs, the goal is to collect and analyze signals and vaccine AEs. In particular, compared with drug products, vaccines are given to large numbers of children (FDA notes on its website that more than 10 million vaccinations are given yearly to children younger than 1 year old). As with all other products, the full safety picture is not known at the time of vaccine approval. Most of the VAERS reports are mild and include fever and injection site reactions, but some 15% are more serious AEs.

The VAERS website (Web Resource 21-58) has sections for consumer and healthcare professional reporting of AEs (Web Resource 21-59) either online, by fax, or by mail.

The VAERS database, unlike the drug database AERS, has a system called CDC WONDER (Web Resource 21-60) for obtaining data and producing tables, maps, charts, and various extracts regarding the incidence of vaccine AEs. For example, one can produce a report grouped by symptoms or medical problems (e.g., gastroenteritis) and various other criteria such as age, gender, manufacturer, U.S. location, date vaccinated, onset interval, seriousness, and outcome. The data are immediately available and are largely up to date. Data downloads are also available. This is a very useful tool. See Chapter 45 on Vaccinovigilance.

■ CDRH (Center for Devices and Radiologic Health)

This is the center that deals with medical devices and radiologics. There are three sections in the CDRH website (Web Resource 21-61) that are worth examining.

The first is the Medical Device Safety section (Web Resource 21-62), which covers alerts and notices, recalls, and emergencies. There is a large section (Web Resource 21-63) on Medical Device Reporting (MDR) of adverse events from manufacturers, importers, and user facilities (e.g., hospitals, nursing homes). Consumer and healthcare professionals report via MedWatch (as with biologics and drugs) using the 3500 voluntary reporting form.

The second is the Device Advice: Regulations & Guidance section (Web Resource 21-64). This is a very useful section that explains the regulations on marketing, standards, guidances, compliance, and postmarket requirements. Note that the entire process of approval, marketing, and safety for devices is markedly different from the processes for drugs and biologics.

The third is the section on medical device databases. There are several, but the key one for safety is MAUDE (Manufacturer and User Facility Device Experience). This database (Web Resource 21-44) contains AE reports for devices and dates back to 1991 for user facilities, to 1993 for distributor reports, and to 1996 for manufacturer reports. It is online and searchable by product problem, product, class, manufacturer, event type (death, injury, malfunction, other), brand name, registration number, and time frame. There is a separate database for reports before 1996. A detailed review of device safety is not in the scope of this manual.

■ OTCs (Over-the-Counter Products)

OTC products are regulated by CDER's Office of Nonprescription Drugs (Web Resource 21-49) and are drug products that can be sold in the United States without a prescription and thus without any medical professional intervention. That is, they are sold without a clear medical diagnosis being made by a medical professional and thus are purchased largely for symptoms as diagnosed by the lay public. Some products are not truly over the counter and are held by the pharmacist "behind the counter" such that the consumer must speak with the pharmacist, who will/should assess the need and appropriateness of the patient and product. OTC products have benefits that outweigh their risks, have low potential for misuse and abuse, can be adequately labeled, and do not require a health practitioner for their safe and effective use.

Drugs can enter the OTC market in several ways. A drug may be approved via the usual NDA process and then may be moved to OTC status through various routes. One is the "Rx to OTC switch." Other drugs that are "generally recognized as safe and effective (GRAS/E)" are listed in the FDA's "OTC monograph(s)" that specify which drugs may be marketed without further studies, FDA review, or approval. There are also so-called negative monographs that limit specific indications for certain drug ingredients. The monographs are very detailed specifications in the Code of Federal Regulations that specify ingredients, doses, formulations, indications, and labeling.

The FDA can act quickly to restrict marketing or remove the product from sale if there is significant risk or lack of evidence for effectiveness, or if the FDA finds that the usual notice and public procedure method are impracticable, unnecessary, or contrary to the public interest. The FDA can thus issue a rule requiring immediate label changes and marketing restrictions. In nonurgent situations, the FDA can use the notice and comment rulemaking mechanism to change marketing status.

In regard to safety reporting, OTC reporting by industry was not required until December 2007 for OTCs that did not have NDAs. That is, there was no requirement for AEs to be collected, analyzed, or submitted by manufacturers. This changed in 2007 when FDA issued a guidance (Web Resource 21-65) that required that serious OTC AEs "associated with the drug" were to be reported via MedWatch by manufacturers, packers, and distributors, using the 3500A form. This essentially means that all serious AEs (whether in the label or not) are reported to FDA within 15 calendar days. Requirements for minimal criteria are essentially the same as for drugs.

■ Drug Safety Oversight Board

Another recent change at the FDA was the creation of the Drug Safety Oversight Board (DSB). The DSB advises the CDER center on handling and communicating important and emerging drug safety issues, especially regarding how such issues impact on federal healthcare systems, as in the armed forces, veterans affairs, the CDC, NIH, and others. Meeting minutes and outcome reports are available online (Web Resource 21-66).

■ Prescription Drug User Fee Act (PDUFA) and FDAAA

In 1992, the Prescription Drug User Fee Act (Web Resource 21-23) was passed and then renewed in 1997, 2002, and 2007. The latest version is known as PDUFA IV. This Act allows the FDA to collect a fee from the manufacturer whenever the manufacturer submits an NDA. In addition, companies pay annual fees for each manufacturing establishment and for each prescription drug product marketed. Previously, taxpayers alone paid for product reviews for NDA approval by the FDA, through congressional budgets. In the new program, industry provides the funding in exchange for FDA agreement to meet drug-review performance goals, which emphasize timeliness. Questions have been raised about the appropriateness of what is, in effect, industry funding of the NDA approval process.

In 2007, PDUFA was actually a part of major new legislation known as the Food and Drug Administration Amendments Act (FDAAA) of 2007 (Web Resource 21-50).

The FDAAA had multiple parts. The ones that deal with postmarketing safety are known as Title IX and give enhanced authority to the FDA in regard to safety. In particular, it created the concept of Risk Evaluation and Mitigation Strategies (REMS), which are outlined in this chapter and in Chapter 30.

Another section strengthened the FDA's power over product labeling. Before 2007, the FDA did not clearly have the power to force labeling changes and most changes were done on a "voluntary" basis, though the FDA, in practice, could force most changes they desired. The act formally empowered FDA to "notify" the sponsor of new safety information that the agency "believes should be included in the labeling." The sponsor then has 30 days to submit an amendment proposing new labeling reflecting FDA's communication or to notify the FDA that it disagrees. FDA may then have discussions with the sponsor that usually last no more than 30 days, after which time the FDA may force the sponsor to make labeling changes the agency "deems appropriate." The FDA has used this new authority on several occasions, including the addition of a black box regarding an increased risk of death in elderly patients treated with antipsychotics for dementia, the addition of a black box regarding an increased risk of tendon injury with fluoroquinolone antibiotics, and the addition of a black box regarding the risk of histoplasmosis and other fungal infections with TNF alpha-blockers.

Other sections dealt with

- A review of proprietary names.
- Information technology.
- Medical devices, including enhancements in the device review program, inspections by third parties, new requirements for certain single-use devices, and user fees.
- Pediatric studies aiming to have sponsors do more studies in children.
- Encouragement of the development of products for tropical diseases and other "neglected" diseases.
- The Reagan-Udall Foundation, made up of senior advisers from outside the federal government, to

advise on innovation and enhanced food and drug safety. (This group has not been funded and is apparently non-functional.)

- Advisory committee conflicts of interest—more transparency regarding possible conflicts is now required.
- The expansion of the clinical trials database (Web Resource 21-45).

Prescription Drug User Fee Act Five-Year Plan

The FDA created multiple action plans and has begun various efforts to enact the requirements of the new law. In particular, FDA issued a "Prescription Drug User Fee Act Five-Year Plan" in 2008 (Web Resource 21-67). This plan includes:

- Assessing current and new methodologies to collect AEs
- Identifying epidemiology best practices
- Acquiring databases for targeted postmarketing surveillance and epidemiology
- Developing and validating risk management and risk communication tools
- Improving postmarket IT systems
- Reducing medication errors associated with name confusion
- Developing three new guidances:
  1. Contents of a complete submission package
  2. Best practices for naming, labeling, and packaging
  3. Proprietary name evaluation best practices

Other FDA initiatives under way are briefly mentioned below. The landscape is changing frequently and FDA's website should be checked periodically for updates and new initiatives.

Sentinel Initiative

The aim of this series of projects is to develop an active electronic safety monitoring system to strengthen FDA's ability to monitor medicinal products on the market and to augment the existing safety monitoring systems. It will enable FDA to access and analyze existing non-FDA healthcare databases by partnering with internal governmental departments (e.g., Defense Department, Medicare, Medicaid, Veterans Affairs) and external or-

ganizations (e.g., insurance companies with large claims databases, owners of electronic health records) to detect signals and evaluate postmarketing safety issues. One of these initiatives is called the Observational Medical Outcomes Partnership (OMOP). This is a combined effort by FDA, PhRMA (the drug industry association), and the Foundation of the National Institutes of Health (FNIH). In addition, there are other ongoing projects with ex-U.S. partners, including:

- European Network of Centers for Pharmacoepidemiology and Pharmacovigilance (ENCePP), to create a network consisting of research and medical-care centers, healthcare databases, electronic registries, and existing networks to strengthen postmarketing monitoring to facilitate the conduct of safety-related postapproval studies
- IMI Topic 6/PROTECT (Europe), to develop and validate tools and methods that will enhance AE data collection and active signal detection, and create standards for pharmacoepidemiology studies and the means to integrate additional data about a product for evaluation of risk–benefit
- European Union-ADR, to design, develop, and validate a computerized system that exploits data from electronic healthcare records and biomedical databases for the early detection of ADRs, which will be complementary to existing systems with more power to detect signals earlier
- Drug Safety and Effectiveness Network (DSEN), to link researchers through a virtual network to assess the risks and benefits of drug products on the market
- Mini-Sentinel, to create a distributed system to access multiple databases and to develop new methodology in drug safety and signal detection strengthening and validation

Thus, the FDA will be able to initiate queries of multiple databases to obtain safety information and to do active and proactive surveillance using current and new techniques. Updates to the initiative are posted on FDA's Sentinel website (Web Resource 21-68).

The Tome

In March 2003, the FDA published its long-awaited proposed new safety rules. See "Safety Reporting Requirements for Human Drug and Biological Products," 68 FR 12405-12497, March 14, 2003, at Web Resource

21-69. The document ran more than 90 pages in the Federal Register. The rules proposed extensive and complex changes to the current IND and NDA safety regulations. Major new obligations on the part of the pharmaceutical industry were proposed.

The FDA invited comments and received many thousands. Many parts are now clearly out of date, especially with regard to electronic transmission, risk management, and requirements of the FDAAA. Some changes and new requirements are still applicable (e.g., ICSRs, SUSARs) and likely to be put in place in some form. In late 2010 the FDA issued new final regulations that cover clinical trial reporting (21CFR312), which went into effect in early 2011. FDA has indicated it will issue updated postmarketing regulations soon also.

One concept in particular from the Tome is worth noting and may be enacted: the "Always Expedited Report." This new category requires submission in 15 calendar days of the ICSR whether expected (labeled) or not: congenital anomalies, acute respiratory failure, ventricular fibrillation, torsades de pointe, malignant hypertension, seizures, agranulocytosis, aplastic anemia, toxic epidermal necrolysis, liver necrosis, acute liver failure, anaphylaxis, acute renal failure, sclerosing syndromes, pulmonary hypertension, pulmonary fibrosis, transmission of an infectious agent by a marketed drug/biologic, endotoxin shock, and any other medically significant SAE that FDA wishes to see.

What Is Expected from Drug Companies by the FDA

The federal regulations noted above describe what the FDA expects to receive from pharmaceutical companies regarding the reporting of drug safety information. In all cases, companies are expected to do follow-up with due diligence to get complete information on (serious) cases:

- Clinical trials—AEs reported to the IND
  - In 7 calendar days: deaths/life-threatening, serious, unexpected, associated with the drug
  - In 15 calendar days: serious, unexpected, associated with the drug
  - In annual periodic reports: summary of all studies, tabular summary of the most serious and most frequent serious AEs, deaths, discontinuations due to AEs, and the 15-day reports submitted since the last report
- Marketed drugs—AEs reported to the NDA

- In 15 calendar days: serious, unexpected. Note that all spontaneous reports are considered to be "associated with the drug." The reasoning is that if the reporter did not believe there was at least some level of association (causality) with the drug, he or she would not have reported it.

- In 15 calendar days: reports from the medical literature that are serious and unexpected.

- In the quarterly or annual periodic reports or PSURs: A narrative summary and analysis of the 15-day alert reports submitted since the last report plus all other reports that are not serious and not unexpected. Foreign nonserious AEs do not have to be reported. In general, clinical trial AEs do not have to be reported to the NDA. Note that currently PSURs are not required by FDA and classic NDA periodic reports (PADERS) are acceptable. FDA has said PSURs will be made obligatory at some point in the future.

- Solicited reports: AEs that are received from disease management programs, patient support programs, and such should be reported as 15-day reports to the NDA if they are serious, unexpected, and associated with the drug. It is the latter causality assessment that differentiates solicited reports from spontaneous reports (FDA Guidance for Industry, August 1997, Web Resource 21-70).

What Is Expected from Consumers and Healthcare Professionals by the FDA

Reporting is purely voluntary but strongly encouraged. Reports may be made to the FDA directly via MedWatch (mail, online, fax, etc.) or to the pharmaceutical company manufacturing, selling, or packing the product.

FDA Publications and Updates

FDA has various publications and feeds available without cost online, such as e-mail alerts and as RSS feeds. "What's New (Drugs)" comes out several times a week with new drug-specific information (Web Resource 21-71). The relevant publications are well worth receiving, particularly the MedWatch and CDER notifications.

Others include (Web Resource 21-72):

- CDER New: New items posted to the CDER website
- Drug Information: Occasional drug information updates on hot topics, frequently asked questions, and more
- Drug Marketing, Advertising, and Communications: Drug marketing, advertising, and communication regulation information; updates to the DDMAC Web pages, which occasionally involve safety matters
- Drug Safety News (Podcast alert): Emerging safety information about drugs, broadcast in conjunction with the release of Public Health Advisories and other drug safety issues
- Drug Safety Newsletter: Postmarket information for healthcare professionals on new drug safety information and reported adverse events
- FDA Patient Safety News (video): TV broadcasts for healthcare professionals about recalls, alerts, and ways to improve the safety of drugs, medical devices, vaccines, and diagnostic products
- MedWatch Safety Alerts: Product safety alerts, Class I recalls, market withdrawals, and public health advisories
- FDA Guidance Documents for the industry
- FDA Warning Letters: FDA Warning Letters issued to companies
- Good Clinical Practice: Information about the development of final rules related to FDA's regulations on good clinical practice and clinical trials

The reports may change from time to time, with new ones introduced and old ones phased out. Check the site for updates. There are other alerts on biologics, CBER, and specific diseases and conditions, including HIV and infectious hepatitis, women's health, devices, research, and cosmetics.

This site offers sign-up for multiple subscriptions at the same time from various health and human services agencies and divisions, including the CDC, NIH, MedLine Plus, and others (Web Resource 21-73).

The FDA, the industry, and nearly everyone else is now struggling with the newly and rapidly arising social media (Twitter, Facebook, LinkedIn, Buzz, blogs, bloginars, eCards, podcasts, widgets, virtual worlds, etc.). As of this writing, FDA had several Twitter feeds and a Facebook page (Web Resource 21-74), and is expanding its use of social media.

The FDA's influence on life in the United States is extensive. The FDA ("The Agency") oversees and regulates drugs, biologics, vaccines, dietary supplements, radiation-emitting devices, food, cosmetics, and now tobacco. They cover both human and veterinary products. FDA's influence outside the United States is obviously less strong than within the United States but nonetheless is felt through direct and indirect actions in international entities (e.g., ICH, CIOMS, where FDA is a major player either directly or indirectly), formal and informal interactions and memoranda of understanding with other health agencies (Europe, Canada, etc.), and as a thought and action leader (e.g., a drug withdrawal in the United States must be addressed, in practice, rather quickly elsewhere).

For those in industries regulated by the Agency, the FDA has an impact on actions every moment of the day in just about all areas of business:

- Approval of INDs and NDAs, 510Ks, and so on
- Regulations covering all aspects of manufacturing (Good Manufacturing Practices), clinical research (Good Clinical Practices), animal research (Good Laboratory Practices), quality systems, drug safety (Good Pharmacovigilance Practices), and so on
- Inspections (often unannounced) of factories, clinical trial sites, safety divisions, clinical trial divisions, and so on
- Drug safety
- Product labeling and packaging
- Product advertising and sales promotion
- Advice to the public

The FDA has multiple "clients" to which it must answer: the Secretary of Health and Human Services (in the President's cabinet), the Congress (which provides funding and oversight), the American public, activist groups (consumer groups, lobbies, etc.), the media (press, TV, internet, blogs, etc.), the pharmaceutical industry, other healthcare players, and, indirectly, foreign health agencies.

Pharmaceutical companies also have multiple clients but different ones: the stockholders (owners) of the company, the American public, activist groups, the media, the FDA, and, if multinational companies, other health agencies, insurance companies, and foreign media.

The FDA's fundamental viewpoint and raison d'être differ from those of pharmaceutical corporations. The FDA's prime concern is protecting the American public (and animals). They are, in theory, not concerned with the viability or profitability of corporations or market share, whereas companies, again in theory, have a primary fiduciary goal of increasing shareholder value. Obviously, a company would not want to increase its stock price at the expense of the public health. But, in practice, decisions on what is good or bad for public health are almost never black and white. Rather, they are the subject of debate on the risks and benefits that fall somewhere in the gray area between the extremes.

Other factors come into play. In general, salaries and bonuses, particularly for professionals, are better in private sector companies than in the FDA or academia. However, benefits, pensions, and retirement packages are often better in government service. Private sector companies tend to have more resources (people, computers, parking spaces, etc.) than government agencies.

As with other federal agencies, there is often a steady flow of personnel leaving the Agency to go to the private sector and, with the FDA, occasionally vice versa. This is generally viewed as a good phenomenon because it allows government workers to understand the functions and pressures in private industry and for private industry personnel to understand how government agencies function. Many people enter the industry or the FDA from academia but primarily just after finishing training (in medicine, pharmacy, nursing, pharmacology, toxicology, statistics, etc.). Others feel this is a bad concept as it binds the regulators and the regulated too closely together and influences the actions of regulators who may want to get a job in industry after leaving the Agency.

There is a continuing debate, which varies in intensity and persistence over time, on whether the FDA works too slowly ("drug approval lag") or too quickly ("releasing dangerous drugs onto the market without adequate evaluation") and whether there are too many regulations ("pharmaceuticals is one of the most regulated or over-regulated industries in the United States").

Most pharmaceutical companies live with a low-level dread of the FDA and other health agencies coming into their safety departments (or other departments) to do an inspection (unannounced as a rule when done by the FDA). The inspection may be routine, done periodically (often every 1 to 2 years) or "for cause" (wherein the FDA has a suspicion that all is not right). The inspection may last from a few days to months if major issues are found. The FDA may go to sites outside the United States if appropriate. Conversely, the EMA and other agencies abroad inspect in the United States (see Chapter 48). However, most companies now understand that building quality management systems (see Chapters 33, 40, and

41) is now obligatory not just in safety but throughout the organization. They also realize that periodic audits (including self-audits) and governmental inspections are now part of the norm and "a cost of doing business."

There has been much controversy after the withdrawal of Vioxx and other products from the U.S. market as well as contaminated products (e.g., heparin) for safety reasons. Some (both from within the FDA and from the outside) have accused the FDA of not sufficiently protecting the American public from "dangerous" drugs, food, and other products. There have been accusations of too rapid approval of drugs, insufficient analysis of data submitted to the FDA, companies' not submitting complete or sufficient data to the FDA, and other charges. Similar controversies have been seen with other regulatory agencies in regard to financial regulation, air transport safety, and so forth. The PDUFA, FDAAA, and other changes are a result of these controversies. More will come.

Drug Safety Inspections

The FDA has an extensive role in doing drug safety PV inspections. This is covered in Chapter 48.

Frequently Asked Questions

Q: Is there too close a relationship between the FDA and the pharmaceutical industry? Are they in bed together?

A: The answer depends on whom you ask.

The FDA would (most probably) say that they are not compromised by maintaining correct and formal communications with the industry. The industry supplies FDA with the large majority of the postmarketing safety data and most of the premarketing safety data. There must be communication between the industry and the Agency to clarify ambiguous points, get further information on critical cases, and so forth. The FDA also encourages (and even requires in some cases) meetings with the industry during the development of drugs (in the IND phases) and in postmarketing situations where safety issues arise. It is a professional-to-professional exchange of information to ensure the safety of the American public.

The industry would say that its influence on the FDA is slight. Companies go out of their way to be sure the FDA gets what it needs (and wants) and companies often submit more than regulations require to be sure that the

FDA gets what it wants and that the companies are not accused of hiding or undersubmitting data. The industry often (privately) believes that the FDA is rather tough and tends to not give the industry a fair shake or a level playing field. Some feel the FDA treats big pharma differently from small pharma or start-up companies, cutting the latter a little more slack and giving them more "hand-holding."

Others claim that there is too much interchange of personnel between the FDA and industry, wherein some people start their careers or spend some time at the FDA and then move on to work for pharma companies, or vice versa, carrying with them their contacts and inner knowledge (which often becomes outmoded quickly) of the other. Some feel that this may influence a person's actions in the company or FDA since his or her next job may be for the "other side."

The consumer groups and activists believe that the FDA is indeed in bed with the industry and point to the various "fiascos" in safety that have occurred, such as Vioxx, Fen-Phen, suicide in pediatric patients on antidepressants, and contaminated heparin, among others (see Chapters 52–54). The FDA and the industry would (probably) counter by saying, quite the contrary, that these episodes have shown that the drug safety system in place is indeed functioning and functioning well and that the challenge is to identify these problems earlier.

These criticisms have been made for many other federal agencies, including regulators of banks, insurance companies, Wall Street, the airline industry, and car manufacturers. This is a fascinating and controversial area that is and will always remain a work in progress.

Q: Should the FDA be broken up into an approving body and a safety body, similar to some other federal regulatory agencies?

A: This proposal has been advanced in the last several years. The argument is that the people who approve a drug have a vested (and emotional) interest in seeing their drug stay on the market and may not act vigorously on safety matters as this might be a tacit admission that their original approval decision was incorrect or too hasty. It is claimed that separate reviewers should oversee safety, as they have no interest in defending an approval decision. Others say that the medical skill set involved in postmarketing safety review is different from that of preapproval safety review. Separating the functions would discount the knowledge the reviewing group has obtained over months and years of review of a product, moving postmarketing follow-up to people unfamiliar with the drug. This also would increase the bureaucracy and be more costly. Clearly, each side has valid points. What will evolve will most likely be a political decision.

22

The European Medicines Agency (EMA, EMEA)

I n 1995, the European Medicines Evaluation Agency (EMEA) was created and based in the Canary Wharf section of London, England. Now, over a decade later, the face of drug regulation in Europe has totally changed. In 2004, a new directive changed the name of the EMEA to the European Medicines Agency (EMA, also called, like the U.S. Food and Drug Administration [FDA] and Central Intelligence Agency [CIA], "The Agency"). See its very extensive website (Web Resource 22-1).

Like the FDA, its main responsibility is the protection and promotion of public and animal health through the evaluation and supervision of medicines throughout the European Union, comprising 27 countries (Member States) and their more than 40 national authorities, as well as the three European Free Trade Area (EFTA) nations of Iceland, Liechtenstein, and Norway. Switzerland also works closely with the EMA, particularly in areas regarding inspections. These 30 countries are also referred to as the European Economic Area (EEA).

The terminology in Europe can be a bit confusing as the European Union/EEA is not the European equivalent of the United States. The European Union/EEA is composed of sovereign nations, which still retain many powers and functions. Some governmental functions are devolved in full or in part to the "central" authority (in Brussels and Strasbourg) and others are retained by the national governments. Not all countries devolve the same functions to the central authority. Thus, the European Union/EEA's handling of drugs and drug safety is similar to but, in many ways, quite different from that of the FDA or other single, national health agencies.

The EMA handles human and veterinary medicinal products (but not food, unlike the FDA). The EMA has the authority to approve the "Marketing Authorisation" (MA) for a product via the "centralized procedure," thus avoiding the need to gain approval in each of the 30 countries. Some products may still be approved by national authorities on a country-by-country basis.

Six scientific committees, with members from all 30 states, handle the main scientific work of the Agency: the Committee for Medicinal Products for Human Use (CHMP), the Committee for Medicinal Products for Veterinary Use (CVMP), the Committee for Orphan

Medicinal Products (COMP), the Committee on Herbal Medicinal Products (HMPC), the Paediatric Committee (PDCO), and the Committee for Advanced Therapies (CAT).

The EMA (with more than 500 employees mainly based in Canary Wharf in London) is headed by an executive director with five reporting divisions, including two that touch on drug safety: the sections on "Human Medicines Development and Evaluation" and the Patient Health Protection. The latter has four subdivisions, including Compliance and Inspection and Pharmacovigilance and Risk Management. The PV and RM group has four subdivisions below it, handling Data Collection and Management, Signal Detection and Data Analysis, Risk Management, and Coordination and Networking. See the organization chart on the EMA website (Web Resource 22-2).

The highest-level committee handling human medicines is the Committee for Medicinal Products for Human Use (CHMP). This committee has created a pharmacovigilance committee called the Pharmacovigilance Working Party (PWP or PVWP) that has experts from each member state. They meet for 2 to 3 days each month (except August) to discuss major safety issues such as standard operating procedures, guidance documents, "points to consider" documents, new procedures, class- or product-specific safety issues, International Conference on Harmonization (ICH) documents, and interactions with other bodies (e.g., the Uppsala Monitoring Centre and non–European Union organizations). In addition, urgent or emergency safety matters may also be brought to the Working Party. Their yearly work schedule is usually published in advance.

The CHMP handles the safety of authorized products via member states' national medicines agencies by monitoring safety concerns (ADRs) and by making recommendations to the European Commission to change, suspend, or withdraw a product's marketing authorization.

Under the CHMP's Pharmacovigilance Working Party is a committee that handles drug safety and has representatives from all member states. Its primary duties include evaluation of potential signals arising from spontaneous reports, advising on risk and risk management (including regulatory options), monitoring regulatory action, setting standards for procedures and methodologies for Good PV Practice, communication and exchange of information between the EMEA and national authorities, and cooperation with ex–European Union agencies (particularly FDA and the World Health Organization). Their domain is largely in the postapproval area, but they do have authority for drugs still under study. They issue work programs in advance of their monthly meetings and publish meeting summaries (Web Resource 22-3), which usually involve safety issues on specific drugs.

In 2001, a European Union-wide central database, called the Eudravigilance System, was created (Web Resource 22-4). This database serves as a "clearinghouse" to ensure that all appropriate cases are transmitted to the appropriate member states. It is used to capture SAEs as Individual Case Safety Reports (ICSRs) both pre- and postauthorization. This allows for a single European database accessible to the member states' HAs. Industry has limited access, primarily to their own cases only. The public does not have access at this time. See Chapter 8 for further details.

The European Union has developed a comprehensive risk management strategy for all products in the European Union. This is a strategy that covers the entire life cycle of a product, and a risk analysis is required for every product upon approval (or during its marketing). The goal is to create a set of pharmacovigilance activities and interventions designed to identify, characterize, prevent, or minimize risks relating to medicinal products, including the assessment of the effectiveness of these interventions. This is discussed in detail in Chapter 30.

In addition to the EMA, each European country has its own national health authority (HA) or authorities that handle drug safety. They are often called "competent authorities (CA)" in European Union regulatory jargon. The European Union is still evolving and the recently enacted Lisbon Treaty has altered some of the basic structures and functions of the European Union governing bodies. The European Union remains still a work in progress. The interplay between the central authority (primarily in Brussels but with various agencies scattered throughout the European Union, such as the EMA in London and the European Central Bank in Frankfurt, Germany) and the individual countries is dynamic and often changing. Note also that the EMA does not have jurisdiction over food. The European Food Safety Authority in Parma, Italy handles those matters.

As noted, for drug safety, some functions are primarily centralized in London and some remain in each member state. Some national authorities are very large and powerful and exert strong influence over smaller member states. This division and, in many cases, duplication of labor, as well as the multitude of languages involved in the European Union, produce a challenge for safety reporting both for the pharmaceutical industry and for the member states themselves. Most of the work in drug safety is done at the international level in English, but, obviously, at the local level the national languages are still used. The comparison with other countries, particularly the United States, where the drug safety function is clearly centralized, is striking. The closest analogy would be if each of the 50 states in the United States had its own mini-FDA and used languages other than English.

In terms of pharmacovigilance the EMA has largely harmonized along the lines of ICH. They have codified the premarketing requirements in a document known as Volume 10 and the postmarketing requirements in Volume 9A. Each is discussed in detail below. Nonetheless, there are still many differences, particularly for clinical trial pharmacovigilance, from country to country.

■ Volume 9A Postmarketing PV

The European Union has issued its postmarketing safety regulations and requirements in a single document known as Volume 9A. The latest version was issued in September 2008. It is available online (Web Resource 22-5) in a PDF file. It is 229 pages long with links in the Annexes (appendices) to multiple other useful documents (e.g., guidelines, ICH documents, the Risk Management Plan template). There is a detailed table of contents and, perhaps more importantly, the document (as a PDF file) is easily searchable using the free Adobe Reader (Web Resource 22-6) or other software, making it easy to find specific references to topics of interest. Unlike the regulations and requirements in other countries, this document is exceptionally readable, clearly written, and comprehensive. It has been updated periodically and will likely be so in the near future.

Here is a brief summary of the contents:

The legal basis for PV in the European Union dates back to 1993 and the Council Regulation (EEC) 2309/93 and Regulation 726/2004. These are all available on Eudralex (Web Resource 22-7). These documents require the EMA, the member states, and others to set up systems to handle the collection, verification, exchange, and presentation of adverse reaction reports within the European Union.

Part I covers guidelines for Marketing Authorization holders (MAHs).

The roles and responsibilities of the MAH are spelled out and require that an appropriate system of PV is put in place by the MAH. All information regarding the benefit–risk profile must be promptly and fully sent to the competent authorities. And most critically, it describes the role of the Qualified Person for Pharmacovigilance

(QPPV or QP), to be appointed by the MAH and to be continuously (24/7) available for safety matters. In brief, the QP establishes and maintains the PV system, has an overview of all the products and safety issues pending, and makes sure all safety functions are handled properly. The QP's roles are discussed in detail in Chapter 23. The QP must ensure that all suspected ADRs are collected, collated, reported, and accessible within the European Union. The MAH must prepare, update, and provide a "Detailed Description of the PV System." This (along with the United Kingdom equivalent, the "Summary of PV Systems") is covered in Chapter 49. This section of Volume 9A further covers the requirements for risk management systems, expedited reporting, PSURs, special situations, databases, documentation, company postmarketing safety studies, and regulatory matters. These topics are covered in detail in this manual in the individual chapters.

Part II covers guidelines for the EMA and health agencies ("competent authorities").

This section covers the obligations of the member states' national health agencies; how PV is to be done; handling of ICSRs, PSURs, signal detection, medication errors, benefit–risk analyses, communication, data exchange, crisis management plans relating to safety matters, inspections, creation, and a rapid-alert and non-urgent information communication system; how referrals to the EMA are to be done; and how the European Union and member states work with the World Health Organization in international PV.

Part III covers the electronic exchange of information.

This section describes the handling, format, transmission, and details of ICSRs and EudraVigilance.

Part IV covers pharmacovigilance communication.

This section describes the principles for communication to healthcare professionals and others.

The Annexes include a glossary, abbreviations, terminology, references to guidelines and templates for the European Union Risk Management Plan, the PSUR sections, and distribution requirements for reporting to competent authorities.

In summary, this is a complete and well-prepared document that is easy to handle and absorb, though it is highly detailed and exacting. The document is rich in explanations and background and anyone in the field of PV, whether in the European Union or not, should read and be familiar with this document. Many of its principles and procedures are used throughout the rest of the world as they are based on the common seminal antecedent documents of PV, namely, the Council for

International Organizations of Medical Sciences (CIOMS) and ICH documents.

Volume 10 Clinical Trial PV

Volume 10 contains six chapters covering multiple aspects of clinical trials. The section covering pharmacovigilance during clinical trials was issued in April 2006 and is entitled, "Detailed guidance on the collection, verification and presentation of adverse reaction reports arising from clinical trials on medicinal products for human use." Unlike Volume 9A for postmarketing safety, this document is short, only 26 pages, and is more limited in its content. Nonetheless, its scope covers all trials (as described in Directive 2001/20/EC) with at least one investigator site in the European Union, whether the product is on the market or not. It is perhaps unfortunate that Volume 10 is not as complete and self-standing as Volume 9A is for postmarketed products. Nonetheless, the information is available here. As with postmarketing requirements, changes are frequent.

The sponsor's responsibilities are described and are the equivalent of those described in Volume 9A for the MAH for marketed products in terms of collecting, recording, handling, and communicating. Additional requirements are explained regarding ethics committees, interactions with the investigators, issues unique to trials (e.g., unblinding), expedited reporting, annual reporting, and other details.

Other sections of Volume 10 refer the reader to other self-standing guidances and documents (including Volume 9A) on quality issues, monitoring, databases (Eudravigilance), inspections, good clinical practices, and so forth. All of these documents are available as PDF files on the Eudralex website (Web Resource 22-8). The contents of many of these documents are described throughout this manual.

The EMA Website

The EMA website (Web Resource 22-1) contains much useful information. The PV guidelines and documents section contains the monthly reports from the PV Working Party, guidelines and documents, presentations, position statements, and Standard Operating Procedures. These are useful to read as there are many of them, and they cover many areas of PV. They give a flavor of how the EMA handles PV on an operational level.

There is a section on European Public Assessment Reports (EPARs), which contain product-specific information (by brand and generic/INN name) on the CHMP opinions in granting Marketing Authorizations. There is often interesting safety information in each document, including the SPC and labeling as well as the scientific reviews (Web Resource 22-9).

There is a very useful section on inspections for GCP, GLP, GMP, and pharmacovigilance. The PV section (Web Resource 22-10) contains information on relevant documents, scope and mission, Inspectors Working Group, and specific procedures and guidances governing inspections. The European Union Risk Management Strategies site is Web Resource 22-11.

There is an up-to-date page of links to the HAs of the European Union and elsewhere, as well as other regulatory agencies and scientific organizations (Web Resource 22-12). The monthly reports of the PV Working Party are available at Web Resource 22-13.

As the EMA is primarily aimed at industry and regulators, there is much less consumer information compared to the FDA website or other national websites within the European Union. The websites of member states vary in completeness and utility. They are in the native language of each country, though many have some sections in English (not always the PV section). Of particular interest is the United Kingdom website, which is examined in Chapter 24. The website of the French HA, the Agence Francaise de Securite Sanitaire des Produits de Sante, is useful but is in French (Web Resource 22-14). The Dutch Agency's website (Web Resource 22-15) has a section on PV in English, as does the German Agency (Web Resource 22-16). However, many of the key documents are in the national languages and are not translated into English.

European Network of Centers for Pharmacoepidemiology and Pharmacovigilance (ENCePP)

ENCePP is a network of centers throughout Europe (not just the European Union) with nearly 100 centers in 21-plus countries, including medical centers, healthcare databases, electronic registries, and other existing networks. Their goal is to further strengthen PV and pharmacoepidemiology in the European Union by facilitating independent postauthorization studies on safety and benefit risk. They are working on several projects, including a checklist of operational research standards, a code of conduct, the means to promote research in PV and pharmacoepidemiology, a European Union resources database with information on data sources and research centers, a study database, and the development of methodology to promote PV research. They are collaborating with the FDA's Sentinel Project and Health Canada's Drug Safety and Effectiveness Network.

The European Union is considering significant changes in pharmacovigilance requirements, which will, if promulgated, produce major changes in the way PV is handled in and for Europe. Under discussion are changes relating to additional reporting of medication errors, misuse and abuse; patient-reported AEs (not all countries accept reports from non-healthcare professionals); making all AEs (not just SAEs), ADRs, or European Union ADRs expeditable; making the PSUR a more analytic document; developing new tools for benefit–risk analysis; proactive drug safety; ENCePP (see below); and more. EMA's high-level thinking on this matter is spelled out in its "Road Map to 2015" (Web Resource 22-17). It is also well worth subscribing to the e-mails from the agencies as well as various blogs and news services to stay up to date on these matters.

■ Newsletters and RSS Feeds

The EMEA has multiple free subscriptions available from its website as RSS feeds (Web Resource 22-18). There are many feeds available, and it is well worth subscribing to several of them. The ones that may contain safety related news are: Ongoing public consultations, European Medicines Agency events, Pending EC decisions and European Public Assessment Reports (EPARs) on human medicinal products and herbal medicinal products, Patient safety news and press releases, Regulatory and procedural guidelines, Inspections, and Scientific guidelines.

■ Comments

The operational issues involved in drug safety in the European Union are far more complex than those in the United States because of the multiplicity of member states and requirements for local submission of certain cases; there is not always a single submission of a case as there is to the FDA in the United States. The closest analogy in the United States would be if there were a requirement to submit AEs to the FDA and some of the AEs to agencies in each of the 50 states, sometimes to several of the states, sometimes to all of the states, and sometimes not in English. The clinical trial PV requirements are markedly less harmonized than the postmarketing requirements at this writing.

Remaining in compliance with all of the ever-changing reporting requirements, new drug approvals, safety issues, and such in the 27 member states plus the EMA plus the affiliated countries presents enormous practical and logistical problems. The European Union, like the United States and Japan, is now undergoing and will continue to undergo changes in many aspects of AE reporting (electronic reporting, new risk management initiatives, a new drug dictionary, etc.). The EMA and the member states are also becoming much more active in inspecting companies' and vendors' drug safety practices, both on a routine basis and on a "for cause" basis, both within Europe and abroad (see Chapter 48).

In practice, what this means now is that any company that does studies or sells (or distributes) products within the European Union must either have subsidiary or affiliated offices within the European Union (and sometimes even within each country in which they sell or study). Failing this, the company needs to engage, with a written contract, a company (i.e., a contract research organization [CRO]) to handle these functions for it. There must be a QP physically living in the European Union, and he or she must have direct and immediate access to the database to deal with the EMA's and individual member states' issues and requests for information on marketed products. Language issues also oblige a company to be sure it has personnel who can deal with local HAs and others in the language of the country. The cost of doing business within the European Union to handle all the regulatory requirements is high. Conversely, European companies wishing to do business in the United States and in Canada must also open offices in these countries, though the United States and Canada still have, to a large degree, "one-stop shopping" at the health agencies.

■ Future Changes

Premarketing

There are currently moves afoot to change the way AEs and safety matters are handled in the European Union both for clinical trials and for marketed products.

For clinical trials, there is a strong possibility of both short-term changes and longer-term changes in the clinical trial directive (after 2011). The guidances that would be affected in the short term include the following:

■ The guidance on the collection, verification, and presentation of adverse reaction reports arising from clinical trials on medicinal products for human use

- The Eudravigilance guidance on the European database of suspected unexpected serious adverse reactions (SUSARs)

The changes would be aimed at making the member state requirements consistent with the clinical trials directive and ICH E2A. This may include a formal requirement for investigators to send SAEs to the sponsor within 48 hours of first knowledge of the event and then follow with a detailed written report. Another change would remove some of the ambiguity in the causality determination requirements for SUSARs. Currently, the investigator or sponsor makes causality determinations, though this is often difficult to do for any particular individual case. The European Union may move toward requiring the sponsor to consult with the investigator to determine a possible causality. If there is disagreement between the sponsor and investigator, then the submitted SUSAR should contain both causalities. Other clarifications include requirements for reporting SUSARs from third countries, the handling of fatal or life-threatening SAEs, reporting to ethics committees, and informing the investigators. In other words, we may see significant clarifications and changes in European Union requirements.

Postmarketing

This legislation came into effect in early 2011 and must be put into national law in each member state by mid to late 2012 though some parts may come into effect in 2011. Some of the things that will change include:

- Fees for pharmacovigilance ranging from €6000 to €72000
- Creation of a PV System Master File which is a detailed description of the PV system used by the MAH and kept on site for inspections
- Electronic submission of PSURs and their storage in a repository
- Single point of reporting to EudraVigilance replacing the complex current system
- Changes in responsibilities for the MAH including more emphasis on off label use, more rapid notification of the CA of any new information on the benefit/risk analysis and any prohibitions or restrictions anywhere in the world, reporting results (good and bad) from all studies anywhere in the world
- Replacement of the CHMP working party with the PV Risk Assessment Committee with membership from member states as well as outside healthcare professionals and patients

- Stronger legal basis for postauthorization Safety Studies (PASS)
- Creation of "conditional" MAs with requirements for postauthorization studies, additional reporting observations, restrictions on use, required postauthorization efficacy studies
- Risk Management Plans for all products subject to inspections by the CA and made available to the public
- Submission of all serious ADRs within 15 days and all non-serious EU ADRs within 90 days. This will include overdoses and medication errors
- Creation of a European Medicines Safety Web Portal with much safety information made public for more transparency: PSURs will be made public
- Changes in the SPC (labeling) with an executive summary in a black bordered box, new text to be bolded for a year, statement that intensive monitoring is underway (where appropriate), use of a symbol like the black triangle for drugs with issues
- QPPVs in each member state (if that state so desires)
- PSURs changed into a benefit-risk analysis not just a safety document. No PSURs required for "low risk" products
- Possible disappearance of Volume 9A

All of this will clearly evolve over the next couple of years. Each member state may handle the items somewhat differently. As noted in various places in this manual, this is a changing target and how it plays out remains to be seen.

■ Frequently Asked Questions

Q: Is it likely that the European Union, the United States, and the rest of the world will "settle down" and stabilize their rules and regulations anytime soon?

A: Probably not. There are several factors at work. First, the entire world of drug safety and risk management is in a state of flux. New technology and regulations are being put in place as a result of many influences, including:

- Consumer awareness
- Political pressures and globalization
- Economic pressures and outsourcing
- Changes in the structure of HAs (e.g., the European Union may expand beyond its current 27 members)

- The evolution of the theory of drug safety, including data mining
- The response to some major drug safety issues in the United States and European Union (e.g., Vioxx)
- Guidelines from international organizations (CIOMS, ICH)
- The emergence of active PV in many other countries outside North America and Europe, including India, China, Brazil, Australia, and others.

It is not clear that collective, global organizations will be any more effective in drug safety as they are in limiting arms proliferation, wars, or climate change.

Q: Does one need to know any other languages besides English if one is doing PV?

A: A delicate question. Obviously, in countries where English is not the official language, one must know the language of that country. Often, some documents, cover letters, local cases, e-mails, and other requirements must be prepared in the local language. In addition, governmental officials, patients, healthcare workers, and company employees are more comfortable in their native language. Having said that, the "official" language of drug safety is English (as much as there can be an official language) and nearly all international documents (e.g., PSURs) are done in English. At a high level and on the international scene (ICH, WHO, CIOMS), the main, or often only, business language is English. Thus, one can often survive rather well knowing only English, but more opportunities are available for those with linguistic skills.

23

The Qualified Person for Pharmacovigilance

For companies with products sold in the European Union, Volume 9A requires that there be a "Qualified Person for Pharmacovigilance" (QPPV or QP). This is a critical role and function within the company and is discussed in detail. The concept of a QP is most interesting. A named individual (and backup) takes corporate and personal responsibility for the functioning of drug safety and pharmacovigilance (PV) for every company that has a Marketing Authorization (MA) in the European Union. There is no direct counterpart in the United States, Canada, or most other countries. This position functions at the European Union level. Some European Union member states also have a national QP (sometimes called by a different title) with similar obligations and responsibilities for that country. This person may or may not also function as the European Union-level QP. The position and requirements are defined in Volume 9A Section 1.2. The QP must be designated (and thus a PV system in place) at the time of submission of an MA. Note that the QP is not responsible for manufacturing issues. There is a separate QP for manufacturing.

Volume 9A notes that:

- Each company must "submit a description of the pharmacovigilance system and proof that the services of a Qualified Person Responsible for Pharmacovigilance (QPPV) are in place."

- The MAH should have permanently and continuously at his disposal a QPPV residing in the European Union or EEA with 24/7 availability.

- One QPPV per system in a company. There should be a qualified deputy also residing in the European Union/EEA. Name and contact information registered with EMEA/member states.

- Some member states require a named person/national QP too. This person may or may not be the same as the European Union QPPV.

- The QPPV should be appropriately qualified,

with documented experience in all aspects of pharmacovigilance. If the QPPV is not medically qualified (i.e., an MD), access to a medically qualified person should be available.

- The QPPV has multiple responsibilities:
  - Establishing and maintaining/managing the MAH's pharmacovigilance
    - Ensuring that all SARs (including literature searches) are collected, collated, and accessible at least at one point within the European Union
    - Ensuring that there is a Detailed Description of PV Systems in place
    - Preparation of ICSRs (PSURs) and company-sponsored postauthorization safety studies (PASS)
    - Continuous overall pharmacovigilance evaluation during the postauthorization period
    - Ensuring that any request from the health agency is answered fully and promptly
  - The QPPV should have oversight of the PV system in terms of structure and performance to ensure the following system components and processes:
    - Establishment and maintenance of a system ensuring that all SARs are collected, collated, and accessible at least at one point within the European Union.
    - Preparation of ICSRs, PSURs, and company-sponsored postauthorization safety studies (PASS)
    - Continuous overall pharmacovigilance evaluation during the postauthorization period
    - Ensuring that any request from the Competent Authorities for additional information is answered fully and promptly, including the provision of information about the volume of sales or prescriptions, benefits and risks, and postauthorization studies
  - Oversight of MAH's PV system includes:
    - Quality control and assurance procedures.
    - SOPs.
    - Database operations.
    - Contractual arrangements.
    - Compliance data (e.g., quality, completeness, and timeliness for expedited reporting and PSURs), audit reports, and PV personnel training.
    - The QPPV and deputy must have a written job description and CV on file.
- MAH Responsibilities:
  - Support the QPPV and ensure appropriate processes, resources, communication mechanisms, and access to all sources of relevant information in place for the QPPV.
  - Ensure full documentation of all procedures and activities of the QPPV.
  - Implement mechanisms for the QPPV to be kept informed of emerging safety and risk-benefit issues including clinical trials and contractual agreements.
  - Ensure the QPPV has the authority to implement changes to the MAH's PV system to maintain compliance.
  - Ensure the QPPV has input into Risk Management Plans and the preparation of regulatory action in response to emerging safety concerns (e.g., variations, urgent safety restrictions, and, as appropriate, communication to patients and healthcare professionals).
  - Ensure the presence of back-up procedures (e.g., in case of non-availability of personnel, AE database failure, failure of other hardware or software with impact on electronic reporting and data analysis).
  - MAH may transfer PV, including the role of the QPPV, to another person or organization.
  - The ultimate responsibility for all PV obligations always resides with the MAH.
  - A detailed and clear documented contract must be in place for this.
  - The contracted person or organization should implement QA/QC and allow auditing by the MAH.

■ Practicalities

The QPPV is a responsible and difficult position. The person must be involved and have real influence in the safety system of the company. He or she must be knowledgeable and able to discuss, at least at a high level, particularly during a governmental inspection, the PV system in place globally, including standard operating procedures (SOPs); working documents; quality assessment/quality control (QA/QC); databases in use for drug safety, privacy, and security issues; all products marketed in the European Union/European Economic Area (European Union/EEA) and where they are sold outside Europe; global licensing; distribution; comarketing; agency agreements; compliance status and key performance indicators (metrics); signal identification; analysis and workup mechanisms in place; specific signals and safety issues pending globally; the risk management system and business continuity/crisis management plans in place; postmarketing trials under way, and new indication trials for marketed drugs; safety training; and issues with health authorities (HAs).

He or she must review and sign Periodic Safety Update Report (PSURs) and other documents submitted to HAs. To succeed in this position, communication is critical—with management, drug safety, the rest of the organization, European Medicines Agency (EMA) and member state HAs, deputy and national QPPVs, and so forth. There must be a formal job description, and many companies also have a formal, written contract with the QPPV. The person, usually a medical doctor (MD), should have senior management's ear.

Many companies, particularly small companies and generic houses, will outsource the QPPV to a Clinical Research Organization (CRO) or consultant. Although this is legal and feasible, the company and the QP must take the job seriously. Some QPs at CROs may be doing this function for 15 or more clients! Whether this is practical and wise is debatable. All delegation, both within the company and outsourced, must be rigidly and carefully documented. The specific delegated functions must be written down and all parties must sign off. Note that all companies with MAs must have a QPPV. This includes generics, over-the-counter products, and so forth. No exceptions.

■ Frequent QP Inspection Findings by the EMA

No QPPV or interim measures (change of QPPV, backup procedures for absence, etc.)

More than one QPPV

Not resident in European Union/EEA

No job description

Failure to notify Competent Authorities of QPPV details

Lack of 24/7 coverage

Inadequate oversight of the pharmacovigilance system (ICSRs, PSURs, PASS, safety profile of products, audits, SOPs, database)

Lack of training or experience

Did not ensure training of drug safety staff

Roles and responsibilities not formally defined (especially important if parts of role are delegated)

Inadequate access to medically qualified personnel.

Penalties can be severe and can include fines of up to 5% of the MAH's European Union sales, with further penalties if the problems are not corrected. Civil and criminal penalties for MAH and QPPV possible.

■ Frequently Asked Questions

Q: Why would anyone want to do this job?

A: Good question, and I'm not sure I have a good answer. Perhaps a combination of responsibility, power, the desire to have a meaningful job that makes an impact, a good salary (though some say they could never be paid enough to do this job), visibility, and the like. For people who like and accept being empowered (and who really are empowered), and who like playing a fascinating role with interactions in all areas and in all levels of the company and with health authorities, this can be a marvelous job. Until something bad happens. Then the stress level rises and it truly becomes a 24/7 job, particularly in the age of the internet, with instant communications and media knowledge of problems.

Q: What do I do if I am QP but not empowered and cannot get management to act on the appropriate needs, resources, and safety issues?

A: Quit. First, do your utmost to convince management that this is serious business and certain things must be done. You may need to get allies to make the case (e.g., the regulatory and legal colleagues in the company or an outside auditor). Point out the key sections from Volume 9A. Document fully in writing everything you have done and everyone notified, all items, actions, resources, and so forth, that you have requested, plus the responses. Always do and say the right thing and document it. Give it a reasonable attempt and length of time to get actions and corrections. It helps to have a forceful type-A personality. If all fails, update your CV and get a new job. You'll sleep better and your gastric acid and blood pressure will return to normal.

United Kingdom Medicines and Healthcare Products Regulatory Agency (MHRA)

The United Kingdom Medicines and Healthcare Products Regulatory Agency (MHRA) is the Competent Authority that handles medicinal products, blood products, advanced therapy products (gene therapy, somatic cell therapy, and tissue-engineered products), and devices for the United Kingdom (England, Wales, Scotland, Northern Ireland). Under the chief executive are five divisions. One, the Vigilance Risk Management of Medicines (VRMMM) Division, primarily handles drug safety matters. Device safety is handled by the Device Technology and Safety Division, inspections by the Inspection, Enforcement and Standards Division, and new approvals by the Licensing Division.

As the United Kingdom is a member of the European Union, safety and pharmacovigilance (PV) are also handled centrally by the European Medicines Agency (EMA) (see Chapter 22). Thus, the United Kingdom operates under Volume 9A and Volume 10 for postmarketing and clinical trial safety as well as the core Directive 2001/83/EC, amended by Directives 2002/98/EC, 2003/63/EC, 2004/24/EC, and 2004/27/EC.

The MHRA has an extensive website (Web Resource 24-1).

The "Medicines" section (Web Resource 24-2) covers drugs, homeopathics, herbals, and licensing (Marketing Authorizations), inspections, names, pediatric medications, labeling, and other topics.

The "Safety" section covers warnings, alerts, and recalls, and has sections for reporting AEs (the Yellow Card Scheme), product-specific advice, and information for healthcare professionals. Drug safety is monitored by multiple methods, including regular (and directed) inspections of manufacturers and suppliers, distributors and storage, clinical trials, laboratories, Notified Bodies (organizations—often private companies—authorized to provide various services, including safety reviews, design examinations, and other aspects of devices in the European Union), and blood establishments. The MHRA also collects reports of AEs via its Yellow Card Scheme, examines advertising, labeling, and promotional material, and can commission research on safety. The MHRA also manages the General Practice Research Database (GPRD) (see Chapter 8).

■ The Yellow Card Scheme

For marketed drug products, the United Kingdom relies on the voluntary spontaneous reporting of AEs by healthcare professionals and consumers as most other countries do. (Industry reporting of AEs is obligatory.) The system is known as the Yellow Card Scheme and is run by the MHRA and the Commission on Human Medicines. The system receives reports of suspected adverse drug reactions (ADRs) from healthcare professionals and consumers/patients. The system was started in 1964, and the original form was a "yellow card."

Patients are encouraged to report all side effects (Web Resource 24-3) while healthcare professionals (Web Resource 24-4) are instructed to report all suspected ADRs on new medicines (which are identified by a black triangle [▲] on the label [see below]) and only serious ADRs for established medicines. This is in contrast to many health authorities (HAs), which instruct healthcare professionals to report all AEs. Reporting may be done online, by downloading the form, filling it in and mailing it, or by e-mailing it to one of several centers around the country. The form is rather simple (and is similar to the MedWatch and CIOMS I forms) and requests data on the patient, the reaction (including its seriousness and outcome), comedications and other relevant information, and the reporter–clinician details. The site contains some basic information on what an ADR is and how to evaluate causality, though the MHRA notes that the healthcare professional should report "if you have the slightest suspicion that there might be an association…do not refrain from reporting simply because you are not certain about cause and effect."

The data from the Yellow Cards are entered into the MHRA's ADR database and used for analysis and signal evaluation. Much of the data from the database is available directly online as "Drug Analysis Printouts" (Web Resource 24-5) (see Chapter 8 and the section below).

■ Black Triangle Products [▲]

Newly approved drugs (usually a new chemical entity, but an older drug if it has a new combination of actives, a new delivery system, a new indication, or a new patient population) are noted by a black triangle. All new biologics have a black triangle. Older drugs, which were black triangle drugs and which moved out of that category but which move back into it ("reinstated") due to new information or a new indication or population, are asterisked: *

The goal is to alert the prescriber and user that this is a new product whose safety profile is not as complete as established drugs and to more intensively monitor and collect safety information. It appears on advertising material. A product will stay on the list for 2 years as a rule but may remain on longer if appropriate. Industry is requested to report all serious cases from the United Kingdom and European Union (not just those not appearing in the Summary of Product Characteristics [SPC] labeling). Black triangle drugs are listed on the website.

■ Regulations

The legislation, guidances, and directives covering drug safety are available through links on the PV Regulatory page of the MHRA website (Web Resource 24-6):

Clinical trials:
- European Union:
  - Directive 2001/83/EC Title IX Articles 101 to 108
  - European Commission guideline on the collection, verification and presentation of adverse reaction reports arising from clinical trials on medicinal products for human use
  - European Commission guideline on the European database of suspected unexpected serious adverse reactions (EudraVigilance-Clinical Trial Module)
  - Volume 10 of Notice to Applicants
- United Kingdom:
  - The Medicines for Human Use (Clinical Trials) Regulations 2004 (SI 2004 no. 1031)

Postmarketing:
- European Union:
  - Directive 2001/83/EC Title IX Articles 101 to 108 PV requirements; Title XI Articles 111, 116 and 117 and Directive 2010/84/EU
  - Regulation (EC) No 726/2004 Title II Ch. 3 Articles 21 to 29 Pharmacovigilance requirements; Title II Ch. 2 Articles 16 to 20 Supervision and Sanctions; Title IV Ch. 1 Article 57 Duties of the EMEA Commission Regulation 540/95: Reporting of non-serious unexpected adverse reactions

- Regulation (EC) No 1394/2007 Specific pharmacovigilance requirements for advanced therapy medicinal products
- Directive 2004/27/EC (amending Directive 2001/83/EC) (external link) and Regulation (EC) No 726/2004
- Volume 9A of Notice to Applicants (the key document for PV)
- United Kingdom:
  - See the United Kingdom regulatory website page: Web Resource 24-6.
  - See also the book published by the MHRA: Good Pharmacovigilance Practice Guide. See below.

The agency puts out a consolidated listing (some 200-plus pages) of its regulations. See Web Resource 24-7.

■ Inspections

The MHRA does extensive PV inspections (Web Resource 24-8). This topic is reviewed in detail in Chapter 48.

■ Pharmaceutical Industry Page: A One-Stop Resource

The MHRA has a page on its website that contains links and key information for the industry on all aspects of drug regulation (Web Resource 24-9). It covers "news and hot topics" as well as how to contact the MHRA, legislation and regulations, clinical trial information, safety and PV and others.

Each major link then goes to a more detailed industry page. The Safety and PV Page (Web Resource 24-10) covers

- Reporting of ADRs/ICSRs. Note that this must be done electronically. Paper submissions are no longer accepted.
- E2B reporting.
- Anonymized single Patient Reports. These are reports received by the MHRA and sent to MAH via an MHRA portal.
- ADR reports received by the MHRA from the medical literature.
- Legislation and guidance.
- Periodic Safety Update Reports (PSURs): Details on how to do them.
- Inspections and good PV practices.

- Defective medicines.
- Letters to healthcare professionals.
- Drug Analysis Prints (see below).

■ Drug Analysis Prints (DAPs)

Drug Analysis Prints are a unique and valuable feature in the world of drug safety. As of this writing, the only other governmental health agency that makes information from its safety database available easily is Health Canada (see Chapter 25). DAPs are listings of ADR reports made to the MHRA from healthcare practitioners and patients via the Yellow Card Scheme. Medicines are listed alphabetically by the name of the active ingredient (not by brand name). See Web Resource 24-11.

The reports are static (not done in real time) but are updated frequently. The reports are immediately available as downloadable PDF files. They are available online and for no charge. Although listings are by active ingredient, the brand names, if reported in the case, are included in the listings. Combo drugs are also included.

The first page shows the drug name, the date the report was run, the period covered (many reports have data starting in the early 1960s), the MedDRA version, the report types (usually spontaneous), the region the reports came from (usually the United Kingdom only), the total number of reactions, the total number of reports (less than the reactions as multiple reactions may be recorded in a single report), the number of fatal reports, and the brand name of products in the report.

The next page is a summary table of the number of reports, broken down by MedDRA SOC for single constituent drug, combination drugs, and total reports. Fatal reports are also listed.

The following pages then give a more detailed breakdown of each SOC down to the Higher Level Term (HLT) and Preferred Term level.

Commonly used products or older drugs may have many thousands of reports (e.g., the cimetidine DAP at this writing has nearly 5400 ADR reports of more than 7700 reactions, of which 96 were fatal).

There is a page that gives the background information about DAPs and describes the limitations of these data. The limitations of spontaneous data are clearly noted: the likelihood (probability, rate, frequency, odds, etc.) cannot be known from these data; causality cannot be judged as these cases are submitted based only on a suspicion of causality (attributability). A natural or chance event cannot be distinguished from a reaction due to the drug or the underlying disease. The comparison of risks between and among medicines cannot be done by looking at the numbers in the DAPs.

Nonetheless, these reports are invaluable in signaling, risk management, PSUR preparation, safety analyses (both for one's own drugs or competitors' products), and getting an overview of safety for a class of drugs.

■ Providing SAE Cases to MA Holders

Anonymized Single Patient Reports from the MHRA are sent to Marketing Authorization (MA) holders. The cases will go to MA holders of the brand if the brand is identified in the case. If the drug is only identified as the active ingredient, all MA holders for that product will receive the case. If the drug is identified at the active substance level, every company holding an MA for the suspected active substance will receive the case. See Web Resource 24-12.

■ E-mail Alerting Service

The MHRA maintains a large number of free e-mail alerts covering a wide range of topics related to all areas of drugs and the MHRA (including job vacancies and conference information) (Web Resource 24-13). For drug safety in particular, the following are available and well worth subscribing to:

■ New items
■ Press releases
■ Drug alerts
■ Safety warnings and messages for medicines
■ Drug safety update
■ Herbal medicine safety news
■ Inspection updates on Good Clinical Practices (GCP), Good Pharmacovigilance Practices (GPVP)
■ Device vigilance

■ Reporting AEs in the United Kingdom

The requirements for reporting AEs, both in clinical trials and for marketed drugs, are similar to requirements in the rest of the European Union and the United States.

That is, clinical trial expedited reports (7- and 15-day) are required as are postmarketing expedited reports (15-day reports). PSURs are required for marketed products. This is different from the U.S. situation, in which New Drug Application (NDA) Periodic Reports (PADERS) or PSURs are allowed, though the United States will move to PSURs (differing somewhat from the European Union PSUR) at some point. Annual reporting of clinical trials is required, though this too differs from the United States (see Chapter 15).

Risk management follows the European Union Risk Management Plan, which differs from the U.S. REMS (see Chapter 30).

■ Good Pharmacovigilance Practice Guide Publication ("The Purple Book")

The reporting requirements, concepts of PV, best practices, recommendations, and details of pharmacovigilance in the United Kingdom are summarized in a superb 200-page book written by the MHRA and published by Pharmaceutical Press. Everyone involved in PV, whether or not they have dealings in the United Kingdom, should read this book. It is intended to be updated periodically. It is known as the "purple book" because of its bright purple cover.

Good Pharmacovigilance Practice Guide. Author: Medicines and Healthcare Products Regulatory Agency (MHRA). Pharmaceutical Press, London and Chicago, 2009. Information available from Web Resource 24-14.

■ Comments

The United Kingdom MHRA is now, as many will say, the best (and some would say the most rigorous, or "toughest") drug regulatory agency in the world. Their regulations and publications are clear, well written, and easily available on their website. The personnel are available for discussions with all stakeholders. Their PV inspections are rigorous, scrupulous, and thorough. Unlike most other agencies around the world, the MHRA makes its safety data easily and freely available to everyone.

Health Canada/
Santé Canada

Health Canada is the federal department in the Canadian government responsible for health matters, including pharmacovigilance. Their remit includes foods, drugs, devices, and many other areas well summarized in an extensive index on their website (Web Resource 25-1), which is fully available in both English and French.

The section "Drugs & Health Products" is also extensive. Canadian Product Monographs are available on the Drug Product Database. The areas that touch on drug safety include "Advisories, Warnings & Recalls," "Compliance & Enforcement," "Drug Products," and "MedEffect Canada" (adverse reactions).

The drug products section includes information on drugs marketed in Canada. Some Summary Basis of Decision (which contain some safety information) documents are available.

The major section on drug safety is the "MedEffect Canada" section (Web Resource 25-2). This section contains information on the voluntary reporting of adverse reactions by consumers and healthcare professionals and the mandatory submission by Marketing Authorization (MA) holders (manufacturers and distributors). Reports from consumers and healthcare professionals may be submitted directly online by filling out a report on the website or by downloading and mailing or faxing the form to a Canada Vigilance Regional Office (there are seven such offices as well as the national center in Ottawa). MA holders must mail or fax reports to the Canada Vigilance National Office in Ottawa.

There is a Q&A section on adverse reactions describing how drug safety is done in Canada (Web Resource 25-3). As in other countries, the foundation for pharmacovigilance is the collection of adverse drug reactions (ADRs) from consumers and healthcare professionals by the seven regional and national adverse reaction centers. Each center performs an initial quality review for transmission and analysis at the national center.

Reporting requirements are summarized in a guidance for Industry on AR reporting (Web Resource 25-4). Expedited reporting for serious ADRs is obligatory for MAHs in Canada. All serious ADRs from Canada and all serious, unexpected ADRs from outside of Canada must be reported within 15 days. A formal annual review of ADRs and serious ADRs must be done and submitted within 30 days of request from Health Canada. Periodic Safety Update Reports (PSURs) are not obligatory but may become so soon. Further detail is available in this guidance.

Signals are identified by a systematic review of the reports and any other information available to Health Canada. The database (see below) is relatively small, and Health Canada is working on initiatives to partner with external agencies with larger databases (e.g., the U.S. Food and Drug Administration).

Inspections are handled by the Health Products and Food Branch Inspectorate, whose goal and function is outlined in a document available on the website (Web Resource 25-5). Inspections are done of manufacturers of pharmaceuticals and biologics and cover Good Manufacturing Practice (GMP) or pharmacovigilance activities. Two ratings are issued following an inspection: (1) C—No objectionable conditions or practices or (2) NC—Objectionable conditions or practices found. A report will be issued with observations. The inspected establishment is expected to correct the deficiencies. When necessary, enforcement actions will be made by Health Canada. From September 2005 to March 2008, 309 inspections were performed in Canada.

Risk management (Web Resource 25-6) plans are being developed in Health Canada. Interim implementation occurred in 2009. This guidance calls for risk management plans in the European Union RMP format, though the U.S. REMS format may be used in some cases. It is expected that formal requirements along the lines of the European Union and U.S. risk management systems will come into effect in Canada within the next few years.

Data from the Canada Vigilance Adverse Reaction Online Database is available free (Web Resource 25-7). This unique service covers data in the Canadian adverse reaction database and is updated four times a year. The information is 3 months behind. After reading the instructions and agreeing to the terms and conditions, one can either do an online search or obtain data extract files in a zip file. The online search allows selection by date, seriousness (type of report, e.g., misuse, spontaneous), gender, outcome, age range, brand or active ingredient name, and AR term (MedDRA). The results are immediate. Cases are from Canada only. Results give a line listing of AR number, MA number, date received, age, gender, drug name, and AR codes. Data may be exported or saved.

The summary of the regulations and guidances in force is available at Web Resource 25-8. Clinical trial and Good Clinical Practices (GCP) regulations and guidances are also available (Web Resource 25-9). The major findings (227 out of 354 findings) were for issues in reporting domestic and foreign ADRs within 15 days. Plans are under way to expand the inspections outside of Canada.

■ E-mail Notifications and RSS Feeds

Health Canada has several publications and new safety information available via free e-mail subscriptions or via RSS feeds, such as the MedEffect e-Notice and the MedEffect Canada RSS Feeds (Web Resource 25-10). The Canadian Adverse Reaction Newsletter (CARN) is also available via these subscriptions. Available in English and French.

26

Australia Therapeutic Goods Administration (TGA)

The Therapeutic Goods Administration (TGA), located near Canberra, is charged with drug and device safety for Australia.

■ AE Reporting

The reporting of adverse events (AEs) in Australia is similar to that in other developed countries. Consumers and patients are encouraged to report AEs to a telephone hotline (1300 134 237) operated by the National Prescribing Service, a nonprofit, independent organization funded by the Australian government. Reports are forwarded to the Therapeutic Goods Administration (TGA). Alternatively, reports may be sent by mail, fax, or e-mail using the "Blue Card" (Web Resource 26-1) similar to the United Kingdom's Yellow Card Scheme. Device information is also available at Web Resource 26-2.

Using the Blue Card, within 15 days sponsors must report all serious reaction cases for prescription drugs that are spontaneous or from company-sponsored Australian postmarketing studies (whether expected or not) that occurred in Australia. All other spontaneous cases from Australia are reported in the Periodic Safety Update Report (PSUR). Ex-Australia cases are not required to be reported unless there is a significant safety issue or action that has arisen from any analysis of foreign reports or that has been taken by a foreign regulatory agency, including the basis for such action. Such reports must be submitted within 72 hours. The TGA also requires that sponsors be able to provide promptly to the TGA clinical details of any foreign adverse drug reactions reports. For over-the-counter (OTC) drugs, the sponsor must report serious reactions that occurred in Australia within 15 days. A summary guideline is available at Web Resource 26-3, and a complete guideline at Web Resource 26-4. There is also a guideline from 2003 on postmarketing surveillance studies (Web Resource 26-5).

Clinical trial guidelines are also available based on the European Union document from 1995, at Web Resource 26-6. There are several other guidances available on all aspects of clinical trials (Web Resource 26-7).

Many European Union guidelines (including directives and regulations) have been adopted in Australia. However, there is a specific disclaimer that such guidelines when relating to prescription medicines are not so adopted (Web Resource 26-8):

Please Note: Where European Union guidelines adopted in Australia include references to European Union legislation (including EC Directives and Regulations), the requirements contained in the referenced European Union legislation are not applicable to the evaluation of prescription medicines by the TGA. The Australian legislative requirements applying to prescription medicines are contained in the Therapeutic Goods Act 1989 and the Therapeutic Goods Regulations 1990, as well as in various legislative instruments such as Therapeutic Goods Orders, Notices and Determinations, see Legislation (Web Resource 26-9).

■ Risk Management

In terms of risk management, the TGA has adopted the European Union Volume 9A Risk Management Plan concept and format. Not all products require an RMP. Those that do are new chemical entities, significant extensions of indications, extensions to pediatric populations, and changes that result in different dosage forms, treatment populations, or changes in the safety profile of a drug. The TGA can request an RMP at any time for an already marketed product. Further details are available at Web Resource 26-10.

The website also lists safety alerts and advisory statements (Web Resource 26-11).

Free subscription to e-mail alerts from the TGA regarding medicine safety is available at Web Resource 26-12. There is also a separate subscription for device information.

The TGA has international agreements with their counterparts in Canada, Europe, Singapore, Switzerland, the United Kingdom, and the United States.

The Uppsala Monitoring Centre

The Uppsala Monitoring Centre (UMC), in addition to maintaining three databases (Vigibase, WHO Drug Dictionary Enhanced, and WHO-ART; see Chapter 14) also provides many services in pharmacovigilance and has done much seminal work in drug safety.

■ WHO Programme for International Drug Monitoring

The UMC is responsible for the WHO Programme for International Drug Monitoring (Web Resource 27-1). This program consists of a network of about 98 National Drug Safety Centers, the WHO in Geneva, and the UMC in Sweden. Its functions include:

- Identification and analysis (including use of data mining) of new adverse reaction signals from the case report information submitted to the national centers, and sent from them to the WHO ICSR database.

- Information exchange between WHO and national

centers, mainly through "Vigimed," an e-mail information exchange system.

- Publication of periodical newsletters (WHO Pharmaceuticals Newsletter and Uppsala Reports), guidelines, and books in the pharmacovigilance and risk management area.

- Supply of tools for management of clinical information, including adverse drug reaction case reports. The main products are the WHO Drug Dictionary and the WHO Adverse Reaction Terminology.

- Training and consulting support to national centers and countries establishing pharmacovigilance systems.

- Computer software for case report management, designed to suit the needs of national centers (VigiFlow).

- Annual meetings for representatives of national centers, at which scientific and organizational matters are discussed.

- Methodological research for the development of pharmacovigilance as a science.

- The UMC has also published many important scientific articles in pharmacovigilance.

■ Publications

Multiple publications are available from the UMC website. Some are free, others are not. Some are published in multiple languages besides English. See Web Resource 27-2.

- UMC Bibliography
- UMC Posters
- Viewpoint: Watching for safer medicines
    - Part 1: Issues, controversies, and science in the search for safer and more rational use of medicines
    - Part 2: International collaboration, research, and resources for the safer and more rational use of medicines
- Guidelines for setting up and running a pharmacovigilance center
- Uppsala Reports: Published several times a year and available free electronically
- Writing on Pharmacovigilance: Selected articles by David J. Finney

- Effective Communications in Pharmacovigilance
- Dialogue in Pharmacovigilance
- Expecting the Worst: Crisis Management
- Pharmacovigilance in Focus
- The Importance of Pharmacovigilance
- The Safety of Medicines in Public Health Programmes
- WHO Pharmaceuticals Newsletter
- Pharmacovigilance: Ensuring the safe use of medicines

The UMC also has multiple conferences and training sessions throughout the year and is heavily involved in drug safety outreach to underdeveloped and developing countries.

The UMC has played a major role in the development and propagation of the concepts and techniques of pharmacovigilance. For many years, it was a lone voice. It has now been joined by others to advance the field of pharmacovigilance. The key publications on its website are well worth reviewing.

28

Data Privacy and Security

Approximately 30 or so years ago, with the advent of enormous changes in communication, personal computers, and medicine and society (greater mobility, the ascent of specialists and subspecialists in medicine), personal privacy and limiting of access to data began to appear as a new and major issue in medicine. With the internet and identity theft, the question of who has access to what data is now in the forefront of people's and governments' minds.

For many years, medical data were believed to be the property of the treating physician or hospital, and they were kept confidential by those parties. In the United States, Europe, and elsewhere, there was no right to privacy as defined by law, and sometimes patients were denied the right to obtain or even see their own medical records. The law that was in place in the United States was state law, which varied from state to state, offering inconsistent levels of protection. Similarly, in Europe and elsewhere, laws were national or local, such as they were.

That viewpoint has largely changed, and a person's health data are now believed to be owned by that individual. There are now clear limitations on what third parties (physicians, hospitals, companies, and governments) can and cannot do with the data. In the United States, the federal government has enacted laws on privacy. The European Union now has rules and regulations that cover all member states (some of which have put forth additional and tougher privacy and security protections). Canada, Australia, Japan, and other countries have also tightened their privacy protections.

For the purposes of drug safety and pharmacovigilance, two major governmental acts, worth studying in detail, largely represent the state of privacy around the world: the U.S. Health Insurance Portability and Accountability Act (HIPAA) and the European Union (EU) Data Privacy Directive. In addition, a brief look at Canada's and Japan's privacy laws are presented. They are reviewed here and the implications and effects on drug safety are discussed.

■ United States Health Insurance Portability and Accountability Act (HIPAA)

Unlike the European Union, the United States does not have one global law for data privacy and security. Rather, different parts, or "sectors," of the country have different approaches. The healthcare sector is covered at the federal level by the Health Insurance Portability and Accountability Act (HIPAA) as well as various other state and local laws, regulations, and court cases. The final HIPAA rule went into effect at the end of 2000.

The regulations cover health plans, healthcare clearinghouses, and those healthcare providers ("covered entities") who conduct certain financial and administrative transactions with paper or electronically. All medical records and other individually identifiable health information held or disclosed by a covered entity in any form, whether communicated electronically, on paper, or orally, are covered. Title I covers healthcare access, portability, and renewability of insurance. Title II requires national standards for electronic healthcare transactions and covers privacy, security, and unique identifiers (National Provider Identifier). Further information on HIPAA can be found on the HHS website (Web Resource 28-1), some of which (the privacy and security features) are summarized here:

- Patient education on privacy protections. Providers and health plans are required to give patients a clear written explanation of how they can use, keep, and disclose their health information.
- Ensuring patients' access to their medical records. Patients must be able to see and get copies of their records and request changes and corrections. In addition, a history of most disclosures must be made accessible to patients.
- Getting patient consent to release information. Patients' authorization to disclose information must be obtained before sharing their information for treatment, payment, and healthcare operations purposes. In addition, specific patient consent must be obtained for other uses, such as releasing information to financial institutions determining mortgages, selling mailing lists to interested parties such as life insurers, or disclosing information for marketing purposes by third parties (e.g., drug companies).
- Consent must not be coerced.
- Providing recourse if privacy protections are violated.
- Providing the minimum amount of information necessary. Disclosures of information must be limited to the minimum necessary for the purpose of the disclosure.

Covered entities are held to the following requirements:

- Adopt written privacy procedures. These must include who has access to protected information, how it will be used within the entity, and when the information would or would not be disclosed to others. They must also take steps to ensure that their business associates protect the privacy of health information.
- Train employees and designate a privacy officer. Covered entities must provide sufficient training so that their employees understand the new privacy protections procedures, and designate an individual to be responsible for ensuring the procedures are followed.
- Establish grievance processes. Covered entities must provide a means for patients to make inquiries or complaints regarding the privacy of their records.
- Psychotherapy. Psychotherapy notes (used only by a psychotherapist) are held to a higher standard of protection because they are not part of the medical record and are never intended to be shared with anyone else.
- Penalties. Failure to comply may lead to civil or criminal penalties, including fines and imprisonment.

Information may be released in the following circumstances:

- Oversight of the healthcare system, including quality assurance activities
- Public health
- Research approved by a privacy board or institutional review board
- Judicial and administrative proceedings
- Certain law enforcement activities
- Emergency circumstances
- Identification of the body of a deceased person or the cause of death
- Activities related to national defense and security

This regulation clearly has implications for pharmacovigilance. Much discussion occurred and the Food and

Drug Administration (FDA) ultimately issued a clarification of the issue.

The FDA fully recognized that pharmaceutical companies are required by law and regulation to maintain databases of adverse events occurring in individuals who have taken their products, reported by health professionals. The data identify the person making the report and may or may not identify the individual. The data come both from clinical trials of new products and from the postmarketing data of drugs already on the market.

Although in such data there is often no specific patient identification (e.g., name and address), there may be sufficient patient data such that it would be possible in many cases, with only minimal effort, to identify the patient based on the known data (e.g., hospital, dates of hospitalization, age or birth date, patient initials, sex, diagnosis, treatment, and hospital course). These data are often required to be submitted to health authorities and are necessary for clinical and epidemiologic evaluation of the adverse event and safety profile of the drug. It is vitally important to know that certain events occur in special populations (e.g., only in children, females, or the elderly). There is a broad consensus in the industry and in the health authorities that these data are vital for maintaining and protecting public health. Removal of these demographic data would make the data much less useful for safety and epidemiologic analyses. Identification of safety problems occurring with both new and old drugs would suffer if the flow of these data were hindered.

The FDA addressed this in the March 2005 Guidance for Industry: Good Pharmacovigilance Practices and Pharmacoepidemiologic Assessment (see Web Resource 28-2). The FDA notes: "It is of critical importance to protect patients and their privacy during the generation of safety data and the development of risk minimization action plans. During all risk assessment and risk minimization activities, sponsors must comply with applicable regulatory requirements involving human subjects research and patient privacy."

It is also clear that "covered entities," such as pharmacists, physicians, or hospitals, are permitted to report AEs without problem from HIPAA. The FDA notes: "The Privacy Rule specifically permits covered entities to report adverse events and other information related to the quality, effectiveness, and safety of FDA-regulated products both to manufacturers and directly to FDA (45CFR164.512(b)(1)(i) and (iii), and 45CFR164.512(a)(1))." See Web Resource 28-3.

In various subsequent initiatives and documents, FDA has reiterated its commitment to protecting privacy.

See, for instance, the Sentinel Initiative (Web Resource 28-4), in which the commissioner notes that all safety safeguards and requirements must be followed in this new drug safety strategy.

Thus, there is a broad understanding that drug safety data may be reported to manufacturers (sponsors) and to the FDA.

■ The European Union and the Privacy Directive

The European Union's approach to privacy is somewhat different from that of the United States. The United States does not really have the equivalent of the pan-European protections that exist in the European Union, where a key directive (95/46) covers data protection and privacy.

In October 1995, the European Commission proposed "Directive 95/46/EC on the protection of individuals with regard to the processing of personal data and on the free movement of such data." All member states in the European Union implemented local laws and regulations covering the contents of this directive. These laws and regulations vary from country to country, and some are stronger (more protective of privacy) than the directive itself. It has had an impact on drug safety, although less than originally feared. A full analysis and history of this effort is well beyond the scope of this book. A brief summary is put forth here, and reference to the directive and various websites is provided. The directive can be found at Web Resource 28-5.

A good summary of the European Union Privacy Directive 95/46 can be found at the website of the European Commission in multiple languages (Web Resource 28-6) including English.

The directive covers all personal data, whether electronic or on paper, and is not limited to health information but broadly covers all other areas of personal data including trade union, cultural, financial, credit card, criminal, and so forth. The directive refers to the "processing" of personal data. Processing refers to "any operation...which is performed...such as collection, recording, organization, storage, adaptation or alteration, retrieval, consultation, use, disclosure by transmission, dissemination...."

Data may not be processed except in the following circumstances:

- The person in question has given consent.
- The processing is necessary for the performance of a contract.

- The processing is necessary to meet a legal obligation.

- The processing is needed to protect the vital interests of the person in question.

- The processing is needed to carry out a task that is in the public interest or is done in exercise of official authority.

Personal data can only be processed for specified explicit and legitimate purposes and may not be processed further in a way incompatible with those purposes. The person (European Union citizen) in question has the right to be informed when his or her data are processed. The person has the right to see all the data processed about him or her as well as the right to changes and corrections to incorrect or incomplete data. The data must be accurate and relevant to the purpose they are collected for, should not contain more information than is necessary, and should not be kept longer than necessary. The person may object at any time to the processing of personal data for direct marketing.

Data may not be transferred to a third country where there is an inadequate level of data protection. The United States is not considered to have adequate levels of protection for European Union data. There are various methods available to transfer data to the United States that meet European Union requirements. See the European Union's data protection page (Web Resource 28-7). A company may implement practices that are consistent with European Union requirements. Another way is the "Safe Harbor."

■ Safe Harbor

Since the United States and the European Union have different approaches to data protection and privacy and the European Union does not feel the American system is adequate, it was necessary to create a mechanism for the United States and the European Union to allow data exchange. To resolve this, the United States and the European Union agreed on the so-called Safe Harbor mechanism. It is under the jurisdiction of the U.S. Department of Commerce (Web Resource 28-8).

The Safe Harbor framework claims to be a simpler and cheaper means of complying with European Union Directive 95/46 than other methods. The Safe Harbor is voluntary for U.S. organizations and is self-certifying. U.S. organizations and companies can join a privacy program that adheres to the requirements or develop their own. There are seven requirements:

- Notice: Organizations must notify individuals about why they collect personal data.

- Transfers to a third party: Organizations can transfer data to a third party if the third party is in the Safe Harbor or is subject to the European Union directive.

- Access: Individuals must be able to access and correct, amend, or delete inaccurate information.

- Security: Organizations must take reasonable precautions to protect data from loss, misuse, disclosure, alternation, destruction, and unauthorized access.

- Data integrity: Personal data must be relevant for the purposes for which it is to be used.

- Enforcement: There must be a mechanism for an individual to have recourse for complaints or issues. There must be procedures to verify that the company is following the safe harbor requirements, and there must be a means to remedy issues.

If companies wish to participate officially in the Safe Harbor program, they must register with the U.S. Department of Commerce. See the website noted above for further information. Many companies establish policies to comply with the European Union directive but do not formally register with the U.S. Department of Commerce. In practice, not many companies have registered and some of the companies that did register failed to comply with the requirements. See one study of the situation (Web Resource 28-9).

Different companies, industries, and countries are approaching data protection and privacy differently. Research (both clinical and epidemiologic) has been affected and "work-arounds" developed. Most large companies in the United States now have "privacy officers" as counterparts to some degree of the European Union-mandated "data controllers." Companies and agencies transmitting data should check with their appropriate personnel to ensure that all privacy and data protection requirements are met. And they should probably recheck periodically because this is a moving target as the requirements change periodically.

In practice, the data protection and privacy acts in the United States, the European Union, and member states have fortunately not had a major effect on pharmacovigilance and signaling. The practical steps that have occurred are as follows:

- MedWatch, CIOMS I, and other paper and electronic means of data and their transmission are "anonymized" or "de-identified" in regard to the patient and the reporter. That is, any information that might allow the reader to identify the patient is removed. This includes patient initials, date of birth (age is okay, however), locale of birth (country is okay but city and postal code are usually not), specifics such as the name of the hospital and date of admission, personal numbers such as telephone or health insurance numbers, and so forth. The reporter is similarly not named but rather his or her occupation is noted (e.g., consumer, physician, pharmacist, healthcare professional, attorney).

■ Attachments such as medical records, laboratory reports, procedure or surgical reports, and autopsy or death certificates must have all identifying information removed or obliterated. This can be tedious and time-consuming but nevertheless must be done. For example, if a multipage narrative report refers to the patient by name in several places and in the headers and footers, all such identifiers must be removed or obliterated.

■ Case report forms (either paper or electronic) and E2B transmissions sent to the drug safety department must also be carefully anonymized, at least concerning the patient information. The reporter information (such as the investigator) may be sent in some cases, because this is part of the clinical trial and agreed to by the investigator.

■ Nonanonymized data may, in general, move within an European Union country or between European Union countries because these countries have (in theory at least) adequate data protection. It is the movement outside the European Union that has caused this concern with the United States. However, some issues of lost personal computers, flash drives, and other security issues in the European Union itself have resulted in many countries rethinking data privacy. Hackers are also periodically attacking various computer systems in Europe, the United States, and elsewhere.

■ Some European Union countries have even more strict data protection rules and laws than the European Union directive, and this makes follow-up and data collection more difficult.

■ The issue of U.S. data's leaving the United States and going to the European Union or elsewhere has not been a significant issue. In general, precautions taken for data entering the United States have been adopted for data leaving the United States. It is generally easier for an organization to treat all data in the same fashion and not make exceptions or "one-offs" for some countries' data.

■ The privacy and confidentiality of MedWatch reporting are protected under U.S. law.

■ Various other requirements for data security and protection, such as electronic signatures, closed systems, and other technical requirements are addressed in various regulations and requirements (including 21CFR11). These are beyond the scope of this manual.

■ New levels of complexity and concern have arisen with the fragmentation and outsourcing of many company functions, including safety. For example, data may be processed in Europe, the United States, and elsewhere. Call centers may be in Mumbai while the servers sit in Latin America. All data, no matter where they sit or are processed, must meet all the appropriate criteria.

■ Canada

At the national level, privacy is protected under the 1983 Privacy Act, which covers how the federal government deals with personal information of Canadians. This act, along with the Personal Information Protection and Electronic Documents Act (PIPEDA), are the basic laws covering the federal government. Each province and territory also has its own privacy legislation. PIPEDA also applies to commercial activities (the private sector) unless a specific exemption is obtained. There is a Privacy Commissioner for Canada (Web Resource 28-10).

Health Canada has addressed information privacy and confidentiality in a policy from 2005 entitled the "Pan-Canadian Health Information Privacy and Confidentiality Framework" (Web Resource 28-11). This document and policy, along with the laws noted above and the Canadian Charter of Rights and Freedoms, are aimed at ensuring data security and privacy at the federal and provincial levels. The provisions are similar to those in the documents above covering the United States and Europe and include privacy of data, notification of the individual of the use or disclosure of information, recourse, consent for certain uses, access of the individual to his or her data, and so forth. As with other measures, however, some uses are allowed without the consent of the individual, including certain forms of research, if disclosure will eliminate or reduce a significant risk of serious harm to a person or group of persons, or if the disclosure is authorized by a governmental enactment.

Pharmacovigilance information relating to the identity of the patient or the reporter that is obtained via MedEffect (Canada's pharmacovigilance system) is protected under the Privacy Act and cannot be made public.

■ Japan

In 2003, the government promulgated the Personal Information Protection Act (PIPA) to cover handling and transmitting personal information and data. Its scope is wide, covering the national and local governments as well as most companies and people.

Any entity handling personal data must

- Clearly specify the purpose for collecting and using the data.
- Obtain the data through legal and fair means, that is, not through fraud or other improper means.
- Ensure the security of the data from loss and unauthorized access or disclosure.
- Notify the subject whose data are held of the purpose for which the data will be used.

- Avoid supplying the data to third parties without prior consent from the person whose data are involved except in certain circumstances.
- Allow for correction and additional data as well as deletion of incorrect data.
- Respond to complaints and requests from the person whose information is in question.
- Companies must have a system to handle data change, alteration, and correction.

Penalties for breaking the law include fines and imprisonment.

Q: This is rather complex. How should companies handle this?

A: Clearly internal expertise must be in place to cover and protect data and patients in all jurisdictions involved If the company cannot handle this internally, external assistance must be used. There is little tolerance, by both governments and individuals, for breaches in data privacy and protection. In addition, attention must be paid to external vendors (e.g., server parks, archiving companies) who also handle the data.

29

The Roles and Interactions of Companies, Governments, Nongovernmental Organizations (NGOs), and Others in the World of Pharmacovigilance

There are many players in the world of pharmacovigilance. The interactions are complex. Alliances are formed and severed as issues or interests change. The groups are active in various causes in the medical and pharmaceutical world, touching not just on safety but on healthcare costs, drug prices, and healthcare availability.

Patients who take medicines and suffer from adverse events (AEs) are the first and primary group involved in drug safety. Healthcare professionals make up the next category and include those who prescribe, sell, or dispense medications and those who must also help deal with the AEs. Other participants in the medical world include pharmaceutical companies, pharmacies, pharmacy/formulation committees (in hospitals, insurance companies, and other institutions in the United States and elsewhere), and drug benefit managers (in the United States) and others who decide which medications are made available or reimbursed and which are not.

Patients suffer the consequences of adverse drug reactions directly and personally, sometimes suffering dearly or even dying. Patients and their families are becoming more sophisticated and research drugs and treatments they take or will take on the internet and through social media, websites, and elsewhere. Some sites and sources, of course, are far more accurate and unbiased than others. Yet patient perceptions are quite variable. Sometimes there may be a perception that every AE that occurs is due to the drug, and, at other times, there is not a real awareness or level of suspicion by the patient that a particular problem could be due to one or more drugs. Many patients believe that if the government agency has approved the drug for marketing it is "safe and effective," using this "buzzword" phrase. This is an unfortunate phrase since it implies absolutes—totally safe and always effective—when in fact its meaning is rather more like: this product has benefits that outweigh the risks (sometimes not by much) when used by the approved patient group, at the approved dosage and route of administration, for the approved length of time; safety is not absolute or guaranteed and is not (ever) fully known, and some patients may have totally unexpected (idiosyncratic) bad side effects. This concept is hard to convey.

It is often presumed (sometimes incorrectly) that a drug cannot produce an adverse reaction if it has been taken safely for months or even years. Drug–drug, drug–food, and drug–alcohol interactions, manufacturing issues, and so on are almost never thought of by patients as explanations of their problem. Patients often do not think of over-the-counter (OTC) products, "health foods," "nutraceuticals," or "herbals" (which may contain drugs or interact with drugs), cosmetics, and illicit drugs as culprits in adverse reactions. Physicians too often forget to ask about them when taking the medical history and investigating medical problems. Many patients who are receiving multiple drugs, particularly the elderly, who are often "polypharmacy" patients, cannot recall the drugs or the doses they take. Moreover, when patients take multiple drugs, it is hard to know or predict drug interactions.

In some societies or cultures, there has been a perception that AEs are the fault of the patient and represent a weakness or a shameful act on the patient's part and that they need to "tough it out." This attitude is changing as the dissemination of information occurs, but is still seen in some older patients.

Healthcare practitioners prescribe, dispense, and administer drugs. When AEs or reactions occur, it may not be the same prescriber, dispenser, or administrator who has to deal with the drug's medical consequences. Emergency rooms may not be able to get immediate access to the patient's medical records or drug history, for example, though it is hoped this will change when and if electronic medical records become widespread.

■ The Pharmaceutical Companies

Pharmaceutical companies play a major role in the world of safety. In the United States, most AEs on marketed drugs are reported to the manufacturers; in other countries, most AEs may be reported to the health agency or other institutions (e.g., medical centers). The companies, through PhRMA and the EFPIA (see below) and the International Conference on Harmonization, have worked with the U.S. Food and Drug Administration (FDA), the European Medicines Agency (EMA), and Japanese regulators to harmonize the safety reporting procedures, requirements, formats, documents, and expectations. This effort has been very successful because the requirements for reporting certain serious AEs from clinical trials and postmarketing situations are clear, consistent, and quite rigorous (7 or 15 calendar days). Major efforts are under way, with varying degrees of harmonization and cooperation between the industry and government, in the areas of electronic transmission and standards (e.g., formats for transmission of healthcare documents, laboratory tests, cardiograms), risk management and minimization, clini-

cal trial standardization, and more. These efforts in regard to "mechanics and operations" may well go beyond the pharmaceutical industry as the FDA and the Department of Health and Human Services standardize the transmission of healthcare data among other entities (hospitals, doctors, pharmacies, laboratories, insurance companies, etc.) and produce significant additional benefits for the public. See HL7, CDISC, and other initiatives in Chapter 8. Most dealings between scientific personnel in the industry and the FDA, EMA, and other agencies are cordial and correct, with the goal of protecting the public health and helping each do his or her job more efficiently and more rapidly, given limited resources.

The reverse of this coin, however, is represented by controversies about specific medical products and safety issues. Some people (consumer groups in particular) believe there is too much cordiality and warmth between the regulators and the regulated, allowing the companies to "get away" with many things to increase profit at the expense of public health. They point out that people move from the government to industry (as in other regulated industries) and vice versa, like revolving doors. They claim that this may compromise the safety of the public because regulators will be hesitant to cross or oppose a company they may shortly wish to work for. There are clearly professional and medical differences between and within the companies and the industry. Many of these "battles" occur behind closed doors or through written (e-mail) or telephonic communications. Most of these communications are privileged and not available to the public.

Pharmaceutical companies play a major role by promoting their products to healthcare professionals and the public (direct-to-consumer advertising in the United States in particular). Sometimes the promotion is not balanced in the eyes of the FDA, and Warning Letters are sent to companies by the FDA's Division of Drug Marketing, Advertising, and Communications. See the Warning Letter section of the FDA's website at Web Resource 29-1. FDA and other health agencies are now struggling with social media in which drugs are publicized, criticized, and commented upon by users, providers, and companies on blogs, tweets, and Facebook without fair balance and often without attribution.

Physicians and other healthcare workers are also "detailed" by pharmaceutical representatives on products for their patients. The detail should contain balanced information and include the AE profile. The approved prescribing information should also be supplied.

■ Governments

In each country or region, there is, of course, the governmental agency or agencies that regulate medicines (the FDA, the EMA, the Medicines and Healthcare Products Regulatory Agency [MHRA], the Agence Française de Sécurité Sanitaire des Produits de Santé [AFSSAPS], etc.). In addition to the agency, its parent organization may exert significant control and pressure (in the United States the Department of Health and Human Services; in other countries the Ministry of Health or Parliament/National Assembly/Congress), and so forth. In the United States, Congress and other federal departments and agencies work in or provide healthcare and medications (e.g., Veterans Affairs, the armed forces, the Centers for Disease Control and Prevention, Medicare, Medicaid, and new agencies that will be created under the U.S. healthcare reform law passed in 2010 and coming into effect over the next several years), as do state/provincial and local health departments, including boards of health. Some countries separate drug safety from drug approval, and some countries, particularly in the European Union, have an overlay at the European level in addition to national- and local-level agencies. In addition, each country may have local institutions that handle various drug safety issues. In France, for example, more than 30 regional centers (often associated with academic/university medical centers) deal with postmarketing AEs.

Government entities involved directly or indirectly in drug safety are complex. In the United States, at the federal level, the executive cabinet-level (ministry-level) Department of Health and Human Services controls the FDA and other health-related agencies and entities. The U.S. Congress controls the budget for the FDA and has legislative oversight of FDA and other health matters. Other federal-level groups with major interests in healthcare and pharmaceuticals include the Veterans Administration, which maintains hospitals, clinics, and pharmacies; the U.S. armed forces, which also maintain hospitals clinics and pharmacies; and the National Institutes of Health, the National Cancer Institute, and the Centers for Disease Control and Prevention. Similar complexities may be seen in many countries around the world, depending on their level of centralization and federalism. Some countries (France in particular) have tight arrangements with academic medical centers in the world of drug safety.

At the state and local level in the United States, there are state and local health departments, Medicaid offices (the program that supplies healthcare to the indigent and certain others at the state level), and state budget and formulation offices. One of the recent controversies has been the push by state and local governments to aid consumers in importing prescription drugs from outside the United States.

Views on drug safety by all of the players may sometimes be simplistic and polarized, especially if they are conveyed in short sound bites. One may hear that the health authority should approve safe drugs only after careful and thorough study. Side effects, if any, should be mild, reversible, and of limited duration. Some supposedly neutral observers refuse to admit a drug to a formulary for cost reasons rather than for medical reasons and justify this with either lack of efficacy or increased safety concerns. Others believe that there should be no more than two or three products in any particular class of drugs because the me-too drugs add no value to the public health. Others disagree. Consumers often believe that, if any really bad side effects occur, someone (somewhere) should be made to pay. At the extreme end, some groups assume malevolence and ill will on the part of the drug companies, whose goal (they say) is only to make money, and helping the ill is a "side effect" of making profit. There are periodic reports of bribery or various illegal actions to get drugs sold, studied, or put on formularies. The FDA encourages whistle-blowers to come forth with information on bad behavior with the inducement of substantial monetary rewards. As rhetoric heats up, the science and clarity disappear.

The controversy and politics tends to cloud some of the very real areas of controversy and concern:

■ How much secrecy should be permitted in the competitive area of drug development and drug safety? How much transparency should there be?

■ What is the role of the industry in patient and healthcare professional education?

■ Is direct-to-consumer advertising a good or bad thing for the public and how does it play regarding drug safety?

■ Is a single-payer system for drugs a good or bad thing for drug safety, and is it too expensive?

■ Is the current drug safety system in the United States, the European Union, and elsewhere adequate?

■ Should the universities be more heavily involved? Should there be a single national formulary?

■ Should me-too drugs be limited? Is the WHO Model List of Essential Drugs (Web Resource 29-2) a good way to handle pharmaceuticals?

■ Should drug safety be separated from the drug agency that approves drugs, as the approvers would be hesitant to "admit" they might have approved a drug with safety issues that appear after marketing?

■ As healthcare is finite and demand infinite, how should rationing be done?

■ Should some level of drug imports by consumers from abroad be tolerated or even encouraged to save money? And how will quality be ensured?

■ How should OTC drug safety be handled? Are consumer reports without any healthcare professional worth collecting and how much effort should be expended in their analysis?

One positive outcome of the controversies of the last several years in drug safety is more availability and transparency of safety information by companies and governments. Detailed information on most clinical trials is now available online at governmental websites (Web Resource 29-3) as well as pharmaceutical companies' individual clinical trial sites.

Postmarketing adverse events are now appearing online or are available as files of variable user-friendliness. Health Canada's safety database is friendly and available for immediate online searching. The United Kingdom's MHRA makes Drug Analysis Prints available, summarizing a drug's cumulative safety profile for many years, and is also easy to use. The FDA puts quarterly files online for downloading (though they are not user-friendly). Anonymized line listings and individual MedWatch reports are available from the FDA for nominal fees or from private companies (for higher costs but with anonymity of the requester).

Much of the older and some of the current clinical trial data are largely proprietary and unavailable to the public or medical profession beyond what is in a drug's labeling, monograph, or record at clintrials.gov. The European Union puts summaries of approvals (EPARs) online, and the FDA has some Summary Bases of Approval (SBOAs) also available online. However, safety data are often limited.

Many countries (United States, United Kingdom) have Freedom of Information laws that allow anyone to obtain nonclassified and nonproprietary data for minimal cost. However, often one must know exactly what one is looking for. "Fishing expeditions" can be hard or not permitted.

Proposals in many countries aim to make far more data available online. The FDA is proposing for marketed products to provide "the public with online access to public information from AE reports about FDA-regulated products submitted to FDA, in a format that is search-able and allows users to generate summary reports of this information, including, if known and as applicable, the trade name and/or established name of the product, dosage, route of administration, description of the adverse event, and the health outcome."

Interestingly, for drugs still unapproved and in use in clinical trials, the FDA is proposing to "disclose relevant summary safety and effectiveness information from an investigational application, or from a pending marketing application" as well as "non-summary safety and effectiveness data from applications submitted to FDA." Whether these are "trial balloons" or changes that will actually be put in place remains to be seen (Web Resource 29-4).

The United Kingdom MHRA also has a freedom of information act and some safety information is available. Interestingly, unlike the U.S. government's published information, which is basically not subject to copyright, there is strict copyright control of information released: "The information below was supplied in response to a Freedom of Information Act request. It is the copyright of MHRA and/or a third party or parties, and is made available for personal use only. You may not sell, resell or otherwise use any information made available via the MHRA FOI Disclosure Log without prior agreement from the copyright holder." See information about "crown copyright" at Web Resource 29-5.

One public venue where differences are aired, often with full media coverage, is represented by public meetings of the FDA advisory committees and similar groups in other countries. See the FDA's website at Web Resource 29-6. See in particular the Drug Safety and Risk Management Advisory Committee (Web Resource 29-7). These are standing committees called by the FDA to discuss and recommend courses of action in controversial or unclear areas in which the agency wishes external advice. Members include the FDA and academia (but not industry). They receive, in advance, data from the FDA and the industry and then meet in public (usually) to discuss the issues involved. The companies are usually well represented in the audience and often make presentations. The discussions are usually scientific and technical but can become adversarial and even quite heated. Some sessions may be held behind closed doors and are not open to the public. Transcripts and presentations of the public sessions are often available shortly afterward on the FDA website. These sessions are often attended by media and Wall Street types when public companies' products are involved. Comments by the committees often influence stock prices of both the company whose drug is discussed and competitors' drugs whose sales might be threatened by a new drug. This is a good example of transparency in the world of pharmaceuticals.

Broadly speaking, professionals working in the drug safety area of government and industry tend to be more aligned and better able and motivated to share ideas than are professionals in other areas of the industry (research, marketing, legal, etc.), because they are less constrained by legal restrictions and by competitive issues. Sharing ideas about "what works" in drug safety, pharmacovigilance, and risk management is common and is seen particularly with operational issues (e.g., drug coding, conventions for the Medical Dictionary for Regulatory Activities coding of AEs). Proprietary drug-specific safety information is not shared. Such alignment and cooperation is now international and facilitated by the web. Data are now being shared on Facebook and other social media.

It is in everyone's interest for AEs to be sent to the FDA and other health authorities in a timely, complete, and correct manner. Companies do, in fact, want their competitors to have well-run and efficient safety departments so that the competition's AEs are sent to the health agencies in a timely and complete manner too!

The Media

The media, including social media, the internet (blogs, websites, RSS feeds, wikis, etc.), and old media (television, radio, newspapers), play active roles from all perspectives of the political and medical scene. This field is evolving, with the health agencies struggling to understand how to use the media themselves as well as how to regulate use by industry.

NGOs and Lobbies

Nongovernmental organizations (NGOs) play major roles in healthcare throughout the world, including the World Health Organization in drug policies and its affiliate, the Uppsala Monitoring Centre in Sweden, in drug safety, pandemics and other public health areas; various foundations that fund healthcare initiatives (e.g., the Gates Foundation); the Drug Safety Research Unit in the United Kingdom; and others.

Lobbies or professional organizations, NGOs from many domains (e.g., Pharmaceutical Research Manufacturers of America [PhRMA], European Federation of Pharmaceutical Industries and Associations (EFPIA), International Society of Pharmacoepidemiology, the Centers for Education and Research on Therapeutics, the American Association of Retired Persons), OTC drug manufacturers, generic manufacturers, hospital groups, vaccine manufacturers, device manufacturers, physician groups, nursing groups, pharmacy groups, consumer groups, disease groups, and advocacy groups, such as Public Citizen (Web Resource 29-8), also play roles in drug safety. The list is growing.

These groups often petition or file position papers to influence legislation, regulatory decisions, and perceptions at the local, state/provincial, and national levels as well as in litigation and in the media. The groups work from all parts of the spectrum, including some who strive to increase profits, speed up or slow down drug approval, and increase or decrease governmental oversight and regulation.

Industry Organizations

The industry organization for pharmaceutical companies in the United States is PhRMA (Web Resource 29-9), and in Europe it is the European Federation of Pharmaceutical Industries and Associations (EFPIA) (Web Resource 29-10). Not all companies are members, especially the smaller companies and those that do not do research. PhRMA, which is based in Washington, DC, has multiple functions, including lobbying for the industry's position on public issues and legislation, outreach to the public, assisting with patient assistance programs, and representing U.S. industry in the ICH. Its goal is to "encourage discovery of important new medicines for patients by pharmaceutical/biotechnology research companies." This is a highly political and controversial area.

The EFPIA is based in Brussels, with an office in Japan. The EFPIA includes national industry associations in Europe as well as pharma companies. Similar organizations exist in other countries and industry associations also exist for vaccines, OTCs, generics, and cosmetics.

In Canada, the industry association is known as Rx&D (Web Resource 29-11).

There are multiple other organizations representing OTC manufacturers, generic manufacturers, and device manufacturers that interact as well as groups representing physicians (American Medical Association in the United States), hospitals (American Hospital Association in the United States), nurses, insurance companies, and so forth. The permutations and combinations of interactions are many, complex, and growing, as groups sometimes work with one another and sometimes against one another. As attributed to Benjamin Disraeli, "There are no permanent allies, no permanent friends, only permanent interests."

Litigation, Lawyers, and Legalities

Litigation plays a major role in safety decisions made regarding drugs in some countries, particularly the United

States. Any significant episode of AEs produces a flurry of lawsuits, often numbering in the thousands. They may take years to resolve, and costs run into the billions of dollars. The issues usually revolve around who in the company and sometimes in the government knew about the drug's toxicity, when it was known, whether it was adequately publicized and labeled, and whether remedial actions were taken in a timely fashion. In the United States (and other countries such as Canada and Italy) the phenomenon of "class action lawsuits" often plays a significant role in drug safety litigation. In these lawsuits, a group of people (sometimes a very large group) will sue a company or companies if their problems are similar. This groups many hundreds or thousands of people into one lawsuit.

To a large degree, litigation and the fear of litigation influences behavior in the drug safety world. Some companies are hesitant to admit in a report sent to the health authorities that their drug might have caused a particular serious AE. Such reports can be used in court cases against the company or against the reporting physician, nurse, pharmacist, and hospital, even if the report only notes the possibility of a causal relationship with the drug (e.g., "a causal relationship cannot be excluded," "possibly related," "probably related"). The United States is the major country where such issues occur, but hesitancy in commenting on causality may be seen in reports to health authorities outside the United States because these reports may be obtained and used in U.S. courts, especially if the reports are easily available in English (e.g., from the United Kingdom, Canada, Australia, New Zealand, Uppsala Monitoring Centre).

Workers in the field of pharmacovigilance should familiarize themselves with the rules (both written and "unwritten") about how much and what sort of statements and conclusions can be made in reports submitted to governments, kept in computers, or on file, and which are "discoverable" (that is, may be obtained by lawyers for use in court cases). If a drug safety case from a company has entered the legal system via a lawyer or lawsuit, the drug safety group will often have to work through the company's legal department to obtain follow-up information and to do its normal drug safety follow-up and due diligence. Some companies also have a legal review of all reports submitted to health authorities (e.g., E2B files, MedWatch and CIOMS I reports, PSURs).

Finally, drug safety personnel may be called on to testify in court and to give long and complex depositions either in individual cases that are on trial (e.g., malpractice, unexpected SAEs, or deaths) or in large lawsuits (such as class action suits in the United States),

particularly those following major drug withdrawals (Baycol, Vioxx, etc.).

Other Groups

Consumer groups, insurance companies, employers paying health insurance, health maintenance organizations, retired persons groups, and others also play roles, sometimes direct and sometimes indirect, in drug safety. Broadly speaking, many or all of these groups favor, to some degree or another, lower-cost (or even "free") drugs, limited formularies ("no need for me-too drugs"), generics, OTC status for many more drugs, and lessening the influence of pharmaceutical companies and increasing the role of regulators, without giving much thought to what this might do (both positively and negatively) to drug safety, or to other unintended consequences. In the United States, many of these groups have strong lobbies in Washington, DC, and at the state levels. Many similar groups exist outside the United States, but their activities and influence on the political systems do not appear to be as strong as in the United States. Nonetheless, the rise of the internet seems to be altering the balance and leveling the playing field to a significant degree.

Organizations for Drug Safety Personnel

There are several organizations that personnel working in the field of drug safety often join:

Drug Information Association (DIA)—The big international organization covers all areas of the drug world, with academia, industry, government, and others joining. They have annual meetings each year in the United States, Canada, Europe, and Asia. They run training programs, publish the DIA Journal, and have an extensive (though hard-to-navigate) website. Annual membership costs are nominal, and if one is joining only one organization, this is usually it (Web Resource 29-12).

International Society for Pharmacoepidemiology (ISPE)—The main organization for pharmacoepidemiology, including pharmacovigilance and risk management. Members are from industry, academia, government agencies, and nonprofit and for-profit private organizations. Members have degrees in a number of fields, including epidemiology, biostatistics, medicine, nursing, pharmacology, pharmacy, law, health economics, and journalism. They hold multiple meetings each year and publish the journal Pharmacoepidemiology and Drug Safety (Web Resource 29-13).

International Society of Pharmacovigilance (IsoP), originally formed as the European Society of Pharmacovigilance—An international nonprofit scientific organization to foster pharmacovigilance both scientifically and educationally and to enhance all aspects of the safe and proper use of medicines in all countries (Web Resource 29-14).

Regulatory Affairs Professionals Society (RAPS)—A global organization of regulatory professionals. A bit peripheral to drug safety, as they cover the full range of regulatory matters. They offer training and hold meetings and have publications of interest to drug safety personnel (Web Resource 29-15).

American Academy of Pharmaceutical Physicians (AAPP)—A global organization of physicians (MD, DO, MBBS, or equivalent degree) that studies drugs, biologics, devices, vaccines, diagnostics, and activities related to research, development, and regulation of these products. Somewhat peripheral to drug safety (Web Resource 29-16).

Pharmaceutical Information and Pharmacovigilance Association (PIPA)—A United Kingdom-based organization of pharmacovigilance professionals (Web Resource 29-17).

European Programme in Pharmacovigilance and Pharmacoepidemiology (Eu2P)—A new organization formed to establish a European private and academic partnership to meet training needs in pharmacovigilance and pharmacoepidemiology for specialists and nonspecialists (Web Resource 29-18).

Institute for Safe Medical Practices (ISMP)—A U.S. nonprofit organization devoted entirely to medication error prevention and safe medication use (Web Resource 29-19).

■ Conclusion and Comments

And finally, there are the unfortunate patients and sometimes unfortunate individual doctors, pharmacists, and nurses who deal on one-to-one levels and who must wade through the controversy, politics, and unclear and equivocal safety information ("the following AEs have been reported with this drug but causality cannot be determined") to come to good decisions for individual patients.

The bottom line is: drug safety is a high-stakes, multiparty, politicized, highly controversial affair with multiple players involved with multiple agendas and multiple millions of dollars, euros, yuan, rupees, and so forth. Data are often soft, incomplete, and skewed in one direction or another. One should look at multiple sources for information and keep an open mind on the ultimate outcome of safety issues with drugs. Usually the "truth will out," although it may take a long time.

■ Frequently Asked Questions

Q: So then how should the individual in the doctor's office, hospital, drug company, health agency, or elsewhere act? What can the individual do to help sort this out?

A: In general, act as a good scientist and citizen, an honest person, and do not judge until there is a good amount of evidence examined from multiple sides. Trust but verify. A good rule of thumb would be whether you or a loved one would take the product in question.

Company safety personnel should always act with the public health foremost in their mind and the company profits secondary. This may be difficult because there are always pressures to "protect the drug" or "hold off on this signal until the data are stronger." Safety workups and signaling should always be done with due diligence and an open mind. Sometimes those terrible-looking serious AEs really do melt away after all the data are in. When the results are bad for the drug, these data must be conveyed to management and to all involved health authorities in a timely and correct manner.

Practitioners, pharmacists, nurses, and patients should maintain a healthy skepticism regarding data, whether they are from the company, academia, the health authority, or the media—especially during the acute controversy when the "fog of war" is at its height and angry words, images, and charges are flying. They should seek out data from all sides and from neutral authorities (if such exist). Healthcare practitioners must always act in the best interest of the patient.

As a person rises in the company or governmental hierarchy in drug safety, the pressures increase as well. More money, more sales, more lives, more consequences (intended and unintended) are in play. This can clearly influence one's judgment in safety and medical matters even unintentionally. To quote the dictum of Lord Acton: "Power corrupts; absolute power corrupts absolutely." Another useful piece of wisdom is from the late Senator Daniel Patrick Moynihan: "Everyone is entitled to his own opinion, but not his own facts" (Web Resource 29-20).

Patients should find honest, caring health personnel and trust them to act in their best interest. Nonetheless, verification (looking at the approved drug labeling, looking on the internet at reliable sites, being treated at major or academic medical centers, etc.) is also well worth doing.

30

Risk: What Is It? Risk Management and Assessment, Risk Evaluation and Minimization Systems (REMS), and Risk Management Plans (RMPs)

Risk is a broad concept and applies to everything in life. We take risks when we drive a car, go to work, eat a meal, and take a drug. Risk analysis of drugs is now very much in vogue to aid the patient and healthcare professional, as well as the health authorities and drug companies, in decision-making. This chapter looks at risk first in a global manner and then as applied to drug therapy in the United States with Risk Management Minimization Systems (REMSs), and in the European Union with Risk Management Plans (RMPs). We are all working on the presumption that these new risk management systems and plans will decrease risk. This, in fact, remains to be seen. Most of the plans require some measure of outcomes and determination of whether risks and suffering have decreased. How this will play out remains to be seen.

Risk can be defined in many ways:

- Exposure to a possibility of loss or damage
- The quantitative or qualitative possibility of loss that considers both the probability that something will cause harm and the consequences of that something
- The probability of an adverse event's resulting from the use of a drug in the dose and manner prescribed or labeled, or from its use at a different dose or manner or in a patient or population for which the drug is not approved
- The exposure to loss of money as a result of changes in business conditions, the economy, the stock and bond markets, interest rates, foreign currency exchange rates, inflation, natural disasters, and war

Over the past 10 years or so, many in the pharmaceutical world (as elsewhere) have been thinking about risk assessment and management. Several documents on risk management have been produced by various groups. Early documents included U.S. Food and Drug Administration (FDA) draft guidances in 2003, ICH E2E

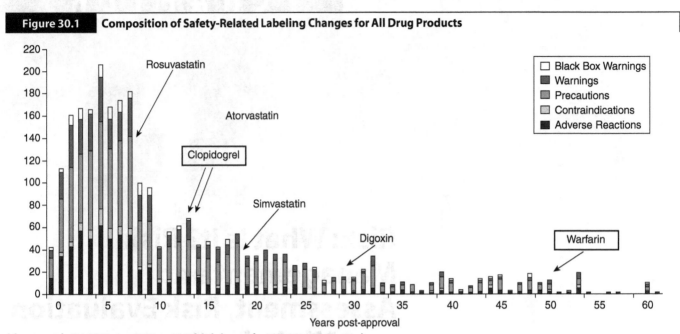

Figure 30.1   Composition of Safety-Related Labeling Changes for All Drug Products

(changes made Oct 2002–Aug 2005, n=2645 label changes for 1601 NDA/BLA entries)

Source: Modified from T Mullin, CDER, Office of Planning and Analysis, OTS presentation, May 2009 (http://www.fda.gov/downloads/Drugs/DevelopmentApprovalProcess/DevelopmentResources/DrugInteractionsLabeling/UCM205986.pdf).

(Web Resource 30-1), finalized in 2005, and a European Medicines Agency (EMA) risk management guidance also in 2005. Risk management during the life cycle of products is now the norm and is expected by FDA, EMA, and other agencies.

The FDA has looked back on labeling changes in the United States over several years and a striking finding is that safety label changes occur years and even decades after a drug has been approved as new safety issues are reported. For example, changes can occur at 50 or 60 years after approval even for such a commonly used and "well-known" drug as warfarin. Figure 30.1 from the FDA illustrates label changes occurring after drug approval.

■ Why Risk Management?

When a drug first reaches the market, its safety profile is not well characterized. Relatively few patients have been studied (especially with orphan drugs), and those who have been studied are usually patients with no other diseases, no or few comedications, not too young or old, with tight inclusion and exclusion criteria in the clinical trials. Thus, "real-world" patients have not taken the drug yet, and rare adverse drug reactions (ADRs) have not been detected. It is only in the postmarketing arena, when large numbers of patients have taken the drug, that the safety profile is better characterized. It is only when data on compliance, use in patients with comorbid conditions,

and multiple other drugs (including over-the-counter) and diets are examined that the real-world safety profile develops. In addition, data from overdose, suicide attempts, unintended pregnancies, and lactation will add to the profile.

Until recently, the primary way to collect such data was from spontaneous reporting systems and periodic aggregate reports (PADERs, Periodic Safety Update Reports, or PSURs, and their various predecessors) and occasional postmarketing studies. Risk management in a formal sense was not done.

Multiple drivers have come into play in pharmacovigilance and risk management:

■ Multiple major safety issues and withdrawals occurred: Fen-Phen, Propulsid, Rezulin, Vioxx, Bextra, Tysabri, Zelnorm, and others.

■ Rising liability costs from litigation and settlements.

■ The medical community was not happy with drug marketing and drug information.

■ ADRs were perceived to be a major health risk, producing death, hospitalization, and significant morbidity. A meta-analysis noted that in 1994 more than 2 million hospitalized patients had serious ADRs and more than 100,000 died, making this the fourth or fifth leading cause of death in the United States (Lazarou, Pomeranz, Corey, Incidence of ADRs in hospitalized patients. *JAMA*

1998;279:1200–1205). Other publications from around the world noted similar findings.

- A public and media perception that drug companies were villainous, greedy, and cared little for public health.

- The internet, bloggers, social media, and other forums' circulating stories, correct or not, on the harm of drugs.

- A perception that the regulators were not doing their job by allowing harmful drugs to reach the market too quickly.

- A perception that the agencies and industry were too closely aligned.

- Media stories highlighting gifts to physicians, slanted continuing medical education, paid speakers bureaus, and multiple conflicts of interest.

- In addition, recent economic issues have brought risk management of money, cars, offshore oil wells, pharmaceuticals, and many other activities in daily life into everyone's mind. One result has been that much of the world has become risk-averse (at least for now).

A consensus developed that risk prediction, evaluation, management, and minimization were not well understood and were rarely done and, when done, were done poorly. Better procedures for risk identification (signaling), characterization, mitigation/minimization, tracking, and communication were needed. And this was necessary for the entire life span of the product, not just after marketing. Companies and health agencies (and in some cases other organizations) needed to be proactive, collect more and better data, put it into electronic databases that were able to "talk to each other," and from which data could easily be extracted for risk evaluation. The benefit–risk analysis (called by the pessimists the risk–benefit analysis) needed to be done in a serious, quantitative, and reproducible manner. It was also understood that the benefit–risk situation will change over the course of a drug and may differ from patient to patient, group to group, indication to indication.

The goals then became:

- Early and better detection of ADRs and characterization of the risk in various patients and settings
- Development and harmonization of data standards and electronic transmission and storage
- Better communication of known and unknown risks
- Minimization of morbidity and mortality—protecting the public health

Many actions on many fronts have occurred already and more are under development. They are summarized below.

■ The FDA

The FDA first published a document on its thinking in May 1999, entitled "Managing the Risks from Medical Product Use and Creating a Risk Management Framework." It addressed pre- and postmarketing risk management and the FDA's role. Further publications have extended and elaborated the FDA's position.

The FDA has published three guidances for industry on risk management (see Chapters 30 and 31):

1. Premarketing Risk Assessment (Web Resource 30-2)
2. Development and Use of Risk Minimization Action Plans (RiskMAPs) (Web Resource 30-3)
3. Good Pharmacovigilance Practices and Pharmacoepidemiologic Assessment (Web Resource 30-4)

The first guidance, on premarketing risk assessment, focuses on measures companies might consider throughout all stages of clinical development of products. For example, a section on special safety considerations describes ways that risk assessment can be tailored for those products intended for use chronically or in children.

General recommended risk assessment strategies include long-term controlled safety studies, enrollment of diversified patient populations, and phase III trials with multiple-dose levels. Some key components of the guidance include:

- Providing specific recommendations to industry for improving the assessment and reporting of safety during drug development trials
- Improving the assessment of important safety issues during registration trials and providing best practices for analyzing and reporting data that are developed as a result of a careful preapproval safety evaluation
- Building on (but not superceding) a number of existing FDA and International Conference on Harmonization guidances related to preapproval safety assessments

The second guidance, on RiskMAPs, describes how industry can address specific risk-related goals and objectives. This guidance also suggests various tools to minimize the risks of drug and biologic products. This guidance has been superseded by a later FDA guidance on REMS (see below). Key components of the guidance include:

- Establishing consistent use and definition of terms and a conceptual framework for setting up specialized systems and processes to ensure product benefits exceed risks
- Broader input from patients, healthcare professionals, and the public when making recommendations about whether to initiate, revise, or end risk minimization interventions
- Evaluating RiskMAPs to ensure that risk minimization efforts are successful

The third guidance, on the postmarketing period, identifies recommended reporting and analytical practices to monitor the safety concerns and risks of medical products in general use. Some key components of this guidance include:

- Describing the role of pharmacovigilance in risk management. Pharmacovigilance refers to all observational postapproval scientific and data-gathering activities relating to the detection, assessment, and understanding of adverse events with the goals of identifying and preventing these events to the extent possible.
- Describing elements of good pharmacovigilance practice, from identifying and describing safety signals, through investigation of signals beyond case review, and interpreting signals in terms of risk.
- Describing development of pharmacovigilance plans to expedite the acquisition of new safety information for products with unusual safety signals.

In September 2007, with the passage of the Food and Drug Administration Amendments Act (FDAAA), the concept of the RiskMAP was superseded by the new REMS. FDA also produced a major new 5-year plan with multiple new initiatives (see Chapter 21).

The concepts behind this plan were that all products need full life cycle risk management, including older and already marketed products. In addition, some products (both new and old) may need specific REMS above and beyond routine postmarketing surveillance. The REMS must be tailored to the product and its known and unknown risks; it must be able to minimize risk in a measurable, quantifiable way; and it must be modified if the risks are not minimized. In addition, effective communication methods are to play a major role in REMS.

In September 2009, the FDA issued a major guidance entitled "Proposed Risk Evaluation and Mitigation Strategies (REMS), REMS Assessments, and Proposed REMS Modifications" (Web Resource 30-5). This important document, which has the REMS template, will be summarized here.

The FDA may require companies submitting New Drug Applications (NDAs), abbreviated New Drug Applications 58 (ANDAs), and biologics license applications (BLAs) to submit a REMS if FDA "determines that such a strategy is necessary to ensure that the benefits of the drug outweigh the risks of the drug." A company may voluntarily submit a proposed REMS if it believes that a REMS would be necessary to ensure that the benefits of the drug outweigh the risks. Companies that had RiskMAPS in place will continue with them and, in some cases, convert them to REMS with or without changes and additions.

The requirement for a REMS is enforceable by law, and if the person responsible for the drug (in the company) fails to comply, the drug is considered misbranded. Penalties of up to $1 million are possible for the first violation and may increase to $10 million for subsequent violations.

The content of a REMS is described. There are two major sections: (1) a proposed REMS and (2) a REMS supporting document (see the appendix).

■ The Proposed REMS

1. Table of Contents
2. Background: The REMS should describe the important risks (e.g., those seen in clinical and preclinical studies), risks seen with similar products or other drugs in the class, and risks expected with the underlying medical problem or disease (e.g., cancer seen with ulcerative colitis). It should also identify subgroups at risk (e.g., certain demographic groups such as the elderly or newborns) and if there are risks seen with similar products (e.g., bleeding with non-steroidal anti-inflammatory drugs [NSAIDs] or rhabdomyolysis with statins).
3. Goals: The goals and objectives of the REMS.

   The goal is a desired safety-related outcome or understanding by patients and providers. It should be clear and absolute, and aim to achieve maximum risk reduction. It should be pragmatic, specific, and measurable. Examples:
   - Patients on Y drug should be aware of the risks of rhabdomyolysis (measurable by the number of serious adverse events, or SAEs, of rhabdomyolysis).

- Patients on X drug should not also be prescribed Y drug (measurable by the number of patients receiving both drugs together).
- Fetal exposures to Z drug should not occur (measurable by the number of fetal exposures).

4. REMS Elements: The REMS may have one or more of the following:

- Medication Guide or Patient Package Insert (PPI)—This will be required if patient labeling could prevent SAEs, if the risks relative to the benefits could affect the patient's decision to use or continue using the drug, or if adherence to directions for use is crucial for effectiveness of the drug.
- Communication Plan to Healthcare Providers—This may be variable and include letters to healthcare providers, and information about REMS elements to encourage implementation or to explain certain safety requirements such as periodic laboratory tests.
- Elements to Assure Safe Use (ETASU)—These will be used if a medication guide and communication plan are not sufficient.
  - Prescribers have certain training experience or certification.
  - Facilities dispensing the drug are certified.
  - Drug is only dispensed to patients in certain settings (e.g., hospitals).
  - Drug is dispensed with documentation of safe-use conditions (e.g., laboratory tests).
  - Patients are subjected to monitoring.
  - Patients enroll in a patient registry.
- Implementation System—If included in the REMS, it should describe the system for implementing, monitoring, and evaluating the intended goals and effects.
- Timetable for Assessments—The assessments should be done no less frequently than at 18 months, 3 years, and 7 years after the REMS is approved.

5. REMS Assessment Plan: What will be done and measured to see whether the goals are achieved and what are the success criteria.

6. Other Relevant Information

Appendix: Supporting documents are included for each section above.

Comments

The goals of the REMS are to continually assess the benefit–risk balance and to ensure that it remains positive, if not globally, for all patients treated, than for some subsets. This may not be clear before marketing, but, where a REMS is required, the best effort must be put into designing a logical and thoughtful REMS, realizing it may change with experience gained after marketing.

Careful thought by a team knowledgeable about the disease and drug in question should work on the REMS. They need to evaluate the patients and disease to determine whether there are measurable early signs, symptoms, or markers that will allow a risk management intervention to prevent a bad outcome or SAE. This will require review of the data available for the drug and similar products, and an understanding of how the drug will be used in the "real world" and whether different populations from those in the clinical trials will be exposed to the drug. Obviously, much of this may not be known before marketing, making it necessary to change the REMS after marketing starts. The tricky question of off-label use (if anticipated) should be considered and possibly incorporated in the REMS.

Some specific examples of ETASUs:

- Prescribers have certain training experience or certification:

  The healthcare professional may be required to have particular training or skills to diagnose the condition being treated, understands the risks and benefits, and to have read the materials provided in the REMS and has particular skills and training to diagnose and treat particular ADRs associated with the product. Training may be by mail or online and should not be too costly to the provider.

- Facilities dispensing the drug are certified:

  This refers to pharmacies, practitioners, or healthcare facilities that may be required to understand the risks and benefits and to have read the materials provided in the REMS, to agree to dispense the drug only after receiving prior authorization, to agree to check lab values or to check for the presence of stickers that providers affix to prescriptions to indicate that the patient has met all criteria for receiving the product ("qualification stickers"), to agree to fill the prescription only within a specified period of time after the prescription is written, and to agree to fill prescriptions only from enrolled prescribers.

- Drug is only dispensed to patients in certain settings:

Settings may include hospitals or physicians' offices equipped to handle specific ADRs, such as allergic reactions or cardiopulmonary resuscitation.

- Drug is dispensed with documentation of safe-use conditions:

  This may refer to checking laboratory tests (e.g., for pregnancy, white blood cell count), receipt of educational materials and demonstration that the patient has understood the risks and benefits, verification by the pharmacy that labs have been checked, or the presence of a physician-qualifying sticker on the prescription.

- Patients be subjected to monitoring:

  Examples include lab tests monitored on a specified periodic basis and contacting the prescriber at specified times after starting treatment.

- Patients enroll in a patient registry:

  Drug access may be contingent on patient enrollment. Data collected may include clinical outcomes, clinical and laboratory data, safety information, compliance data, and impact of tools on ensuring compliance and outcomes.

- Other postmarketing actions may be taken, such as "enhanced surveillance" (often this is ill-defined and turns out to be just a bit more due diligence on spontaneously reported cases), targeted safety studies, Large Simple Safety Studies (LSSS), epidemiologic studies (e.g., comparative observational studies), and drug utilization studies.

- ETASUs should not be confused with postmarketing commitments (studies or other procedures promised to FDA after NDA approval and as a condition of the approval), which may or may not be part of a REMS.

Implementation System: Details may be required and include a description of the distribution system of the contents of the REMS and certification of wholesalers and distributors to ensure they comply. Examples of implementation methods include the maintenance of a validated database to track certified prescribers/dispensers, and periodic audits of pharmacies, practitioners, and others to ensure compliance with ETASUs. The assessments should be done at least at 18 months, 3 years, and 7 years. Changes along the way to improve the REMS are encouraged if the goals are not being met. All changes must be approved by the FDA.

Further details and an example of a mock REMS are found in the FDA draft guidance cited above.

REMS that are in place are available for review on FDA's website. This site is worth reviewing for anyone involved in REMS preparation or review. The drug name, date of REMS approval, and contents (as PDF files) are available (Web Resource 30-6).

As of this writing, the most REMS are limited only to medication guides. A few also have communication plans and a handful also have ETASUs. Some are rather extensive, such as the REMS developed by a joint FDA/industry working group on opioids (Web Resource 30-7).

■ Classwide REMS

Beginning in 2009, the FDA began requiring all products in certain classes of drugs to have REMS. The first group in this category was for botulinum toxin products, which had safety issues such as muscle weakness, loss of bladder control, and breathing problems. All such products are mandated to have a medication guide, communication plan, and a timetable for assessments, but there were no other ETASUs required. Other products with classwide REMS include testosterone gel drugs and extended-release oral opioid products. In addition, if a branded product has a REMS it is likely that the generic versions of the product will also require a REMS. The generic's REMS is often the same as that of the branded product. Sometimes all the companies producing a drug may work together on a single REMS, though this is not common.

REMS Template

As noted above, the template is available at "Proposed Risk Evaluation and Mitigation Strategies (REMS), REMS Assessments, and Proposed REMS Modifications" (Web Resource 30-5).

Comments

In theory, a REMS should be short, compact, and not burdensome on patient access or the healthcare delivery system. In practice, many are complex and must be designed with the European Union and other countries' risk requirements in mind. Ideally, a company would like to develop one risk plan for all markets, but the practicalities and requirements for local content often render this difficult or impossible. Nonetheless, REMS and risk plans need to be thought about throughout a product's life cycle by the appropriate personnel either inside the company or outside as consultants. Review of the publically available REMS should be done frequently.

There is a continuous and, for now, unresolvable debate that many companies go through when submitting a new drug/biologic approval (NDA/BLA). The question is whether one should offer up a REMS voluntarily or let FDA "force" one on the company. The case for a REMS up front and voluntarily is that, if it is good for the public health and the correct thing to do, it should be done without having to be told to do it. It will allow the company to prepare a thoughtful, reasonable, cost-effective program rather than finding out at the last moment (e.g., just before approval) that the FDA wants a REMS and perhaps an aggressive one that contains more than the company feels appropriate. Negotiations and research on REMS components at the last minute before approval in a pressured atmosphere where the company may feel obliged to commit to a large program just to get the drug on the market quickly is usually not a good idea. However, some companies are willing to take the risk and not propose REMS in the hope that the FDA won't require one. This avoids, from their point of view, unnecessary expense and effort. Others argue that the company should propose a REMS but that it should always be minimalist (e.g., just a medication guide and maybe a communication plan to the healthcare providers) to show "good faith" but not to "overcommit." The obvious answer to all of this is that one should do the right thing for the patients. It is also hoped that the company's and the health agencies' views on what constitutes an appropriate REMS will not differ too much. Unfortunately, the right thing is not always clear, and economics and politics often enter into the decision.

■ European Union Risk Management Plans (RMPs)

The fundamental documents establishing pharmacovigilance (PV) and RMP concepts for the European Union are Directive 2001/83/EC and Volume 9A. A guideline was published by the EMEA in 2005 and was based to a large degree on ICH E2E. It has since been incorporated in Volume 9A.

All companies must have a PV system. The PV system that a company maintains is different from a Risk Management Plan (or system), which is defined as a set of pharmacovigilance activities and interventions designed to identify, characterize, prevent, or minimize risks relating to medicinal products, including the assessment of the effectiveness of those interventions. For some or many drugs, the usual "routine" drug safety/PV activities (spontaneous reporting, PSURs, etc.) will suffice. For others, certain conditions or restrictions on supply or use of the product may be appropriate and required (for both centrally and nationally authorized products).

An RMP is a "set of pharmacovigilance activities and interventions designed to identify, characterize, prevent or minimize risks relating to medicinal products." The terminology becomes confusing as Volume 9A states: "The description of a risk management system should be submitted in the form of an European Union-RMP." This RMP has two parts: Part I is a safety specification and a PV plan, and Part II is an evaluation of the need or risk minimization activities and, if needed, nonroutine risk minimization activities, known as a risk minimization plan.

Part I is derived from ICH E2E and covers life cycle PV management. It includes a "safety specification," which is a "summary of the important identified risks of a medicinal product, important potential risks, and important missing information. It should also address the populations potentially at risk (where the product is likely to be used), and outstanding safety questions which warrant further investigation." See "The Safety Specification" below.

Part II represents a review by the Market Authorization (MA) holder to determine whether any of the risks of the product require additional "nonroutine" activities and which go beyond the usual PV system described above. If only routine risk minimization activities are required, then no RMP need be submitted. If yes, however, then the activities should be submitted in Part II. See the RMP below.

Bottom line: All drugs need a Risk Minimization System. This is summarized in Part I of the document and covers the usual and routine PV activities a company performs. If the MA (and health authorities) feels that more actions are needed to control risk for a particular product, then Part II (a Risk Minimization Plan) is submitted. Thus, all drugs need a Safety Specification and Risk Minimization System and some drugs need a Risk Minimization Plan.

■ When Is an RMP Needed?

At any point in a drug's life cycle, an RMP may be needed. The health authority and/or the MA applicant may determine an RMP is needed

- At the time of application for a new MA or a new active substance
- For "a similar biological medicinal product"
- For certain generic/hybrid products
- For an application for pediatric use
- For a significant change in marketing: new dosage form, new route of administration, new manufac-

turing process of a biotech product, significant new indication, new pediatric indication
- For certain other situations, including fixed combination products

The Safety Specification (Part I)
The Nonclinical Section

This section should include a discussion of findings not adequately addressed by clinical data, such as:

- Toxicity, including repeat-dose, reproductive and developmental toxicity, nephrotoxicity, hepatotoxicity, genotoxicity, carcinogenicity
- General pharmacology, including cardiovascular, QT prolongation, nervous system
- Drug interactions
- Discussion of the relevance to drug use in humans

The Clinical Section

This section should start with "limitations." That is, limitations

- Of the size of the safety database and the patients not studied due to inclusion/exclusion criteria in the clinical trials
- With regard to patients expected to be exposed to the drug after marketing
- Regarding the ability to detect infrequent ADRs
- In regard to finding long-term risks (e.g., cancer)
- Regarding populations not studied in the premarketing period (e.g., pediatric, pregnancy, comorbid conditions, more severe, subpopulations)

The next section covers clinical postmarketing experience (if any) and should address any information obtained from countries in which the drug has already been marketed. It should discuss exposure data (amount sold, use by particular populations such as children, market research information, etc.), as well as the actual way the drug is prescribed and used (off-label) compared with the approved labeling. This section should discuss any new safety concerns and whether any regulatory actions were taken for safety matters.

Risks that require further evaluation should be identified and discussed, in particular more frequent or more serious/severe ADRs. The possible mechanism, risk factors, risk groups, reversibility, and estimated frequency should be discussed.

Risk data, where available, should then be presented. This data should be study or epidemiologic data, which allows for quantitative risk estimation, including excess risk (vs. placebo and comparators), risk by various populations studied, time-to-event data (survival data), stratification by drug, placebo, age, gender, dose, and so forth.

If pharmacokinetic or pharmacodynamic interactions are suspected, any possible further studies should be detailed.

The impact of the key actual and potential risks should be addressed using strength of evidence, plausibility, nature of evidence, potential public health burden, morbidity, and mortality. Special attention should be paid to at-risk, susceptible patient groups. A structured format and classification by dose, time, and risk factors should be used.

The epidemiology, as known, should be discussed, including incidence, prevalence, mortality, and comorbidity with stratification by sex, age, race, ethnicity, and region (European Union in particular). Background incidence rates of the AEs in question should be included if possible.

The RMP should also discuss other risks where appropriate:

- Known or suspected class effects
- Potential for overdose, especially if there is a narrow therapeutic window
- Potential for transmission of infectious agents
- Potential for misuse for illegal purposes and what steps will be taken to limit misuse (e.g., added flavoring, dose pack size limit)
- Potential for off-label use, particularly pediatric use

Finally, a summary of identified and potential risks, missing information, and a PV plan should be included.

The PV Plan

The plan should propose actions to take in addition to usual safety reporting and signal detection:

- If no special concerns seen, routine PV is sufficient.
- If additional concerns, further activities should be done that can include (note that these are additional surveillance activities and are different from minimization actions [similar to U.S. ETASUs] noted below):

- Safety studies.

- Active surveillance (e.g., formal follow-up of patients filling a prescription for drug X with a survey and telephone contact later on).

- Sentinel sites of selected prescribers interviewed and medical record review.

- Intensive monitoring schemes where case data are collected from prescribers or hospitals on a specific drug or problem.

- Prescription event monitoring (especially the United Kingdom). Identify patients electronically and send follow-up questionnaires periodically to find course and outcome.

- Registries by drug, disease/outcome with follow-up questionnaires.

- Epidemiologic studies:

  - Comparative observational studies to validate signals—prospective or retrospective.

  - Cross-sectional studies or surveys to collect data on patients at a single point in time or over an interval regardless of exposure or disease status.

  - Cohort studies of a population on drug X at risk for a specific AE to be followed over time (prospectively or retrospectively) for the occurrence of that event, allowing the calculation of an incidence rate.

  - Case-control studies where patients with a specific AE already seen are selected and a control group without the AE also chosen. Exposure to the drug is then searched for.

  - Occurrence of disease studies of the specific AE to better characterize the patients at risk, the clinical course, and so forth.

  - Novel designs to be worked out with the health authorities.

- Clinical trials particularly with the subgroups at risk: children, elderly, and so forth.

- Large simple safety studies, or LSSS (randomized trial but minimal data collection and follow-up).

- Drug utilization studies of the marketing, prescribing, and use in a population and how this influences outcomes.

- Medication errors should be discussed if there is risk of such a problem.

Next, risk minimization activities (similar to the U.S. REMS ETASUs) should be detailed, and they may include one or more of the following:

- Providing information (Summary of Product Characteristics [SPC], Patient Leaflet, other)

- Additional educational material for patients, practitioners, and others that could include special training, use of checklists, or guides

- Restrictions on availability ("legal status change") with use only in hospitals or prescribing only by a specialist

- Controls at the pharmacy level

- Control of prescription size or time the prescription is valid

- Informed consent

- Restricted access

- Patient registries

- Special risk communication using other media for key messages.

Direct, periodic measurement of the effectiveness of the activities should be done by looking at measureable metrics, such as the incidence of a particular SAE or outcome, such as pregnancy with the drug in question or a survey of whether leaflets are actually read.

The PV plan must be a written document covering the safety concerns, objectives and rationale of the proposed actions, monitoring of the plan, and milestones for evaluation. After the HA(s) accept the RMP, periodic updates to the EMA or HAs should be done, usually in the PSURs.

The instructions for the Risk Management System and Plan are found in Volume 9A. There is a very specific and useful template that should be followed when preparing the document. The template is referenced in Volume 9A. A guidance describing the RMP (Guideline on Safety and Efficacy Follow-Up—Risk Management of Advanced Therapy Medicinal Products/November 20, 2008 Doc. Ref. EMEA/149995/2008) is found at Web Resource 30-8.

◼ Practicalities, Coordination, and Other Comments

Risk management strategies in the United States, European Union, and elsewhere have been in use in their current form for only a short time. U.S. REMS really began in earnest in April 2008 and the 18-month analyses are now under way. The instruction documents on risk management are guidances, not regulations, though they are functioning, de facto, as obligatory regulations. It is likely that, after review of their effectiveness, some changes in content and requirements will occur. The role of REMS, RMPs, and postmarketing commitments is also ill-defined and likely to be clarified over time.

There are significant differences between risk requirements in the United States and the European Union:

- In the United States, only some products will have a REMS. In the European Union, all new products and old products upon reapproval need some level of a risk plan.
- Formats and some content are different in the United States and European Union.
- Attention should be paid to local risks. That is, country- or region-specific risks should be addressed in the European Union and United States.
- In the European Union, the Qualified Person is clearly identified and has ownership of PV in a company. Ownership is less clear in the United States.

Although there is a large degree of overlap in the goals and content for risk plans in various jurisdictions (the United States, European Union, and Japan in particular), the format, timing, and implementation can be quite different. That is, there is not much harmonization yet. Companies and agencies are still debating how to use risk plans both strategically and tactically, and, to a degree, companies are debating how much to offer up voluntarily and how long to wait for a mandate from the HA. Evaluation groups are studying risk handling in the agencies in the United States, the European Union, and elsewhere. It is expected that updates and changes will be made in the United States and the European Union requirements. The reader should pay attention to new guidances and regulations from the FDA and European Union and member states, in particular to updates to Volume 9A. The European Union is expected to make significant changes in the next few years. Subscribing to the FDA's, European Union's, and other agencies' RSS feeds or e-mail alerts is free and worthwhile. Another good RSS feed to subscribe to is that of the European Federation of Pharmaceutical Industries and Associations (EFPIA) at http://www.efpia.org.

It is also hoped, perhaps less optimistically, that there will be international coordination and harmonization at some point to avoid duplication of efforts and excess use of limited resources. However, for many reasons, risks in one country may be quite different from those in other countries, and tailored country- or region-specific plans may still be needed.

■ Risk Management within Pharma Companies

As with most things in life, there is no single best way to do something (or if there is, it is never clear whose way is the best!). Broadly speaking, the fragmentation of risk evaluation at each stage of drug development has changed. For example, in the past it was often common for the clinical team to develop phase I trials based on preclinical data without significant input from the group handling later-stage development, marketing, and safety. Now, the tendency is to develop teams with broad cross-functional representation to meet periodically, evaluate the data to date, and outline broad and sometimes specific areas to be examined to evaluate and minimize risk.

In practice, this means several ways of doing business must change:

- There needs to be clear responsibility and governance in risk evaluation, minimization, management, and change management.
- Cross-functional risk teams with clearly delineated responsibilities need to be in place, need to be empowered, and need to act throughout the life cycle of the drug.
- The global players (or stakeholders) include senior management, pharmacology, toxicology, manufacturing, medical research teams, regional/affiliate/subsidiary personnel, legal, regulatory, finance, drug safety/PV, epidemiology, labeling, risk management (in the financial/insurance sense), marketing, sales, corporate communications, and so forth. That is, at some point, most if not all company groups will be involved in a large or small way. A smaller, practicable working group will usually need to be formed that reports periodically to a senior risk team.
- Tools and processes need to be developed so that each team in the company doing risk does not work "one-off" or ad hoc.
- Realistic budgets and personnel must be allocated. Resources will be needed for the team (operational and subject-matter experts), not all of whom will do "risk management" in addition to their day job, for data collection from external sources and databases, epidemiologists, surveys and drug utiliza-

tion studies, postmarketing commitments, external consultants, communication, and so forth.

- From the IT point of view, it will be necessary for all the data needed for the risk function to be easily accessible. This has broad implications in terms of normalization and standardization of data, timing of data preparation and delivery, accessibility and data security, operational planning, task and responsibility tracking, and planning. There should also be good tools available for signaling and document preparation. The agencies expect this and use these tools themselves.

- Quality management systems are an integral part of risk evaluation and management.

- Understand that for innovative companies and even generic and OTC houses, the old model of spontaneous reporting and PSURs is ending.

- Understand that health agencies talk to one other and that a company cannot say one thing to one agency and another thing (or nothing) to another agency. The world is becoming more risk-averse and more and more will be asked for in terms of risk management.

- Agencies are doing inspections, looking at postmarketing safety commitments and REMS/RMPs in addition to the classic PV inspection. Commitments must be taken seriously.

- Expect that all safety problems and data will become public rapidly both through the formal outlets (release of data by health agencies) and by the blogosphere and social media.

- The world is flat and global. A core risk plan should be developed that will be moldable and thus useful throughout all jurisdictions.

Many of the large multinational pharmaceutical companies and CROs are now investing heavily in setting up large, international structures and teams to handle risk, REMs, RMPs, and the like.

■ Comments and Suggestions

- Determine whether your company can handle risk management internally. If not, outsource the function but realize that this is not turnkey. The pharma company must maintain clear and continuous oversight and input into the vendor's actions.

- Create a risk function in the company with a designated chief and team. It may not be a full-time task

for the participants but the function is now absolutely necessary.

- Understand that "lack of evidence is not evidence of lack." That is, risks and safety data will accrue over time. The drug's best profile is on the day of launch. It is "downhill" from there.

- Do periodic (e.g., yearly) internal audits of the risk and PV functions.

- Prepare and keep up-to-date a risk plan using the European Union and U.S. template and E2E principles, which is then tailored as necessary to national or regional requirements. Prepare and keep up-to-date a Summary of PV Systems document (Medicines and Healthcare Products Regulatory Agency, or MHRA) and a Compliance Report (MHRA). See Chapter 49.

- Appoint and empower a chief safety officer. In the European Union, this is obligatory and is the Qualified Person. Elsewhere this role is often less clearly defined. Nevertheless, this person should be a medical doctor (or have close access to an empowered MD) with true and real engagement in the company's PV activities. If outsourced, the outsourced QP should be an engaged and serious participant in the company's PV activities. Beware of someone who is a PV for multiple companies. It's hard enough to do it for one company.

- Create a system of internal company communication to be sure safety and risk issues in faraway (from the home office) areas are carefully followed by a local responsible person (whether in-house or outsourced). This refers to specific drugs as well as regulatory and risk requirements from the local HA.

- Keep all labeling up to date (U.S. PI, CCSI, SPC, Investigator Brochures, etc.) and easily available electronically.

- Prepare PSURs for all marketed drugs whether required or not. This document in a sense forces periodic signaling and safety/risk evaluations.

- Ensure adequate resources (money, personnel, IT, etc.) for risk evaluation needs and management, including outsourced functions, epidemiologic studies, and so forth.

- Appoint someone to pay attention to risk management, attend national and international meetings, interact with the key players, and get "intelligence."

31

The United States FDA's Three Risk Guidances of 2005

In March 2005, the U.S. Food and Drug Administration (FDA) issued three guidances, which were years in the making, summarizing the agency's views on risk management. These documents are critical to conveying how the FDA (and other health agencies) views risk. The guidances can be found at the links below and are briefly summarized in this chapter.

1. Premarketing Risk Assessment (Web Resource 31-1)
2. Development and Use of Risk Minimization Action Plans (RiskMAPs) (Web Resource 31-2)
3. Good Pharmacovigilance Practices and Pharmacoepidemiologic Assessment (Web Resource 31-3)

◼ The First Guidance: Premarketing Risk Assessment

The FDA begins by noting that routine risk assessment is already being done. It notes that this guidance is not aimed at use on all products but rather only on those that "pose a clinically important and unusual type or level of risk."

The adequacy of assessment of risk depends on quantity (number of patients studied) and the data quality ("the appropriateness of the assessments performed, the appropriateness and breadth of the patient populations studied, and how results are analyzed").

"Providing detailed guidance on what constitutes an adequate safety database for all products is impossible." Each product is weighed on its own merits.

Size of the Safety Database

The number of patients studied depends on the novelty of the drug, the availability and safety of alternate therapies, the intended population, the condition being treated, and the duration of use.

The FDA does not give safety database size advice for products for the short term (<6 months use) but does make suggestions for products aimed at treatment longer than 6 months. For these, the FDA and the International Conference on Harmonization (ICH) recommend 1500 subjects, with 300 to 600 exposed for 6 months and 100 exposed for 1 year using doses in the therapeutic range. Higher numbers of patients may need to be studied if:

- Specific safety issues arise from animal studies.
- Similar drugs or the class of drugs suggest a specific problem.
- Pharmacokinetic or pharmacodynamic properties of the drug are associated with certain adverse events (AEs).
- It is important to quantitate the occurrence of low-frequency AEs.
- The benefit from the product is small, and one wants to be sure there are no rare AEs that will not be picked up unless large numbers of patients are studied.
- The benefit is experienced by only a fraction of the treated patients (i.e., the benefit is "rare" and thus the same reason as above to look for rare AEs).
- The benefit is unclear (e.g., surrogate endpoints used).
- Statistical power requires larger a number of patients to show that an already high background rate of safety issues will not be unduly raised even more because of the drug.
- The proposed treatment is for healthy populations (e.g., preventive vaccines).
- A safe and effective alternate treatment is available.

In practice, this has been done for quite some time. The ICH/FDA figures above are somewhat arbitrary and may need to be higher, depending on the drug and population being studied. Often, statistical needs for power or significance for the efficacy endpoints drive sample size and are usually insufficient for statistical safety conclusions. What is noteworthy is the requirement for longer-term exposure (6 months and 1 year) for drugs that are used for 6 months. Even these suggestions may be conservative, and some drugs have had much longer follow-ups (e.g., Adriamycin, diethylstilbestrol), where chronic toxicity is expected or suspected to occur.

Long-Term Controlled Safety Trials

The FDA notes that, in many clinical programs, uncontrolled, single-arm, long-term safety studies are done.

Although useful, the use of a control or placebo (if possible) is preferable, especially when the AEs in question are relatively common in the treated population (e.g., sudden death in patients with ischemic heart disease), or when the AE might mimic the disease being treated, such as asthma exacerbations due to inhalation treatments given for asthma (see fialuridine and hepatitis, Chapter 52). Long-term safety studies are also useful if the toxicity worsens with cumulative exposure.

Uncontrolled studies are useful in picking up certain AEs that (essentially) never occur spontaneously. The FDA gives the examples of aplastic anemia and severe hepatocellular injury (though not stated, one presumes they mean noninfectious hepatic injury).

This section highlights an issue that has been around for many years but is changing: the use of placebo-controlled trials. Historically, the FDA felt that placebo-controlled trials are the gold standard for characterizing a drug's safety and efficacy. However, such trials are becoming more difficult to perform as the ethics of placebo use have evolved. Most placebo studies are frowned upon. The World Medical Association's Declaration of Helsinki states:

> Extreme care must be taken in making use of a placebo-controlled trial and that in general this methodology should only be used in the absence of existing proven therapy. However, a placebo-controlled trial may be ethically acceptable, even if proven therapy is available, under the following circumstances:
>
> - Where for compelling and scientifically sound methodological reasons its use is necessary to determine the efficacy or safety of a prophylactic, diagnostic or therapeutic method; or
> - Where a prophylactic, diagnostic or therapeutic method is being investigated for a minor condition and the patients who receive placebo will not be subject to any additional risk of serious or irreversible harm (Web Resource 31-4).

In addition, sponsors often avoid head-to-head trials for fear of unexpected bad results against a competitor or even against the sponsor's own comparator (e.g., an older drug the sponsor wishes to discontinue). This too is changing as comparative effectiveness requirements are established around the world. The United Kingdom has done this for some years (see The UK National Institute for Health and Clinical Excellence at Web Resource 31-5). Clinical effectiveness and comparisons are expected to be established in the United States within the next several years. Hence, many studies now are done against the "standard of care" (SOC—do not confuse this abbreviation with the MedDRA SOC, meaning System Organ Class), which often means that these studies are not able to show superiority (one treatment is better than the other) but only noninferiority. Medical practitioners generally prefer to see trials against the current SOC, arguing that practitioners do not treat with placebo in the real world but rather with something already out on the market.

Diversity

The premarketing safety database (mainly in phase III studies) should represent, as much as possible, the expected target population. The FDA argues that, where possible, inclusion criteria should be fairly broad to include elderly patients (and, in particular, "the very old") with concomitant diseases and patients taking concomitant medications.

Another fundamental area of potential conflict is between sponsors (companies) and the FDA. Sponsors generally like "very clean" studies in homogeneous patients so that efficacy (and safety) can be evaluated without extraneous "noise" (confounders) and that sample size can be kept "reasonable." The FDA, knowing that the drug will be used in the general population, only some of which resembles the test population, would like to see a much broader selection of patients tested before marketing.

Exploring Dose Effects

Normally, if one is skilled and lucky, the phase II trials establish the clinical dose that is then studied in large numbers of patients in phase III studies. The FDA argues for the study, in phase III, of more than one dose. They indicate that many efficacy and safety data can be obtained from these trials. This may or may not be feasible.

Drug Interactions

It is not possible to study all potential drug or other interactions. Those studies that are done should focus on the following:

- Drug–drug interactions should be looked at using those drugs that might be expected to produce safety issues resulting from known metabolic pathways (e.g., certain cytochrome P450 enzymes). Logical choices of test drugs should be made (e.g., for a new cholesterol-lowering treatment, examin-

ing the consequences of concomitant use of HMG CoA reductase inhibitors).
- Drug–demography interactions should be sought where gender, age, race, or other demographics might play a role.
- Drug–disease interactions should be examined if necessary.
- Drug–dietary supplement interactions may need to be evaluated (e.g., interactions between an antidepressant and St. John's wort).

The FDA recommends that pharmacokinetic assessments be built into some late-phase clinical trials to see whether unexpected interactions can be picked up.

Drug–drug interactions in particular remain a difficult nut to crack. Certain standard studies looking at the key cytochrome P450 enzyme pathways or drugs known to have many interactions (e.g., Coumadin, anticonvulsants) are straightforward and generally done routinely, as are drug–food and drug–alcohol studies. It is only after marketing that "surprise" interactions are seen (e.g., St. John's wort and human immunodeficiency virus drugs). Sometimes pharmacokinetic interactions are seen but with no pharmacodynamic or clinical implications. It may not be feasible, safe, or ethical to treat normal subjects with two drugs to see whether the drugs interact. Similarly, it may not be feasible, safe, or ethical to treat a cohort of patients already on a drug (e.g., acquired immunodeficiency syndrome patients, asthmatics) with the new drug to see whether there is an interaction.

Comparative Safety Data

The FDA next comments on safety data and comparators in clinical trials. They note that "much of the safety data in an application may be derived from placebo-controlled trials and single-arm safety studies, with little or no comparative safety data." Placebo-controlled trials may no longer be feasible in most cases. The FDA notes that active controls or a placebo arm if possible would be useful in the following circumstances:

- The background rate of AEs is high. Using a single-arm study might show an alarmingly high rate of AEs, which would be of less concern if a placebo arm showed a similarly high rate.
- There is a well-established treatment already. A single-arm trial would likely be uninformative and a placebo control unethical. Thus an active comparator is the usual choice.
- A superiority claim for safety or efficacy is desired. A control then is obviously needed.

Certain special circumstances require a tailored approach:

- Chronically used, long-half-life drugs or drugs with dose-related toxicities should have studies to determine whether a lower dose or less frequent dose is appropriate.

- If a specific titration schedule is needed, this schedule should be based on specific studies to determine the best titration scheme.

- If certain AEs are not likely to be detected or reported without special attention or tests, studies should include these. As an example, the FDA cites a new drug with central nervous system effects and notes that it should have assessments of cognitive function, motor skills, and mood.

- In pediatric studies, special attention should be paid to effects on growth and neurocognitive development if the drug is used in the very young, to excipients, and to immunization recommendations.

- The sponsor should evaluate whether and when the collection from some or all patients of blood or other bodily tissues or fluids during phase III studies for analysis at a later time should be done. This might be useful for analyzing unusual signals or for retrospective analyses at a later date.

Large Simple Safety Studies

These are usually randomized controlled studies done to assess limited specific safety outcomes in large numbers of patients. Rarely, they may be uncontrolled if the event being assessed is uncommon. The FDA notes these are usually done as formal phase IV commitments, although they could be done occasionally earlier in development. Another place for a large study is a product developed for preventive use in at-risk subjects who are otherwise healthy and where the benefits may be small.

Medication Errors

Although, historically, medication errors were not a part of drug safety or pharmacovigilance, they are now a high FDA priority in risk management. The FDA now wants sponsors to pay close attention before marketing to possible areas of medication error such as packaging, drug name, and labeling. Should medication errors or potential for errors be noted in the premarketing clinical trials, they should be acted on to remove potential for errors.

The FDA recommends drawing from the experience of Good Manufacturing Practice and device development by

- Conducting a failure mode and effects analysis
- Using expert panels
- Using computer-assisted analysis
- Using direct observation during clinical trials
- Using directed interviews of consumers and medical and pharmacy personnel to better understand comprehension
- Using focus groups
- Using simulated prescription and over-the-counter use studies

Assessing Safety During Product Development

During the development of all new small-molecule drugs, the following should be addressed as part of the New Drug Application (NDA):

- Drug-related QTc prolongation (to exclude arrhythmic potential)
- Drug–drug interactions
- Polymorphic metabolism

These experiments are conducted with "normal" doses in humans and are now known as safety pharmacology, in contrast to animal toxicology, which consists of increasing dosages until some untoward effect occurs:

- Drug-related liver toxicity
- Drug-related nephrotoxicity
- Drug-related bone marrow toxicity

Not all drugs require studies looking at all of these issues. The FDA has issued various other guidances and requirements for premarketing testing. Refer to the FDA website for specific information.

Biologic products may require additional testing:

- Immunogenicity: "both the incidence and consequences of neutralizing antibody formation and the potential for adverse events related to binding antibody formation."
- Transfection of nontarget cells and infection transmissibility to close contacts should be evaluated for gene-based products.
- "For cell-based products, assessment of AEs related to distribution, migration and growth beyond the initial intended administration are important as are AEs related to cell survival and demise."

Data Analysis and Interpretation

The FDA refers the reader to three ICH guidances on preparing NDAs, clinical study reports, and the common technical document. The FDA notes that the later phases of product development are primarily aimed at efficacy, with endpoints identified in advance and with statistical calculations based on these endpoints. In contrast, the safety measures are usually not addressed with any prespecified level of statistical sensitivity. Thus, premarketing safety data are often only exploratory and useful primarily for signal development.

Describing AEs to Identify Signals (Coding): The FDA recommends use of a single coding system (e.g., MedDRA), with a standardized coding convention and without updates throughout the program.

Coding Accuracy: Care should be taken with investigators and coders such that the reported verbatim terms are accurately reflected in the MedDRA codes used for these reported AEs. Severity and magnitude should not be exaggerated (e.g., coding acute liver failure when all that occurred was isolated transaminase elevation without elevated bilirubin, coagulopathy, or encephalopathy) or masked (using a nonspecific and "unimportant" term to describe a serious AE). The sponsor may "recharacterize" an AE code when appropriate but with an audit trail and with FDA consultation.

Verbatim terms from investigators should be captured, verified to be accurate, and mapped to the appropriate MedDRA term (e.g., the verbatim term "suicidal ideation" should not be captured as "emotional lability"). The sponsor should ensure that verbatim terms are consistent across studies and individual coders. The FDA also suggests that the sponsor "consider a coded event in conjunction with other coded events in some circumstances" and may define certain entities as "an amalgamation of multiple coding terms." They give as an example "acute liver failure," which could be used if it is based on recognized definitions of this term. The FDA does not, however, come down squarely on one side or the other in the "lumpers versus splitters" debate (i.e., combine terms or report them separately). This is an area of continued controversy, with various coding conventions proposed.

Coding Analysis: The FDA cautions about how analyses can be altered or obscured by the way coding is done. They urge the sponsor to pay attention and use coding (whether lumping or splitting) to obtain the best signals:

- Splitting: Using multiple terms may at times be more useful than combinations. They give the

example that "dyspnea, cough, wheezing and pleuritis" is more sensitive and useful than "pulmonary toxicity" but warn that "constipation" might include and hide cases of "toxic megacolon."

- Splitting may, however, falsely decrease the incidence of AEs. "Fluid retention" may give a better signal and truer incidence than dividing the AEs into "pedal edema, generalized edema, peripheral edema."

- Prospective grouping may be useful in clinical programs where appropriate: serotonin syndrome, parkinsonism, and drug withdrawal are useful and "not well characterized by a single term." Other groupings may be done retrospectively, although the FDA should be consulted.

Analyzing Temporal and Other Associations: The FDA next gives a high-level discussion of factors that need to be considered in analyzing signals. They note that simple comparisons of frequency may not be sufficient to analyze a signal and that temporal associations may aid in evaluating causality. This includes duration of exposure to a product, time to onset, and so on. Various statistical methods, including the Kaplan-Meier approach, may be useful for evaluating risks of AEs. The product's pharmacokinetic and pharmacodynamic profiles as well as "an appreciation of physiologic, metabolic and host immune responses may be important in understanding the possible timing of treatment-related AEs." Concomitant medications, the initiation or withdrawal of other therapies, and changes in the preexisting conditions over time should also be considered.

Analyzing Dose Effect: AEs should be analyzed as a function of dose. That is, are there different AE responses at different doses? It may be useful to consider weight or body surface area-adjusted doses. Subgroup analysis by dose may also be useful. The FDA also makes the important point that "the likelihood of observing false positive signals increases with the number of analyses conducted." Consistency across studies should be investigated to help validate such findings.

Data Pooling: The FDA notes that "data pooling is performed to achieve larger sample sizes and data sets because individual clinical studies are not designed with sufficient sample size to estimate the frequency of low incidence events or to compare differences in rates or relative rates between the test drug (exposed group) and the control (unexposed group)." Further, "pooled analyses can enhance the power to detect an association between product use and an event and provide more reliable estimates of the magnitude of risk over time…and can also provide insight into a positive signal observed in a single study by allowing a broader comparison." The FDA discusses issues for and against use of such pooled data.

The FDA next notes that all placebo-controlled trials should be considered for data pooling. The patient populations should be relatively homogeneous and have similar methods of AE and dropout ascertainment. Phase I trials should generally be excluded. Risks should not just be expressed in event frequency (e.g., AEs per 100 persons) but also in time-event analyses when appropriate.

Rigorous Ascertainment of Reasons for Withdrawals from Studies: The FDA emphasizes that all participants dropping out must be followed up to fully understand why they did so. Some reasons may be irrelevant and trivial (e.g., moved away) or very important in regard to safety (e.g., had a stroke, was intolerant to adverse reactions). Terms like "withdrew consent," "failed to return," "administratively withdrawn," or "lost to follow-up" are too vague to be useful. These reasons should be followed up for more specific causes, especially if safety issues are involved. Dropouts because of abnormal laboratory tests, vital signs, or electrocardiographic findings may not be always characterized as AEs but should be followed up and accounted for. Follow-up on safety issues should be done until the AE is resolved or stabilized.

Long-Term Follow-Up: In some instances (e.g., the drug has a very long half-life, is deposited in bone or brain, or might cause irreversible AEs such as cancer) patients should be followed to the end of the study or even after the study ends. This may mean follow-up long after the drug treatment ends. This is especially true in long-term treatment and outcome studies. The FDA recommends discussions with the agency for these special cases.

Important Aspects of Data Presentation: Finally, the FDA makes several comments on data presentation in the NDA integrated summary of safety and elsewhere:

- AE rates should be presented from more restrictive (e.g., myocardial infarction) to less restrictive (e.g., myocardial ischemia).
- AEs for the drug that are important and seen for other drugs in the class should be discussed.
- Analyses of pooled data looking at gender, age, extent of exposure, concomitant medical conditions, and concomitant medications should be included.
- Differential discontinuation rates (e.g., placebo-treated patients may drop out of a trial earlier than drug-treated patients) must be accounted for.
- Case report forms submitted for patients who died or discontinued should have relevant hospital records, biopsy reports, and so forth included.

- Narrative summaries of important AEs should be sufficiently detailed to allow the case to be understood and analyzed.

Most of the concepts introduced in this document remain true and reflect FDA's thinking. However, some areas are evolving, especially in light of further ICH, CIOMS, and EU activities. Nonetheless, this document is still worth reading.

■ The Second Guidance: Development and Use of Risk Minimization Action Plans

This guidance has largely been superseded by the REMS concepts put forth in the 2007 Food and Drug Administration Amendments Act (FDAAA) and Prescription Drug User Fee Act (PDUFA) documents. The elements and actions in the RiskMAPs are very similar to those in REMS, and several RiskMAPs were converted to REMS without much difficulty. Only a very brief summary is given here.

This document advises industry on initiating and designing plans, called Risk Minimization Action Plans (RiskMAPs), to minimize identified product risks selecting and developing tools to minimize those risks, evaluating RiskMAPs and monitoring tools, communicating with the FDA about RiskMAPs, and recommending components of a RiskMAP submission to the FDA. The FDA references the International Conference on Harmonization E2E document on Pharmacovigilance Planning in designing a RiskMAP.

Goals: The RiskMAP should state its goal(s) in "absolute terms" to achieve maximum risk reduction. Examples include "patients on X drug should not also be prescribed Y drug" or "fetal exposures to Z drug should not occur."

Objectives: The objectives should be pragmatic, specific, and measurable. For the goals stated above of "patients on X drug should not also be prescribed Y drug" or "fetal exposures to Z drug should not occur," the objective could be, "lowering physician coprescribing rates and/or pharmacist codispensing rates."

Tools: In this example, possible tools include targeted education and outreach to healthcare professionals and patients, reminder systems or forms, and limiting access.

When to Develop a RiskMAP: Anytime during a product's life cycle. It may be done by the company or proposed by the FDA and should consider the types, magnitude, and frequency of risks and benefits; the populations at greatest risk or those likely to derive the most benefit; the existence of treatment alternatives and their risks and benefits; the reversibility of the adverse events observed; the preventability of the adverse events in question; and the probability of benefit. Examples include all schedule II controlled substances, teratogens, and drugs requiring specialized healthcare skills, training, or facilities to manage the therapeutic or adverse effects of a drug.

Tools to minimize risk include:

- Targeted education and outreach, such as letters, training programs, continuing medical education, "prominent professional or public notifications," patient medication guides and Package Inserts, direct-to-consumer advertising highlighting the risks in question, and disease management/patient access systems with patient–sponsor interactions
- Reminder systems, such as consent forms, prescriber and testing, special data collection systems, limiting the amount of product dispensed, forbidding refills, and special packaging
- Performance-linked access systems, such as obligatory laboratory testing before drug prescribing

The FDA also has mechanisms to minimize risk, including product recalls, warning and untitled letters, import alerts, safety alerts, guidance documents, and regulations and judicial enforcement procedures such as seizures or injunctions.

Tools and programs must be assessed to measure their effectiveness using either direct measurements (e.g., if the goal is to prevent a particular AE, the measurement of the AE rate could be used), surrogate measurements (e.g., emergency room visits), process measurements (e.g., performance of a laboratory test or signature on an informed consent), and assessments of comprehension, knowledge, attitudes, and behavior changes (e.g., of the prescriber, pharmacist, or patient). RiskMAP tools should be evaluated before implementation where possible. A timetable of evaluations should also be conveyed to FDA.

■ The Third Guidance: Good Pharmacovigilance Practices and Pharmacoepidemiologic Assessment

In this guidance, the FDA discusses pharmacovigilance and how a product is marketed, noting that pharmacovigilance must be very active after New Drug Application approval. The FDA takes a broad definition of pharmacovigilance: "All scientific and data gathering activities relating to the detection, assessment, and understanding of adverse events. This includes the use of pharmacoepidemiologic studies."

Identifying Signals: Good Reporting Practice

The FDA also defines "signal" as "a concern about an excess of adverse events compared to what would be expected to be associated with a product's use...(though) even a single well-documented case report can be viewed as a signal... Signals generally indicate the need for further investigation, which may or may not lead to the conclusion that the product caused the event."

Sponsors make "reasonable" attempts to get complete information on safety reports they receive at the initial contact and at follow-ups, especially for SAEs. The "detective work" should be done by experienced healthcare professionals. The greatest efforts should be made to obtain follow-up information for serious cases, particularly ones that are not already known to occur with the drug in question. For consumer reports, an attempt should be made to obtain corroborative details from the consumer's healthcare practitioner and to obtain medical records.

Case reports should contain all of the following elements:

- Description of the AEs, including time to onset
- Suspected and concomitant medication details (i.e., dose, lot number, schedule, dates, duration), including over-the-counter medications, dietary supplements, and recently discontinued medications
- Patient demography (e.g., age, race, sex), baseline medical condition before product therapy, comorbid conditions, use, relevant family history, and risk factors
- Documentation of the diagnosis and procedures done regarding the AEs
- Clinical course of the event and outcome (e.g., hospitalization or death)
- Relevant therapeutic measures and laboratory data at baseline, during, and after therapy
- Information about response to dechallenge and rechallenge

Medication errors should also be captured in detail.

Developing a Case Series

If a signal is noted from spontaneous reports, the sponsor should develop a case series by looking for additional similar cases in its safety and clinical trial databases, the FDA's AERS database, published literature, and elsewhere. Formal written case criteria/standards should be developed to ensure that similar cases are chosen for the series. Next, each case in the series should be evaluated with emphasis on unlabeled SAEs. Incomplete cases should have follow-up done. Duplicate cases should be removed.

During the evaluation of each case, causality should be evaluated. This causality is not needed for sending expedited 15-day reports to the NDA. Rather, the causality is needed for the signal analysis. There are, as the FDA notes, no internationally accepted standards for causality, especially for events with a high background or spontaneous incidence in the population. "FDA does not recommend any specific categorization of causality, but the categories probable, possible, or unlikely have been used previously." If different categories are used, the criteria should be clearly spelled out.

The FDA suggests using the following criteria for causality reviews:

- Occurrence of the AE in the expected time frame (e.g., type 1 allergic reactions occurring within days of therapy; cancers developing after years of therapy)
- Absence of symptoms related to the event before exposure
- Evidence of positive dechallenge or positive rechallenge
- Consistency of the event with the established pharmacological/toxicologic effects of the product (medical and pharmacological plausibility)
- Consistency of the event with the known effects of other products in the class
- Existence of other supporting evidence from preclinical, clinical, or pharmacoepidemiologic studies
- No other alternative explanations for the event

After this review, "unconfounded" cases, that is, "clean cases" where no other explanation seems possible, should be evaluated separately. If, following this exercise, the case series suggests that additional investigation be done, the case series data should be assembled as a chart as follows:

- The clinical and laboratory manifestations and course of the event
- Demography (e.g., age, gender, race)
- Exposure duration
- Time from initiation of product exposure to the AE

- Doses used and lot numbers, if available
- Concomitant medications taken
- The presence of comorbid conditions, particularly those known to cause the AE
- The route of administration
- Changes in event reporting rate over calendar time or product life cycle

Data Mining

The FDA gives a brief description of data mining, or the use of statistical or mathematical tools to derive additional information on excess AEs (signals) in a database containing AE reports, such as the FDA's AERS database. The FDA notes that these techniques are "inherently exploratory and hypothesis generating" and that caution should be used with them because of incomplete data, duplicate reports, underreporting, stimulated reports due to publicity or litigation ("secular effects"), and other biases.

The FDA describes proportionality analyses (see Chapter 19) and that other data-mining methods (such as the neural network and proportional reporting ratios) are referenced in the FDA's guidance (see the document for full details). The FDA notes that the use of data-mining techniques is not obligatory, but if submitted to the FDA, it should be done in the context of a larger clinical and epidemiologic evaluation. Note: This is still true to an extent though, now, several years after the publication of this guidance, the expectations for quantitative signal analysis using various data-mining techniques are growing. They are not clearly obligatory yet, but as research and development in drug safety proceeds, they may well become so.

Safety Signals That May Warrant Further Investigation

Once a signal is identified, a decision must be made by the sponsor and/or the FDA about doing further investigation. Signals that generally warrant further workup include:

- New unlabeled AEs, especially if serious.
- An apparent increase in the severity of a labeled event.
- Occurrence of serious events thought to be extremely rare in the general population.
- New product–product, product–device, product–food, or product–dietary supplement interactions.
- Identification of a previously unrecognized at-risk population.

- Confusion about a product's name, labeling, packaging, or use.

- Concerns arising from the way a product is used (e.g., AEs seen at higher than labeled doses or in populations not recommended for treatment).

- Concerns arising from potential inadequacies of a currently implemented risk minimization action plan (RiskMAP) (e.g., reports of serious AEs that appear to reflect failure of a RiskMAP goal). Now REMS rather than RiskMAPs.

Reporting Rates Versus Incidence Rates

The FDA next discusses a chronically vexing issue in pharmacovigilance: reporting rate calculations. Clearly, in epidemiology risk assessment, it is worth calculating the number of new cases of an event that occurs in the exposed population (the incidence rate). In clinical or epidemiologic studies, this is doable.

However, for spontaneously reported AEs, problems arise in both the numerator (reports of an AE) and in the denominator (population exposed). In regard to the numerator, there is always underreporting by a variable and unknown amount. In regard to the denominator, it is difficult to get accurate estimates of the number of patients exposed to the product and of the duration of treatment. In addition, the data may be unreliable because it is often difficult to exclude patients who are not at risk, or a product may be used in different populations for different indications.

Given all these limitations, the FDA still believes it is worthwhile to calculate the reporting rate using reported cases divided by estimates of national (i.e., United States) exposure of patients or patient-time. Only if this is not available should surrogates be used for exposure, such as prescriptions filled or kilograms of product sold.

The FDA then notes that comparisons of reporting rates and their temporal trends may be useful and may be done but with caution. Reporting rates can never be considered as incidence rates, however, and should never be compared with them.

It is also useful to obtain estimates of background occurrence rates in the population or in subpopulations (e.g., diabetics, premenopausal women) from published literature and from health statistics from databases or studies. Cautious comparisons of these data with reporting rates may be useful in some situations.

The FDA then comments on the interpretation of reporting rates. Because underreporting is often substantial, if the reporting rate is higher than background expectations, this may be a strong indicator of a high true incidence rate. Conversely, a lower-than-background reporting rate does not necessarily mean the product is not associated with an increased risk for the AE in question. Nor does it imply that the drug protects against this AE, as has been claimed by some sponsors!

Epidemiologic Studies

The FDA encourages sponsors to consider the use of nonrandomized observational studies, particularly if randomized trials are not possible or feasible. Three categories of observational studies are discussed: (1) pharmacoepidemiologic studies, (2) registries, and (3) surveys.

Pharmacoepidemiologic Studies

Several types of epidemiologic studies are possible, including prospective or retrospective cohort studies, case-control studies, nested case-control studies, case-crossover studies, or others. A clinical trial is not feasible in the following situations:

- The AE in question is uncommon (e.g., 1:2000–3000), and clinical trials are not practical because of the very large number of patients needed.
- Exposure to the product is chronic.
- Exposure to the product is done in patients with significant comorbid conditions.
- Patients are taking multiple comedications.
- The study is meant to identify risk factors for an AE.

Pharmacoepidemiologic studies, however, have their own set of problems, including confounding (other conditions produce the same outcome or AE), effect modulation (the association between the drug and the AE is altered by another factor, e.g., ethnic background), and other biases. There is no "one-size-fits-all" set of criteria to allow an easy choice of which study type to use. Each situation should be considered individually, with the best choice being the one that minimizes these biases. Sometimes more than one study is needed. Each study should have a detailed description of the methodology used, including:

- The population to be studied
- The case definitions to be used
- The data sources to be used (including a rationale for data sources if from outside the United States)
- The projected study size and statistical power calculations

■ The methods for data collection, management, and analysis

The choice of the database for the study also entails some careful analysis. Many studies are now done in automated (insurance) claims databases (e.g., health maintenance organizations, Medicaid). The choice of the database should be based on

■ Demography of the patients enrolled in the health plans (e.g., age, geographic location)
■ Turnover rate of patients in the health plans
■ Plan coverage of the medications of interest
■ Size and characteristics of the exposed population available for study
■ Availability of the outcomes of interest
■ Ability to identify conditions of interest using standard medical coding systems (e.g., International Classification of Diseases)
■ Access to medical records
■ Access to patients for data not captured electronically

The results should be validated by review of some or all the medical records of the patients in the database. The FDA recommends discussions between the sponsor and the agency during the development of such trials.

Registries

The FDA defines registries in this context as "an organized system for the collection, storage, retrieval, analysis, and dissemination of information on individual persons exposed to a specific medical intervention who have either a particular disease, a condition (e.g., a risk factor) that predisposes [them] to the occurrence of a health-related event, or prior exposure to substances (or circumstances) known or suspected to cause adverse health effects." When possible, a control or comparison group should be included. They may be used when such data are not available in automated databases or when collection is from multiple sources (e.g., medical doctors, hospitals, pathologists) over time.

The FDA suggests that all registries have written protocols describing objectives; a literature review; plans for systematic patient recruitment and follow-up; methodology for data collection, management, and analysis; and registry termination conditions. Again, the FDA suggests collaboration between the sponsor and agency in the development of the registry.

This definition is more extensive than the classical definition of a registry, which was basically a file of data

without control groups, analysis objectives, formal protocols, and termination plans. This definition is much closer to a true "study."

Surveys

Surveys of patients or healthcare providers can provide information on signals, knowledge of labeled AEs, actual use of a product, compliance with RiskMAP (now REMS) requirements, and confusion over sound-alike or look-alike products. As with registries, the FDA suggests a written protocol with details on the methodology, including patient or healthcare professional recruitment and follow-up, projected sample size, and methods of data collection, management, and analysis. Validation should be done against medical or pharmacy records or through interviews with healthcare providers. Where possible, validated or piloted instruments should be used. And again, discussion between the sponsor and the FDA is encouraged.

Interpreting Signals

After identifying a signal, studying the individual cases in the series, using as needed data mining, reporting rate calculations, a literature review, and possibly other data (e.g., animal studies), the sponsor should consider whether a study should be done to determine whether a safety risk exists.

Whenever in the process the sponsor concludes that there is a potential safety risk, a submission to the FDA should be made of all available safety information and analyses (from preclinical data on). The submission should include:

■ Spontaneous and published cases with denominator or exposure information
■ Background rate for the event in general and specific patient populations, if available
■ Relative risks, odds ratios, or other measures of association derived from pharmacoepidemiologic studies
■ Biologic effects observed in preclinical studies and pharmacokinetic or pharmacodynamic effects
■ Safety findings from controlled clinical trials
■ General marketing experience with similar products in the class

The sponsor should make a benefit–risk assessment for the population as a whole and for identified at-risk groups and propose, if appropriate, further studies or risk minimization actions. The FDA also makes its own evaluation. These analyses should be done iteratively in an ongoing logical sequence and manner as the data become available.

Items that the sponsor and the FDA should consider in their evaluations include:

- Strength of the association (e.g., relative risk of the AE associated with the product)
- Temporal relationship of product use and the event
- Consistency of findings across available data sources
- Evidence of a dose response for the effect
- Biologic plausibility
- Seriousness of the event relative to the disease being treated
- Potential to mitigate the risk in the population
- Feasibility of further study using observational or controlled clinical study designs
- Degree of benefit the product provides, including availability of other therapies

Developing a Pharmacovigilance Plan

Depending on the situation, the sponsor may wish to develop a pharmacovigilance plan above and beyond the usual postmarketing spontaneous AE collection and analysis. The FDA refers to the guidance on RiskMAPs issued in March 2005 (refer now to REMS; see Chapter 30). The need for a plan should be based on

1. The likelihood that the AE represents a potential safety risk
2. The frequency with which the AE occurs (e.g., incidence rate, reporting rate, or other measures available)
3. The severity of the event
4. The nature of the population(s) at risk
5. The range of patients for whom the product is indicated

6. The method by which the product is dispensed (through pharmacies or performance-linked systems only)

In general, RiskMAPs should be developed for products with serious safety risks that have been identified or where at-risk populations have not been adequately studied. Such a plan could include the following:

- Submission of specific serious AEs in an expedited manner beyond routine required reporting (i.e., as 15-day reports).
- Submission of AE report summaries at more frequent prespecified intervals (e.g., quarterly rather than annually).
- Active surveillance to identify AEs that may or may not be reported through passive surveillance. Active surveillance can be (1) drug-based, identifying AEs in patients taking certain products; (2) setting-based, identifying AEs in certain healthcare settings where they are likely to present for treatment (e.g., emergency departments); or (3) event-based, identifying AEs that are likely to be associated with medical products (e.g., acute liver failure).
- Additional pharmacoepidemiologic studies.
- Creation of registries or surveys.
- Additional controlled clinical trials.

The sponsor should periodically reevaluate the plan's effectiveness. The FDA will also do so and may choose to bring questions to its Drug Safety Risk Management Advisory Committee or an FDA advisory committee dealing with the specific product.

This document basically describes how to do pharmacovigilance in the United States circa 2005. Although some practices have changed and globalized, the methodology described in this document remains largely valid and appropriate. Nonetheless, expect further developments and changes in risk management.

32

Data Management Committees and IRBs/ Ethics Committees

■ Data Management Committees

Over the years, in addition to Investigational Review Boards (IRBs), the concept of a separate and additional independent group to monitor the safety of clinical trials has developed. This group or function is known under several names, including Data Monitoring Committee (DMC), Data Safety Monitoring Committee (DSMB), Data Safety Board, Clinical Trial Safety Monitoring Committee/ Board, and others. This was codified as a draft guidance by the U.S. Food and Drug Administration (FDA) in 2001 (Web Resource 32-1) and by the European Medicines Agency in 2003 (Web Resource 32-2).

As stated in the FDA document: "A DMC is a group of individuals with pertinent expertise that reviews on a regular basis accumulating data from an ongoing clinical trial. The DMC advises the sponsor regarding the continuing safety of current participants and those yet to be recruited, as well as the continuing validity and scientific merit of the trial."

The EMA definition is similar: "A group of independent experts external to a study assessing the progress, safety data and, if needed, critical efficacy endpoints of a clinical study. In order to do so a DMC may review unblinded study information (on a patient level or treatment group level) during the conduct of the study. Based on its review the DMC provides the sponsor with recommendations regarding study modification, continuation or termination."

The sponsor or creator of the DMC can be the holder of the IND or equivalent, a company or government agency, or any individual or group to whom the sponsor delegates authority for decision-making, including the study steering or executive committee, the contract research organization (CRO), or the principal investigator. The presence of a DMC, however, is additive to the safety precautions in the trial. All legal and regulatory obligations in all jurisdictions must still be carried out by the investigator (patient protection, AE reporting, etc.) and sponsor (expedited reporting, signaling, etc.).

The DMC must be independent, meaning that no member has any personal basis for preferring the trial outcome to be in one or the other direction, and no member has any ability to influence the trial conduct in a role other than that of a DMC member.

The committees should contain at least three members and include such expertise as

■ Clinical medicine (appropriate specialty)
■ Biostatistics

- Biomedical ethics
- Basic science/pharmacology
- Epidemiology/pharmacovigilance—drug safety
- Clinical trial methodology
- Legal
- Patient advocate/community representative

Ideally, there should be geographic representation, especially in international trials, demographic representation on the committee relevant to the trial (race, gender, age), personalities amenable to consensus development, reliability and time to attend meetings, and prior DMC experience. The appointment to the committee should be made by the sponsor, and, for government-sponsored trials, members should be acceptable to the health agency and the investigators. Expenses and honoraria should be paid by the sponsor, and the members should be independent and free of conflicts of interest. The DMC should not have any representation from the industry sponsor, study investigators, or individuals who stand to gain or lose financially from the study outcome, such as major consultants or investors in the sponsor or a competitor.

A DMC is needed in general for (FDA criteria):

- Large, randomized multisite studies that evaluate treatments intended to prolong life or reduce risk of a major adverse health outcome such as a cardiovascular event or recurrence of cancer
- Any controlled trial of any size that will compare rates of mortality or major morbidity
- When DMC review is practical
- When DMC review helps ensure the scientific validity of the trial

EMA criteria:

- In case of life-threatening diseases, usually the implementation of a DMC is indicated from an ethical point of view.
- Certain patient populations (even if trial is in a noncritical indication): pediatric and mentally disabled patients.
- Prior knowledge or strong suspicion that a treatment under consideration has the potential to harm patients (even though it will be eventually more effective than other available treatments).
- Preplanned interim analyses for early stopping (either for futility or for positive efficacy) or in case of complex study designs in which a possible modification of the study design based on unblinded interim data is intended. In such a situation, the use

of an independent DMC gives more credibility to the process.

Some trials should almost always have a DMC:

- If more than one investigational drug is being used in a trial
- Trials where early stopping for efficacy is considered
    - Treatment reduces mortality or major morbidity
    - Treatment reduces toxicity, cost, or other important secondary factors while maintaining efficacy against mortality/major morbidity
- Trials raising special safety or ethical concerns
    - Early AIDS vaccine trials
    - Gene therapy trials
    - Trials in especially vulnerable populations
- International and multicenter trials
- Phase III confirmatory trials
- Phase IIb test-of-concept trials
- Trials where review by independent experts would optimize patient safety and the scientific integrity and credibility of the trial
- Politically sensitive or highly emotional trials

When a DMC is generally not needed:

- Not required or recommended for most clinical studies (FDA)
- Trials at early stages of product development, for example, phase I (FDA)
- Trials addressing lesser outcomes, such as relief of symptoms, unless the trial population is at elevated risk of more severe outcomes (FDA)
- A clinical study that can be performed in a short time frame that does not allow for appropriate preparation of information for a DMC (EMA)
- Clinical studies in noncritical indications where patients are treated for a relatively short time and the drugs under investigation are well characterized and known for not harming patients (EMA)

The DMC will have several functions during a trial, including the rapid identification of any safety problems; of logistical problems, such as inadequate accrual, undesirable distribution of baseline characteristics, excess dropouts, or noncompliance; of the continued feasibility of the trial as designed; and of whether the trial objectives have been met and the trial terminated early.

The committee must maintain full confidentiality, as they will usually receive unblinded data. Health agencies typically expect that confidentiality of the interim data will be maintained even if the DMC interacts with the sponsor or trial investigators to clarify issues relating to the conduct of the trial, potential impact on the trial of external data, or other topics.

To these ends, the DMC will review and approve the study protocol, assess the study conduct, evaluate accumulating data for both safety and efficacy, recommend termination or continuation of the study, recommend modifications of the study (including the informed consent), and recommend additional safety or efficacy analyses if appropriate.

The DMC must have a written charter that is drafted and approved by the sponsor and DMC members. The health agency may in some cases also be involved in the drafting and approval. The charter must include the schedule and format for meetings, including unscheduled meetings if a safety problem occurs, the format for presentation of data, the specification of who will have access to interim data and who may attend all or part (closed sessions) of the DMC meetings, procedures for assessing conflict of interest of potential DMC members, the method and timing of providing interim reports to the DMC from the sponsor or data-gathering group, the definition of a quorum for decision-making, and details on how the committee will meet (webinars, teleconferences, etc.; see DAMOCLES Study Group, *Lancet* 2005;365:711–722).

A key component (though not "officially" a member) of the DMC is the statistician or statistical group, who prepares, analyzes, and presents interim trial results to the DMC. The statistician may be from the company or sponsor or may be from an external CRO or independent consulting firm. The statistician will usually have the blinding key and will unblind study results (see below).

Each DMC meeting usually has an initial open session, followed by a closed session and then a wrap-up open session. At the initial "open" session with DMC and the sponsor, nonconfidential matters are discussed, including the clinical trial program, the status of recruitment, baseline patient characteristics, ineligibility rate, accuracy and timeliness of data submissions, and other administrative data and plans. The closed session is attended by only the DMC members and the (sponsor or outside) statistician who prepared and is presenting the interim analyses to the DMC. After the closed session, a wrap-up open session may be held with the sponsor to relay any recommendations from the DMC. The DMC has the option of conducting an "executive" session with no participants other than DMC members (that is, no sponsor representatives at all), though this is usually not needed.

There has been controversy over whether the DMC should see blinded or unblinded data. Most feel that DMC members should have access to unblinded data to ensure their ability to make accurate risk–benefit assessments. If this is the case, then printed reports of unblinded interim analyses should be supplied to the DMC members several days (at least) before the meeting to allow for adequate review of the information. Sometimes a partial unblinding is done, whereby treatment codes are given for each treatment group (e.g., drug X, drug Y, rather than the names of the drugs). The sponsor should supply the data in a reviewable form. For large studies, some sponsors provide the DMC with listings of individual patients' data, often in a very non-user-friendly way. When there are hundreds or thousands of patients each with multiple labs, exams, and so forth, totaling millions of data points over thousands of pages, it is hard to "eyeball" the data and find trends or issues. Excellent software is available for examining trends and outliers. Many DMCs also want to see the CIOMS I/MedWatch forms for all serious cases or at least all expedited cases.

There is a "statistical downside" to multiple reviews of interim data that the sponsor may perform in some studies, namely, that repeated statistical comparisons of event rates between the treated and control groups increases the "false-positive" rate if P values are not adjusted for multiple testing. To put it another way, the more interim data reviews that are done, the more likely that a type I error will be found. At the $P < 0.05$ level, the probability of nominally significant results occurring with three interim analyses is about 10% greater, and with 10 interim analyses about 20% greater (see McPherson, Statistics: the problem of examining accumulating data more than once. *New Engl J Med.* 1978;290:501–502). To get around this problem, there are various options available that basically increase the P value required for significance (e.g., requiring a level of 0.018 at each interim and final analysis or 0.001 at each interim analysis and 0.05 at the final analysis). No matter what statistical techniques are used, the DMC must not rely on statistical analyses alone to reach a conclusion. Clinical judgment must also be used to evaluate the safety and efficacy of information.

The DMC will compare AE rates in each treatment arm to see whether there are any major imbalances of concern and which seem to be due to the intervention rather than the disease or confounding factors (e.g., all the patients in some Northern Hemisphere centers come down with a seasonal influenza). The DMC may also want to see specific patient information for critical or important cases (e.g., SUSARs, acute liver failure, all patients where the blind is broken by the sponsor or investigator for safety reasons). Again, this calls for good software and reporting tools to allow the DMC to see the data it needs.

The DMC has three options after each meeting. All meetings are minuted.

1. Continue the trial unmodified.
2. Modify the trial:
   - Drop a treatment arm or subgroup.
   - Modify the treatment dose/schedule.
   - Add additional safety tests (e.g., electrocardiograms) at screening or during the trial.
   - Modify consent/investigators' brochure.
3. Terminate the trial early due to:
   - Serious safety issues.
   - The efficacy question has been answered and the results are truly compelling, with the risk of a false-positive conclusion acceptably low.
   - The hypothesis is no longer relevant or the hypothesized benefit cannot be achieved.

There are no rigid stopping rules. Rather, the committee must exercise judgment. General rules of thumb have developed. It is usually appropriate to demand less rigorous proof of harm to justify early termination than would be appropriate for a finding of benefit.

Interestingly, there is an ongoing and probably unanswerable ethical conflict with DMCs, namely, where does their primary responsibility lie?

- Perspective 1: The DMC's primary responsibility is to the specific patients enrolled in the trial. This implies that the DMC should stop the trial early if further results are unlikely to change the conclusion based on interim data. That is, do not put the individual patients at further risk or subject them to placebo for longer than the minimal time necessary.
- Perspective 2: The DMC's primary responsibility is to the entire "patient horizon" and the practice of medicine in general. In this case, the DMC would stop the trial early only if the results are sufficiently persuasive to effect changes in medical practice based on limited data.

No correct answer fits all cases.

The DMC is usually advisory to the sponsor, and the sponsor may reject the DMC's comments, though this will obviously produce controversy and multiple ethical issues. The DMC results must be communicated to the health agency and the IRBs in any case.

In practice, for large multiyear, multicenter studies, DMCs have proved very useful when well constituted and well run. Logistics can be costly and complex if there are thousands of patients and several studies going on at the same time. It is likely that more and more DMCs will be used. Some are even considering DMCs or their equivalent in the postmarketing setting, looking at the spontaneous data coming into the sponsor or Marketing Authorization (MA) holder. Some have used DMCs in early phase I trials also.

Investigational Review Boards/Ethics Committees

Clinical trials require formal, external, neutral committees to review the protocol and course of the study as well as other aspects of the study. These are called either Investigational Review Boards or Ethics Committees. The rules are fairly complex and vary a bit in different regions, but the concepts are all the same: patient protection and good science. These committees may be attached to medical institutions (e.g., hospitals, medical schools) or may be unattached and free-standing, which has led to some controversy. Some may be "central" (e.g., in the European Union covering all sites in one country or in the United States covering all sites) or local. Some studies use a mixture of both local and central IRBs.

ICH addressed the issue in their document E6(R1) Good Clinical Practice Guidance (Web Resource 32-3).

The EU addressed Ethics Committees in several places, including Directive 2001/20/EC and Volume 10 Clinical Trials Guidelines (Web Resource 32-4). There are extensive FDA regulations and guidances for IRBs to follow regarding their requirements and obligations in clinical studies. In particular, see the "Detailed guidance on the application format and documentation to be submitted in an application for an Ethics Committee opinion on the clinical trial on medicinal products for human use" at Web Resource 32-5.

The key U.S. regulations are found at 21CFR56.109 IRB on the review of research. Other requirements include 21 CFR 50.25, which covers protection of human subjects. An FDA summary page of guidances for IRBs, clinical investigators, and sponsors can be found at the FDA Web site (Web Resource 32-6).

Finally, in January 2010, the FDA issued a draft Guidance for IRBs, Clinical Investigators, and Sponsors IRB Continuing Review after clinical investigation approval. See Web Resource 32-7. This is an extensive document updating original, somewhat outdated regulations as trials become more complex. The IRB is now expected to be sure that:

- Risks to the subjects are minimized.
- Risks to subjects are reasonable in relation to anticipated benefits, if any, to subjects, and to the importance of the knowledge that may be expected to result.
- Selection of subjects is equitable.
- Informed consent will be sought and appropriately documented.
- Where appropriate, the research plan adequately provides for monitoring the data collected, to ensure the safety of subjects.
- Where appropriate, there are adequate provisions to protect the privacy of subjects and to maintain the confidentiality of data.
- Appropriate additional safeguards are included to protect vulnerable subjects.
- Where the study involves children, the research complies with 21 CFR 50, Subpart D.

The IRBs and Ethics Committees must review and approve clinical trial protocols to ensure the maximum possible patient protection. This includes a review of the protocol, informed consent, and other aspects of the safety procedures in these trials before the trial starts, as well as maintaining ongoing monitoring of the conduct and results of the trial at least yearly. These requirements oblige investigators and sponsors to submit certain serious AEs to the IRBs/Ethics Committees either as they occur or in aggregate summary reports. The key current controversy revolves around what data are to be sent to the IRBs and Ethics Committees. In the past, every expedited report and follow-up case was sent. This proved to be logistically problematic for the investigators and IRBs as follow-up reports often contained trivial data (correction of height or weight). The health agencies have clarified this situation to a degree and now recommend aggregate reporting and line listings sent periodically. Individual expedited cases are still required but follow-up reports are usually not sent unless they are medically important. It is useful to discuss with the IRBs and Ethics Committees before starting the study what they wish to receive.

For further information, the reader is referred to these documents as well as documents in each country where a trial is being held. This is a complex and changing area as health agencies and the public are becoming increasingly concerned about patient protection.

33

Product Quality Issues

In the past several years, it has been realized that many other issues in addition to bad reactions to the active chemical entity in the product play a significant role in drug safety and pharmacovigilance, because of the realization that a safety issue may be related to more than just the active ingredient (moiety). Excipients (see Chapter 5), residues from the manufacturing process, quality control (or lack thereof), the container and packaging, storage issues in the pharmacy or home, tampering, counterfeiting, and other adventures that occur before and after the product has left the factory can produce bad effects. So an adverse event (AE) is more than just a bad reaction to the active chemical entity. This chapter summarizes briefly issues that revolve around quality and manufacturing.

Patient or healthcare professional product complaints can revolve around the following:

- The drug did not work (lack of efficacy).

- The drug produced an AE (safety issue).
- The drug looked, tasted, or smelled funny or different. It was crumbling. There was a powder on the pill and so forth (product manufacturing or quality issue).
- The drug was a tablet in the past, but this time it was capsules (quality issue in packaging, dispensing, etc.).
- I want my money back or I am suing.
- I ordered these pills on the internet from a pharmacy supposedly in Canada (possible counterfeit or quality issue).
- I saw on the internet that this pill should….
- Others ("My dog accidentally ate the pills.").

Frequently, one sees multiple issues with a single phone call: "The pill was the wrong color, and when I took it, I developed chest pain, and I want my money back or I'll sue." Part of the issue here involves getting the correct people within the pharmaceutical company (or health authority or call center if they are the first to receive the call) to act on each of the issues involved: the AE component, the product quality component, and the monetary/legal component. In this chapter, we address product quality issues.

Manufacturing is regulated in most countries and regions by a set of regulations, directives, laws, and guidances that go under the general rubric of "Good Manufacturing Practices," or GMP. The International Conference on Harmonization (ICH) has addressed manufacturing issues in a series of "Quality Guidelines" (Web Resource 33-1), covering such topics as stability, analytical validation, impurities, and so forth. The key document is Q7: Good Manufacturing Practices. Each country or region has enacted its own requirements for GMP.

- In the United States in the Code of Federal Regulations section 21CFR211, Current Good Manufacturing Practice for Finished Pharmaceuticals
- In the European Union in Directive 2003/94/EC (Web Resource 33-2) for the United Kingdom in guidances and legislation (Web Resource 33-3)
- In Canada multiple guidances (Web Resource 33-4)

To a large degree, the GMP requirements are quite similar around the world, and one factory will frequently produce products sold in many (or all) global markets, thus meeting all standards.

In the United States, the specific section covering product quality issues is 211.198 Complaint Files:

(a) Written procedures describing the handling of all written and oral complaints regarding a drug product shall be established and followed. Such procedures shall include provisions for review by the quality control unit, of any complaint involving the possible failure of a drug product to meet any of its specifications and, for such drug products, a determination as to the need for an investigation in accordance with Sec. 211.192. Such procedures shall include provisions for review to determine whether the complaint represents a serious and unexpected adverse drug experience which is required to be reported to the Food and Drug Administration (21CFR211.198).

This section obliges the manufacturer to maintain written procedures on the handling of all complaints and specifies that a review must be done for serious and unexpected AEs. The U.S. Food and Drug Administration (FDA) performs inspections (more than 22,000 in 2004 but dropping to 15,000 in 2008). The FDA has committed to increasing its inspections, and product quality issues are often cited. An example follows from a Warning Letter to a pharmaceutical company:

2. Failure to follow established Standard Operating Procedures regarding the handling of written and oral drug product quality complaints [21 CFR 211.198(a)]

Your firm's QCU failed to follow established written Standard Operating Procedures (SOP) for investigating drug product quality complaints received by your firm. Specifically, your firm's SOP states that it is the responsibility of the support departments (e.g., Quality Assurance, Quality Control, etc.) to complete their part of the complaint investigation "usually within 30 days." Yet, our Investigator observed incomplete complaint investigations lasting as long as 247 and 301 days after receipt of the complaint (Warning Letter to Koss Pharmaceuticals, December 29, 2003; Web Resource 33-5).

The responsibility for investigating product complaints generally falls within the competence of one of the quality units in a company. The drug safety department usually becomes involved when there is a product quality complaint, a medical error, or an AE. That is, even though there was an issue with the manufacturing or quality of the product, the subject took the product and had an AE. Sometimes, of course, the quality issue is only discovered or noted after the use of the product (e.g., the patient had an AE and went back to look at the package and noted the tablets smelled funny and were off-color—a quality issue).

Within the pharmaceutical company, this is a "double issue," with an evaluation of the AE by the drug safety group and an evaluation of the product complaint by the quality unit and the manufacturing unit concerned. There are several critical operational issues:

- All units (e.g., drug safety, manufacturing, and quality control) must be informed that the other units are involved in the same case if the case was received and triaged elsewhere (e.g., in Medical Affairs or Medical Communications). Each unit follows its procedures and does its evaluation, usually simultaneously.
- The units must communicate their findings to each other because one or both will likely be required to submit the findings to the health authorities. A mechanism must be developed to request that the patient who filed the complaint return any unused product to the company for analysis. Some companies do this for all complaints, whereas others set up specific criteria for requests for return of

product. The quality workup may include reviewing batch records, testing the retained sample, and testing the sample returned by the patient.

- The results of this testing must be conveyed to the drug safety unit to include in the report to the FDA and any other concerned health authorities. If this is an expedited report, the quality unit must get the new information to the drug safety unit so that the follow-up to the agencies is done within the required time (often 15 calendar days or less for serious issues). The quality unit must not delay sending the information to the drug safety group. Similarly, relevant clinical follow-up information (e.g., lot numbers) from the drug safety unit should be forwarded immediately to the quality unit on the case.

- The case may have two or more different identification numbers—one in the drug safety unit and the other in the quality unit. If the computer system(s) cannot handle the two numbers for the same case, then another method of tracking must be developed to ensure that the case does not fall through the cracks. For large companies, the volume of such investigations may be quite high, with many data flowing back and forth between the departments. In addition, a third or even fourth department may be involved if the case involves a refund of money to the patient or a possible legal or police action (e.g., a lawsuit or police investigation for tampering).

- Now that the manufacture of many products is outsourced and sometimes done in more than one factory (e.g., one for raw materials and another for finished product and packaging), coordination and investigation may become complex and require careful and meticulous coordination and tracking.

- AEs and product quality complaints are now considered "two sides of the same coin." That is, if an AE occurs after taking a drug, it is not always evident that the event is due to the active ingredient. It might be due to an excipient or a problem in manufacturing, storage, or shipping, or perhaps the product is a counterfeit. It is good pharmacovigilance practice for the drug safety group or the pharmacovigilance or risk management group to examine product quality issues on a regular basis to determine whether a clue or suggestion indicates that quality issues have produced AEs. The methodology for this evaluation (the relationship of quality issues to AEs) has not been fully harmonized yet

and remains a methodology of "global introspection." Some of the newer safety databases are now able to capture product quality issues for cases in addition to the usual AE data. The analysis should attempt to see whether there are similar cases (AEs and product complaints) seen with that product's lot, batch number, or geographic area. (Mail-order pharmacy systems distributing drugs from centralized locations to all parts of the United States now make geographic tracking much harder and less useful. The days when a particular batch of a drug was used in a localized geographic area are disappearing in the United States but less so in smaller countries or regions).

- Significant and severe product quality issues, in particular those that risk patient health or produce serious AEs or suggest tampering, must be acted on immediately. The pharmaceutical company must have a mechanism in place to recognize such issues, investigate them, and bring the information in a timely fashion to the responsible levels of the company and the health agencies. If necessary, a product may need to be withdrawn immediately, public and internet/social media announcements made, protocols stopped, and so forth. The company should have a procedure whereby the team that would need to perform these actions is easily mobilizable for action.

- Many of the AE/product quality issues are often small and noncritical. Examples include the discovery that a part of the packaging (e.g., vials or stoppers) was obtained from a new vendor and looked or acted differently, or late stability testing showed problems. Sometimes it is discovered that a part or procedure was slightly but clearly out of specification. The determination of how far to proceed in terms of analysis and recall of products is often a difficult decision that requires the assistance of multiple departments within the company and the concerned health agencies. Complications can arise if one health agency wants or demands a recall and another does not. A formal written procedure must be developed and used.

The definitions of recalls and withdrawals in the United States are as follows:

- Class I recall: a situation in which there is a reasonable probability that the use of or exposure to a violative product will cause serious adverse health consequences or death.

- Class II recall: a situation in which use of or exposure to a violative product may cause temporary or medically reversible adverse health consequences or where the probability of serious adverse health consequences is remote.
- Class III recall: a situation in which use of or exposure to a violative product is not likely to cause adverse health consequences.
- Market withdrawal: occurs when a product has a minor violation that would not be subject to FDA legal action. The firm removes the product from the market or corrects the violation. For example, a product removed from the market due to tampering, without evidence of manufacturing or distribution problems, would be a market withdrawal.
- Medical device safety alert: issued in situations in which a medical device may present an unreasonable risk of substantial harm. In some cases, these situations are considered recalls.

Examples of recalls, withdrawals, and safety alerts can be seen at the FDA's website (Web Resource 33-6), including a partial listing of some of the recalls in early 2010 for drugs (Web Resource 33-6) and biologics (Web Resource 33-7) in the following two sections.

Drugs

- Alli 60 mg capsules (120-count refill kit): Counterfeit product
- Atlas Operations, Inc.: Recall of sexual enhancement products
- Avandia (rosiglitazone): Ongoing review of cardiovascular safety
- Benadryl Extra Strength Itch Stopping Gel: Packaging changes to reduce use errors
- Camolyn eye drops, Fisiolin nasal drops: Voluntary recall due to nonsterility
- Erythropoiesis-Stimulating Agents (ESAs): Procrit, Epogen, and Aranesp: Drug safety communication
- Exjade (deferasirox): Boxed warning
- GnRH Agonists: Safety review of drug class used to treat prostate cancer
- Heparin: Change in reference standard
- Invirase (saquinavir): Ongoing safety review of clinical trial data
- Long-Acting Beta-Agonists (LABAs): New safe use requirements
- Maalox Total Relief and Maalox Liquid Products: Medication use errors

- MasXtreme Capsules (Natural Wellness): Product contains undeclared drug ingredient
- McNeil Consumer Healthcare Over-the-Counter Infants' and Children's Products: Recall
- McNeil Consumer Healthcare Over-the-Counter Products: Recall
- Meridia (sibutramine hydrochloride): Follow-up to an early communication about an ongoing safety review
- Metronidazole injection 500 mg/100 mL: Voluntary recall due to nonsterility
- MuscleMaster.com Products Sold on Internet as Dietary Supplements: Recall
- Oral Bisphosphonates: Ongoing safety review of atypical subtrochanteric femur fractures

Biologics

- Important Notice RabAvert Rabies Vaccine (Rabies Vaccine for Human Use) Kits
- Important Information Regarding Influenza A (H1N1) 2009 Monovalent Vaccine Live, Intranasal Expiration Dating
- Recall of AMICUS Ancillary PL2410 Plastic Storage Container 4R2350
- Recall of Prevnar Pneumococcal 7-valent Conjugate Vaccine, Wyeth
- Market Withdrawal of Chiron RIBA HCV 3.0 SIA
- Recall of Influenza A (H1N1) 2009 Monovalent Vaccine
- Field Correction of Influenza A (H1N1) 2009 Monovalent Vaccine in Prefilled Syringes
- Recall of Y-Type Blood Solution Sets
- Field Correction of Influenza A (H1N1) 2009 Monovalent Vaccine Live, Intranasal Expiration Dating

Generally, most countries have mechanisms for emergency recalls or withdrawals from the market of products that have severe or dangerous or high-risk quality problems. This may be for the entire drug or only for certain formulations, lots, or other subgroups. These may be handled as expedited, reports or "rapid alerts" in the European Union. Although the safety group may be closely involved, the operational issues of the withdrawal or alert will involve multiple groups, including manufacturing, regulatory, legal, and communications (if the public has to be contacted).

■ Counterfeiting

Counterfeit, fake, specious products are now a major concern. This is especially true for certain high-margin, highly desired drugs on the market (e.g., erectile dysfunction drugs, narcotics). Many companies and health agencies are confronting this issue. Warnings are issued almost weekly by health agencies to consumers and medical personnel regarding fake products that can be harmful to patients. FDA has issued a guidance on mechanisms companies can implement to identify counterfeit products: "Incorporation of Physical-Chemical Identifiers into Solid Oral Dosage Form Drug Products for Anticounterfeiting" (see Web Resource 33-8).

See also the World Health Organization's information on drug counterfeiting (Web Resource 33-9).

Every company marketing or distributing a product should have an SOP dealing with counterfeit or suspected counterfeit products. It should set up procedures for drug safety, corporate quality/manufacturing, legal, and regulatory to deal with matters in their domains. The manufacturing/quality groups should determine that the product is fake, ideally by requesting that it be sent to the company (in a postage-free mailer). Unfortunately for drug safety, the case usually arrives as a "normal" SAE or nonserious AE and must be handled as such even if it is suspected to be from a counterfeit medication. Such suspicions should be noted in the narrative of the initial report if present, and a note made that follow-up verification is being pursued. The physical product should be requested immediately, including the packaging, and

forwarded to manufacturing/quality for testing upon receipt. Obviously, all communications and receipt must be well documented in the database.

If a case turns out to be due to a counterfeit and not due to the company's product, this should be notified in a follow-up to all concerned health authorities. How it is handled in the database in periodic reports (PSURs) is tricky and not standardized. As a rule, the case should not be included (necessarily) in the tables, listings, and analyses of the company's product, but rather addressed in a separate section of the report. It may be difficult to handle this within the safety database. Drug safety may want to work with the legal and regulatory departments as well as manufacturing to set up a coordinated system to handle this. Some companies are now setting up security departments just to deal with counterfeits.

■ Frequently Asked Questions

Q: This doesn't seem fair. Why should a company have to report and waste time and resources on tracking down safety matters concerning counterfeit drugs?

A: Well, of course, life is not fair. But this is still an important public health issue and the company will serve both the public health and its own interest (to protect its products) by pursuing and resolving issues around counterfeits. In practice, it is not always clear whether a drug is or is not a counterfeit, especially if the original packaging is no longer available.

34

Drug Labeling

L abeling is a general term encompassing many things about a drug. Labeling is divided for pharmacovigilance purposes into several different documents. For drugs that are not yet on the market (approved for sale), labeling used for adverse events (AE) reporting and all other "official" considerations is the "Investigator Brochure" as prepared by the sponsor and submitted to the health authorities (e.g., U.S. Food and Drug Administration, Health Canada). After a drug is approved for marketing (e.g., New Drug Application or Marketing Authorization granted), the labeling that is used for regulatory reporting of AEs now changes to that document prepared by the sponsor and submitted to, negotiated with, and approved by the health authority for that jurisdiction: the "Package Insert" (PI) in the United States, and the Summary of Product Characteristics (SPC or SmPC) in the European

Union. The other key labeling document is the Clinical Core Safety Information (CCSI). All are discussed below.

■ Investigator Brochure (IB)

The requirements for the IB are listed in ICH E6 Guidance on Good Clinical Practices (Web Resource 34-1), which has been adopted in most jurisdictions. It is a compilation of clinical and nonclinical data on the study product that is relevant to the investigators performing the trial, allowing them to understand the rationale and key features of the drug. It is the sponsor's responsibility to prepare the IB and keep it up to date. It summarizes the chemical, physical, and pharmacologic properties of the drug; nonclinical studies; effects in humans; including absorption, distribution, metabolism, and excretion (ADME) data, as well as clinical studies in volunteers and patients covering both efficacy and safety. Marketing experience, if available, is also included.

The IB should contain summaries of safety across multiple trials with indications in subgroups using tabular summaries of ADRs. Important differences in ADR patterns/incidences across indications or subgroups should be noted if present. The IB should provide a description of the possible risks and ADRs to be anticipated on the basis of prior experiences with the product and with related products. Any precautions or special monitoring to be done should also be noted. The IB can be dozens of pages long and should be more inclusive rather than less inclusive. It is not a marketing document and will be reviewed by investigators, Investigational Review Boards/Ethics Committees and data safety management committees.

The IB should be updated yearly or more often if new information, particularly about safety, becomes available. This document is used in the preparation of 7- and 15-day expedited (alert) reports to the health authorities and for investigational new drug annual reports (e.g., Development Safety Update Reports, or DSURs).

After a drug is approved for marketing and if it is also in clinical trials, it will have both an IB and postmarketing labeling (e.g., SPC, U.S. PI).

■ Clinical Core Safety Information (CCSI)

The "Core Safety Information" (CSI), or "Company Core Safety Information" (CCSI), which is part of the larger "Company Core Data Sheet" (CCDS), contains the key safety data for the marketed product. This document was defined originally by the CIOMS III and CIOMS V documents (Web Resource 34-2). The CCSI contains (only) basic safety information that should appear in the safety labeling for the product in all countries where the product is used. It should not contain speculation or safety information that might appear in only one country's labeling for some local reason. Thus, the information in the CCSI represents the minimal safety data that should appear globally in all local or national labeling. Additions may be made in local labeling beyond what is in the CCSI if the local health authority or company so chooses. Marketing considerations should not play a role in preparing the CCSI. AEs due to excipients should be included, but those that have no well-established relationship to the drug should not be included. The CCSI is used to determine which AEs are considered "listed" when preparing the Periodic Safety Update Reports (PSURs). It is not used for expedited reporting expectedness (the approved, postmarketing label is used).

Other safety documents used in various countries include the Development Core Safety Information, Development Core Data Sheets, and Target Product Profiles. They all are similar to the CCSI and contain key

safety information used for clinical trials, periodic reporting, and so forth. It is likely that the DSUR—the parallel to the PSUR used for marketed drugs—will formalize the safety reference document to be used.

■ United States Safety Labeling for Marketed Products

The U.S. requirements for labeling are summarized in 21CFR1. The official definition of labeling for a marketed product is 21CFR1.3(a) (see Web Resource 34-3):

(a) Labeling includes all written, printed, or graphic matter accompanying an article at any time while such article is in interstate commerce or held for sale after shipment or delivery in interstate commerce.

(b) Label means any display of written, printed, or graphic matter on the immediate container of any article, or any such matter affixed to any consumer commodity or affixed to or appearing upon a package containing any consumer commodity.

Thus, it includes the FDA-approved written material describing a drug, such as the Package Insert and the packaging and box that a drug is shipped or sold in. Synonyms for labeling include "Package Insert," "professional labeling," "direction circular," "approved labeling," and "package circular." It also includes the FDA-approved patient labeling (called "Medication Guides") where this exists (see Web Resource 34-4 for approved patient medication labeling).

In 2003, the FDA introduced the new requirements for the electronic formatting of labels, called the "Structured Product Labeling" (SPL), using a document markup standard approved by HL7 (see Chapters 8, 19, and 20). See FDA's website for further information on this labeling initiative (Web Resource 34-5).

The specific requirements for drug labeling are found in 21CFR201.57 (Web Resource 34-6). These labeling requirements, which were revised in 2006, include:

Highlights section, drug names, dosage form, route of administration and controlled substance symbol (if such a drug), initial US approval, boxed warning (if any), recent major changes, indications and usage, dosage and administration, dosage forms and strengths, contraindications, warnings and precautions, adverse reactions, interactions, use in specific populations (including pregnancy, teratogenicity, geriatric and pediatric use), patient counseling information, revision date, drug abuse/dependence, overdosage, clinical pharmacology, non-clinical toxicology, clinical studies, references, how supplied, patient counseling information.

Note that the highlights section, is a short summary (1/2 to 2 pages) of the rest of the labeling. Labels before 2006 have largely the same sections, though there is no highlights section, and the safety sections are much shorter in many cases.

FDA issued a guidance covering the new requirements in more detail, entitled "Labeling for Human Prescription Drug and Biological Products —Implementing the New Content and Format Requirements" (Web Resource 34-7). Several other guidances covering the various sections of the labeling were also issued and are available at Web Resource 34-8.

The guidance covering the adverse reaction section will be discussed briefly here (Web Resource 34-9).

- The goal is to include only information useful to practitioners making treatment decisions and monitoring patients. Exhaustive lists of AEs should be avoided.

- The Adverse Reactions (ARs) section should contain those that occur with the drug itself and ARs from the class if appropriate. Clinical trial and spontaneous reports must be listed separately.

- All serious and otherwise important ARs should be listed and cross-referenced (e.g., Boxed Warning, Warnings and Precautions).

- ARs that resulted in a significant rate of discontinuation or other clinical intervention, such as dose change in clinical trials.

- ARs from clinical trials is the major component of the AR section and should include the most commonly occurring ARs (e.g., all ARs >10% and 2 × placebo rate). This section should describe the clinical trial database in terms of exposure, number of patients, demographics, types of studies, doses, and so forth. Data should be presented in a table to allow side-by-side comparisons. The best available data should be used—placebo-controlled and dose response studies.

- Less common ARs should be presented if there is a basis to feel that a causal relationship to the drug exists.

- Additional information should be given for the most clinically significant ARs (i.e., most common,

cause discontinuation, or dose change or require monitoring).

- Dose response, demographic, and subgroup information should be included if important.

- If there are multiple indications and/or multiple formulations, a discussion about these issues in regard to safety should be included.

- A separate listing of spontaneous ARs should be included, particularly those that are serious, frequent, or seem to be causally related ARs.

- When reporting rates are included, all cases of that AE should be used rather than just those the reporter feels are related.

- Comparative safety claims (frequency, severity, or character of the AR) must be based on data from adequate and well-controlled studies.

- Negative findings, if convincingly demonstrated in an adequate trial, may be included.

- Data may be pooled from studies when the studies are appropriate to pool (similar design, populations, etc.).

- Data should be coded meaningfully and grouped as appropriate (e.g., sedation, somnolence, and drowsiness should be grouped as a single AR). Syndromes should be used where appropriate (e.g.. hypersensitivity).

- ARs should be categorized by body system, by severity (in decreasing frequency), or by a combination of both. An appropriate frequency cutoff may be specified.

- Quantitative data (e.g., labs, vital signs, ECGs) should be presented as rates of abnormal values, with a cutoff for inclusion (e.g., five times the upper limit of normal) rather than a grading system.

- If the AR rate is less than it is for the placebo, this information should not be included unless there is a compelling reason to do so.

- Statistical significance should not be included unless based on an adequately designed and powered study.

- The label should be reviewed at least annually to be sure all appropriate data are included.

For an example of this labeling, see the Zyprexa (olanzpine) label (May 2010) at Web Resources 34-10 and 34-11. The label is 32 pages long, and the Warnings and Precautions section runs about 7 pages and includes 7 tables. The AR section runs 9 pages and contains 14 tables, and the Interactions section runs 2 pages. From a practical point of view, if a practitioner has a question, such as "Does this drug cause headache?" and if it is not listed in the summary, the most expedient way to find this is to load the document onto a computer or handheld device as a PDF file and search for that term. Multiple hits may occur, leading to listings in several tables from which the practitioner can draw his or her conclusions. One might observe that this is not necessarily a quick or practical way to find out whether a specific AE or problem has occurred with the product in question.

Many drug labels and patient information for specific drugs can be found at the FDA website (Web Resource 34-12). In addition, most pharmaceutical companies have posted their product labeling on their websites. If the drug is sold in multiple countries, each local company website usually posts the local labeling.

In the United States, many, but not all, prescription drug labels are printed in the reference book known as the Physicians' Desk Reference (PDR), published yearly by Thomson. It is about 3000 pages long and has photos of many of the products as well as the product information. There are other editions for over-the-counter (OTC) products, veterinary products, and so on. See Web Resource 34-13. An electronic version is available free to medical professionals at Web Resource 34-14. Other countries have the equivalent publications with drug labeling.

European Union Safety Labeling for Marketed Products

The requirements for labeling in the European Union (which is called the Summary of Product Characteristics [SPC, or sometimes SmPC]) is found in Volume 2C, which includes the requirements for submitting the dossier for a new product (Web Resource 34-15). This includes the September 2009 European Union Guidance on SmPCs (Web Resource 34-16).

The SPC "sets out the agreed position of the medicinal product as distilled during the course of the assessment process." It cannot be changed without agreement by the health authorities. If a drug is approved centrally in the European Union, or if the labeling is harmonized, then there should only be one SPC per product, though there may be additional SPCs for the same chemical entity if there are different forms or strengths. Drugs that are not approved or harmonized may have a different SPC in each member state. The SPC will usually be in the local language of the country.

Similar to other country labeling, the SPC includes the name, strength, pharmaceutical form, composition, indications, dosing (called "posology"), method of administration, special populations (renal, hepatic impairment, elderly, genotype-particular patients, pediatrics), contraindications, special warnings, precautions (including ARs to which healthcare professionals need to be alerted), interactions, fertility, pregnancy and lactation, effects on driving and machine use, undesirable effects (adverse reactions), overdose, pharmacological properties, preclinical safety data, pharmaceutical details, including excipients, incompatibilities, shelf life, storage, appropriate container, disposal instructions, and registration and update information.

The adverse reaction section should include all ARs from clinical trials, postauthorization safety studies, and spontaneous reports "for which a causal relationship between the medicinal product and the adverse event is at least a reasonable possibility." ARs should not be listed if there is no suspicion of a causal relationship. The section should contain the following:

- A summary of the safety profile containing information on the most serious and/or most frequent ARs.
- A tabulated list of ARs with frequency. It should be a single table in general though separate tables may be used in exceptional circumstances (e.g., using a product in different indications or dosages). In general, MedDRA Preferred Terms (PTs) should be used. If appropriate, data from several trials may be pooled.
- A description of selected ARs that "may be useful to prevent, assess or manage the occurrence of an adverse reaction in clinical practice."

For further detail, see Volume 2C. As an example, the olanzapine Pliva SPC (cf. Zyprexa above) is 11 pages, and the safety section is approximately 6 pages with 2 tables. See Web Resource 34-17.

Other Countries

Most countries of the world have fairly similar registration and approval systems, involving a multidisciplinary review of all the submitted data and labeling based on the submitted data. The approvals may vary significantly from country to country; however, they are based on different data submitted or emphasized, different indications requested, different formulations, different patient populations treated, and local customs. Thus, the labeling may be somewhat different from country to country. In addition, in non-English-speaking countries, the labeling is, of course, in the local language.

In the European Union, the approved labeling is known as the Summary of Product Characteristics (SPC, or SmPC). There is a curious use of terminology by some people. In the United States, the generic term labeling (sometimes called the "Package Insert," or "PI") is used to refer to the official FDA-approved U.S. product information. The word "labeling" is also used in the United States for the SPC when referring to European labeling. Some in the European Union, conversely, use the term SPC (or SmPC) when they are referring to their own official labeling or to the U.S. labeling. Thus, one might hear a reference to the U.S. SPC—a concept that does not really exist in the United States. This refers, in practice, to the U.S. official labeling and not the European Union SPC.

In terms of pharmacovigilance, sections of labeling of most interest include the AEs, warnings, drug interactions, precautions, and pregnancy information. In particular, the labeling is used to determine whether a particular AE that is reported for that product is "labeled"/"listed" (expected; see Chapter 1). In general, if an AE is expected, it does not have to be reported to the health authority as an expedited report. Class labeling of a particular AE/AR is not considered expected or labeled for the purposes of expedited reporting in most jurisdictions.

Changes, additions, removals, "variations," and alterations to product labeling must usually be approved by the health authority concerned (the FDA for U.S. labeling). In many jurisdictions, the sponsor (NDA holder, MAH) may change the labeling to add an urgent safety warning without prior approval by the health agency. In the United States, this is known as "Changes Being Effected." This is permitted

> to add or strengthen a contraindication, warning, precaution, or adverse reaction for which the evidence of a causal association satisfies the standard for inclusion in the labeling…to add or strengthen a statement about abuse, dependence, psychological effect, or overdosage…to add or strengthen an instruction about dosage and administration that is intended to increase the safety of the use of the product.

See, for example, 21CFR601.12 Changes to an approved application for biologics. Similarly, in the European Union, "urgent safety restrictions" are permitted. See the European Union document SOP/H/30752 (Web Resource 34-22).

Note that drug labels do not always use MedDRA terms for AEs. Many drugs are quite old and date back many years to pre-MedDRA days. Thus, terms used are from other dictionaries, such as COSTART or WHO-ART, or the terms may be non-standardized. This can clearly produce issues when one attempts to determine whether a term (e.g., a MedDRA term) is considered labeled or listed if a similar but not quite exactly matching term is found. Presumably, all labels will eventually be "MedDRA-ized."

In Canada, the equivalent of the PDR is called the Compendium of Pharmaceuticals and Specialties (Web Resource 34-18), available in English and French. In France, it is called the "Vidal" (this website is in French, Web Resource 34-19) and in Germany, the "Rote Liste" (this website is in German, Web Resource 34-20). In the United Kingdom, SPCs and Patient Information Leaflets (PILs) are available at Web Resource 34-21.

■ OTC Labeling in the United States

The labeling for OTC products in the United States is usually different from the labeling of prescription products. With most OTC drugs, labeling is derived from "monographs" (the CFR sections dealing with these products and specifying which products may be sold without an NDA or Abbreviated New Drug Application [ANDA]). OTC drugs are used by patients and consumers without a healthcare intermediary (physician, pharmacist, nurse) to explain the product, its use, its adverse events, and so forth. The labeling is what is written on the package (box) in the section marked "Drug Facts." This is a lay version of a Package Insert but is often very skimpy regarding AEs. Sometimes none is listed at all. This is often most surprising because certain products that had extensive lists of AEs (e.g., loratadine, nonsteroidal anti-inflammatory drugs) in the Package Insert when they were prescription drugs now have minimal safety information in the OTC Drug Facts.

Some OTC products may be sold under an NDA or ANDA, and these products may have a classic Package Insert. These drugs do not fall under the monographs and were previously prescription drugs with an NDA or ANDA that remains in effect.

Similarly, for food supplements, there is a label marked "Supplement Facts." Many companies that sell OTC products sell supplements, drugs, devices, and sometimes even cosmetics, making for very complicated AE collection and reporting.

This labeling situation complicates AE reporting to the FDA. A product may be an OTC through (usually) two mechanisms: (1) an approved NDA or ANDA that was originally for a prescription product that has been moved to OTC status or (2) through the OTC drug monograph process. Safety reporting obligations depend on which route was used. For products with an NDA or ANDA the requirements are the same as for prescription products (e.g., expedited reporting, approved labeling, Periodic Reports/PSURs). Until 2007, there was no obligatory safety reporting for monograph products, though some companies voluntarily submitted safety reports, usually for SAEs. The Dietary Supplement and Nonprescription Drug Consumer Protection Act of 2006 and a subsequent guidance in 2009 clarified the situation.

The reporting requirements are as follows:

- Manufacturer, packer, or distributor whose name is on the label (called the "responsible person") must submit to FDA all SAEs with a copy of the label within 15 business days.
- All follow-up information received within 1 year of the initial report must be submitted within 15 business days. Note that the law says states only 1 year of follow-up, but FDA has indicated that it wants no time limit. That is, report all follow-ups forever.
- MedWatch (3500A) form or E2B to be used for reporting.
- The NDA definitions for minimum criteria, reportability, and so forth, are in effect here.
  - For brand families, it is necessary to know the active ingredient to have a reportable drug
  - If multiple suspect drugs, submit Individual Case Safety Report (ICSR) to FDA and to other manufacturers
- No aggregate reporting requirements
- Signaling is required for the NDA/ANDA products but is not specifically stated to be required for monograph products, though it would be wise to do so.

In the European Union, there are no OTC products without MAs, so all prescription drug reporting requirements apply to OTC products. In practice, many companies treat all OTC products the same and do expedited reporting, periodic reporting, and signaling. Some countries have multiple and more complex rules, including "over-the-counter" and "behind-the-counter" products, which do not require prescriptions but which may (in the latter category) require the customer's talking to the pharmacist before being able to purchase the product.

The pharmacovigilance worker in a company or health agency should be sure to receive updated labeling by the group in charge of preparing these documents. Though obvious, this is not always routine. Groups other than those that deal with pharmacovigilance usually prepare labeling, and preparers may not always remember to distribute new labeling to drug safety and other groups that need it.

For pharmacovigilance professionals, knowledge of the labeling for the drugs for which they are responsible is absolutely necessary. For drugs with many AEs, it is generally a good idea to prepare a separate table either on paper or in a spreadsheet as a reference, listing the AEs, to aid when determining labeledness/listedness (expectedness). These AEs may, in fact, appear in multiple sections and at varying levels of specificity. They should be harvested and grouped appropriately so that a ready reference (known as a "cheat sheet") can be consulted when evaluating and coding AEs. It may be useful to list the corresponding MedDRA terms and level (verbatim, preferred term, lower-level term). Some computer safety databases are able to mechanize the specific MedDRA terms that are considered labeled/listed, obviating the need for such "cheat sheets."

Many drugs have multiple labeling documents if there are different preparations (e.g., different labeling for intravenous and oral preparations of the same active ingredient). The AEs in the two labels may differ because some will be route-specific (e.g., injection site reactions or those related to a first-pass effect after oral intake).

Frequently Asked Questions

Q: This seems rather duplicative and wasteful. In general, wouldn't the safety profile be the same worldwide? Wouldn't one label be sufficient for a marketed drug?

A: In theory, both questions should be answered with a "yes." However, labeling is quite complicated and each health authority wants to reserve its right to review and change the labeling. The CCSI is the common worldwide label, and this concept seems to work well and could reasonably be extended to full official labeling. That said, there are situations in which a drug might work differently in one group or region. Thus, regional differences requiring different labels may be justified in some cases. Nonetheless, all differences and subgroups could still be listed in one single global label. One, two, or perhaps three countries at most could be responsible for a drug and its labeling, safety profile, and updates. This probably is feasible but, given the geopolitical situation in the world, is unlikely to come about anytime soon.

Pregnancy and Lactation

Testing pregnant animals is done as part of the usual preclinical development of new drugs, but a drug that is not teratogenic (leading to congenital malformations) in some or all animal species tested may sometimes, unfortunately, still be noxious in women. For obvious reasons, clinical testing is almost never done in pregnant women during the development of new drugs unless the drug is developed expressly for use in pregnancy. Thus, the safety and efficacy of drugs in pregnant women is largely unknown at the time of marketing, and only a little additional information is gained from spontaneous reporting of adverse events (AEs).

Some drugs are used and, to some degree, tested in pregnancy, usually in situations in which treatment is obligatory for either the mother or unborn child (e.g., hypertension, asthma, rheumatoid arthritis, epilepsy). These studies are usually not blinded and are prospective or retrospective observational or surveillance studies.

Pregnancy registries are now required for manufacturers and Marketing Authorization/New Drug Application holders for most marketed drugs. That is, every use of the drug that the company becomes aware of in a pregnant woman or by a pregnant woman's partner is recorded and followed to outcome (birth, miscarriage, etc.).

■ Situation in the United States

The U.S. Food and Drug Administration's current pregnancy categories are as follows:

A: Adequate, well-controlled studies in pregnant women have not shown an increased risk of fetal abnormalities to the fetus in any trimester of pregnancy.

B: Animal studies have revealed no evidence of harm to the fetus; however, there are no adequate and well-controlled studies in pregnant women.

Or

Animal studies have shown an adverse effect, but adequate and well-controlled studies in pregnant women have failed to demonstrate a risk to the fetus in any trimester.

C: Animal studies have shown an adverse effect, and there are no adequate and well-controlled studies in pregnant women.

Or

No animal studies have been conducted, and there are no adequate and well-controlled studies in pregnant women.

D: Adequate, well-controlled, or observational studies in pregnant women have demonstrated a risk to the fetus. However, the benefits of therapy may outweigh the potential risk. For example, the drug may be acceptable if needed in a life-threatening situation or for a serious disease for which safer drugs cannot be used or are ineffective.

X: Adequate, well-controlled, or observational studies in animals or pregnant women have demonstrated positive evidence of fetal abnormalities or risks. The use of the product is contraindicated in women who are or may become pregnant.

■ Proposed Changes by FDA

In 2008, the FDA issued proposed changes in the rules for pregnancy and lactation labeling. The proposed rule would remove the letter categories noted above and would replace them with three new sections:

1. The "Fetal Risk Summary" section would describe what is known about the effects of the drug on the fetus, and if there is a risk, whether this risk is based on information from animals or humans. A risk conclusion would be made, such as "Human data indicate that (name of drug) increases the risk of cardiac abnormalities," followed by a summary of the data.

2. The "Clinical Considerations" section would include information about the effects of the use of the drug on the mother and fetus if it is taken before a woman knows she is pregnant.
   - Inadvertent exposure
   - Risk from the disease
   - Dosing adjustments during pregnancy
   - ARs unique to pregnancy with this drug
   - Interventions needed (e.g., monitoring)
   - Complications associated with the drug
   - Effects during labor and delivery

3. The "Data" section would describe in more detail the available data.

Information on the pregnancy registry would also be included. See FDA's pregnancy/lactation section for further information (Web Resource 35-1).

The lactation section of the labeling would use the same format as the pregnancy section noted above.

This change in label presentation does not change or alter the data collected; it is simply a better way to present the known data.

■ FDA Guidance for Industry—2002

In August 2002, the FDA issued a guidance for industry on establishing pregnancy registries. In this guidance, the FDA gives a specific definition of a birth registry to differentiate it from a teratology registry:

A pregnancy exposure registry is a prospective observational study that actively collects information on medical product exposure during pregnancy and associated pregnancy outcomes.

This type of registry is not a pregnancy prevention program. The FDA does not recommend a registry for all drugs:

We recommend that a pregnancy exposure registry be seriously considered when it is likely that the medical product will be used during pregnancy as therapy for a new or chronic condition.

A medical product may also be a good candidate for a pregnancy exposure registry when one of the following conditions exists:

- Inadvertent exposures to the medical product in pregnancy are or are expected to be common such as when products have a high likelihood of use by women of childbearing age.

- The medical product presents special circumstances, such as the potential for infection of mother and fetus by administration of live, attenuated vaccines.

Pregnancy exposure registries are unlikely to be warranted in the following situations: (1) there is no systemic exposure to the medical product, or (2) the product is not, or rarely, used by women of childbearing age.

A registry can be established at any time during the life of a drug. The sponsor or the FDA may initiate the request. The design of the registry is a function of the objective. It may be an open-ended surveillance to the specific testing of a hypothesis-using standard.

Good Epidemiologic Practices

The guidance then details critical elements of a registry, including objectives, exposure, sample size, eligibility requirements, data source and content, fetal anomalies sought, use of an independent data monitoring committee, an investigational review board, and informed consent. The reader is referred to the guidance for these epidemiologic details.

A few points of note:

When estimating the number of exposed pregnancies to be enrolled prospectively, it is important to be aware that approximately 62 percent of clinically recognized pregnancies will result in a live birth, 22 percent will end in elective termination, and 16 percent will result in fetal loss (i.e., spontaneous abortions and fetal death/stillbirth (Ventura, Mosher, Curtin, et al., Vital Health Stat 2000;21:56).

Birth defects occur "spontaneously" in a high number of women. The March of Dimes Birth Defect Foundation, Fact Sheet 2001, available on its website (Web Resource 35-2), reports the following rates for various pregnancy outcomes and fetal abnormalities:

- Spontaneous abortions/miscarriage (loss before 20 weeks): 1 in 7 known pregnancies
- Low birth weight (<2,500 grams): 1 in 12 live births
- Fetal death/stillbirth (loss after 20 weeks): 1 in 200 known pregnancies
- Any major birth defect: 1 in 25 live births
- Heart and circulation defects: 1 in 115 live births
- Genital and urinary tract defects: 1 in 135 live births
- Nervous system and eye defects: 1 in 235 live births
- Club foot: 1 in 735 live births
- Cleft lip with or without cleft palate: 1 in 930 live births

The guidance also notes that other types of studies, such as case-control studies, may be useful to evaluate rare adverse birth outcomes and to identify whether the drug in question is an associated risk factor. They are useful when long-term follow-up is needed. They can be nested within other existing pregnancy registries.

Automated database studies (e.g., health maintenance organizations, Medicaid) may be useful also.

Regulatory Reporting Requirements

Registries are considered solicited information and thus must be reported as if they were clinical trial AEs: the cases must be serious, unexpected, and have a reasonable possibility that the product caused the AE. See 21 CFR 310.305(c)(1), 314.80(c)(2)(iii) and (e), and 600.80(c) (1), (c)(2)(iii) and (e)). Congenital anomalies are considered serious AEs (21 CFR 314.80(a) and 600.80(a)). Registries that are run independently of sponsors holding New Drug Applications are not subject to postmarketing reporting requirements.

The sponsor must submit an annual status report to the FDA on any registry being run. A registry may be discontinued if

- It has accumulated sufficient data to meet the registry objectives.
- The feasibility of collecting sufficient information diminishes to unacceptable levels due to low exposure, poor enrollment, or loss to follow-up.
- Better methods are developed.
- Termination criteria should be listed in the original protocol.

In conclusion, sponsors who are studying or marketing drugs that may pose a pregnancy/teratology threat must give careful and early consideration to adequate data gathering to determine whether a safety problem exists or whether it is already known to exist in order to quantify and track safety problems. The obvious aim is risk minimization using the various means available.

Situation in the European Union

Volume 9A Section 5.4 addresses pregnancy and lactation. The Marketing Authorization holder (MAH) should follow up all reports from healthcare practitioners of drug use in pregnancy and make "reasonable" efforts when received from consumers. If an AE or abnormal outcome occurs, this should be an expedited report. This includes congenital anomalies, fetal death or spontaneous abortion, and serious adverse reactions. The health authority may require exposure (even without ill effects) for certain products, such as those with high teratogenic potential.

The MAH is encouraged to collect complete data and report even normal outcomes, as this is useful information. This is, in effect, a pregnancy registry and such reports should be included in the Periodic Safety Update Reports along with aggregate data on exposure and outcomes. Formal prospective pregnancy registries should also be included.

Further details are available in the 2005 European Union Guideline on the Exposure to Medicinal Products During Pregnancy (Web Resource 35-3). This document notes the issues to be addressed in Risk Management Plans, data sources, and types of studies (e.g., case series from spontaneous reports, record linkage, pregnancy registries, birth-defect registries, clinical and observational studies, and nongovernmental sources of data). There is also a discussion of data quality and data standardization. This excellent overall review of drugs and pregnancy is worth reading.

Labeling in the European Union (the SPC) should include, per the 2005 European Union Guideline (Web Resource 35-4):

- Clinical data from human experience in pregnancy with the frequency when appropriate.
- Conclusions from developmental studies that are relevant for assessing risk associated with exposure during pregnancy. Only malformative, fetotoxic, and neonatal effects should be mentioned in this paragraph.
- Recommendations on the use of the medicinal product during the different periods of gestation, including a sentence on the reasons for these recommendations.
- Recommendations for managing exposure during pregnancy when appropriate (including relevant specific monitoring, such as fetal ultrasound and specific biological or clinical surveillance of the neonate).

■ Lactation

In general, no breast-feeding infant should be exposed to products the mother takes. In practice, it is not always feasible for the mother to stop certain critical drugs. Fortunately, contrary to pregnancy studies, lactation studies are relatively easy to do and are done routinely in the study of new drugs. The FDA issued a guidance in October 2004, "Guidance for Industry, Pharmacokinetics in Pregnancy—Study Design, Data Analysis, and Impact on Dosing and Labeling" (see Web Resource 35-5).

As the World Health Organization (WHO) states in its publication, "Breast Feeding and Maternal Medication.

Recommendations for Drugs in the 11th WHO Model List of Essential Drugs": "There are very few kinds of treatment during which breastfeeding is absolutely contraindicated. However, there are some drugs which a mother may need to take which sometimes cause side effects in the baby." See its website for the document (Web Resource 35-6). This publication gives specifics for many drugs, with specific recommendations such as "compatible with breastfeeding," "avoid if possible," "avoid breastfeeding," and "no data available."

In the United States, under the new proposal as noted above, the lactation section of the product labeling would include the same three sections:

- Risk summary: Effects of the drug on milk production, whether the drug is present in milk and, if so, how much and the effect on the breast-fed child
- Clinical considerations: How to minimize exposure to the child (e.g., timing, pumping, discarding milk), potential drug effects in the child and monitoring for the effects, dose adjustments.
- Data summary.

In the European Union, the 2005 guideline noted above covers lactation, briefly noting:

If available, clinical data should be mentioned, including studies on the transfer of the active substance or its metabolite(s) into human milk. Information on AEs in nursing neonates should be included if available. Recommendations should be given to stop or continue breast-feeding or to stop or continue treatment. Data on animal studies should be given only if no human data are available.

■ AEs in Pregnant Partners of Males Taking a Drug

This is an area with little information. Reproductive studies in animals are done to determine the effects of new drugs on the testes and sperm. Thus, there are often animal data in regard to whether a drug is toxic to the male reproductive system. There are few data, however, on toxicity in the female and the fetus due to transfer of the drug into the female from the male's semen or other body fluids. In general, advice is given to avoid use. An example:

PegIntron and Ribavirin is an antiviral used in combination with interferon-alpha used for treating hepatitis C and which should clearly not be used in pregnant women,

women who may become pregnant, and male partners of women who are pregnant. The FDA-approved Package Insert notes as follows:

> PegIntron Monotherapy: Pregnancy Category C: Nonpegylated interferon alfa-2b has been shown to have abortifacient effects in Macaca mulatta (rhesus monkeys) at 15 and 30 million IU/kg (estimated human equivalent of 5 and 10 million IU/kg, based on body surface area adjustment for a 60-kg adult). PegIntron should be assumed to also have abortifacient potential. There are no adequate and well-controlled studies in pregnant women. PegIntron therapy is to be used during pregnancy only if the potential benefit justifies the potential risk to the fetus. Therefore, PegIntron is recommended for use in fertile women only when they are using effective contraception during the treatment period.
>
> Use with Ribavirin: Pregnancy Category X: Significant teratogenic and/or embryocidal effects have been demonstrated in all animal species exposed to ribavirin. REBETOL therapy is contraindicated in women who are pregnant and in the male partners of women who are pregnant [see Contraindications (4) and the REBETOL Package Insert].
>
> A Ribavirin Pregnancy Registry has been established to monitor maternal-fetal outcomes of pregnancies in female patients and female partners of male patients exposed to ribavirin during treatment and for 6 months following cessation of treatment. Physicians and patients are encouraged to report such cases by calling 1-xxx-xxx-xxxx. (Package Insert for PegIntron Web Resource 35-7)

The area of female exposure to drugs or teratogenic effects from male partners taking the drugs requires significant additional study. However, the methodology for such work is and will remain exceedingly difficult.

■ Other Resources

From a practical point of view, the critical issue for healthcare practitioners, consumers, and health authorities is to determine what drugs may be safely taken before and during pregnancy (including the weeks after conception and before diagnosing the pregnancy) and lactation.

Perinatology.com

An excellent website is perinatology.com (Web Resource 35-8). This site has multiple links as well as information on specific drugs, their effects in the various trimesters (if known), lactation information, neonatal AEs, and a literature search.

■ Motherisk

A major center in the world for information on pregnancy and drugs, called Motherisk, is located at the Hospital for Sick Children in Toronto, Canada. See its excellent website (Web Resource 35-9). Its goal is as follows:

> The Motherisk Program at The Hospital for Sick Children in Toronto is a clinical, research and teaching program dedicated to antenatal drug, chemical, and disease risk counseling. It is affiliated with the University of Toronto. Created in 1985, Motherisk provides evidence-based information and guidance about the safety or risk to the developing fetus or infant, of maternal exposure to drugs, chemicals, diseases, radiation and environmental agents.

Further, its web page (Web Resource 35-10), devoted to drugs, includes the following:

> Pregnancy, whether planned or a pleasant surprise, brings with it important concerns about prescription and over the counter drugs. Not every medication poses a risk to your unborn baby. However, some do. If you are already pregnant, Motherisk's published research can help you and your doctor make informed decisions about possible drug therapy. Since 1985, Motherisk has reviewed data from around the world, conducting controlled, prospective studies to determine the potential risks of therapeutic drugs during pregnancy. It is now clear that there are many drugs that are safe for use in pregnancy.

> They list several classes of drugs with references, including anticonvulsants, antihistamines, anti-infectives, anti-inflammatories, antirheumatics, psychotropics, cardiovascular agents, chemotherapeutic agents, contraceptives, gastrointestinal agents, herbal products, nausea/vomiting and treatment, radiation, recreational/social drugs, vitamin A, and congeners. The reader is referred to this website for specific references and studies.

Important: This information represents the opinion of Motherisk and is not necessarily the same as that of the approved drug labeling in the United States, the European Union, Canada, or elsewhere. This is not an approval, guarantee, or clearance that a particular drug is safe to use in a pregnant woman. Others may disagree about the safe use of these drugs in pregnancy. This question should always be one between the woman and her physician.

Teratology Registries and Organizations

Given the scarcity of information, it is now recognized that tracking the pregnancy and its outcome in women who have taken products either accidentally (not knowing they were pregnant) or knowingly is an important way to understand the potential toxicity (and efficacy) of drug products.

- An umbrella organization for the teratology agencies is The Organization of Teratology Information Services, covering the United States, Canada, the United Kingdom, and Israel. See its website at Web Resource 35-11. This organization serves as a clearinghouse for information and research on drug therapies. It often maintains (retrospective) teratology registries of reported birth defects from hospitals in its catchment area.
- A European counterpart is the European Network of Teratology Information Services, at Web Resource 35-12. There are also various teratology and mutagenicity societies around the world in the pharmaceutical and chemical industries, among others.
- Eurocat is a European network of population-based registries for the epidemiologic surveillance of congenital anomalies, covering 43 registries in 20 countries and 29% of the European birth population. See its website at Web Resource 35-13.

One center of particular interest is the Swedish Medical Birth Registry, at Web Resource 35-14, which is a part of the Centre for Epidemiology at the National Board of Health and Welfare in Sweden. What makes this center of unique interest is that it aims to collect prospective gestation and pregnancy data on all births in Sweden—between 86,000 and 120,000 per year. Data collected include information on previous gestation, smoking habits, medication, family situation, hospital, length of gestation, type of delivery, diagnoses of mother and child, operations, type of analgesia, sex, weight, length, size of head, birth conditions, place of residence, nationality, and outcome, delivery, and infant information.

To this end, many health agencies around the world now urge or require pharmaceutical companies, hospitals, and so on to track all known pregnancies.

Finally, the extraordinary and tragic situation with diethylstilbestrol (DES) deserves mention. This was a drug taken by pregnant women to prevent miscarriages. A major AE (vaginal carcinoma) was found to be produced many years later by DES in daughters of women who took DES. The possibility that ingestion of a drug during pregnancy could produce an AE years later in the patient or even the offspring is a challenge to medical research that does not seem solvable with the existing state of the art.

■ Frequently Asked Questions

Q: What about the more complex areas of drug–drug, drug–food, or drug–alcohol interactions in the pregnant and lactating woman?

A: This is really an unknown area. Because gold-standard, prospective, blinded studies are rare to impossible with pregnant women, data are difficult to obtain even in the "simpler" situations of a single drug taken by a pregnant woman. The complexities of interactions, particularly with agents known to be toxic (e.g., alcohol) are not able to be studied adequately (if at all) at this time. The critical issue is the inability to test hypotheses other than those suggested by epidemiologic studies. That is the state of the art today.

Q: Is there not a paradox of sorts here? If a pregnancy registry is done for a drug that is known or strongly suspected to be harmful to the mother or fetus, doesn't the success of the registry in answering whatever question is asked indicate the failure of the warning and risk management program?

A: Indeed, a successful risk management program, or REMS/RMP, to avoid pregnancies with a known teratogen will theoretically make the registry unnecessary and undoable. It is one of the tragedies in medicine today that women who are pregnant knowingly or unknowingly take drugs that are clearly known to be teratogens. Much more attention is now being paid to risk management programs to prevent pregnancies in women taking these drugs. Whether this will be successful remains to be seen. This is an area of public health that also requires "good pregnancy behavior" by the mother (and father) in terms of smoking, alcohol, eating, medications, and drugs (both licit and illicit).

36

CIOMS

This chapter summarizes the functions of the Council for International Organizations of Medical Sciences (CIOMS) and the reports issued by working groups created by CIOMS. These reports have been crucial for the International Conference on Harmonization (ICH) and the development of safety regulations in North America, Europe, Japan, and elsewhere. They are worth reviewing. Keep in mind that not all proposals from the CIOMS reports were adopted, and those that were adopted were not necessarily adopted directly and without change by ICH and national regulatory authorities.

From the CIOMS website (Web Resource 36-1): "CIOMS is an international, non-governmental, non-profit organization established jointly by WHO (World Health Organization) and United Nations Educational, Scientific and Cultural Organization (UNESCO) [Web Resource 36-2] in 1949." The membership of CIOMS includes 60 international member organizations,

representing many of the biomedical disciplines, national academies of sciences, and medical research councils. The main objectives of CIOMS are

- To facilitate and promote international activities in biomedical sciences, especially when the participation of several international associations and national institutions is deemed necessary

- To maintain collaborative relations with the United Nations and its specialized agencies, in particular with WHO and UNESCO

- To serve the scientific interests of the international biomedical community in general

CIOMS has several long-term programs, including one on drug development and use. Starting in the early 1980s, working groups composed of experts from industry and governments have been examining key issues in drug safety. They have issued many reports, several of which have served as seminal documents for procedures and regulations that ICH, the U.S. Food and Drug Administration (FDA), the European Union, Japan, and other drug safety authorities have issued. The key documents are summarized below.

■ CIOMS I (1990): International Reporting of Adverse Drug Reactions

The goal of this working group was "to develop an internationally acceptable reporting method whereby manufacturers could report post-marketing adverse drug reactions rapidly, efficiently and effectively to regulators." It noted the fact that postmarketing surveillance is necessary because premarketing studies in animals and humans have "inherent limitations." It noted the need for standardization internationally.

The report established several conventions that have largely been adopted, including the following:

■ The concept and format of a report ("a CIOMS I report") from the manufacturer receiving the event to the regulators.

■ "Reactions" are different from "events." "Reactions" are reports of clinical occurrences that have been judged by a physician or healthcare worker as having a "reasonable possibility" that the report has been caused by a drug. "Events" have not had a causality evaluation made, and thus may or may not be related to or associated with the drug.

■ Causality is discussed. No particular method of assessing causality is recommended. The report recommends that manufacturers not separate out those spontaneous reports that they receive into those that seem to be drug-related and those not seemingly drug-related. The physician, by making the report to the manufacturer, indicates that there is some level of causality possible in the report. This is a "suspected reaction." This has become a fundamental concept in most spontaneous reporting systems around the world, wherein all spontaneous reports from physicians (now extended to all healthcare providers, and in some countries, such as the United States and Canada, to consumers) are to be considered possibly related to the drug; that is, they are "reactions," not "events."

■ Because labels for marketed drugs differ from country to country, it is recommended that all reactions be collected at one point and then submitted to local authorities on a country-by-country basis based on whether the reactions are labeled locally.

■ The report discusses the four minimum requirements for a valid report: (1) an identifiable source (reporter), (2) a patient (even if not precisely identified by name), (3) a suspect drug, and (4) a suspect reaction.

■ The report recommends that all reports be sent in as soon as received and no later than 15 working days after receipt, to create a common worldwide deadline. This concept has been adopted, but the 15 working days has been changed to 15 calendar days because of differences in the designation of "working days" and nonworking days (holidays) around the world. The reporting clock starts the date the report is first received by anyone anywhere in the company.

■ The CIOMS I form was created. It is essentially the same form still used now. This form is to be used for reporting to regulatory authorities.

■ Reactions are to be reported in English.

■ CIOMS II (1992): International Reporting of Periodic Drug-Safety Update Summaries

This working group proposed a standard for Periodic Safety Update Reports (PSURs) of reactions received by manufacturers on marketed drugs. This standard, with modifications from the ICH and other organizations, has been widely adopted. The document defined several key terms:

■ CIOMS Reportable Cases or Reports: "serious, medically substantiated, unlabeled ADRs with the 4 elements (reporter, patient, reaction, suspect drug)."

■ Core Data Sheet (CDS): A document prepared by the manufacturer containing all relevant safety information, including adverse drug reactions (ADRs). This is the reference for "labeled" and "unlabeled." This concept, which has been widely accepted, has since gotten more complex, and one must distinguish labeling from listing (e.g., unlabeled and unlisted).

■ International Birth Date (IBD): The date that the first regulatory authority anywhere in the world has approved a drug for marketing.

■ Data Lock-Point (Cut-Off Date): The closing date for information to be included in a particular safety update.

■ Serious: Fatal, life-threatening, involves or prolongs inpatient hospitalization.

The sections of the PSUR include the following:

Scope
1. Subject drugs for review

2. Frequency of review and reporting

Content

1. Introduction
2. CDS
3. Drug's licensing (i.e., marketing approval) status
4. Review of regulatory actions taken for safety, if any
5. Patient exposure
6. Individual case histories (including a "CIOMS line listing")
7. Studies
8. Overall safety evaluation
9. Important data received after the data lock-point

Other fundamental concepts were established:

■ Reports should be semiannual and not cumulative (unless cumulative information is needed to put a safety issue into context).

■ The same report goes to all regulatory authorities on the same date irrespective of the local (national) approval date of the drug.

■ Reactions reported should be from studies (published and unpublished), spontaneous reports, published case reports, cases received from regulatory authorities, and other manufacturers. Duplicate reports should be eliminated.

■ The manufacturer should do a "concise critical analysis and opinion in English by a person responsible for monitoring and assessing drug safety."

A sample simulated PSUR is included based on a fake drug, "Qweasytrol."

■ CIOMS III (1995 and 1998/1999): Guidelines for Preparing Core Clinical Safety Information on Drugs (1995), Including New Proposals for Investigator's Brochures (1998/1999)

The CIOMS III guideline is now out of print but established and extended several fundamental concepts now in use in much of the world. The idea of the CDS introduced in CIOMS II was extended to the Core Safety Information (CSI). The CDS contains all of the key core data (not just safety data) on a drug. The CSI contains (only) core

safety information and is a subset of the CDS. Several fundamental concepts were introduced:

■ The CSI is the core safety information that should appear in all countries' labeling for that drug. Additional information could be added at the national level, but the core information should be included in all countries' labels. The CSI (and national labels) are guides for healthcare professionals and contain the most relevant information needed for the drug's use.

■ Marketing considerations should not play a role in preparing the CSI.

■ The CSI was proposed primarily as a medical document and not as a legal or regulatory document.

■ Every drug should have a CSI prepared and updated by the manufacturer.

■ Adverse events (AEs) due to excipients should be included.

■ AEs that have no well-established relationship to therapy should not be included.

■ The CSI should include important information that physicians are not generally expected to know.

■ As soon as relevant safety information becomes sufficiently well established, it should be included. The specific time when it is included occurs when the safety information crosses the "threshold for inclusion," which is defined as the time when "it is judged that it will influence physicians' decisions on therapy."

■ Thirty-nine factors were proposed that can be ranked and weighed for an AE for a particular drug to see whether the information has crossed the threshold. An extensive discussion on the threshold is given:

1. The threshold should be lower if the condition being treated is relatively trivial, if the drug is used to prevent rather than to treat disease, if the drug is widely used, or if the ADR is irreversible.

2. Hypersensitivity reactions should be noted early.

3. Substantial evidence is required to remove or downgrade safety information.

■ Ten general principles were proposed:

1. In general, statements that an adverse reaction does not occur or has not yet been reported should not be made.

2. As a general rule, clinical descriptions of specific cases should not be part of the CSI.

3. If the mechanism is known, it should be stated,

but speculation about the mechanism should be avoided.

4. As a general rule, secondary effects or sequelae should not be listed.

5. In general, a description of events expected as a result of progression of the underlying treated disease should not be included in the CSI.

6. Unlicensed or "off-label" use should be mentioned only in the context of a medically important safety problem.

7. The wording used in the CSI to describe adverse reactions should be chosen carefully and responsibly to maximize the prescriber's understanding. For example, if the ADR is part of a syndrome, this should be made clear.

8. The terms used should be specific and medically informative.

9. The use of modifiers or adjectives should be avoided unless they add useful important information.

10. A special attribute (e.g., sex, race) known to be associated with an increased risk should be specified.

- Where possible, frequencies should be provided, although it is admitted that this is very difficult with spontaneous safety data. A proposed classification is:
  - Very common: ≥1/10 (≥10%)
  - Common (frequent): ≥1/100 and <1/10 (≥1% and <10%)
  - Uncommon (infrequent): ≥1/1000 and <1/100 (≥0.1% and <1%)
  - Rare: ≥1/10,000 and <1/1000 (≥0.01% and <0.1%)
  - Very rare: <1/10,000 (<0.01%)

Many of these recommendations have been adopted in one form or another around the world, though not in their totality. The revised edition (1998/1999) of this document appeared as CIOMS V (see below).

■ CIOMS IV (1998): Benefit–Risk Balance for Marketed Drugs: Evaluating Safety Signals

From the preface of the report: "CIOMS IV is to some extent an extension of CIOMS II and III. It examines the theoretical and practical aspects of how to determine whether a potentially major, new safety signal signifies a shift, calling for significant action in the established relationship between benefits and risks; it also provides guidance for deciding what options for action should be considered and on the process of decision-making should such action be required."

The report looks at the general concepts of benefit–risk analysis and discusses the factors influencing assessment, including stakeholders and constituencies, the nature of the problem (risk), the indication for drug use and the population under treatment, constraints of time, data and resources, and economic issues. It recommends a standard format and content for a benefit–risk report:

- Introduction
  - Brief specification/description of the drug and where marketed
  - Indications for use, by country, if there are differences
  - Identification of one or more alternative therapies or modalities, including surgery
  - A very brief description of the suspected or established major safety problem
- Benefit evaluation
  - Epidemiology and natural history of the target disease(s)
  - Purpose of treatment (cure, prophylaxis, etc.)
  - Summary of efficacy and general toleration data compared with
    - Other medical treatments
    - Surgical treatment or other interventions
    - No treatment
- Risk evaluation
  - Background.
  - Weight of evidence for the suspected risk (incidence, etc.).
  - Detailed presentations and analyses of data on the new suspected risk.
  - Probable and possible explanations.
  - Preventability, predictability, and reversibility of the new risk.
  - The issue as it relates to alternative therapies and no therapy.
  - Review of the complete safety of the drug, using diagrammatic representations when possible (risk profiles); when appropriate, focus on selected subsets of serious AEs (e.g., the three most common and three most medically serious adverse reactions).

- Provide similar profiles for alternate drugs.
- When possible, estimate the excess incidence of any adverse reactions known to be common to the alternatives.
- When there are significant adverse reactions that are not common to the drugs compared, highlight important differences between the drugs.
- Benefit–risk evaluation
  - Summarize the benefits as related to the seriousness of the target disease and the purpose and effectiveness of treatment.
  - Summarize the dominant risks (seriousness/severity, duration, incidence).
  - Summarize the benefit–risk relationship, quantitatively and diagrammatically if possible, taking into account the alternative therapies or no treatment.
  - Provide a summary assessment and conclusion.
- Options analysis
  - List all appropriate options for action.
  - Describe the pros and cons and likely consequences (impact analysis) of each option under consideration, taking alternative therapies into account.
  - If relevant, outline plans or suggestions for a study that could provide timely and important additional information.
  - If feasible, indicate the quality and quantity of any future evidence that would signal the need for a reevaluation of the benefit–risk relationship.
  - Suggest how the consequences of the recommended action should be monitored and assessed.

Several examples of benefit–risk analyses are given (quinine and allergic hematologic events, felbamate and blood dyscrasias, dipyrone and agranulocytosis, temafloxacin and renal impairment and hypoglycemia, remoxipride and blood dyscrasias, clozapine and agranulocytosis, sparfloxacin and phototoxicity).

No example of a real benefit–risk report is given using this format. This type of report seems eminently possible in situations where the risk is small and there is no urgent or immediate action needed to protect the public health. However, in situations in which immediate action is needed, usually in multiple markets around the world, the preparation of such a report is probably not feasible.

Since this CIOMS IV report, several other guidelines and documents on benefit–risk analysis have been published by the FDA, European Medicines Evaluation Agency, ICH, and others (see Chapters 30–31). Most of these documents use similar conceptual frameworks for benefit–risk analyses but do not follow or propose the rigid CIOMS IV format. Clearly, however, this document served as a stimulus to a much closer and intense examination of benefit–risk analyses around the world. The document is worth reading, in particular for the specific case studies noted above.

■ CIOMS V (2001): Current Challenges in Pharmacovigilance: Pragmatic Approaches

The CIOMS V report is a 380-page document that covers a wide variety of current issues in drug safety. A summary of some of the proposals follows. Not all these recommendations are universally accepted or required.

The sources of individual case reports are recommended as follows:

Traditionally, the primary source of safety information on marketed drugs was spontaneous reports, with occasional literature reports also appearing. New types of reports are now appearing, including internet reports, solicited reports from patient support programs, surveys, epidemiologic studies, disease registries, regulatory and other databases, and licensor and licensee interactions. Consumer reports were often not analyzed unless medical validation was obtained.

The CIOMS V report makes various recommendations, some of which are noted below:

- Consumer reports
  - Consumer reports should be scrutinized and should receive appropriate attention.
  - The quality of a report is more important than its source.
  - Spontaneous reports are always considered to have an implied causal relationship to the drug.
  - Respect privacy and the laws and regulations governing it.
  - If a report is received from a third party, that party should be asked to encourage the consumer to report the information to his or her physician or to authorize the sponsor/authority to contact the physician directly.
  - All efforts should be made to obtain medical

confirmation of serious unexpected consumer reports. The regulators may be in a better position to get this information if companies have been unsuccessful.

- If an event is considered not to be drug related, it should be retained in the company database but not reported.
- Even in the absence of medical confirmation, any ADR with significant implications for the medicine's benefit–risk relationship should be submitted on an expedited or periodic basis.
- Consumer reports should be included in PSURs in an appendix or as a statement indicating they have been reviewed and do or do not suggest new findings.

- Literature
  - Cases may appear in letters to the editor.
  - There may be a long lag time between the first detection of a signal by a researcher and his or her publication of it.
  - Publications may be a source of false information and signals.
  - Companies should search at least two internationally recognized literature databases using the International Normalized Nomenclature name at least monthly.
  - Broadcast and lay media should not ordinarily be monitored. If such information is made available to the company, it should be followed up.
  - Judgment should be used in regard to follow-up, with the strongest efforts made for serious unexpected ADRs.
  - If the product source or brand is not specified, a company should assume it was its product. The company should indicate in any report that the specific brand was not identified if this is the case.
  - If there is a contractual agreement between two or more companies (e.g., for comarketing), the contract should specify the responsibility for literature searches and reporting.
  - English should be the standard language for literature report translations.
  - Regulators should accept translation of an abstract or pertinent sections of a publication.
  - References cited in a publication on apparently unexpected/unlisted and serious reactions should be checked against the company's existing database of literature reports. Articles not

previously reported should be retrieved and reviewed as usual. Routine tracking down of all such sources is unrealistic unless faced with a major safety issue.

- The clock starts when a case is recognized to be a valid case (reporter, patient, drug, event).

- The internet
  - Protection of privacy is particularly important regarding internet cases.
  - A blank ADR form should be provided on a website to facilitate reporting.
  - A procedure should be in place to ensure daily screening of a company's or regulator's website(s) to identify potential case reports.
  - Companies and regulators do not need to routinely surf the net beyond their own sites other than to actively monitor relevant special home pages (e.g., disease groups) if there is a significant safety issue.
  - The message should be consistent around the world because the internet does not respect geographic (or linguistic) boundaries.

- Solicited reports
  - Solicited ADR reports arising in the course of interaction with patients should be regarded as distinct from spontaneous unsolicited reports.
  - They should be processed separately and so identified in expedited and periodic reporting.
  - To satisfy postmarketing regulations, solicited reports should be handled in the same way as study reports: causality assessments are needed. Serious unexpected ADRs should be reported on an expedited basis.
  - Serious expected and nonserious solicited reports should be kept in the safety database and reported to regulators on request.
  - Signals may arise from solicited reports, so they should be reviewed on an ongoing basis.

- Aspects of clinical trial reports
  - In general, safety information reported expeditiously to regulatory authorities should be reported to all phase I, II, and III investigators who are conducting research with any form of the product and for any indication.
  - It is less important to notify phase IV investigators; they will ordinarily use the available up-to-date local official data sheet as part of the investigator's brochure.

- Quality of life studies should be handled like clinical trial data.
- Epidemiology: observational studies and use of secondary databases
  - Structured epidemiologic studies should have the same reporting rules for suspected ADR cases as clinical trials.
  - For epidemiologic studies, unless there is specific attribution in an individual case, its expedited reporting is generally not appropriate.
  - If relevant, studies should be summarized in PSURs.
  - Promptly notify regulators (within 15 days) if a study result shows an important safety issue (e.g., a greater risk of a known serious ADR for one drug versus another).
  - For manufacturers, expedited reports from comparator drug data should be forwarded to the relevant manufacturer(s) for their regulatory reporting as appropriate.
- Disease-specific registries and regulatory ADR databases
  - A registry is not a study. Cases should be treated as solicited reports (causality assessment required).
  - Although there are numerous ADR databases created by regulatory authorities, it is unnecessary to attempt to routinely collect them for regular review. If a company possesses data from a regulatory database, it should review those data promptly for any required expedited reporting. Careful screening should be done to avoid duplicates.
  - It is advisable to mention in the PSUR that the databases have been examined even if no relevant cases have been found.
- Licenser–licensee interactions
  - When companies codevelop, comarket, or copromote products, it is critical that explicit contractual agreements specify processes for exchange of safety information, including timelines and regulatory reporting responsibilities.
  - The time frame for expedited regulatory reporting should normally be no longer than 15 calendar days from the first receipt of a valid case by any of the partners.
  - The original recipient of a suspected ADR should ideally conduct any necessary follow-up; any subsequent follow-up information sent to the regulators should be submitted by the same company that reported the case originally.
- Clinical case evaluation
  - The company or regulatory authority staff can propose alternate clinical terms and interpretations of the case from those of the reporter, but unless the original reporter alters his or her original description in writing, the original terms must also be reported.
  - When a case is reported by a consumer, his or her clinical description should be retained even if confirmatory or additional information from a healthcare professional is obtained.
  - There is an important distinction between a suspected ADR and an "incidental" event. An incidental event occurs in reasonable clinical temporal association with the use of the drug product but is not the intended subject of the spontaneous report (it did not prompt the contact with the company or regulator). There is also no implicit or explicit expression of possible drug causality by the reporter or the company's safety review staff. They should be included as part of the medical history and not be the subject of expedited reporting. Incidental events should be captured in the company database.
- Assessing patient and reporter identities
  - When cases do not meet the minimum criteria (patient, reporter, event, drug) even after follow-up, the case should be kept in the database as an "incomplete case."
  - The regulatory reporting clock starts in the European Union at the first contact with a healthcare professional, but in the United States and Canada, it starts when the case is initially reported to the company, even by a consumer.
  - One or more of the following pieces of information automatically qualify a patient as identifiable: age, age category (e.g., teenager), sex, initials, date of birth, name, or patient number.
  - Even in the absence of such qualifying descriptors, a report referring to a definite number of patients should be regarded as a case as long as the other criteria for validity are met. For example, "Two patients experienced..." but not "A few patients experienced...."
  - For serious, unexpected, suspected reactions, the threshold for reporting in the absence of confirmatory identity should be lowered.

- Criteria for seriousness
  - Hospitalization refers to admission as an inpatient and not to an examination or treatment as an outpatient.
  - All congenital anomalies and birth defects, without regard to their nature or severity, should be considered serious.
  - There is a lack of objective standards for "life threatening" and "medical judgment" as seriousness criteria; both require individual professional evaluation that invariably introduces a lack of reproducibility.
  - Within a company, the tools, lists, and decision-making processes should be harmonized globally.
- Criteria for expectedness
  - The terminology associated with expectedness depends on which reference safety document is being used and for what purpose:
    - "Listed" or "unlisted" refers to the ADRs contained in the CSI for a marketed product or within the development CSI (DCSI) in the investigator's brochure.
    - "Labeled" or "unlabeled" refers to the ADRs contained in official product safety information for marketed products (e.g., summary of product characteristics in the European Union or the package insert in the United States).
  - Determining whether a reported reaction is expected is a two-step process: first, is the reaction term already included in the CSI? Second, is the ADR different regarding its nature, severity, specificity, or outcome?
  - Expectedness should be strictly based on inclusion of a drug-associated experience in the ADR section of the CSI. Special types of reactions, such as those occurring under conditions of overdose, drug interaction, or pregnancy, should also be included in this section.
  - Disorders mentioned in "contraindications" or "precautions" as reasons for not treating with the drug are not expected ADRs unless they also appear in the ADR section.
  - If an ADR has been reported only in association with an overdose, it should be considered unexpected if it occurs at a normal dose.
  - For a marketed drug CSI, events cited in data from clinical trials are not considered expected unless they are included in the ADR section.

- For expedited reporting on marketed drugs, local approved product information is the reference document for expectedness (labeledness).
- For periodic reporting (PSUR), the CSI is the reference document for expectedness (listedness).
- Disclaimer statements for causality (e.g., "X has been reported but the relationship with the drug has not been established") are discouraged; however, even if used, the reaction X is still unexpected.
- Class labeling does not count as "expected" unless the event in question is included in the ADR section.
- Lack of expected efficacy is not relevant to whether an AE is expected.
- If the treatment exacerbates the target indication, it would be unexpected unless already detailed in the CSI.
- Unless the CSI specifies a fatal outcome for an ADR, the case is unexpected as long as there was an association between the reaction and the fatality.
- Case follow-up approaches
  - Highest priority for follow-up are cases that are serious and unexpected; followed by serious, expected; and nonserious, unexpected.
  - Cases "of special interest" (e.g., ADRs under active surveillance at the request of the regulators) also deserve high priority, as do any cases that might lead to a labeling change.
  - For any cases with legal implications, the company's legal department should be involved.
  - When the case is serious and if the ADR has not resolved at the time of the initial report, it is important to continue follow-up until the outcome has been established or the condition stabilized. How long to follow up such cases requires judgment.
  - It is recommended that collaboration with other companies be done if more than one company's drug is suspected as a causal agent in a case.
  - Follow-up for unexpected deaths and life-threatening cases should be done within 24 hours.
  - If a reporter fails to respond to the first follow-up attempt, reminder letters should be sent as follows:
    - A single follow-up letter for any nonserious expected case.

- For all other cases, a second follow-up letter should be sent no later than 4 weeks after the first letter.
- In general, when the reporter fails to respond or is incompletely cooperative, the two follow-up letters should reflect sufficient due diligence.

- Role of narratives
  - A company case narrative is different from the reporter's clinical description of a case, though the reporter's comments should be an integral part of the company narrative. The reporter's verbatim words should be included for the adverse reactions.
  - Alternate causes to that given by the reporter should be described and identified as a company opinion.
  - The same evaluation should be supplied to all regulators.
  - Narratives should be prepared for all serious (expected and unexpected) and nonserious unexpected cases but not for nonserious expected cases.
  - Narratives should be written in the third person past tense. All relevant information should be in a logical time sequence.
  - In general, abbreviations (except laboratory parameters and units) and acronyms should not be used.
  - Time to onset of an event from the start of treatment should be given in the most appropriate time units (e.g., hours), but actual dates can be used if helpful to the reader.
  - If detailed supplementary records are important to a case (e.g., autopsy report), their availability should be mentioned in the narrative.
  - Information may be supplied by more than one person (e.g., initial reporter and supplementary information from a specialist); all sources should be specified.
  - When there is conflicting information provided from different sources, this should be mentioned and the sources identified.
  - If it is suspected that an ADR resulted from misprescribing (e.g., wrong drug or wrong dose) or other medication error, judgmental comments should not be included in the narrative because of legal implications. Only the facts should be stated (e.g., "four times the normal dose was administered," "the prescription was misread and a contraindicated drug for this patient was given").

- The narrative should have eight sections that serve as a comprehensive stand-alone "medical story":
  - Source of the report and patient demography.
  - Medical and drug history.
  - Suspect drug(s), timing and conditions surrounding the onset of the reaction(s).
  - The progression of the event(s) and their outcome in the patient.
  - If the outcome is fatal, provide relevant details.
  - Rechallenge information, if applicable.
  - The narrative preparer's medical evaluation and comment.

- PSURs: content modification
  - For reports covering long time periods (e.g., 5 years), it is more practical to use the CSI current at the time of PSUR preparation.
  - Clinical trial data should be supplied only if they suggest a signal or are relevant to a possible change in the benefit–risk relationship.
  - If there are more than 200 individual case reports, submit only summary tabulations and not line listings (which may be supplied on request by the regulator).
  - For 5-year reports, follow-up information on cases described in the previous report should be provided only for cases associated with new or ongoing safety issues.
  - Inclusion of literature reports should be selective and cover publications relevant to safety findings, independent of listedness.
  - For PSURs with large numbers of cases, discussion and analysis for the overall safety evaluation should be by system organ class rather than by listedness or seriousness.
  - An abbreviated PSUR saves time and resources if little or no new safety information is generated during the time period covered. Criteria for an abbreviated report:
    - No serious unlisted cases
    - Few (e.g., ≤10) serious listed cases
    - No significant regulatory actions for safety
    - No major changes to the CSI
    - No findings that lead to a new action

- PSURs: a bridging report
  - A summary bridging report is a concise document that provides no new information and integrates two or more previously prepared PSURs to cover a specified period.
  - Its format follows that of a regular PSUR, but the content should consist of summary highlights of the reports being summarized.
- PSURs: an addendum report
  - This report is prepared on special request of the regulators to satisfy regulators who require reports covering a period outside the routine PSUR reporting cycle (e.g., if the reports are based on the local approval date in that country rather than on the IBD).
  - It updates the most recently completed PSUR.
  - It follows the usual PSUR format.
- PSURs: miscellaneous proposals
  - A brief (e.g., one-page) stand-alone overview (executive summary) should be provided.
  - Manufacturers should be allowed to select the IBDs for their old products to facilitate synchronization of PSURs.
  - If there is no CSI for an old product, the most suitable local labeling should be considered for use.
  - The evaluation of cases in a PSUR should focus on unlisted ADRs, with analyses organized primarily by system organ class (body system).
  - Discussion of serious unlisted cases should include cumulative data.
  - Complicated PSURs and those with extensive new data may require more than 60 days to prepare adequately and the regulators should be flexible.
  - The possibility of "resetting" the PSUR clock (from annual to semiannual reports as the result of a new indication or dosage form) should be allowed by the regulators.
- PSURs: population data
  - Detailed calculations on exposure (the denominator) are ordinarily unnecessary, especially given the unreliability of the numerator; rough estimates usually suffice, but the method and units used should be explained clearly.
  - Drug exposure data are approximate and usually represent an overestimate.
  - For special situations, such as dealing with an important safety signal, attempts should be made to obtain exposure information covering the relevant covariates (e.g., age, gender, race, indication, dosing details).

CIOMS VI (2005): Management of Safety Information from Clinical Trials

The CIOMS VI working group focused on clinical trial safety, which represents a departure from the focus of the earlier working groups that concentrated primarily on postmarketing safety issues. The report, available from the CIOMS office in Geneva, like the CIOMS V report runs some 300 pages. The most important points are summarized here. The reader is referred to the report for further detail. Keep in mind that these recommendations are quite new and have not been put into regulations in all jurisdictions.

General Principles and Ethical Considerations

- The concepts of pharmacovigilance presented here apply to trials in phases I through IV.
- Any study that is not scientifically sound should be considered unethical.
- Informed consent is the cornerstone of human subject research, but there are situations in which it is either not possible or appropriate (such as in anonymous tissue sample studies, epidemiologic research, or emergency treatment protocols).

Systematic Approach to Managing Safety Data

- The concepts of pharmacovigilance, risk management, assessment, and minimization should be applied to the study phases and the postmarketing period. Sponsors must have in place a well-defined process to readily identify, evaluate, and minimize potential safety risks. The process should start before the first phase I study. A formal development risk management plan should be developed.
- A dedicated safety management team should be formed for each development program to review safety information on a regular basis so that decisions can be made in a timely manner. The review

should be at least quarterly, and the team should consider changes to the investigator's brochure, informed consent, and protocol as needed.

- When licensing partners are involved, a joint safety committee should be created, with clear roles and responsibilities. This should ideally be defined in the initial contract. A project management function should be set up to ensure scheduling, tracking, and timelines.

- All pertinent data must be readily available from the clinical trial and safety databases as well as preclinical toxicology, mutagenicity, pharmacokinetic, pharmacodynamic, and drug interaction data.

- Epidemiology should be incorporated into the planning process.

- Certain toxicities should be considered for all new drugs, including abnormalities of cardiac conduction, hepatotoxicity, drug interactions, immunogenicity, bone marrow toxicity, and reactive metabolite formation.

■ Data Collection and Management

- The investigator should report to the sponsor (immediately if judged critical) any information considered to be important in regard to safety even if the protocol does not call for it. The sponsor must carefully train the investigative site in this matter.

- The collection of "excessive" data can have a negative impact on data quality. Case report form fields should collect only those data that can be analyzed and presented in tabular form. All other data should be collected as text comments.

- Safety monitoring in phase IV studies may not require the same intensity as for phase I–III trials, but the same principles and practices should apply.

- If a company provides any support for an independent trial it does not sponsor (investigator-initiated studies/trials), the company should still obtain at a minimum all serious suspected adverse reactions. The company should do its own causality assessment and, if appropriate, report it to the health authorities, even if the investigator has already done so.

- In the early phases of drug development, it is often necessary to collect more comprehensive safety data than in postmarketing studies. Some studies may require longer follow-up.

- Phase I data are especially important because these data are collected in healthy volunteers and are critical to the future development of the drug.

- There is no definitive way to determine causality of a particular AE. That is, its attribution to the drug or to a background finding with only a temporal association cannot be definitively done. Thus, the following is recommended:

- All AEs, both serious and nonserious, are collected whether believed to be related or not. This applies to the experimental product, placebo, no treatment, and active comparators.

- Similarly, studies initiated during the immediate postapproval period should continue this practice. Once the safety profile is judged to be well understood, it may be possible to collect less data (e.g., omitting nonserious AEs believed not to be due to the drug).

■ Other Points

- The use of herbal and other nontraditional treatments should be sought when data are being collected in all studies.

- Although causality assessments based on aggregate data or case series are usually more meaningful than those based on individual cases, the investigator causality assessment should be done and may play a role in the early detection of significant safety events, especially rare ones.

- The investigator should be asked to use a "simple binary decision" for drug causality of serious AEs: related or not related, reasonable possibility or no reasonable possibility, and so on. The use of the words "unknown" or "cannot be ruled out" should be avoided.

- Causality for nonserious AEs should not be requested from investigators routinely.

- Where appropriate, the investigator should supply a diagnosis rather than signs and symptoms. However, when a diagnosis is supplied for a serious AE, the accompanying signs and symptoms should be recorded.

- Before starting a study, AEs of special interest and anticipated AEs (if known) should be communicated to the investigator. This is less critical for nonserious AEs unless they are prodromes of more serious conditions (e.g., muscle pain and creatine phosphokinase elevation as a possible prodrome of rhabdomyolysis).

- Medically serious clinical events recorded in a trial as clinical efficacy outcomes or endpoints should be reviewed by the sponsor and data monitoring committee even though they are not considered AEs.

- It is preferable to frame questions to patients in general terms rather than suggest that the study treatment was responsible for reported AEs. Although a "laundry list" of AEs should not be read to the patient, patients should be alerted to known issues of medically important suspected or established AEs so they can alert the investigator as soon as possible.

- Data collection should start from the time the informed consent is signed.

- Safety data event collection should continue after the last dose of the drug for at least an additional five half-lives of the experimental product.

General rules for data quality:

- Cases should be as fully documented as possible.
- There should be diligent follow-up of each case.
- The reporter's verbatim terms should be captured and retained.

- If the reporter's terms are considered inaccurate or inconsistent with standard medical terminology, attempts should be made to clarify them. If disagreement continues, the sponsor should code the AE terms according to its judgment but identify them as distinct from the reporter's terms and note reasons for differences.

- Primary analyses of the data should be done using the reporter's terms. Additional analyses may be done using the sponsor's terms. Any differences must be noted and explained.

- Individual case safety reports should be categorized and assessed by the sponsor, using trained individuals with broad experience. Investigators should obtain specialist consultation for clinically important events that fall outside their expertise.

- AE tables may display both the reported investigator's verbatim term and the sponsor's terms.

- The sponsor (as well as health authorities) may wish to consider the use of a listing of event terms always regarded as serious and important. Such events then routinely trigger special attention and evaluation.

- Cases should not be "overcoded" using more terms than minimally necessary to ensure retrieval of the cases. Similarly, cases should not be "undercoded," where the terms chosen downgrade the severity or importance of events.

■ Risk Identification and Evaluation

- Ongoing safety evaluation
  - Sponsors should develop a system to assess, evaluate, and act on safety information on a continuous basis during drug development to ensure the earliest possible identification of safety concerns to allow risk minimization.
  - The integrity of the studies should not be compromised by the safety monitoring and analysis.
- Safety data management
  - Safety data should be handled using consistent standards and criteria, with care and precision.
  - Safety evaluations must be individualized for each product because there are no standard approaches to evaluating or measuring "an acceptable level of risk."
- Review of safety information
  - Safety data analysis should involve both individual case reports as well as aggregate data. Individual cases should be reviewed within specified time frames and aggregate data on a periodic basis.
  - The evaluation should be done in the context of the patient population, the indication studied, the natural history of the disease, and currently available therapies.
  - Causality determinations should be done for all reported cases. The investigator causality assessment should be taken into account when the sponsor is reviewing the safety information.
  - AEs of special interest should be identified in the protocol and handled as if they are serious even if they do not meet the regulatory definition of serious.
  - Nonserious AEs should be reviewed to see whether there are events of special interest, with particular attention paid to those associated with study discontinuation.

■ Frequency of Review of Safety Information

- Safety review of all data should be done frequently:
  - Ad hoc for serious and special interest AEs
  - Routine periodic review of all data whose frequency varies from trial to trial or program to program

- Reviews triggered by specific trial or program milestones
- At the time of study completion and unblinding

Analysis and Evaluation

- Subgroup analysis, though possibly limited by small sample size, should be done for dose, duration, gender, age, concomitant medications, and concurrent diseases.
- Data pooling should include studies that are of similar design. This can include all controlled studies, placebo-controlled studies, studies with any positive control, studies with a particular positive control, and particular indications.
- If the duration of treatment varies widely among participants, data on the effect of treatment duration should be analyzed.

Statistical Approaches

- The techniques for use of statistics for analyzing safety data are less well developed than for efficacy.
- Statistical association (probability values) alone may or may not be of clinical value. Examination of both statistical and clinical significance must involve a partnership between the statistical and clinical experts.
- It may be necessary to acknowledge when the data are insufficient to draw conclusions on safety: "Absence of evidence is not evidence of absence."
- There are several large sections of this report devoted to specific statistical situations and techniques, and the reader is referred to the report for further detail.

Regulatory Reporting and Communications of Safety Information from Clinical Trials

The working group notes, in bold type, that these recommendations are only proposals and do not supersede current regulations. They represent proposals for discussion.

- The group endorses ICH Guideline E2A (see Chapter 26) and recommends the harmonization of criteria for expedited reporting, whereby such reporting to authorities should include only suspected ADRs that are both serious and unexpected. Only under exceptional circumstances should other cases (i.e., expected cases) be submitted as expedited reports. If reporting without regard to causality is required, it should be done on a periodic basis with clearly defined timelines and format.
- The regulators should adopt the phrase "a reasonable possibility of a causal relationship" and not use the ICH E2A phrase of "a causal relationship cannot be ruled out" in regard to suspected ADRs.
- Once a drug is marketed, the company CSI (CCSI) document should be used as the reference safety document for determining expectedness for regulatory reporting of phase IV trials. For new indication trials, the DCSI document should be used. The two documents should be aligned as much as possible.
- As with spontaneous reports, reportability for case reports from trials should be determined at the event level. That is, a case would be expedited if there is a suspected adverse reaction that is serious and unexpected.
- Suspected ADRs that are serious and unexpected and thus are expedited reports should, in general, be unblinded. There may be certain circumstances where this should not occur, however (e.g., serious AEs that are also efficacy endpoints). Such exceptions should be agreed on by the regulatory authorities and be clearly described in the investigator brochure and the protocol.
- Unblinded placebo cases should not be reported to regulatory authorities as expedited cases. Unblinded (and open-label) comparator drug cases should be reported to the regulatory authorities or the company owning the comparator on an expedited basis, whether or not expected.
- Seven-day reports should be limited to cases from clinical trials and not spontaneous reports. This should apply both in countries where the drug is approved and where it is only under clinical study.
- The sponsor should develop clear standard operating procedures for the expedited or prompt reporting of other safety issues, with special attention to when the clock starts for
  - Nonclinical safety issues that might have implications for human subjects
  - A higher incidence of a serious AE for the drug compared with the comparator or the background rate in the general population

- An increased frequency of a previously recognized serious adverse reaction
- A significant drug interaction in a pharmacokinetic study
- AEs that are deemed not to be drug-related but are considered study-related

- Contrary to established regulations, the working group recommends that routine expedited cases reported to investigators and Investigational Review Boards (IRBs)/ethics committees (as opposed to reports to regulatory authorities) be eliminated and replaced with regular updates of the evolving benefit–risk profile highlighting new safety information.

- For unapproved products, the reports to investigators and IRBs should include a line listing of unblinded clinical trial cases that were expedited to regulatory agencies during this time period, a copy of the current DCSI with an explanation of changes, and a brief summary of the emerging safety profile. Quarterly updates are the "default" with other frequencies as appropriate.

- For approved products, the reports to investigators and IRBs should be quarterly if the product is in phase III trials. For well-established products, a less frequent interval would be acceptable. At some point, only investigators and IRBs would need to be updated for significant new information. For phase IV investigators and IRBs, only changes to the CCSI would be needed.

- The reports, whether for approved or unapproved products, should include in the line listings only unblinded expedited reports from trials and include only interval data (i.e., changes since the last update). A summary of the emerging safety profile should be included with cumulative data as needed. MedDRA should be used. The listings should not include spontaneous reports, which should be described in narrative form in the update.

- Should a significant safety issue be identified (i.e., an issue that has a significant impact on the course of the clinical trial or program or warrants immediate update of the informed consent), the sponsor should promptly notify the regulatory authorities, investigators, IRBs, and, if relevant, data safety monitoring committees.

- A safety management team should review all safety data on a regular basis: quarterly before approval and coordinated with the PSUR schedule postapproval. Ad hoc meetings would occur as needed to address urgent safety issues and signals. They would review the overall evolving safety profile to make changes to the DCSI, informed consent, and protocol as needed.

- A single Development Safety Update Report (DSUR) should be submitted to regulators annually. The format and content would be defined and would cover the drug product, not just a single study.

- For marketed products with well-established safety profiles and for which most trials are in phase IV in the approved indications, the PSUR would replace the DSUR.

- Sponsors should incorporate the DCSI into every investigator brochure, either as a special section of the investigator brochure or as an attachment. The sponsor should clearly identify the events for which the company believes there is sufficient evidence to suspect a drug relationship. These events would be considered expected ("listed") for regulatory reporting criteria.

- The investigator brochure and DCSI should be reviewed and updated at least annually.

- If the developer or manufacturer of a product is not the sponsor of a particular trial but rather supports an external clinical or nonclinical investigator-sponsored study, a provision of any agreement should be the prompt reporting to the company of all serious suspected ADRs in humans or significant findings in animals.

- As with the CCSI for marketed drugs (see CIOMS III/VI), the same threshold criteria should be applied to the DCSI and informed consent in preapproval drugs.

- Informed consent should be renewed with the subjects whenever there is new information that could affect the subjects' willingness to participate in the trial. In certain circumstances, a more immediate communication may be appropriate.

■ CIOMS VII (2006): Development Safety Update Report (DSUR)

This working group has created the concept of the DSUR, which will be the premarketing equivalent of the Periodic Safety Update Report for marketed products. Its report has been published and it will likely be adopted throughout the world as the PSUR has been. A brief summary of the report follows.

There should be one DSUR for one chemical entity. The goal is to include all new, pertinent, clinical, and non-clinical safety information, that is, the drug's safety profile. It will include both cumulative and interval summaries of key safety data and will attempt to evaluate safety data to patient exposure. It will describe new safety issues, summarize known and potential risks, and give an update on the status of the clinical development program. It will note any urgent or emerging issues and will note changes to clinical trial protocols, consent forms, and the IB. It is not meant to be a signal detection tool or a means to document or discuss individual cases. The DSUR should be prepared in parallel to the PSUR if the drug is already on the market. The first authorization anywhere in the world to conduct a clinical trial will be the developmental international birth date, in the same way that the first approval anywhere in the world creates an international (marketing) birth date. It will be prepared annually by the sponsor and submitted to the regulatory agencies within 60 days of the data lockpoint. An executive summary plus line listings of serious ADRs will be sent to IRBs and ethics committees. The reference labeling document will be the investigators' brochure in place at the beginning of the reporting period. It may contain some proprietary information, which may need to be redacted if the document is sent to places other than regulatory agencies.

The contents include:
a. Title Page
b. Table of Contents
c. Executive Summary
d. Introduction
e. Worldwide Marketing Authorization Status
f. Update on Actions Taken for Safety Reasons
g. Changes to Reference Safety Information
h. Inventory and Status of Ongoing and Completed Interventional Clinical Trials
i. Estimated Patient Exposure in Clinical Trials
j. Presentation of Safety Data from Clinical Studies
k. Significant Findings from Interventional Clinical Trials
l. Observational and Epidemiological Studies
m. Other Information
n. Information from Marketing Experience
o. Late-Breaking Information
p. Overall Safety Evaluation
q. Summary of Important Risks
r. New Actions Recommended
s. Conclusions
t. Appendices to DSUR

■ CIOMS VIII (2010): Signal Detection (Points to Consider in Application of Signal Detection in Pharmacovigilance)

This working group has developed and published a consensus document on signaling for consideration by sponsors, health agencies, and others who deal with drug safety. It takes a life cycle view of signaling. This is a well-written summary of the state of the art of signaling. It is not prescriptive in the sense of mandating a "one-size-fits-all" policy but rather comes forward with conclusions and recommendations to be tailored to the particular product and situation. The sections include:

- Background—pharmacovigilance and key definitions

- Overview of approaches to signal detection including the traditional approaches, and statistical data mining methods including their interpretation within an integrated overall approach to signaling

- Spontaneously reported drug safety-related information and its use and limitations in signaling

- Databases that support signal

- Traditional methods of signal detection including case and case series review and the analyses of larger databases

- More complex quantitative signal detection methods including disproportionality analysis, Bayesian methodologies, frequentist versus Bayesian approaches, evaluating data-mining performance, and potential conflict of interest

- How to develop a signal detection strategy

- Overview of signal management, including prioritization, evaluation, options analysis of potential and identified risks, reporting and communicating risks

- Future directions in signal detection, evaluation, and communication, including new algorithms and use of non-spontaneous report databases

■ Other Areas

CIOMS is or has worked on vaccine vigilance, standardized MedDRA queries, drug development and pharmacovigilance in resource-poor countries, and other areas in drug development.

37

International Conference on Harmonization (ICH)

This chapter summarizes the purpose of the International Conference on Harmonization (ICH) and the reports issued by the various working groups related to drug safety. These reports have been used as the basis for creating certain safety regulations in North America, Europe, Japan, and elsewhere. They are worth taking the time to review online or in this chapter. Keep in mind that not all proposals from the ICH were adopted nor were the adopted proposals necessarily taken directly and without change by national regulatory authorities.

The documents in question are:

- E2A: Clinical Safety Data Management: Definitions and Standards for Expedited Reporting

- E2B(R3): Maintenance of the Clinical Safety Data Management, including the Maintenance of the Electronic Transmission of Individual Case Safety Reports Message Specification

- E2C: Clinical Safety Data Management: Periodic Safety Update Reports for Marketed Drugs

- E2CA Addendum to E2C: Periodic Safety Update Reports for Marketed Drugs

- E2D: Postapproval Safety Data Management: Definitions and Standards for Expedited Reporting

- E2E: Pharmacovigilance Planning

They can be found at Web Resource 37-1.

■ E2A Clinical Safety Data Management: Definitions and Standards for Expedited Reporting

E2A combines many concepts from the Council for International Organizations of Medical Sciences (CIOMS) I and CIOMS II documents covering the development of standard definitions and terminology for safety reporting and the appropriate mechanism for handling expedited (alert) reporting. This document was originally developed to cover primarily the investigational phase of drug development, but its concepts have been extended to cover postmarketing (approved) drugs also (see document E2E below).

The definitions and recommendations for expedited reporting developed in this document have largely been accepted throughout the world. However, some of the recommendations have been tried and withdrawn (e.g., increased frequency reporting in the United States), inconsistently applied (e.g., breaking the blind), or never applied (reporting an expedited case to all open Investigational New Drug Applications [INDs]).

Definitions

Adverse event or adverse experience (AE): "Any untoward medical occurrence in a patient or clinical investigation subject administered a pharmaceutical product and which does not necessarily have to have a causal relationship with this treatment."

Adverse drug reaction (ADR): "In the pre-approval clinical experience with a new medicinal product or its new usages, particularly as the therapeutic dose(s) may not be established: all noxious and unintended responses to a medicinal product related to any dose should be considered adverse drug reactions. For marketed products: A response to a drug which is noxious and unintended and which occurs at doses normally used in man for prophylaxis, diagnosis, or therapy of disease or for modification of physiological function."

Unexpected ADR: "An adverse reaction, the nature or severity of which is not consistent with the applicable product information (e.g., Investigator Brochure for an unapproved investigational medicinal product)." Note that this applies to nonmarketed drugs. This definition was extended to marketed drugs in E2E (see below).

"Serious" and "severe": The terms serious and severe are differentiated. The term "severe" is often used to describe the intensity (severity) of a specific event (as in mild, moderate, or severe myocardial infarction); the event itself, however, may be of relatively minor medical significance (such as severe headache). This is not the same as "serious," which is based on patient/event outcome or action criteria usually associated with events that pose a threat to a patient's life or functioning. Seriousness (not severity) serves as a guide for defining regulatory reporting obligations.

Serious: "A serious adverse event (experience) or reaction is any untoward medical occurrence that at any dose results in death, is life-threatening, requires in-patient hospitalization or prolongation of existing hospitalization, results in persistent or significant disability/incapacity or is a congenital anomaly/birth defect."

"Medical and scientific judgment should be exercised in deciding whether expedited reporting is appropriate in other situations, such as important medical events that may not be immediately life-threatening or result in death or hospitalization but may jeopardize the patient or may require intervention to prevent one of the other outcomes listed in the definition above. These should also usually be considered serious." Note that "cancer" and "overdose" have been removed. These terms appeared in various pre-1995 definitions of "serious."

What Should Be Reported to Regulatory Authorities as Expedited Reports?

All ADRs that are both serious and unexpected are subject to expedited reporting. This applies to reports from spontaneous sources and from any type of clinical or epidemiologic investigation, independent of design or purpose.

- Note that this means all adverse reactions (i.e., causally related to the drug) that are serious and unexpected. Thus, it requires all three categories (causality, seriousness, and unexpectedness) for clinical trial cases. Although not explicitly stated in this document, for postmarketing cases the causality is implied (i.e., all spontaneous reports are presumed to be causally related), and thus only two criteria need to be examined: seriousness and expectedness.
- No international standard exists for causality classification.
- An increased frequency of a known serious ADR should be reported in an expedited fashion.
- A significant hazard to the patient population, such as lack of efficacy with a medicinal product used in a life-threatening disease.
- A major safety finding from a newly completed animal study.

Reporting Time Frames

- Fatal or life-threatening ADRs: 7 calendar days by phone or fax followed 8 calendar days later with an expedited 15-day report.
- Other serious unexpected ADRs: 15 calendar days after the first knowledge by the sponsor that the case meets the minimum criteria for reporting.

Minimum Criteria for Reporting

- An identifiable patient
- A suspect medicinal product
- An identifiable reporting source
- An event or outcome that is serious and unex-

pected and, for clinical trial cases, a reasonable suspected causal relationship

Follow-up information should be sought and reported as soon as it becomes available. The CIOMS I form should be used to report the cases. (Note: Now with electronic transmission E2B transmissions are required in most jurisdictions).

Managing Blinded Cases

This report recommends that, although it is advantageous to retain the blind for all patients before study analysis, when a serious adverse reaction is reportable on an expedited basis, the blind should be broken only for that specific patient by the sponsor even if the investigator has not broken the blind. The blind should be maintained where possible for the personnel in the company responsible for the analysis and interpretation of the results. There may be circumstances where not breaking the blind is desirable, and in these circumstances, an agreement with the regulatory authorities should be pursued.

Other Issues

- For reactions with comparators, the sponsor is responsible for deciding whether to report the case to the other manufacturer or to the appropriate regulatory agencies. Placebo events do not normally need to be reported.
- When a drug has more than one presentation (e.g., different dosage forms, formulations, delivery systems) or uses (different indications or different populations), the expedited report should be reported to or referenced to all other product presentations and uses.
  NOTE: This is generally not the case currently. Reporting is usually to only one IND or premarketing dossier in most countries should multiple INDs or dossiers exist.
- Poststudy AEs are usually not collected or sought by sponsors but may nonetheless be reported to the sponsor by the investigator. These events should be treated as if they were study events and reported as expedited reports should they qualify to be such.

Two working groups were set up in the ICH to develop the means for the electronic transmission of individual case safety reports between or among companies and regulators, regulators and regulators, and companies and companies. This system would allow the (theoretical) replacement of paper-based submissions using MedWatch or CIOMS I forms. To do this, the data elements, fields, and contents of the electronic report needed to be rigidly standardized. There are two series of documents in question.

The first is the E2B documents, which were prepared by the medical representatives and specified data elements for the transmission. The second is the M2 documents, prepared by the informatics representatives, which provide technical specifications for structured messaging; electronic data interchange; data definitions to incorporate structured data formats (e.g., SGML); security to ensure confidentiality, data integrity, authentication, and nonrepudiation; documents to handle heterogeneous data formats; and physical media for storage and transferability of data.

Several documents were issued and the nomenclature is a bit confusing.

■ The E2B(R2) and M2 Documents

The terminology here has been confusing as there have been multiple other names for earlier versions of these documents, including E2B(R), E2B(M), and others. The documents were first developed in 1997 and finalized (more or less) in 2001. The R3 document includes experience gained over the last several years but has not been formally adopted by all countries.

There are several initiatives under way that aim to standardize data transmission of health data, including individual case safety reports (ICSRs), of which E2B is the current standard. Ultimately, it is expected that the HL7 requirements will encompass ISO, local regional requirements, and ICH requirements. The other groups include ISO (International Standards Organization) and HL7 (see Chapter 8). The R2 document is the current document used globally.

- E2B(R3): Revision of the E2B(R2) ICH Guideline on Clinical Safety Data Management: Data Elements for Transmission of Individual Case Safety Reports
- E2B(R2): Maintenance of the Clinical Safety Data Management, including Data Elements for Transmission of Individual Case Safety Reports (previously called E2B(M))
- M2: Electronic Standards for the Transfer of Regulatory Information (ESTRI)

Personnel involved in drug safety should be familiar at a high level with the E2B documents; in addition, the informatics personnel supporting them should be familiar with M2. The contents of the E2B transmissions determine to a certain degree how data are handled and stored in a company's database. For example, decisions must be made on whether to code laboratory data as free text or as structured fields.

We briefly review here the data elements of the E2B documents. The goal of the E2B document is to provide all the data elements needed to comprehensively cover complex reports regardless of source, destination, and databases at either end of the transmission. Not all cases have all data elements. Thus, simple cases have few elements transmitted, and complex cases have many or most of the elements transmitted. The E2B transmission concepts can be used for pre- and postapproval AEs/ADRs. Currently, E2B is primarily used for expedited reporting.

Structured data are strongly recommended and are available for AE terms and other elements using the Medical Dictionary for Regulatory Activities (MedDRA). However, structured vocabularies for other elements (e.g., drug names) are not yet available, finalized, or agreed on. The E2B document also allows for unstructured text (e.g., narratives) to be transmitted and, in some cases, allows data to be transmitted as structured or unstructured data (e.g., laboratory values).

There are two sections to a transmission. The first is the header, which contains technical information, and the second is the data elements, in two parts: first, the administrative and identification information, and, second, the case information. The data elements are described briefly here.

A1. Identification of the case safety report
- Case unique identifier number and MedDRA version
- Source country; country where the AE occurred
- Date of transmission
- Type of report (spontaneous, study, other)
- Seriousness
- Date of latest information
- List of other documents held by sender
- Expedited report?
- Other identifying numbers for the case (e.g., local health authority numbers)

A2. Sources
- Reporter name, address, profession
- Literature reference
- Clinical study information (name, type, study number)

A3. Sender Information

- Type: company, regulatory authority, healthcare professional, World Health Organization, and so on
- Sender identifier, address, e-mail, and so on

B1. Patient characteristics
- Identifier, age, date of birth, age at reaction onset, weight, height, sex
- Medical and drug history and concurrent conditions (either structured or as free text)
- Death information
- Parent–child report information

B2. Reaction(s)/event(s): This is a repeating section so that a new section can be created for each reaction/event.
- Verbatim term, MedDRA lower-level term, term highlighted by reporter
- Seriousness criterion
- Start and stop dates and outcome

B3. Tests and procedures (and their results) done to investigate

B4. Drug information
- Drug type (suspect, concomitant, interacting, blinded, etc.)
- Drug name, active ingredient
- Authorization (New Drug Application) holder and (New Drug Application) number
- Dose, start date, route of administration, indication for use, action taken
- Drug-reaction matrix for causality (to capture causality at the event level and a reporter and company causality)

B5. Narrative (clinical course, therapeutic measures, outcome, and additional relevant information)
- Reporter comments
- Sender's diagnosis/syndrome and comments

■ E2C(R1) Clinical Safety Data Management: Periodic Safety Update Reports for Marketed Drugs

This was adopted by ICH in November 1996. An addendum was published in 2003 and is summarized below. These documents give guidance on the format and content of safety updates, which need to be provided at intervals to regulatory authorities after products have been marketed. The guideline is intended to ensure that the worldwide safety experience is provided to authorities at defined times after marketing with maximum efficiency and avoiding duplication of effort.

PSURs have been adopted by many countries, including those in the European Union, Japan, Canada, and others. In the United States, they are not yet obligatory, but most NDA holders submit PSURs rather than the older NDA Periodic Reports. FDA is expected to make PSURs obligatory at some point soon. Companies wishing to submit PSURs in place of New Drug Application periodic reports must contact the FDA to obtain U.S. requirements and FDA consent for their submissions.

The general principles are as follows:

- One report for one active substance. The PSUR should cover all dosage forms, formulations, and indications. There may be separate presentations of data for different dosage forms or populations if appropriate. The PSUR should be a "stand-alone" document.

- For combination products also marketed individually, safety information may be done as a separate PSUR or included in the PSURs prepared for one of the components, with cross-referencing.

- The report should present data for the interval of the PSUR only, except for regulatory status information, renewals, and serious unlisted ADRs, which should be cumulative.

- The report should focus on ADRs. All spontaneous reports should be assumed to be reactions (i.e., possibly related). Reports should be from healthcare professionals. For clinical trial and literature reports, only those cases believed by the reporter and sponsor to be unrelated to the drug should be excluded.

- Lack of efficacy reports (which are considered to be AEs) should not be included in the tables but should be discussed in the "other information" section.

- Increased frequency reports for known reactions should be reported if appropriate.

- If more than one company markets a drug in the same market, each Marketing Authorization holder (MAH) is responsible for submitting PSURs. If contractual arrangements are made to share safety information and responsibilities, this should be specified.

- Each product should have an international birth date (IBD), usually the date of the first Marketing Authorization anywhere in the world. This date should be synchronized around the world for PSUR reporting such that all authorities receive reports every 6 months or at multiples of 6 months based on the IBD.

- The report should be submitted within 60 days of the data lock-point.

- The reference document for expectedness ("listedness" as opposed to "labeled-ness," which refers to national data sheets such as the U.S. Package Insert) should be the company core data sheet (CCDS), the safety section of which is known as the company core safety information (CSI).

- The verbatim reporter term as well as standardized coding term (i.e., MedDRA, which was approved after E2C was finished) should be used.

- ADR cases should be presented as line listings and summary tabulations. That is, individual CIOMS I or MedWatch forms are not included.

The sections of a PSUR are as follows:

- Introduction
- Worldwide market authorization status
  - A table with dates of Market Authorization and renewals, indications, lack of approvals, withdrawals, dates of launch, and trade names
- Update of regulatory authority or MAH actions taken for safety reasons
- Changes to the Reference Product Information
  - The version of the CCDS in place at the beginning of the PSUR interval as the reference document. If there is a time lag between changes to the CCDS and local labeling, this should be commented on when submitting to that local health authority.
- Patient exposure
  - The most appropriate method should be used and an explanation for its choice provided. This includes patients exposed, patient-days, number of prescriptions, and tonnage sold.
- Presentation of individual case histories from all sources (except nonmedically confirmed consumer reports)
  - Follow-up data on previously reported cases should be presented if significant.
  - Literature should be monitored and cases included. Duplicates should be avoided. If a case is mentioned in the literature, even if obtained also as a spontaneous or trial case, the citation

should be noted.

- If medically unconfirmed cases received from consumers are required to be submitted in the PSUR, they should be submitted as addenda line listings and summary reports.

- Line listings should include each patient only once. If a patient has more than one adverse drug experience/ADR, the case should be listed under the most serious adverse drug experience/ADR, with the others also mentioned there. If appropriate, it may be useful to have more than one line listing for different dosage forms and indications. The headings for the listings are:

  - MAH reference number
  - Country where the case occurred
  - Source (trial, literature, spontaneous, regulatory authority)
  - Age and sex
  - Daily dose, dosage form, and route of suspected drug
  - Reaction onset date
  - Treatment dates
  - Description of the reaction (MedDRA code)
  - Patient outcome at the case level (resolved, fatal, improved, sequelae, unknown)
  - Comments (e.g., causality if manufacturer disagrees with reporter, concomitant medications)

- Line listings should include the following cases:
  - Spontaneous reports: all serious reactions, nonserious unlisted reactions.
  - Studies or compassionate use: all serious reactions (believed to be serious by either the sponsor or the investigator).
  - Literature: all serious reactions and nonserious unlisted reactions.
  - Regulatory authority cases: all serious reactions.
  - If nonserious, listed ADRs are required by some authorities, they should be reported as an addendum.

- Summary tabulations
  - Each line listing should have an aggregate summary that will normally contain more terms than patients. It may be broken down by serious and nonserious and listed and unlisted, as well as other breakdowns as appropriate. There should also be a summary for nonserious listed

spontaneous reactions.

- Data in summary tabulations should be noncumulative except for ADRs that are both serious and unlisted, for which a cumulated figure should be provided in the table.

- MAH analysis of individual case histories
  - This section may contain brief comments on individual cases. The focus here is on individual cases (e.g., unanticipated findings, mechanism, reporting frequency) and should not be confused with the global assessment as described below.

- Studies
  - All completed studies (nonclinical, clinical, epidemiologic), planned or in-progress studies, and published studies yielding or with potential to yield safety information should be discussed.

- Other information
  - Lack of efficacy information should be presented here.
  - Late-breaking information after database lock should be presented here.

- Overall safety evaluation
  - The data should be presented by system organ class and should discuss
    - A change in characteristics of listed reactions
    - Serious unlisted reactions, placing into perspective the cumulative reports
    - Nonserious unlisted reactions
    - Increased frequency of listed reactions
    - New safety issues
    - Drug interactions
    - Overdose and its treatment
    - Drug misuse or abuse
    - Pregnancy and lactation information
    - Experience in special patient groups
    - Effects of long-term treatment

- Conclusion

This section should indicate which safety data do not remain in accord with the previous cumulative experience and with the company CSI:

- Any action recommended or initiated
- Appendix: Company Core Data Sheet (CCDS)

The Addendum provides clarification and guidance on PSURs and addresses some new concepts not in E2C but reflecting current pharmacovigilance practice needs, including Proprietary Information (Confidentiality), Executive Summary, Summary Bridging Report, Addendum Reports, Risk Management Program, and Benefit–Risk Analysis.

- International Birth Dates (IBDs)
  - PSURs should be based on IBDs. To transition to a harmonized IBD, the MAH may submit its already prepared IBD-based PSUR plus (1) line listings and/or tabular summaries for the additional period (≤3 months if submitting a 6-month PSUR or ≤6 months if submitting a longer PSUR) with comments, or (2) an Addendum Report (see below) with the same duration limits as in (1).
  - In attempting to harmonize IBDs, it is possible that a drug will be on a 5-year cycle in one country and a 6-month cycle in another. If harmonization is not possible, the MAH and regulators should try to find a common birth month and day so that reports can be submitted on the same month and day whether every 6 months, yearly, or every 5 years. (Note that many regions have changed the frequency from 5 years to 3 years.)

- Summary Bridging Reports
  - A summary bridging report integrates two or more PSURs to cover a specific time period for which a single report is requested. Thus, two 6-month PSURs could be used to create a summary bridging report to cover the full year or 10 6-month reports to cover a 5-year PSUR. The bridging report does not contain new data but briefly summarizes the data in the shorter reports. The report should not contain line listings but may have summary tables.

- Addendum Reports
  - An addendum report is used when it is not possible to synchronize PSURs for all authorities requiring submissions. The addendum report is an update to the most recently completed PSUR. It should be used when more than 3 months for a 6-month PSUR and more than 6 months for a longer PSUR. It is not intended as an in-depth report (which will be done in the next regularly scheduled PSUR). It should contain an introduction, any changes to the CSI, significant regulatory actions on safety, line listings, and summary tabulations and a conclusion.

- Restarting the Clock

- For products in a long-term PSUR cycle (e.g., 5 years), the return to a 6-month reporting schedule may occur if a new clinically dissimilar indication is approved, a previously unapproved use in a special population is approved, or a new formulation or route of administration is approved. Restarting the reporting clock should be discussed with the regulatory authorities.

- Time Interval Between Data Lock-Point and the Submission
  - The MAH has 60 days to prepare a submission after the data lock-point. An issue that arose was review and comment by the regulatory authority(ies), which took a long time to do and was sent back to the sponsor at a date very close to the submission of the following PSUR. If this review contains new requirements or other obligations for the MAH, the MAH may not be able to adequately complete the additional analyses requested in time for the next PSUR. Hence, the Addendum notes that the regulatory authority will attempt to send comments to the MAH
    - As rapidly as possible if any issues of noncompliance with format and content are noted.
    - As rapidly as possible and before the next data lock-point if additional safety issues are identified that may require further analysis in the next PSUR. Such analyses could also be submitted as a separate stand-alone report instead of in the next PSUR.

- Additional Time for Submissions
  - In rare circumstances, the MAH may request an additional 30 days to submit a PSUR. This might occur if there is a large number of case reports and there is no new safety issue, if issues are raised by the authorities in the previous PSUR for which additional time is needed for further analysis for the next PSUR, or if issues needing further analysis are identified by the MAH.

- Reference Safety Information
  - The MAH should highlight differences between the CSI and the local product-labeling in the cover letter accompanying the PSUR.
  - For 6-month and 1-year PSURs, the CSI in effect at the beginning of the period should be used as the reference document.
  - For PSURs longer than 1 year, the CSI in effect

at the end of the period should be used as the reference document for PSURs and Summary Bridging Reports.

- Other Issues
  - The title page of the PSUR should have a confidentiality statement because proprietary information is contained in the report.
  - An executive summary should be included right after the title page in each PSUR.
  - Patient exposure data
    - It is acknowledged that these data are often difficult to obtain and not always reliable. If the exposure data do not cover the full period of the PSUR, extrapolations may be made. A consistent method of exposure calculations should be used over time for a product.
  - Individual case histories
    - Because it is impractical to summarize all cases as narratives, the MAH should describe the criteria used to describe the cases summarized.
    - The section should contain selected cases, including fatalities, presenting new and relevant safety information and grouped by medically relevant headings or system organ class.
  - Consumer listings
    - If required by regulators, consumer listings should be done in the same way that other listings and summary tabulations are prepared.
  - The "comments" field
    - This field should be used only for information that helps to clarify individual cases.
  - Studies
    - This section should contain only those company-sponsored studies and published safety studies (including epidemiology studies) that produce findings with potential impact on safety. The MAH should not routinely catalogue or describe all studies.
  - The "other information" section
    - Risk management programs may be discussed in this section.
    - When a more comprehensive safety or risk–benefit analysis has been done separately, a summary of the analysis should be included here.
    - Discussion and analysis for the "Overall Safety

Evaluation" section should be organized by system organ class and not by listedness or seriousness.

■ E2D: Postapproval Safety Data Management: Definitions and Standards for Expedited Reporting

This guideline was finalized in 2003 and provides a standardized procedure for postapproval safety data management, including expedited reporting to the relevant authority. It parallels and adds to the E2A document, which covered preapproval (clinical trial) safety data management, by covering postmarketing safety data management. This document standardizes data management of cases from consumers, literature, internet, and other types of postmarketing cases.

Definitions

AE: The definition is nearly identical to the E2A version, leaving out the reference to clinical trials. "An AE is any untoward medical occurrence in a patient administered a medicinal product and which does not necessarily have to have a causal relationship with this treatment. An adverse event can therefore be any unfavorable and unintended sign (for example, an abnormal laboratory finding), symptom, or disease temporally associated with the use of a medicinal product, whether or not considered related to this medicinal product."

ADR: This definition is similar to the preapproval definition (E2A) but defines the causality component in the postmarketing setting ("at least a possibility" of a causal relationship). "All noxious and unintended responses to a medicinal product related to any dose should be considered adverse drug reactions. The phrase 'responses to a medicinal product' means that a causal relationship between a medicinal product and an adverse event is at least a possibility (refer to ICH E2A). A reaction, in contrast to an event, is characterized by the fact that a causal relationship between the drug and the occurrence is suspected. If an event is spontaneously reported, even if the relationship is unknown or unstated, it meets the definition of an adverse drug reaction."

Serious AE/ADR: This definition is the same as the one in E2A for preapproval issues. "Any untoward medical occurrence that at any dose that results in death, is life-threatening, requires inpatient hospitalization or results in prolongation of existing hospitalization, results in persistent or significant disability/incapacity, is a congenital anomaly/birth defect, is a medically important event or reaction. Medical and scientific judgment should be exercised in deciding whether other situations should be considered as serious such as important medical events that may not be immediately life-threatening or result in death or hospitalization but may jeopardize the patient or may require intervention to prevent one of the other outcomes listed in the definition above. These should also be considered serious."

Unexpected ADR: The definition of expeditedness is somewhat different from that in E2A for preapproval cases because the reference documents are different (Investigator Brochure for preapproval and the local labeling for marketed drugs). In addition, class labeling is discussed. This is summarized briefly:

> An ADR whose nature, severity, specificity, or outcome is not consistent with the term or description used in the official product information should be considered unexpected. An ADR with a fatal outcome should be considered unexpected, unless the official product information specifies a fatal outcome for the ADR. In the absence of special circumstances, once the fatal outcome is itself expected, reports involving fatal outcomes should be handled as for any other serious expected ADR in accord with appropriate regulatory requirements.

The term "listedness" is not applicable for expedited reporting (refer to ICH E2C for definition in which listedness refers to whether the reaction is noted in CSI for PSURs). "Class ADRs" should not automatically be considered to be expected for the subject drug. "Class ADRs" should be considered to be expected only if described as specifically occurring with the product in the official product information.

Healthcare professional: "Any medically-qualified person such as a physician, dentist, pharmacist, nurse, coroner, or as otherwise specified by local regulations."

Consumer: "A person who is not a healthcare professional, such as a patient, lawyer, friend or relative of the patient."

Sources of Individual Case Safety Report

- Unsolicited sources: spontaneous reports
    - These are unsolicited communications by healthcare professionals or consumers to a company, regulatory authority, or other organization (e.g., World Health Organization, Regional Centers, Poison Control Center) that describe one or more ADRs in a patient who was given one or more medicinal products, and that does not derive from a study or any organized data collection scheme.
    - "Stimulated reporting may occur in certain situations, such as a notification by a 'Dear Healthcare Professional' letter, a publication in the press, or questioning of healthcare professionals by company representatives. These reports should be considered spontaneous." (Note this contradicts to a certain degree the FDA's guidance of August 1997 [Web Resource 37-2], which requests that such cases be considered as if they were obtained from a postmarketing study and thus requires the triple criteria of seriousness, causality, and expectedness.)
    - Consumer reports should be handled as spontaneous reports irrespective of any subsequent "medical confirmation," a process required by some authorities for reportability. Emphasis should be placed on the quality of the report and not on its source. Even if reports received from consumers do not qualify for regulatory reporting, the cases should be retained in the database.
- Unsolicited sources: literature
    - The MAH is expected to regularly screen the worldwide scientific literature by accessing widely used systematic literature reviews or reference databases according to local requirements or at least every 2 weeks. Cases of ADRs from the scientific and medical literature, including relevant published abstracts from meetings and draft manuscripts, might qualify for expedited reporting.
    - The regulatory reporting time clock starts once it is determined that the case meets minimum criteria for reportability.
    - If the product source, brand, or trade name is not specified, the MAH should assume that it was its product, although reports should indicate that the specific brand was not identified.
- Unsolicited sources: the internet
    - MAHs are not expected to screen external websites for ADR information. However, if an MAH becomes aware of an adverse reaction on a website that it does not manage, the MAH

should review the case and determine whether it should be reported.

- Unsolicited cases from the internet should be handled as spontaneous reports.
- Regarding e-mail, identity of the reporter needs to be evaluated to see whether it refers to the existence of a real person. That is, it is possible to verify that the patient and reporter exist.

- Unsolicited sources: other sources
  - Cases from nonmedical sources, such as the lay press, should be handled as spontaneous reports.
- Solicited sources
  - This refers to cases from organized data collection systems, which include clinical trials, postapproval named patient use programs, other patient support and disease management programs, surveys of patients or healthcare providers, or information-gathering on efficacy or patient compliance. AE reports obtained from any of these should not be considered spontaneous. For safety purposes, reporting solicited reports should be handled as if they were study reports and therefore should have an appropriate causality assessment.
- Contractual agreements
  - If companies make contractual arrangements to market a product in the same or different countries or regions, explicit agreements must be made to specify the processes for exchange of safety information, including timelines and regulatory reporting responsibilities, though the MAH is ultimately responsible. Duplicate reporting should be avoided.
- Regulatory authority sources
  - Individual serious unexpected ADR reports originating from foreign regulatory authorities are always subject to expedited reporting. Resubmission of serious ADR cases without new information to the originating regulatory authority is not usually required, unless otherwise specified by local regulation.

Standards for Expedited Reporting

- Serious ADRs
  - Serious and unexpected cases of ADRs are subject to expedited reporting.
  - For reports from studies and other solicited

sources, all cases judged by either the reporting healthcare professional or the MAH as having a possible causal relationship to the medicinal product qualify as ADRs. This now parallels the FDA's 1997 guidance on expedited reporting of solicited reports.

- For reporting purposes, spontaneous reports associated with approved drugs imply a possible causality.

- Other observations
  - Any significant unanticipated safety findings, including in vitro, animal, epidemiologic, or clinical studies, that suggest a significant human risk and could change the benefit–risk evaluation should be communicated to the regulatory authorities as soon as possible.
  - Lack of efficacy observations should not be expedited but should be discussed in PSURs unless local requirements oblige their being expedited.
  - Overdoses with no associated adverse outcome should not be reported as adverse reactions. The MAH should collect any available information on overdose related to its products.
  - Minimum criteria for reporting include an identifiable reporter, an identifiable patient, an adverse reaction, and a suspect product. The MAH is expected to exercise due diligence to collect missing data elements.
  - Reporting time frames for expedited reports are normally 15 calendar days from initial receipt of the minimal information by any personnel of the MAH. This is day 0. Additional medically relevant information for a previously submitted report restarts the clock.
  - Nonserious ADRs are not normally expeditable whether expected or not.

Good Case Management Practices

- Assessing patient and reporter identifiability
  - One or more of the following automatically qualifies a patient as identifiable: age (or age category, e.g., adolescent, adult, elderly), gender, initials, date of birth, name, or patient identification number. In the event of secondhand reports, every reasonable effort should be made to verify the existence of an identifiable patient and reporter.

- All parties supplying case information or approached for case information should be identifiable.

- In the absence of qualifying descriptors, a report referring to a definite number of patients should not be regarded as a case until the minimum four criteria for case reporting are met.

- The role of narratives

  - The objective of the narrative is to summarize all relevant clinical and related information, including patient characteristics, therapy details, medical history, clinical course of the event(s), diagnosis, and ADR(s), including the outcome, laboratory evidence, and any other information that supports or refutes an ADR. The narrative should serve as a comprehensive stand-alone "medical story." The information should be presented in a logical time sequence; ideally, this should be presented in the chronology of the patient's experience rather than in the chronology in which the information was received. In follow-up reports, new information should be clearly identified.

  - Abbreviations and acronyms should be avoided, with the possible exception of laboratory parameters and units.

- Clinical case evaluation

  - An ADR report should be reviewed by the recipient for the quality and completeness of the medical information. This should include, but is not limited to, the following: Is a diagnosis possible? Have the relevant diagnostic procedures been performed? Were alternative causes of the reaction(s) considered? What additional information is needed?

  - The report should include the reporter's verbatim term (and, in the case of consumer reports, the consumer's description of the event). Staff receiving reports should provide an unbiased and unfiltered report of the information from the reporter. Clearly identified evaluations by the MAH are considered acceptable and, for some authorities, required.

- Follow-up information

  - The information from ADR cases when first received is generally incomplete. Efforts should be made to seek additional information on selected reports.

- The first consideration should be prioritization of case reports by importance: cases that are (1) both serious and unexpected, (2) serious and expected, and (3) nonserious and unexpected. In addition to seriousness and expectedness as criteria, cases "of special interest" also deserve extra attention as a high priority (e.g., ADRs under active surveillance at the request of the regulators), as well as any cases that might lead to a labeling change decision.

- Follow-up should be obtained by a telephone call, a site visit, or a written request. The MAH should provide specific questions it would like answered. The MAH should tailor the effort to optimize the chances of obtaining the new information.

- Written confirmation of details given verbally should be obtained whenever possible. Ideally, healthcare professionals with thorough pharmacovigilance training and therapeutic expertise should be involved in the collection and the direct follow-up of reported cases.

- Pregnancy exposure

  - MAHs are expected to follow up all reports, from healthcare professionals or consumers, of pregnancies where the embryo/fetus could have been exposed to one of its medicinal products.

- How to report

  - The CIOMS I form has been widely accepted. Whatever form is used should have all the appropriate elements included.

  - MedDRA should be used for coding.

  - E2B should be implemented for electronic transmission of individual cases.

- Recommended key data elements

  - The reader is referred to the Appendix of the E2D report for a list of recommended key data elements that should appear in all expedited reports.

■ E2E: Pharmacovigilance Planning

This guideline was finalized in 2004 and is intended to aid in planning pharmacovigilance activities, especially in preparation for the early postmarketing period of a new drug. The main focus of this guideline is on a Safety Specification and Pharmacovigilance Plan that might be submitted at the time of the application for marketing.

Background and Scope

All three regions of the ICH (United States, European Union, and Japan) have been turning their attention to risk management and pharmacovigilance planning throughout the life cycle of a drug. This document reflects ICH's views.

The guidance is proposed for new chemical entities, biotechnology-derived products, and vaccines, as well as for significant changes in established products (e.g., new dosage form, new route of administration, or new manufacturing process for a biotechnology-derived product) and for established products to be introduced to new populations or for new indications, or where a new major safety concern has arisen.

It is recommended that company pharmacovigilance experts get involved early in product development. Planning and dialogue with regulators should also start long before license application. A safety specification and pharmacovigilance plan can also be developed for products already on the market (e.g., new indication or major new safety concern). The plan could be used as the basis for discussing pharmacovigilance activities with regulators in the different ICH regions and beyond.

For products with important identified risks, important potential risks, or important missing information, the pharmacovigilance plan should include additional actions designed to address these concerns. For products for which no special concerns have arisen, routine pharmacovigilance should be sufficient for postapproval safety monitoring, without the need for additional actions (e.g., safety studies). During the course of implementing the various components of the plan, any important emerging benefit or risk information should be discussed and used to revise the plan.

The following principles underpin this guidance:

- Planning of pharmacovigilance activities throughout the product life cycle
- Science-based approach to risk documentation
- Effective collaboration between regulators and industry
- Applicability of the pharmacovigilance plan across the three ICH regions

■ The Sections of a Pharmacovigilance Plan

A pharmacovigilance plan for a product has three sections: (1) Safety Specification, (2) Pharmacovigilance Plan, and (3) Annex—Pharmacovigilance Methods.

The safety specification is a summary of the important identified risks of a drug, important potential risks, and important missing information. It should also address the populations potentially at risk (where the product is likely to be used) and outstanding safety questions that warrant further investigation to refine understanding of the benefit–risk profile during the postapproval period.

The format and contents should focus on the identified risks, important potential risks, and important missing information. It should refer to the three safety sections in the Common Technical Document. The following elements should be considered for inclusion.

- Nonclinical
  - This section should present nonclinical safety findings that have not been adequately addressed by clinical data, for example, toxicity (including repeat-dose toxicity, reproductive/developmental toxicity, nephrotoxicity, hepatotoxicity, genotoxicity, carcinogenicity, etc.), general pharmacology (cardiovascular, including QT/QTc interval prolongation, nervous system, etc.), drug interactions, and other toxicity-related information. If the product is intended for use in special populations, consideration should be given to whether specific nonclinical data need to exist.

- Clinical
  - Limitations of the human safety database (e.g., related to the size of the study population, study inclusion/exclusion criteria) should be considered and discussed. Particular reference should be made to populations likely to be exposed during the intended or expected use of the product in medical practice.
  - The worldwide experience should be briefly discussed, including the extent of the worldwide exposure, any new or different safety issues identified, any regulatory actions related to safety, and populations not studied in the preapproval phase (children, elderly, pregnant or lactating women, patients with relevant comorbidity, such as hepatic or renal disorders, patients with disease severity different from that studied in clinical trials, subpopulations carrying known and relevant genetic polymorphism, patients of different racial or ethnic origins).
  - AEs/ADRs: This section should list the important identified and potential risks that require further characterization or evaluation. Discussion of risk factors and potential

mechanisms should draw on information from the Common Technical Document and other relevant information, such as other drug labels, scientific literature, and postmarketing experience.

- Identified risks that require further evaluation:
  - More detailed information should be included on the most important identified AEs/ADRs, which would include those that are serious or frequent and that also might have an impact on the balance of benefits and risks of the product. This information should include evidence bearing on a causal relationship, severity, seriousness, frequency, reversibility, and at-risk groups, if available. Risk factors and potential mechanisms should be discussed. These AEs/ADRs should usually call for further evaluation as part of the pharmacovigilance plan (e.g., frequency in normal conditions of use, severity, outcome, at-risk groups).
- Potential risks that require further evaluation:
  - Important potential risks should be described and the evidence that led to the conclusion that there was a potential risk should be presented. It is anticipated that for any important potential risk, there should be further evaluation to characterize the association.
  - Identified and potential interactions, including food–drug and drug–drug interactions, should be discussed with consideration of the evidence, and potential health risks posed for the different indications and in the different populations should be discussed.
- Epidemiology
  - The epidemiology of the indication should be discussed, including incidence, prevalence, mortality, and relevant comorbidity, and should take into account whenever possible stratification by age, sex, and racial or ethnic origin. Differences in the epidemiology in different regions should be discussed (because the epidemiology of the indication(s) may vary across regions), if this information is available.
  - For important AEs that may require further investigation, it is useful to review the incidence rates of these events among patients in whom the drug is indicated (i.e., the background incidence rates).

- Pharmacologic class effects
  - The safety specification should identify risks believed to be common to the pharmacologic class.
  - Summary: This should include the important identified risks, potential risks, and missing information on an issue-by-issue basis.

Pharmacovigilance Plan

The pharmacovigilance plan should be based on the safety specification and developed by the sponsor. It can be discussed with regulators during product development, before approval of a new product (i.e., when the marketing application is submitted), or when a safety concern arises postmarketing. It can be a stand-alone document.

For products for which no special concerns have arisen, routine pharmacovigilance should be sufficient for postapproval safety monitoring, without the need for additional actions (e.g., safety studies). However, for products with important identified risks, important potential risks, or important missing information, additional actions designed to address these concerns should be considered. It should be updated as important information on safety becomes available and milestones are reached.

The format and content should include the following:

- Summary of ongoing safety issues, including the important identified risks, potential risks, and missing information.
- Routine pharmacovigilance practice should be conducted for all medicinal products, regardless of whether additional actions are appropriate as part of a pharmacovigilance plan. This routine pharmacovigilance should include the following:
  - Systems and processes that ensure that information about all suspected adverse reactions that are reported to the personnel of the company are collected and collated in an accessible manner.
  - The preparation of reports for regulatory authorities, including expedited ADR reports and PSURs.
  - Continuous monitoring of the safety profile, including signal detection, issue evaluation, updating of labeling, and liaison with regulatory authorities.
  - Other requirements, as defined by local regulations.
- Action plan for safety issues:
  - The plan for each important safety issue should be presented and justified according

to the safety issue, objective of proposed action, action proposed, rationale for proposed action, monitoring by the sponsor for safety issue and proposed action, and milestones for evaluation and reporting. Any protocols for specific studies may also be provided.

- Summary of actions to be completed, including milestones:
  - An overall pharmacovigilance plan for the product, bringing together the actions for all individual safety issues, should be presented and organized in terms of the actions to be undertaken and their milestones.
  - It is recommended that milestones for completing studies and for submitting safety results be included in the pharmacovigilance plan. The milestones should reflect when exposure to the product will have reached a level sufficient to allow potential identification/characterization of the AEs/ADRs of concern or resolution of a particular concern and when the results of ongoing or proposed safety studies are expected to be available.
  - These milestones might be aligned with regulatory milestones (e.g., PSURs, annual reassessment, and license renewals) and used to revise the pharmacovigilance plan.
- Pharmacovigilance methods
  - The best method to address a specific situation can vary, depending on the product, the indication, the population treated, and the issue to be addressed. When choosing a method to address a safety concern, sponsors should use the most appropriate design.
- Design and conduct of observational studies
  - Carefully designed and conducted pharmacoepidemiologic studies, specifically observational (noninterventional, nonexperimental) studies, are important tools in pharmacovigilance.
  - A protocol should be finalized and experts from relevant disciplines (e.g., pharmacovigilance experts, pharmacoepidemiologists, and biostatisticians) should be consulted. It is recommended that the protocol be discussed with the regulatory authorities before the study starts. A study report after completion, and interim reports if appropriate, should be submitted to the authorities according to

the milestones within the pharmacovigilance plan.

- The sponsor should follow good epidemiologic practice for observational studies and internationally accepted guidelines, such as the guidelines endorsed by the International Society for Pharmacoepidemiology.
- Annex

A detailed discussion of pharmacovigilance methods is appended to the document to which the reader is referred for further details.

■ E2F: Development Safety Update Report

This document is now being formally adopted in most jurisdictions. The contents of the DSUR in E2F are very similar to those in the CIOMS DSUR report.

The DSUR is intended to be the common standard for annual clinical trial safety reporting and would replace the U.S. IND Annual Report and the European Union Annual Safety Report, among others. It will present an annual review and evaluation of pertinent interval safety information (1) to summarize the current understanding and management of identified and potential risks, (2) to describe new safety issues that could have an impact on the protection of clinical trial subjects, (3) to examine whether the information obtained during the reporting period is in accord with previous safety knowledge, and (4) to provide an update on the status of the clinical investigation/development program. The contents proposed are:

Title page
Executive Summary
Table of Contents
1. Introduction
2. Worldwide Marketing Authorization Status
3. Update on Actions Taken in the Reporting Period for Safety Reasons
4. Changes to Reference Safety Information
5. Status of Clinical Trials Ongoing and Completed During the Reporting Period
6. Estimated Exposure
   6.1 Cumulative subject exposure in clinical trials (Phase I–IV)
   6.2 Patient exposure from marketed setting
7. Presentation of Safety Data from Clinical Trials
   7.1 General considerations

This is similar to the CIOMS proposal. Full details on the contents can be found in the document on the ICH website (Web Resource 37-1).

38

Pharmaceutical Companies

There are many types of companies and institutions in the pharmaceutical world with responsibilities regarding drug safety. A summary of various types of institutions follows.

There are many large drug companies in the world that sell billions of dollars of product each year. Although the number has decreased through mergers and acquisitions, there still remain more than 50 publicly traded companies with annual sales of more than $1.5 billion per year and roughly another 400 with sales less than $1 billion per year. The largest public company has sales of more than $60 billion per year (*Fortune* magazine, Morningstar). In addition, there are several very large and many other small and midsized companies that are privately held (not traded on the stock exchange). As noted throughout this book, companies are obligated to report animal and human safety data (among other information) to health authorities, ethics committees, investigational review boards, and so on.

■ Big and Somewhat Big Pharma

Big pharma generally refers to the dozen or so large, "full-service" companies with revenues in the billions of dollars. These companies are multinational, with head-quarters in the United States or Europe primarily but with some located in Japan and elsewhere (India or Israel). They usually have scientists doing drug discovery in an attempt to come up with new patentable drugs that will, it is hoped, become "blockbusters" (drugs with sales of more than a billion dollars a year by some definitions). The companies have the capacity to do their own preclinical studies (pharmacology and toxicity) and clinical trials (phases I–IV). Many now also have generic divisions that develop and market generics, both of their own branded products and of other companies' products that are off patent. They have large marketing and sales divisions with hundreds to thousands of "representatives," "sales reps," or "detailers." The big pharma company does some of its own manufacturing in factories throughout the world as well as outsources production from other countries, including India and China in particular. There are large departments to handle regulatory issues, legal issues, and patents. Many have subsidiaries in the major markets (50 or more) throughout the world. Some are only sales organizations, whereas others are staffed to do clinical research as well. Some functions may be located outside the mother country (e.g., home office in the United States but a phase I clinical research unit in the United Kingdom or Asia, or vice versa).

Of course, there is a large drug safety department. The safety department is often, but not always, located in the corporate headquarters in the mother country. This is the major center for drug safety, with receipt of some or all of the individual case safety reports for data entry as well as preparation of MedWatch and CIOMS I forms, Common Technical Documents (eCTDs), Marketing Authorizations, PSURs, NDA periodic reports, IND annual reports, European Annual Safety Reports, clinical trial reports, and other aggregate reports.

The servers for the safety database are located at a central location as a rule, with backup servers at a different location. There are usually drug safety departments in most or all subsidiaries to receive local safety reports (in the local language) and make submissions (sometimes in English, sometimes in the local language) if electronic E2B reporting is not done centrally.

These subsidiaries, depending on size and function, may have a separate physician serving as safety officer or have the medical director (often the only medical doctor in the local company) also serve as the safety physician. The subsidiaries often serve as "pass through" points for AEs to be sent to central or regional data centers for data entry into the safety database. Sometimes a subsidiary (or regional center) will have expanded functions covering multiple countries. For example, some companies (e.g., whose headquarters are located in the United States or Japan) will set up a major center in the European Union to do data entry and to prepare PSURs and other documents for submission to the European Medicines Agency and national health authorities. In other situations where the corporate headquarters are located in a smaller country (e.g., Switzerland), one of the "subsidiaries" may become the dominant center for drug safety (e.g., in the European Union or United States). There is a tendency for safety departments to now be located in major English-speaking countries, such as the United States or the United Kingdom, which, coincidentally or not, are the regulatory sites for the two major world pharmaceutical markets (the United States and the European Union).

Things are changing, however, in biggish pharma. The large companies are getting larger, following mergers and acquisitions (e.g., Merck, Pfizer). There is now a trend in the very big companies to have some functions remain centralized for the entire corporation, such as IT and the safety database, but for the drug safety functions to be separate. That is, there may be several relatively independent drug safety groups (one for prescription products, another for OTC, another for vaccines, etc.) doing individual case processing and aggregate reporting but sharing IT, epidemiology, risk management, and certain other common functions. Thus, big companies may function as "holding companies" for multiple smaller

subunits. Others remain rigidly monolithic. There is no single model applicable to all.

There are several trends evident. One is that drug discovery has been somewhat slow of late in big pharma, with fewer new blockbusters and many old blockbusters going off patent ("the patent cliff"). Many firms, both large and midsized, are now "rightsizing" or downsizing" (i.e., firing workers and replacing them, if at all, with temporary workers and consultants). Thus, they tend to do less research and more development as "R&D" is now becoming distinct. Research is, to a significant degree, being left to the small biotech companies that do the early development and then sell the product to the bigger pharmas for the late phase II and III development for submission of the New Drug Application (NDA) or Marketing Authorization (MA) dossier.

Another trend is the use of generics in the developed world as well as in developing countries. More than half of the drugs sold in the United States are now generics and this trend will continue as many older drugs go off patent. Europe is following this trend too. Some national and multinational companies are devoted only to generic products and thus have little or no drug discovery or clinical research capacity. They may do small studies to show bioequivalence. Occasionally, they do formal phase II, III, or IV clinical trials but usually outsource them. The generic companies create safety departments according to the functions needed, but they tend to be less involved with critical issues than the companies that deal with new chemical entities. By the time a drug is generic, most of the safety issues have been addressed and AE reporting and pharmacovigilance tends to be a "maintenance function," with few new data or signals appearing. Many of the safety reports are, in fact, literature cases with few spontaneous AEs received. In addition, because it is often hard to identify the manufacturer of a generic product, the AEs tend to get reported to the originating company that first created and sold the product whether the actual AE occurred with that product or not.

Some big pharma companies have generic divisions in addition to the innovator divisions. This is done to make money selling generics but also to be in the position to manufacture generics to the branded products they sell after these products go off patent. That is, a company may sell a branded and a generic version of the same product.

We are now beginning to see biosimilar products. These are in a sense "generic biologics" but clearly are not. Many biologics are complex proteins that cannot be created, assembled, and "folded" except in living organisms. Regulatory agencies and companies realize these biosimilars cannot be handled like generic drugs of small molecules. The rules are evolving, and it is likely that pharmacovigilance ("biovigilance") will need to be done at the level of innovator products.

Another trend is the outsourcing and offshoring of many functions that formerly remained entirely within the company. Drug safety falls into this category. The operational aspects of drug safety are usually strong candidates for this. Processing individual case safety reports has now become something of a commodity ("a good or service whose wide availability typically leads to smaller profit margins and diminishes the importance of factors [like brand name] other than price"—*Merriam-Webster's Collegiate Dictionary*, Web Resource 38-1), whereby the place and personnel who do the case processing, data entry, and follow-up are chosen almost entirely on the basis of lowest cost. Thus, much of the drug safety work is now being done in India, China, Brazil, the Philippines, and elsewhere. Manufacturing, toxicology, computer programming, and other services are also following this route. The major business, risk–benefit, and epidemiologic and management decisions tend to remain in the home office.

Midsized and Small Pharma

Some pharmaceutical companies are midsized (sales in the hundreds of millions of dollars) and are sometimes located in a single country. They thus do not have to establish worldwide expertise in the safety department and can concentrate on the safety analysis and reporting in their one or two markets only. These companies range from those that have significant sales figures (e.g., hundreds of millions of dollars) down to small biotech start-up companies with only one product in clinical research, no marketed products, and no sales. These companies usually establish a safety function either as a stand-alone unit with a handful of people if the volume warrants it or combine the function with the medical/clinical research group or the regulatory affairs group. Sometimes the drug safety department is one single person, often with other functions! The trend is to outsource some or all of the function (e.g., data entry, aggregate report writing) to clinical or contract research organizations (CROs) or other outsourcing firms, though the pharma company will retain the final say on the cases.

Sometimes these companies have contractual agreements for research or sales with other companies both inside and outside their home country. These contracts oblige the company to conform to safety and regulatory requirements if the partner is outside the home country.

That is, they must send AEs and other safety information to the contracting business partner in a timely manner and in the proper format so that the business partner can remain in compliance with its local laws and regulations. These safety functions may be kept inside the company or outsourced.

Clinical Research Organizations, Also Called Contract Research Organizations (CRO)

CROs are companies that handle some or all clinical and regulatory functions that pharmaceutical companies do, including phases I–IV studies, regulatory submissions, safety data, pharmacovigilance, IT matters, eCTD, IND, NDA preparation, and so forth. There are large "full-service" CROs that are almost mini-pharmaceutical companies, and there are "niche," or "boutique," CROs that specialize in one or two functions in the pharma world, such as drug safety/PV CROs.

These CROs usually set up whatever safety system(s) are needed for their functions. If they are doing primarily clinical research, they often set up a database for entering or uploading the individual case safety reports that are either sent to the sponsoring company or to the U.S. Food and Drug Administration directly (either by paper or electronic data capture [EDC], also called electronic case report forms [eCRFs]). They may prepare IND or European Union annual reports or handle investigator notification, IRBs/Ethics Committees, and so on. Others that handle safety as their primary function may set up multiple safety databases so that they are able to use the same ones that the sponsoring company(ies) use, both for clinical trials and postmarketing data. Many of the CROs will have to support multiple databases as their clients may use different safety databases and do not want their data transferred to a new system. Other CROs will use one single database for drug safety and arrange for data imports or data reentry between their database and the clients' databases.

There are multiple other types of service organizations that serve the pharmaceutical industry. A listing in the Drug Information Association's publication "Contract Service Organization Directory" includes companies providing the following services: abstract preparation; advertising; specific types of trials (e.g., AIDS); analytic laboratories; bibliography preparation; contract management; validation of assays and laboratories; specimen storage; preparation of NDAs, Biologic

License Applications, CANDAs, PSURs, clinical study reports, investigator brochures, expert reports, publications, drug master files; cardiovascular monitoring; case report form preparation; central laboratories; chemistry–manufacturing–control issues; studies: phases I–IV, investigator-initiated trials, compassionate use trials, epidemiology trials, pharmacoepidemiology trials, claims support studies, safety studies; information technology services (server management, programming and software development, data migration, data management, validation); clinical pharmacology; clinical packaging; clinical supply management; study management; focus groups and consumer testing; auditing; ethics committees and investigational review boards; data safety monitoring boards; digitized QTc analysis; dissolution testing; DNA diagnostics; document imaging; paper and electronic data management; translations; environmental assessments; formulation development; compliance with Good Clinical Practices, Good Manufacturing Practice, Good Laboratory Practice, Good Pharmacovigilance Practices; home infusions; intranet, internet, and website development; investigational site finding; setting up investigator meetings; licensing and acquisitions; market research; medical communications; call centers; medical science liaisons; microbiology testing; nursing; patient compliance, education, recruitment; preparation of labeling and patient information leaflets; process validation; project management; quality assurance and quality control; quality of life assessment; randomization; regulatory affairs; registries; remote data entry; prescription to over-the-counter switch; stability testing; standard operating procedure development; statistical services; toxicology; training; transportation; and reengineering and process redesign. New to the game are social media niche companies that deal in Twitter, Facebook, blogs, and the other new and evolving communication methods. Not all these organizations deal with safety or pharmacovigilance issues, although occasionally issues do come up, and the drug safety department may need to work with these companies on safety-related projects.

The business models in the pharmaceutical world are changing. Some of the bigger CROs are actually becoming pharma companies as they in-license or purchase early or even late-stage drugs and then continue the development on their own. Innovation is tending to come now from small start-ups and biotechs as well as from large pharmaceutical companies. The large pharma companies are now downsizing in some areas and outsourcing many functions to CROs and other vendors that they formerly kept in-house. They are thus transforming into development and marketing companies, leaving much of the innovative discovery to the smaller companies. Similarly, when large pharmas purchase small biotechs they often inadvertently (or expressly) transform the smaller innovator into a more classic company, destroying the innovation atmosphere. Any acquisition will force changes in the handling of safety data as one or both companies must adapt to the new products and procedures.

■ Mergers, Acquisitions, and Bankruptcies

For better or worse, the pharma world is one where companies join, split, merge, and occasionally go bankrupt. No matter what happens in such situations, the responsibility for drug safety and pharmacovigilance remains in place.

When a corporate change occurs, it is the responsibility of the company (in the European Union of the QPPV) to ensure that a clear transition of responsibilities occurs and that all drug safety activities are maintained. Specifically, there must be clarity on who will be the new QPPV and when, what database(s) are in place, and, if more than one is in use at one time, how is compliance assured? Are all safety exchange agreements still in place and valid with other companies? If the MA or NDA changes ownership, how is this handled to ensure that all clinical trial and postmarketing SAEs, PSURs, IND safety, or annual reports are submitted correctly and on time? In other words, there must be a smooth transition to ensure that no safety issues or responsibilities are missed. The transition teams (both internal and external consultants) must ensure the turnover and make it a very high priority. The concerned health authorities should be kept informed and assured that all issues have been successfully dealt with. As the merger or acquisition is usually done for financial and business reasons, safety and PV are often an afterthought and may not be addressed until very late in the negotiations, or sometimes not until after the deal is concluded. This can produce operational challenges for all parties.

Expect a governmental inspection from one or more of the health authorities after the merger to ensure that all the requirements and systems for drug safety are in place and functioning well.

Bankruptcies (also called liquidations) can be tricky if the company ceases to exist. Legal counsel should be obtained where necessary and the health agency contacted as needed. As always, the safety functions must continue uninterrupted.

39

Universities and Academic Medical Centers

Universities and academic medical centers have multiple areas in which they interact with the drug safety world:

- Discovery and licensing
- Specialized clinical research units (CRUs) that run studies
- Other clinical divisions that run studies
- Training medical students, pharmacists, nurses, epidemiologists, and other healthcare professionals
- Ethics Committees/Investigational Review Boards (IRBs)
- Data safety monitoring committees and adjudication committees
- Consultation to the industry
- Reporting ADRs that occur in the hospital

■ The Bayh-Dole Act in the United States

The Bayh-Dole Act, or Patent and Trademark Law Amendments Act, was passed in 1980 (35USC200-212

and 37CFR401). See Web Resource 39-1. Among other provisions, it gave universities the right to hold patents for discoveries from research that they performed that also had federal funding. Government agencies had been hesitant about letting universities and small businesses obtain or license government-held or government-sponsored patents. This act encouraged universities and small businesses to move discoveries into the marketplace. Examples now abound:

- New York University: Professor Jan Vilcek and colleagues at the New York University School of Medicine developed the drug infliximab (Remicade), from which many millions of dollars in royalties were made. Professor Vilcek donated $105 million to the medical school (*New York Times*, August 12, 2005).

- Emory: Emory University receives significant sums of money from the sales of emtricitabine (Emtriva) (Source: Emory University; Web Resource 39-2).

- University of California: "A Drug's Royalties May Ease Hunger" (*New York Times*, March 7, 2004).

- Northwestern University: "Royalty Pharma Buys Portion of NWU's Royalty Interest in Lyrica for $700M" (Web Resource 39-3).

In the American setting, the development of university-held patents has, of course, produced lawsuits over royalties.

- In 1999, Glaxo Wellcome agreed to pay the University of Minnesota royalties on the company's worldwide sales of Ziagen, an antiviral AIDS drug, to settle a lawsuit brought by the university over royalties for patents held by a College of Pharmacy professor and subsequently licensed to Glaxo (Source: University of Minnesota; Web Resource 39-4).
- Princeton "University and the drug manufacturing company Eli Lilly filed a lawsuit last week against Barr Laboratories, alleging that Barr was infringing on a University patent covering the active chemical in the cancer drug Alimta. The suit aims to prevent Barr from manufacturing a generic version of the drug that brought in more than $1 billion in revenue for Lilly last year" (*The Daily Princetonian*, May 11, 2009, Web Resource 39-5).

If universities and medical centers conduct clinical studies, they also have the usual obligations of the investigator to report certain safety information to health authorities, ethics committees, and IRBs, as well as to contractual partners.

Clinical Research Units

Many universities have established clinical research units, including the University of Chicago, University of Buffalo, University of Medicine and Dentistry of New Jersey-New Brunswick, Duke University, University of Miami, University of Pennsylvania, University of Arizona, and University of Kentucky. In addition, there are units in the United Kingdom, Belgium, Canada, Germany, and other countries. Duke University, in fact, runs a clinical research organization, which they note is the largest academic clinical research organization (CRO) in the world, with more than 3500 studies in over 60 countries.

These units may perform both inpatient and outpatient studies in phases I, II, III, and IV. When functioning as sponsors, the CRU takes on all sponsor responsibilities as outlined in the laws and regulations (and local institutional policies) for the study as if it were a pharmaceutical company or a large consortium running trials (e.g., cancer trials, National Institutes of Health). When it functions as a study site for a pharmaceutical company, its safety functions revolve primarily around sending AEs (particularly serious ones) to the sponsor and notifying the

IRB of serious cases. Thus, such units may take on some or all of the safety functions in the trial.

Frequently, individual investigators within universities or medical centers contract with pharma companies, CROs, consortia, the National Institutes of Health, and others to run studies or participate in multicenter clinical trials. These trials are run separately from the CRU (if such a unit exists in the institution). In such a case, the investigator is responsible for complying with all safety obligations under the regulations and local university policies. Many universities now set up offices within the administration that handle such "extramural" research activities. They offer assistance to the investigators and ensure that the university collects the appropriate fees for use of their facilities. Doing clinical trials may serve as a significant source of revenue for academic centers. Some pharma companies encourage their medical staff to remain in contact with medical centers, and physicians in companies often hold academic appointments in academia. Some controversy has arisen where academic physicians and researchers form for-profit companies that aim to discover, market, or do further research on drugs. Universities in the United States and elsewhere are now attempting to create clear "firewalls" between companies and academia even to the point of forbidding company detailers (reps) from coming on site. Some academic centers do not allow their staff to use pens with drug or company logos.

Some countries have much tighter ties between academia and government. The French health authority (AFSSAPS; Web Resource 39-6, in French) has a network of 31 academic medical centers that collect ADRs and train physicians and other health professionals on drug safety matters. They also provide consultative work for the agency upon request.

Drug Safety Training in Academia

Academia in the United States and Canada plays a surprisingly small role in drug safety, unlike the situation in France and elsewhere. There are at most a handful of departments of pharmacology, medicine, or epidemiology in North America that play major roles in the drug safety world. Although academics sit on advisory committees for health authorities (FDA, European Union member states, Japan), many more make speeches (for a fee paid for by the pharmaceutical companies' "speakers bureaus") around the country regarding drug therapy, though this is now changing as conflicts of interest are being actively sought out and, in theory, stamped out (if that is possible) or at least minimized. In addition, many academics perform clinical trials paid for by the pharmaceutical companies, thus removing them as neutral observers or consultants on safety. Pharmacology departments in medical schools have historically played only a minor role in pharmacovigilance. Much of the drug safety interest and research is coming from IT and biostatistical departments in universities looking at data mining, electronic health records, and such.

Pharmacovigilance is rarely taught to medical or nursing students in North America. On the positive side, pharmacy schools seem to be incorporating more drug safety concepts into their curricula, and some universities are now developing academic certification and degree (MS, PhD) programs in pharmaceutical medicine. See the Biopharma Educational Initiative at the University of Medicine and Dentistry of New Jersey (Web Resource 39-7). They offer a master's degree and a "certificate" and hope to offer a PhD program in the future.

The training that does occur usually involves classical pharmacology and treatment with minimal (if any) discussion of the pharmaceutical industry, the FDA or Health Canada, and the subjects addressed in this book. Similarly, nursing and other allied medical programs also have little emphasis on drug safety. Some pharmacy schools and public health training programs cover drug safety and epidemiology in their curricula and may establish rotations through industry or health agencies during the training of the students. The rudiments of epidemiology (though not pharmacoepidemiology) are taught to medical students.

This is in marked contrast to Europe, where academic institutions play a major role in drug safety, often working with the government and health authority. In several western European countries, drug safety teaching seems to be well integrated in those university hospitals where a pharmacovigilance reporting center, a drug information center, a poison control center, or a pharmacoepidemiology or epidemiology department exist. See the European Programme in Pharmacovigilance and Pharmacoepidemiology (Web Resource 39-8). Eu2P will develop an educational curriculum with a high level of excellence, including innovative and interactive e-learning tools (Web Resource 39-9). See also the Innovative Medicines Initiative (Web Resource 39-10). It is likely that academia in the United States will "discover" pharmacovigilance and the other functions of the industry and incorporate them into training healthcare professionals and others.

Obviously, it is in everyone's interest for drug safety and pharmacovigilance to become topics in which all healthcare professionals are trained and skilled.

■ Academic Consultation

When academic researchers (physicians primarily) and healthcare workers consult to the pharmaceutical industry, much controversy results. This can include giving (for a fee) opinions on clinical trial programs, protocols, clinical development, and drug safety issues. In particular, a sponsor may ask one or more academic clinicians or pharmacologists to review one or more case reports of AEs reported with the use of a drug. The review would help determine whether the AE is related to the drug.

Various reports in the news and online have indicated that some physicians involved in clinical trials have been consulting with Wall Street financial analysts (for a fee) and it appears that the analysts wanted some indication of how the particular drug was faring in the clinical trials, usually in matters of safety as the efficacy data were blinded. Trouble can ensue. In one case a physician was charged with leaking insider information on a clinical trial to a hedge fund ("Bail Set For Doctor in Insider-Trading Case," *Wall Street Journal*, November 26, 2010).

Consultation also includes giving "scientific marketing talks" (discussions of diseases or particular drugs) to other physicians and healthcare workers on marketed drugs that the sponsor makes. The controversy here revolves around the independence and impartiality of consultants who are also receiving sums of money for scientific marketing activities. Some believe that full disclosure of all financial ties, even remote, permits objectivity. Others believe that objectivity in such a circumstance is never truly possible and that comments on clinical trial efficacy or drug safety are not unbiased. Because this practice is fairly widespread, it has produced, in some cases, difficulties in finding consultants with no industry ties to serve on FDA advisory committees and data safety management boards. The companies are now publishing online detailed lists of the names and sums of money the consultants receive. The NIH is proposing tougher conflict-of-interest rules (Web Resource 39-11). It is likely that transparency in these areas will become greater over time.

Much has been written on this topic in the United States. See articles by Marcia Angell, MD, and Jerome Kassirer, MD, both formerly editors of the *New England Journal of Medicine*, and, in particular, Brennan, et al., Health industry practices that create conflicts of interest:

a policy proposal for academic medical centers. *JAMA* 2006;295:429–433; Steinbrook, Controlling conflict of interest—proposals from the Institute of Medicine (Web Resource 39-12); and Okike, Kocher, Wei, Mehlman, Bhandari, Accuracy of conflict-of-interest disclosures reported by physicians. *New Engl J Med* 2009;361(15): 1466–1474.

The Pharmaceutical Research Manufacturers of America (PhRMA), the organization of the pharmaceutical companies, has put out several codes and guidances on industry actions and behavior in research, marketing, and sales. The Code on Interactions with Medical Professionals has been signed by some 50 companies and sets certain voluntary standards on drug marketing (see also Chapter 50 and Web Resource 39-13).

Universities and medical centers are placing more and more limits on what drug company representatives ("reps") can say and do in their institutions. In the United States, many institutions are limiting samples, free lunches, detailing, and other pharma company activities in their centers. In France, limits have been placed on what reps can say and how many free samples are dispensed to physicians, and it is claimed that these requirements are now stricter than those in the United States and Canada (Silversides, Tight regulation of French drug reps mean French doctors get more balanced information than doctors in the US. *BMJ* 2010;341:c6964).

The Joint Commission (Web Resource 39-14) standard COP.11.6 requires organizations to monitor the effects of medications on patients. However, the requirement is not explicit on reporting adverse drug reactions (or medication errors) to the FDA, although this is encouraged by the FDA via the MedWatch Program. Thus, hospitals must develop some level of drug safety expertise, usually via the pharmacy department or the formulary committee (the group that decides which drugs will be kept on formulary and which will not). Requirements outside the United States vary from country to country.

■ RADAR (Northwestern University)

Northwestern University in Chicago is home to a group known as RADAR. Their aim is "to disseminate safety reports for serious ADRs and to identify barriers to identification and reporting of these events." Investigators note that they have developed a system to compile case report information on ADRs and to identify milestones associated with ADR information. This ADR identification system allows the collection of ADR information from a diverse set of data sources in order to identify and report ADRs in a timely and thorough manner. The RADAR methodology relies on initial recognition of these "sentinel" cases that then prompts hypothesis-driven inquiries as to whether an unrecognized adverse drug event signal is present in the patients exposed to that drug. Hypothesis-driven active surveillance of small but thorough sets of safety reports serves as the underlying conceptual framework of RADAR pharmacovigilance. Fewer than 20 individual ADR reports led to RADAR investigators' identifying safety signals for the majority of the ADRs described to date (see Web Resource 39-15). Other academic work in medicine, pharmacology, and informatics is expected to change how drug safety is done.

Organization of a Typical Drug Safety Department

T his description covers a "standard" safety department found in a large or midsized (multinational) pharmaceutical company. Some functions and divisions do not exist in smaller companies or in companies that do not have international or research functions. Some functions are combined with others. Some functions may work with other divisions in the corporation in addition to the safety department.

regulatory affairs or clinical research. In some companies, the QP is different from the senior medical officer and is sometimes not a physician.

There is also a functional head of drug safety, who ensures that the department runs in a timely, orderly, and professional manner. In smaller companies, the chief safety officer and the functional head may be the same person. That person is usually a healthcare professional. In larger companies, they tend to be separated, especially if the company has several major safety units around the world.

■ Management

Generally, companies have a physician who is designated "chief safety officer," "chief medical officer," or "qualified person for pharmacovigilance (QP or QPPV)" who is (usually) a senior-level physician (e.g., executive or senior vice president) and is responsible for the final decision on medical issues for the corporation. This job includes decisions on product withdrawals, stopping clinical trials, amending protocols, changing product labeling, and so forth, for safety reasons. This person is either in the senior management of the company or in

■ The Qualified Person

This is a critical role for companies with marketing authorizations in the European Union and is discussed in detail in Chapter 23.

■ Triage Unit

The triage unit is responsible for receiving and reviewing, often at a single central point, all incoming adverse events (AEs), plus, in many cases, product complaints, requests for information from consumers and healthcare professionals, requests for reimbursement, and other medical information functions. Each incoming contact is routed to the appropriate department for handling. Decisions have to be made if a single incoming contact has several components: "I took your pill, which was red instead of its normal blue color; I had chest pain after I took it—is that normal? And I want my money back." This is a product quality complaint, an AE, a question, and a request for reimbursement. In general, the priority should go to the AE and quality issue. Routes of entry of AEs are changing. Formerly, phone calls and letters were predominant. Now, phone calls, e-mail, websites, social media, and other electronic avenues bring in many postmarketing AEs. "Snail mail," case reports of clinical trial AEs, reports from the Food and Drug Administration (FDA) and other health authorities, medical literature screening, lawsuits, and other assorted sources also supply AEs. Some drugs have more AEs reported by healthcare practitioners and others by consumers and patients. Triage must be rapid and in real time because expedited (7- and 15-day) reports need to be acted on immediately. Serious AE cases should generally be reviewed more quickly than nonserious cases.

The triage is usually made up of both professional and clerical personnel whose job is to do the first-level screening of all incoming contacts. Telephone calls are usually screened initially by call centers with or without medically trained personnel (pharmacists, nurses) as the initial responders. E-mail, website information, and other electronically arriving AEs may first be seen by clerical or IT staff but must be routed rapidly to medical professionals to perform the medical triage. Mail with possible AE information must be handled rapidly by personnel in the mailroom.

In multinational companies, there is usually a triage group locally to handle phone calls and written communications arriving in the local language. U.S. phone centers often are able to handle calls in English and Spanish and sometimes other languages. In Canada, English and French are required. Many companies are now moving call centers "offshore," especially to India, the Philippines, and other English-speaking countries, as well as to Latin America for Spanish-language calls. Cost savings can be substantial, though time zone and cultural differences may also be significant. Obviously, these centers must function at the same level and under the same regulatory requirements as if they were in the United States. The FDA will hold them to U.S. standards if they receive calls from American patients and physicians. Similarly, other health agencies will require domestic standards to be applied to external centers as well.

■ Case Assessment and Prioritization

A medical professional should rapidly review the cases for seriousness, expectedness (labeledness), and causality (for clinical trial cases). Priority then goes to AEs that are 7- and 15-day expedited reports. The personnel must have all the needed tools (computer access and training, latest labeling and investigator brochures, etc.).

■ Data Entry Unit

After triage, cases must be medically evaluated (if not already done) and entered into the safety database. Cases that come in electronically, such as from clinical trial electronic data capture programs or postmarketing cases from online data entry forms, partner databases, and so forth, usually do not need to be reentered unless the sending database and the receiving safety database cannot "talk" to each other. Rather, these cases may sit in an electronic "holding area" and must be screened by the triage or medical personnel for minimum criteria, correct drug identification, duplicates, and so forth, before being uploaded into the safety database. Uploading is normally instantaneous when done electronically and has implications for the "clock start date." Some companies may allow direct upload into their safety database from trusted, validated, and virus-free sources, such as partner companies or CROs.

Paper cases (including faxed, PDF, or other "paper cases" that arrive electronically but not in files that are directly uploadable) must be manually entered into the database. Cases that are identified at triage to be expedited reports are usually prioritized for immediate data entry. Cases that are not expedited reports are put into a queue for handling and data entry. Serious cases that are to be manually entered are usually "databased" within 7-15 days and nonserious cases within 30 days. Companies' procedures vary widely.

The initially received information is entered into the drug safety database after screening for the four minimum criteria, the correct drug, and duplicates is done. Data entry is usually performed by clerical personnel who have been trained on how to enter cases into the company's safety database and sometimes after training in medical terminology. Some companies do manual data entry at a single site or at multiple sites (e.g., one on each continent). Most data, though not all, are entered in English. Source documents may also be entered (either summarized or scanned in or both), catalogued, and stored in the database. Some data may need to be anonymized or redacted to remove personal information. See Chapter 28 on data privacy.

Case Processing Unit

This unit is made up of health professionals, usually nurses and pharmacists, but occasionally also podiatrists, dentists, and other healthcare professionals. This group does the initial evaluation for expedited cases (as noted above, usually before data entry) and then reviews and/or prepares the case medical information. In particular, this involves the creation of the "narrative" (which is a stand-alone text summary of the case that appears in the electronic case [E2B] or on the MedWatch and CIOMS I forms), and the verification of drug names, dosages, past medical history, and so on. The case-processing group also prepares medical queries (with the assistance of the physicians) to be sent to the reporter or investigator to obtain further information if the initial data are incomplete, including the final outcome for ongoing cases.

Medical Case Review

This group is usually composed of physicians with expertise in drug safety and case review. They generally review the assessment, the AE coding, and the medical content of the narrative to ensure that the medical story is cogent and that it is a true reflection of the source data supplied. These physicians may also handle other work, including the preparation and review of signals, aggregate reports, and ad hoc queries.

Transmission Unit

This group ensures that the appropriate cases are sent to the appropriate recipients. Expedited reports either go directly to the health agencies (usually by electronic E2B transmission or paper) or to the regulatory department for transmission to the health authorities. Cases may also be sent within the company to other interested parties (e.g., clinical research, legal) and to associated business partners who market or study the drug. This function may be assumed by a unit that handles all "traffic" matters, including triage, routing, and transmission. If the transmission is via E2B there may not be a separate transmission unit, though someone must still track what goes where.

Regulatory Unit

Usually, this unit is not a part of drug safety but is a separate division, at least in larger companies. In some companies, expedited cases are reviewed by the regulatory group before transmission to the health authority as a final quality check. Many companies prefer to have all communications to and from the health authorities handled by the regulatory division rather than by drug safety and other groups to ensure tight tracking of all governmental contacts.

Legal Unit

This unit is never a part of drug safety. The legal unit interacts with drug safety in three primary areas. First, in some companies, the legal department reviews all cases that are sent to health agencies to ensure that "troublesome" statements will not be included that may produce difficulties for the company. (This is controversial, as it may mean that the company cannot make a causality assessment on cases, as that might mean admitting the drug and the company are "guilty" of causing that ADR.) The second area involves litigation or potential litigation based on AEs. In these cases, the drug safety and legal areas work tightly together in defending the litigation and in obtaining any follow-up from the suing party. Such follow-up is often done via the attorneys rather than directly from drug safety. The legal unit may also be a source of AEs that arise in lawsuits against the company that first arrive in the legal department. The third area is in negotiating agreements with external parties for in- or out-licensing, outsourcing, comarketing, and so forth. The two groups work together to ensure that all safety obligations to all health authorities and other companies are met.

Signaling, Pharmacovigilance, Pharmacoepidemiology, Medical Information or Medical Affairs Unit

Although this function may be called many things, as noted in the heading, its primary job is to look for new signals. This unit is made up of physicians and other healthcare workers. Their main function is to review the safety data (AEs, medical errors, and product quality complaints) collected by the company and to evaluate whether new signals are popping up or old ones are resolving or worsening. They may use tools available commercially or developed in-house for data mining (see Chapters 8 and 19). When an issue is found, they begin an initial safety investigation that includes a review of the published literature, the company's clinical research database (if different from the safety database), external databases, medical literature (which must be searched weekly under

European Union Volume 9A requirements), toxicology, pharmacology, and any other relevant information, to prepare a summary report for presentation to the decision-makers (e.g., the senior corporate safety committee) for resolution.

They may handle other functions, including review of individual cases, preparation of Investigational New Drug Application (IND) annual report, New Drug Application (NDA) periodic reports, annual safety reports, Development Safety Update Reports (DSURs), Periodic Safety Update Reports (PSURs), integrated safety summaries, responses to queries from health authorities, pharmacoepidemiology studies and analyses, advertising review for medical content, review of communications to the public ("Dear Doctor" or "Dear Healthcare Professional" letters), review of labeling and Package Inserts, medical testimony in litigation, and consultation on drug withdrawals. Some of these functions may be split into separate groups, such as a PSUR preparation group, a pharmacoepidemiology group, and so forth, particularly in large companies.

This group may also handle the preparation of risk management documents such as REMS or RMPs (see Chapter 30).

■ Aggregate Report Preparation

This unit, comprising physicians and other healthcare professionals, sometimes separate from the pharmacovigilance unit, prepares aggregate or summary reports of data derived from individual case safety reports. These reports include IND annual, NDA periodic reports, annual safety reports, DSURs, PSURs, ad hoc and PSUR-derived queries from health authorities, and other corporate departments. They will sometimes prepare white papers or literature reviews for internal and external scientific requests for information.

■ Labeling Review and Update for Safety

This function is sometimes done within drug safety and sometimes separately by the labeling group or regulatory affairs. It involves the continuous monitoring of the labeling of the company's products to ensure that all the safety information is fully up to date and the transition to new labeling format and content requirements in various countries is being performed (see Chapter 34). This includes examination of the core safety information document (CCSI) as well as local labeling sheets (e.g., U.S. Package Insert, Summary of Product Characteristics) and patient information leaflets. Areas of interest include AE, warnings, precautions, contraindications, pregnancy and lactation, overdose, and drug interactions. This may be a very substantial task if the company sells multiple drugs with multiple formulations in many countries around the world.

It may also require the monitoring of the safety labeling of products of other companies' drugs in the same class as well as drugs that may have interactions with the company's drugs. For example, if company B adds a statement to its drug's labeling stating that there is a drug interaction between the company B drug and a company A drug, company A should determine whether it should add a similar statement to its labeling.

■ Archive/File Room

Archiving involves several issues. First, there is now an enormous amount of electronic information, including e-mails, electronic case reports, lab data, and computer files and programs. This is critical data that must be backed up and archived. This is usually an IT function, which is transparent to the drug safety group. This has become, with the advent of electronic storage and data security and privacy rules, a very complicated matter.

In terms of paper, although there is a trend toward the so-called paperless office, the amount of paper and the number of photocopy machines used do not yet appear to be decreasing. The safety department must make sure they have an adequate archive/file room system such that all safety information is saved in the appropriate place and is readily available for immediate review whether by the company or during a health authority inspection. In terms of electronic data, secure server parks with backup and all appropriate privacy and data protection must be in place. If multinational data are stored in a server then all applicable laws and requirements from the data's source country must be in place.

Several logistical decisions need to be made for both paper and electronic archiving concerning such things as:

- The storage of documents in a multinational company where serious AE reports may come in multiple languages: Should they be kept in the country where they are received (and are able to be read) or centrally or both? What should be translated? And if translated, what must be "officially" translated and what can be translated using a fast but inaccurate computer translation program?

- Are the storerooms adequately protected from fire, flood, and other hazards? Should sprinkler systems specifically not be installed but rather an alternative system used for fire protection?

- Storing paper charts for tens of thousands of cases per year (in a large company) can require large physical storage areas. Should these cases be kept on site or archived in a document storage facility off-site?

- What tracking system will be used? Should bar codes or chips be used for paper files, and, if so, for the folder jacket or for every document inside? If a case has some parts stored as paper and some as electronic files, should they be merged and all stored electronically? How should they be indexed and tracked? How will follow-up data be stored and indexed?

- How long should documents and electronic files be retained? Note that retention rules differ for various jurisdictions. In general, documents should be retained for the longest time required by any country whose documents are stored in that archive. Some companies keep all safety data forever.

- Who has access to and control of the file room and electronic files?

- What backup methods are used (e.g., in case of fire or water damage) for paper and electronic records?

- Are all privacy and anonymization regulations being followed?

- If contract facilities (outside vendors) are used, who supervises them and ensures the safe keeping of the files and the ability to retrieve needed files (e.g., for a health authority audit) within 24 hours?

■ Information Technology/ Informatics Liaison

Almost all drug safety departments use a commercial or homegrown database to store safety data and produce MedWatch, CIOMS I forms, CIOMS II line listings, annual safety reports, PSURs, and so forth. There is usually a dedicated informatics/information technology (IT) support and development group that works with drug safety ("the business owners") to support the database and handle changes, bugs, new hires and access levels, upgrades, MedDRA and other dictionaries, testing, and validation. Sometimes the IT support person(s) report directly to the drug safety group and sometimes not.

Usually, the IT group is fully versed in the IT aspects of the database but needs business input from a "superuser" or drug safety expert who understands the safety business and issues and who can speak the "IT language" to facilitate communication. This IT liaison function has various titles from company to company but is found in nearly all companies because the need to bridge the gap between the computer experts and the safety experts is real and ongoing.

In large companies, the 24/7 maintenance of the multiple databases involved in safety in one way or another (clinical trial database, ePRO-electronic patient recorded outcomes, safety database, telephone call tracking database, product complaint database, labeling database, etc.) requires IT departments of scores or even hundreds of persons all around the world (wherever someone has a computer, iPhone, Blackberry, etc.). Linking databases and ensuring database-to-database communications (E2B), as well as keeping up to date on other data standardization matters, is now a major operation in most companies (see Chapter 20).

■ Standard Operating Procedure (SOP) Creation and Maintenance

Written formal SOPs, working documents, and guidances are obligatory in drug safety departments under Good Clinical Practices (GCP) requirements from the International Conference on Harmonization (ICH), the FDA, the European Medicines Agency (EMA), and other agencies and bodies. In addition, there may be manuals, guidances, and job aids that accompany the SOPs (e.g., a data entry manual). The first thing an FDA, EMA, or internal company inspector will ask for at the start of an inspection or audit is a copy of the organizational chart of the safety department and list of the SOPs in place. The SOPs govern the handling of everything in pharmacovigilance: safety data, report preparation, training, database and computer issues, crisis management, and so forth. It is not uncommon for a company to have 50 or more such SOPs and guidances. The creation, review (yearly at least), maintenance, and updating of SOPs is a function that must be ensured in a safety department. The issue of version control of SOPs must also be addressed so that everyone has access to and is working from the latest versions of the SOPs and guidances. This means controlled distribution of electronic (or paper copies) of the latest and applicable SOPs.

Training

Another requirement of GCP and quality systems is that training be done and documented *before* the SOP or process is put in place or the person starts work. The training, based on the SOPs, guidances, and working documents, covers:

- The concepts of drug safety, pharmacovigilance, and risk management
- The laws, guidances, and regulations in place
- The specific procedures in that organization or division and others if appropriate (e.g., clinical research)
- The computers and software

In addition, there is the more general training the organization offers on corporate values and workplace behavior, equality issues, physical safety in the workplace, and so on.

There is usually a formal training function or department within drug safety with a dedicated trainer (sometimes "certified" by some training body or organization either internal to the company or outside) who develops formal curricula and courses for the various people (based on job function) who need to be trained. This applies to both new hires and update training for current employees. The training involves the drug safety department workers as well as others in the organization who might receive AEs in the course of their own jobs (e.g., in clinical research, regulatory, legal, telephone operators, customer relations). Each person in the safety department should have an up-to-date and accurate training folder documenting all training that person has had. This will often need to be produced during a health authority audit.

Much training is now done online with elegant self-pacing and self-testing modules, allowing the individual to do the training at his or her own pace and timing (though by a certain due date). There are multiple organizations that offer courses both in-house and externally.

Quality Assurance/Control

The concept of "quality assurance/control and quality systems" is relatively new to drug safety and GCP compared with their use in the manufacturing and laboratory areas. Quality is broadly broken up into two phases.

The first is quality assurance (QA), which, as we refer to it in drug safety, refers to actions taken during the process of handling safety data to ensure that the work is correct and complete. During the preparation of an ICSR for submission to a health authority by a pharmacist, the QA might be done by his or her supervisor. This is quality that must be built in up-front and during the process. The view is that, if something bad has to be picked up at the end of the workflow when everything is completed, it is too late. Corrections should be made during the process and in real time.

The second phase is quality control (QC), which usually refers to a review of the (final) deliverable. This is done to ensure that the deliverables (e.g., the completed MedWatch or CIOMS I form or PSUR) were correctly and completely prepared and that no data are lost or changed along the way. QC may include formal audits by third parties from outside or inside the company or organization. Such audits are routinely done at the end of the process. The difference from QA is that the review is usually done after the case is completed. Note that confusion exists since some use QA and QC interchangeably or use QA to mean "after-process quality" and QC to mean "in-process quality". Others consider quality assurance to be a component of the overall quality control system. In any case, quality must be done both during and after no matter what we label it!

Organizations should have both quality functions in place. During the processing and analysis of safety data, quality checks should be performed at the appropriate stages in the process. After the work is done, a review or an audit may be done on selective cases routinely or periodically (e.g., monthly) to see that the entire process is done correctly. Key performance indicators (KPIs) and other metrics should also be built in. Many safety departments in companies have a yearly audit done by their corporate quality group (separate from the drug safety group) or by an external PV auditor/consultant. Of course, the health agencies (the FDA, EMA, and Medicines and Healthcare Products Regulatory Agency [MHRA] in particular) do periodic pharmacovigilance inspections to check the quality of the safety department's work (see Chapter 48).

Safety (AE) Exchange Agreement Function: Creation and Maintenance

Many pharmaceutical companies, both large and small, now enter into agreements with other companies to outsource or share certain responsibilities, such as comarketing in the same country, marketing in other countries, clinical trials (including development, monitoring, and data analysis), manufacturing, and safety data handling.

As with other business arrangements, it is obligatory that all parties involved have written contracts specifying the safety functions and requirements of all partners. The contract should set specific terms for the exchange of all needed safety data, both individual case safety reports and aggregate reports such as PSURs and NDA periodic reports as well as labeling, investigator brochures, advertising, and regulatory communications. This must be done so that all partners are able to stay in full compliance with all regulations and laws (see Chapter 47). In the European Union, the QPPV must ensure that this function is done completely and correctly (see Chapter 23).

■ Literature Review

United States and European Union regulations, as well as those elsewhere, require periodic review of the worldwide literature to ensure that published reports of safety information on a company's products are found and reported to health authorities. This involves a computerized literature search (weekly as required by the European Union in Volume 9A) of large databases that scan hundreds to thousands of medical journals and then report on "hits" (i.e., citations containing the drug in question or any other keywords designated in the search). Once a safety case is found that meets reporting criteria (drug, AE, patient, reporter), the usual reporting requirements (e.g., 15 calendar days for an expedited report) apply. The safety department must ensure that this function, usually done in conjunction with the corporate library or an outside vendor, is performed in a correct and timely manner. This can be a complex task as it is required that both branded and generic cases be included in the literature search and reported in PSURs. Issues of timing, clock start, and translation must be worked through.

Interestingly, the regulations (United States and European Union) do not clearly specify which literature cases should be sought. It is clear that expedited cases (serious ADRs) must be reported. In regard to serious expected and nonserious cases, there is no clear mention in the literature section of Volume 9A or the U.S. regulations, but the PSUR section of Volume 9A (see section 6.2.6.c and 6.3.7.a) refers to the line listings and summary tabulations of serious cases and non-serious unlisted cases, thus implying that the MA holder should collect all serious cases and (at the very least) all nonserious unlisted cases. Companies handle this in various ways. Some only database serious unexpected cases for expediting, choosing not to record other serious and nonserious cases. Other companies database all serious cases and others all serious and nonserious cases. Based upon the Volume 9A requirements, companies would be wise to database all serious cases and at the very least all nonserious unlisted cases. In practicality it may be logistically easier to database all nonserious cases whether listed or not.

■ Data Dictionary Maintenance

In this sense of the word, a "dictionary" is a listing of standardized and fixed terms that companies and regulators agree to use. This is particularly important when data are exchanged electronically. If an unknown term is used in sending a case from one company or health authority to another, the receiving computer system often rejects (or at least notes, or "flags") the case for attention.

MedDRA is the standard dictionary used for the coding of AE terms. Other (now largely outmoded) AE dictionaries include COSTART, WHO-ART, and HARTS. Dictionaries exist for the standardization of drug names (e.g., WHO Drug Dictionary), abbreviations, laboratory measurements and units, and so forth.

A more global dictionary now being used primarily in the United States and the United Kingdom is SNOMED CT (see Web Resource 40-1 and Web Resource 40-2). SNOMED CT stands for Systematized Nomenclature of Medicine–Clinical Terms and is claimed to be the most comprehensive multilingual clinical healthcare terminology in the world. The U.S. Department of Health and Human Services is using SNOMED to build "a national electronic healthcare system that will allow patients and their doctors to access their complete medical records anytime and anywhere they are needed, leading to reduced medical errors, improved patient care, and reduced healthcare costs" (see Chapter 14). It is likely that at some point SNOMED will be used with or instead of MedDRA. It is also likely that a mapping of MedDRA into and out of SNOMED will be done at some point.

■ Coding Unit

Again related to dictionaries, in particular to MedDRA, the use of a standardized coding dictionary also implies the use of this dictionary in a standardized manner. That is, every member of the drug safety staff (and any other unit that does coding, such as clinical research) should be taught to code in the same manner using the same methodology and conventions to achieve internal consistency. This is done through a central coding unit (within or outside of drug safety) that either does the actual coding or verifies the coding done by the drug safety personnel. Not all companies have this function and those that do not will often suffer through coding reconciliation at the end of a study or at the time aggregate reports are prepared.

Planning and Project Management/Operations

Many pharmaceutical companies are now integrating project planning directly into the drug safety unit to oversee and facilitate the multiple and ongoing changes that now seem to be a part of daily life in drug safety. This includes ensuring a smooth integration of ongoing safety work by introducing new procedures, software and hardware, and dictionaries. For example, regulations change frequently around the world and all of them must be adhered to—even though they may sometimes be contradictory. Other usual occurrences include MedDRA upgrades twice a year, safety database upgrades or transfer to a new platform, and new contracts signed with business partners. To coordinate the successful implementation of these ever-changing requirements, a solid operations and project planning/management function must be in place to manage contingencies, timing, personnel, and communications. Many of these functions are being combined with or handled by the life cycle risk management groups so that they address global planning for all aspects of a drug's "needs," including drug safety and PV.

Risk Management

Risk management throughout the entire life cycle of a drug is now obligatory. Companies now form an internal (or use an external) function to handle risk management analysis and planning. At the early stages of a drug's life cycle the risk management functions may be small. However, as the drug enters clinical testing, real-time serious risk management must be done at all stages to ensure that patients are protected, that the drug is developed rationally, and that no major risks that could have been found earlier are discovered at the last minute. Risk management and minimization is now obligatory in the United States, the European Union, and elsewhere (see Chapter 30).

Liaison to External Organizations/Drug Safety Intelligence

Many companies and health authorities regularly attend meetings held by international organizations that examine and develop new guidances and procedures. These include the ICH, CIOMS, Pharmaceutical Research Manufacturers of America (PhRMA), EFPIA, CDISC, HL-7, the International Society of Pharmacoepidemiology, the Drug Information Association, and many others. Pharmaceutical companies send personnel from their drug safety units to these meetings. Attendees are either employees whose sole or primary function is to represent the company at external organizations or ad hoc representatives chosen because of the duties they perform in their companies.

Participation in these meetings is critical for the future of pharmacovigilance because these organizations continue to spearhead the changes and advances in drug safety. ICH has produced many guidances that now form the basis for pharmaceutics in the United States, the European Union, and Japan. CIOMS developed the "CIOMS I form" and "CIOMS II line listings," among others.

This group may also serve as a "safety intelligence unit," gathering information on new laws, regulations, and guidance that touch drug safety. They then disseminate this information to relevant departments in the company. If this function is not done here, it must be done elsewhere in the company to be sure that the company is up to date and in full compliance with all rules and requirements.

How an Individual Case Safety Report (ICSR) Is Handled from Start to Finish

This chapter traces an adverse event (AE) through its course in a company from start to finish. The focus of this chapter is on process. Below a typical case handling process is outlined. They vary from company to company, but all such processes must have written procedures for data receipt, case assessment for expedited reporting, data entry, coding and data review by medical professionals (initially often by a nurse or pharmacist), and a final data review by a physician. The processes illustrated here are not necessarily better than other processes used in the industry. Nor is there a mandated process from the U.S. Food and Drug Administration (FDA), European Medicines Agency (EMA), Medicines and Healthcare Products Regulatory Agency (MHRA), or any other health authority. Rather, whichever process is implemented, it should ensure a smooth workflow and full compliance with all laws, regulations, and directives.

The mission of the AE processing unit is to ensure that all complaint cases (defined as AEs, product quality problems, tampering, packaging problems, counterfeits, etc.) are processed in a timely and accurate manner such that all cases are of high quality and sent to the appropriate departments within the company, to other companies, and to health authorities on time. The goals are to ensure prompt handling and submission of expedited reports, periodic premarketing (e.g., annual safety reports) and postmarketing (e.g., Periodic Safety Update Reports, or PSURs) reports and any other obligatory reports. Because late reports to health agencies and business partners are usually easily and immediately noted, this statistic tends to be the one that drug safety groups, management, and health authorities look at to "grade" companies. The goal is 100% compliance all the time, but reality tends to suggest that, in an imperfect world, 100% is not always attained. However, nobody will officially write or say this or give an acceptable error rate. More importantly, cases that are late should not be late by very long or for the same reason twice. A root cause analysis to find errors, failures to follow the standard operating procedures, and so on should be performed and corrective actions put in place.

Many companies put maximal effort into keeping the expedited report score around 100%, often at the expense of case quality or delays in the processing of nonexpedited cases—even though no one ever admits to decreases in quality. Companies often build up backlogs of unprocessed or partially processed cases when resources are insufficient to be fully compliant with both expedited and nonexpedited cases. Sooner or later, this situation produces a disastrous result unless corrective actions are applied and processes are put in place that are workable and actually followed. Everything has to be done correctly.

There are many ways to handle cases. In some companies, there is ownership by an individual drug safety specialist (e.g., a nurse or pharmacist), who is responsible for the completion of the case from start to finish, making sure that any other personnel involved in the case (e.g., medical reviewers) handle the case and return it to the specialist who "owns" it. Other companies have less individual ownership of a case and instead move a case from task to task in the workflow, with a separate "pool" of workers responsible for a particular step, such as one group that just performs data entry, another that just does coding, and another that just writes narratives.

■ AE Sources and Arrival in the Safety Department

Serious adverse events (SAEs) and non-SAEs may arrive in a company from multiple sources (feeder groups). Standard operating procedures must be in place to ensure that these AEs arrive in a timely manner (usually 1–2 days) in the drug safety department if they first arrive elsewhere in the company or at a partner company.

Spontaneous SAEs and nonserious cases arrive by telephone (the most common route of arrival in many companies); websites; electronically; e-mail; snail mail; fax; reports to sales representatives; reports to other company employees, agents, or contractors; the legal department; health authorities (e.g., FDA, MHRA, Health Canada); other companies who receive AEs on their own drugs in which one of their drugs is involved; and other miscellaneous sources such as newspaper, social media, or TV stories. They are received primarily from consumers, healthcare professionals, and lawyers. It should be kept in mind that such AEs may arrive at any location in the company such as the manufacturing facilities (especially if the product package says something to the effect of, "Manufactured by XXX Pharma in YYY City, Ohio," or if an address or phone number is on the package or patient information), subsidiaries and affiliates, contrac-

tors, outsourcers, and business partners with whom safety exchange agreements are in place.

Safety department call centers are usually staffed to receive phone calls from a particular region. Usually, they cover a whole country but not more than one country, because labeling, indications, precautions, and warnings may differ from country to country and the appropriate information must be given to residents of the appropriate country. There may also be language issues. For example, any phone center covering Canada must be able to respond in English or French. In the United States, though not required by law, many phone centers have Spanish-speaking personnel available in addition to English speakers. Phone centers may be available Monday through Friday during business hours or sometimes 24 hours a day, 7 days a week. Multiple time zones must also be taken into account for geographically large countries (e.g. Canada, United States). Call centers may be kept in-house or outsourced to companies that specialize in handling medical phone calls. These call centers may be within the country or far away (e.g., India, Philippines, and other English-speaking countries are now handling calls from the United States and Canada in many cases). Interestingly, some call centers covering English language callers are now being placed in non-native English speaking countries.

Call centers should be set up to receive calls from consumers, patients, physicians, and other healthcare providers. They usually cover questions about the products; requests for reimbursement; and reporting of AEs, product quality defects, and problems and emergencies regarding the drug, including tampering, counterfeiting, and overdoses. For clinical trial (nonmarketed) products, the call center may need to have an emergency code break to handle an acute AE. The call center must be set up to ensure that all AEs and quality complaints are captured and sent to the appropriate departments for handling (e.g., the AEs to drug safety and the quality complaints to manufacturing). In addition, any questions or requests for reimbursement must be handled rapidly and correctly. Callers who are complaining or agitated must also be handled carefully and diplomatically. Thus, a clear protocol must be set up to ensure that customers are served quickly and well, that their requests are met, and that all AEs and complaints are captured. The call should be picked up on the first or second ring, the caller should not be kept on hold for any significant length of time, and the caller should not have to give his or her name, address, and product issue more than once. The caller should not be bounced to multiple departments. Professional call centers are able to track very precise metrics measuring all of these factors.

All this requires a well-thought-out system to handle all issues (especially when a caller has multiple issues: "I took your pill, which was supposed to be red but was blue; it smelled bad; I developed a headache; I want my money back; and I have a question."). The decision about when to have medically trained personnel take the call must be clarified: should all calls come directly to a nurse or pharmacist or should there be some level of nonmedical screening before sending the call to the healthcare professional? If nonmedical professionals are used, an algorithm or script is often used to ensure that no incorrect information is given to the caller. In addition, the priorities must be considered: should the AE and quality complaint be handled first (most drug safety people would say yes to this but marketers might not)? Because there are multiple company stakeholders involved (drug safety, information technology, product quality, marketing, reimbursement, medical information, etc.), the development of the call center is complex and expensive.

Other sources of AEs (and follow-up) include the following:

- Clinical studies: Clinical study events may come in from the company's clinical research and clinical pharmacology departments as well as any other group that might (often unbeknown to the drug safety department) run studies. Such groups might be in marketing, subsidiaries, affiliates, market research, pharmacoepidemiology, pharmacoeconomics, or other companies that are studying the drug with your company or are studying the drug without your company's consent and knowledge. AEs may also arrive from contract research organizations. Often, much to the chagrin of the safety group, the first awareness that a study is being run in some far-off outpost of the company is the arrival of an SAE. In the most egregious of such cases, an event may arrive for a drug that the safety department does not even know to be owned, studied, or sold by the company. It might, for example, be studied (or marketed) only in one subsidiary, affiliate, or partner far away.

- Legal: Lawsuits are sometimes the unfortunate first notification to a company that there is an SAE. These cases usually come in through the legal department, which should be sensitized to the fact that they must not only defend a lawsuit but also report the AEs to the drug safety department. These AEs are usually on marketed products but may sometimes involve clinical trial patients. Rarely, a company may be notified of an issue by the arrival of a subpoena to provide evidence in a lawsuit to which the company is not a party, such as a malpractice case in which there is also a drug issue. Normally, the receipt of AEs via lawsuits is limited, but in certain circumstances, such cases may be voluminous, especially in class action lawsuits in the United States.

- Health agencies: Many health authorities send to or allow companies (and sometimes the public) access to specific AE cases. The FDA has a program (MedWatch to Manufacturer) in which it sends copies of spontaneously received MedWatch reports of SAEs on newly approved products (new molecular entities or "important new biologics") to the manufacturer of the product. The drug must be a new chemical entity. This program lasts 3 to 4 years and is done at the request of the manufacturer (see Web Resource 41-1). These reports do not have to be resubmitted to the FDA by the company unless additional information is obtained but may have to be submitted to health authorities outside the United States if the drug is marketed elsewhere. Health Canada allows everyone to search their database, and the MHRA publishes "Drug Analysis Prints" with SAEs by drug (see Chapters 8 and 24). In addition, various agencies, including the MHRA and AFSSAPS, have mechanisms whereby the Marketing Authorization holder (MAH) may obtain certain SAEs on their own products.

- Literature reports: U.S. and European Union regulations require that companies periodically (weekly, per Volume 9A) search the medical literature for SAEs. Such publications are usually on marketed products but may occasionally include SAEs from clinical trials of new uses for old drugs unknown to the company. Once a drug is on the market, anyone may do a clinical trial using the drug (following, of course, regulations, consent, ethics committee approval) without telling the company. Reports in the literature may be of SAEs or nonserious AEs, though the former predominate. In oncology, cooperative groups may use marketed drugs in clinical trials for new indications or at different doses or schedules from the approved labeling.

- Stimulated reports: Many companies have patient support programs in which company or outside service companies' representatives (e.g., nurses, physicians) contact patients to encourage them to continue to take their medications and give support in regard to dosing, AEs, and so forth. During the course of discussions, AE reports may be obtained. If the company is involved in these support programs (internally or outsourced), a mechanism must be created to ensure that all AEs reach the company in a timely manner and are handled appropriately. Other programs such as speaker programs, named-patient programs, and compassionate use may also stimulate reports.

- Other sources of AEs include poison control centers and company and external internet sites (blogs, social media, etc.). In general, the company is not required to troll the internet looking for such AEs, though it must track and capture AEs from its own websites. If a drug is reported to another company either by mistake or expressly (e.g., a marketing competitor, another company doing a trial with your drug or in which your drug is a suspect medication in an ICSR), SAE reports may arrive unannounced from other companies on your drug. These cases may be problematic as they may arrive as completed, anonymized MedWatch forms from the other company. Because of the anonymization, follow-up will be impossible.

Electronic receipt of ICSRs by E2B (or customized) formats is common and the company should have systems in place allowing receipt (and transmission) of such cases. Note that follow-up information may arrive by a different means from the original report (e.g., an initial phone report may be followed by a written e-mail/PDF or snail mail communication).

■ Triage

Upon arrival, by whatever route, of the case data in the drug safety department, it must be properly classified for processing. If the report does not arrive electronically, it must be date-stamped upon entry into the drug safety department. For paper cases, this is a manual rubber stamp with the date and time of arrival. For electronic reports, presumably whatever system is used automatically date stamps the information. Note that this then forces day 0 to be the electronic time stamp. In "the old days," if a case is delivered on Saturday but not opened in the mailroom until Monday, the date stamp and day 0 are Monday. In the "modern electronic world" if the case arrives by fax or other electronic means and is date-stamped electronically as Saturday, that is day 0. Follow-up information must also be handled expeditiously.

The initial triage should be to determine whether the report needs urgent processing to be transmitted to the health authorities, others in the company (e.g., manufac-

turing for quality issues), or business partners as an expedited report. The triage should be done by someone with a medical skill set to make an accurate determination. Many companies have nurses and pharmacists in this critical role. Triage or case assessment should be standardized and trainable. Some companies use dedicated personnel for this function and others rotate staff in to do the triage. For difficult or controversial cases, the triage personnel may request assistance from the drug safety physicians.

Triage should cover, at the least, the following:

- Which drug(s) involved?
- Case type: spontaneous, clinical trial, stimulated, other
- Are the four elements of a valid case (reporter, patient, AE, drug) present and identifiable?
- Serious or nonserious
- Causality (for serious clinical trial cases, not for spontaneous cases)
- Expectedness (labeledness) for serious and nonserious cases
- Determination of which reports are expedited reports, using this algorithm:
  - 7-day clinical trial report: serious and death/life-threatening, unlabeled, and associated (possibly caused by) with the drug in question
  - 15-day clinical trial and solicited report: serious, unlabeled, and associated with (possibly caused by) the drug in question
  - 15-day postmarketing report: serious and unlabeled (no causality determination required)
  - Other reports requiring urgent processing, such as those cases requested by the health agency ("heightened surveillance") to be transmitted to them in an expedited fashion, but that do not meet the formal criteria above or where contracts with a business partner require rapid transmittal
- Pregnancy cases (some companies examine for pregnancy cases at triage and others do it later on in the case processing)
  - With an accompanying AE/SAE
  - No accompanying AE/SAE
- Product quality complaints (if handled in drug safety)—urgent or non-urgent

These criteria may be built into an electronic algorithm in the workflow in the safety database or may be handled with a paper log and tracking form for each case. Some databases have "portals," or desktop displays, of all new and ongoing cases, which can be customized for each employee so that a person knows which cases he or she owns as well as their workflow status. Manager-level screens may show all the cases in the staff reporting to that manager. Some companies also log all cases into a spreadsheet to track them and ensure that they are not lost in transit within the safety department or at the time of "hand-offs" at each step of the case. In particular, "incomplete cases," or those that do not yet have the four required elements of a case but may later on, should be tracked to ensure they are not forgotten or do not "slip through the cracks." A case number should be assigned at this point. This may be a screening case number or the definitive case number assigned by the safety database. Note that if an "informal" spreadsheet is used to track cases or potential cases, it is subject to audit or inspection and should be secured so that it cannot be altered or changed inappropriately. In general, using such informal spreadsheets or non-secure databases is not a good idea.

After triage, each case should be assigned to the appropriate work channel. Each company develops various channels. They should roughly run along these lines:

- Rapid processing of the death/life-threatening clinical trial cases for submission to the health authorities within 7 calendar days from first receipt by anyone in the company, business partners, CROs, and so forth. This usually means completing the case within approximately 5 calendar days. Attempts should be made immediately to get needed follow-up information, which would be included in a follow-up report to the agencies.

- Processing of 15-day expedited reports for clinical trial or marketed products. These are serious cases for which processing must be completed by calendar day 15 but preferably sooner to allow quality review, transmission to business partners, and transmission to the agencies. Many companies develop workflow such that all cases are completed by, say, calendar day 10 after initial receipt. Completion dates tend to range from 8 to 12 calendar days in companies, though most companies pick one time frame for all cases and stick to it. This makes for simpler processing and tracking within the drug safety group. CROs and companies that work with multiple partners may (unfortunately) have to tailor their processing procedures for each partner.

- Processing of other serious cases that are not expedited reports. These cases do not have to be sent to the health agencies within 15 calendar days. Rather they are sent in periodic reports at intervals that vary from 3 months to several years, depending on the status of the drug and the regulations in that country. Thus, there is usually the potential for a longer time frame for processing the case if needed. Some companies will use the same processing system for all serious cases, whether expedited or not.

- Serious cases that are to be sent to subsidiaries, business partners, and others may also require rapid processing if contractual arrangements require this. Many companies exchange all serious cases within 10 calendar days whether expedited or not.

- Sometimes a case is not an expedited report in one country but is an expedited case in other countries (e.g., the local labeling or reporting regulations are different there). This case must be transmitted to the subsidiary or business in time to meet 15-day reporting rules there. It is often the situation, especially in large multinational companies, that the sending company (e.g., drug safety in the home office) is not able to know whether any particular serious case is an expedited report or not in all countries where the drug is sold. Thus, many companies process these cases as if they were expedited reports and use a completion date of about 10 calendar days (as noted above).

- Nonserious cases may be processed more slowly (e.g., 30 days) because they are not reportable at all or are reportable only in aggregate reports. Nevertheless, it is wise to screen nonserious cases rapidly upon receipt, especially if they come from "less than reliable sources," to ensure that no serious cases are misclassified (presumably not intentionally) as nonserious cases. This could lead to late expedited reports.

- Similarly, the "other" cases, such as literature, legal, and cases received from health authorities, should be processed as appropriate for the company's needs. It is a general rule of thumb that the process should be kept as simple as possible and that "exceptions to the rule" be kept limited. As few as three fundamental procedures could serve: 7-day cases, all serious cases (handled as if they are all expedited cases), and all nonserious cases.

■ Database Entry

At this point, the case should be entered into the computerized safety database. If the case is received electronically, it should be reviewed in a "holding area" before it is officially uploaded into the safety database unless it comes from a trusted source where such review is deemed unnecessary. For example, clinical trial cases uploaded from a dedicated electronic data collection system for a company's studies may be uploaded directly if the case is entered in sufficient detail and with quality checks at the investigational site.

If the case arrives manually using a standardized paper data collection form, then manual data entry should be fairly easy to do. If not, the data may arrive in any sort of form: case report forms, handwritten notes, CIOMS I or MedWatch forms, hospital records, physicians' notes, telephone reports, and so forth. Sometimes data entry is easy; sometimes it is not. Some companies have an initial review by a medical professional who highlights items for data entry; other companies have the source documents sent directly to the data entry group (nonmedical professionals) and have medical review only after that is completed.

If a case number (also called a "control number" or "medical reference number") has not been assigned to the case at the triage or logging level, it is assigned now. MedDRA coding of AEs, medical history, and other required MedDRA fields is done either by the drug safety group or by a dedicated coding group. Drug coding using a standardized dictionary is also done. The case narrative is usually written at this point. The narrative may be difficult and complex if the case is long and complicated. There are standard ways that narratives should be written in terms of format, content, follow-up information, etc. The narrative is the key summary of the case and should usually be a good "stand-alone" summary of the case. Much care should be taken in its preparation.

■ Quality Review

At this point, a drug safety specialist (usually a nurse or pharmacist) reviews the data entry against the source documents and prepares or reviews the case narrative. Any changes or additions to the case are made at this time. A clear methodology on the quality check should be developed so that it is done in a standardized and repeatable way. Those fields, if any, that are not reviewed (e.g., height) should be defined in the methodology up front in addition to those fields that are. The quality review should look at content, grammar, and format. In general, one does not need to be a perfectionist regarding grammar; however, sentences that are unclear or do not convey the desired meaning should be corrected. Short simple sentences should be used because many of the readers may not be native English-language speakers.

■ Follow-Up

Follow-up information should be requested when the initial case is incomplete or unclear. Rarely does a case have complete information, especially if the AE just happened or is ongoing. Thus, it is usually required that follow-up queries be sent to the reporter to complete the case data. The need for follow-up is also mentioned in 21CFR312.32(d) for IND reports and 314.80(c)(1)(ii) for NDA reports. Volume 9A also notes that follow-up is necessary: "The Marketing Authorisation Holder is expected to follow-up all reports of serious adverse reactions to their medicinal product(s) to obtain comprehensive information where available. Additional information not available at the time of the initial report should be provided in the form of follow-up reports" (Section 4.4). Follow-up data should be entered into the database using a procedure similar to the one used for initial data. Care must be taken to ensure that the data are not mistaken for a new case but rather are clearly identified as follow-up to a case already received.

■ Medical Review

At this point in the case, after it has been completed and reviewed by the drug safety specialist and after it has undergone a quality review, some or all cases should be reviewed by the drug safety physician. Historically, physician review was limited to serious cases, but many companies are now having all cases undergo physician review to ensure that no serious cases are misclassified as nonserious. The medical review should generally cover the medical content of the case, with particular attention paid to the narrative, the suspect and concomitant drugs (including dosages), the past medical history, and coding. It is generally not the role of the physician to do a source document quality review unless he or she needs to refer to the source documents for clarification of a medical point. This varies from company to company, however. In certain critical cases, it is often desirable that the physician review all source documents even if this is not routine policy.

■ Case Closure

In one sense, a case is never really closed, as new information could arrive weeks, months, or even years later, requiring the case to be updated. But for practical purposes, once the above steps are concluded and follow-up requested, a case may be considered closed or completed for operational purposes. If and when follow-up arrives, the case can be reopened and processed. The distinction between closure (or locking) of a version and closure or completion of a case should be noted. A company may, for practical operational reasons, "lock" each case a certain number of days after the receipt of the information so that the case can be processed properly without new data arriving and being entered into the case just when it is in medical review or ready to be transmitted to the health authorities. For example, if data are received on day 0, the case is processed and locked on, say, calendar day 7 and sent to the health authorities on calendar day 14. Any additional follow-up data on this case that arrive after day 7 is put into a follow-up version of the case. This prevents the staff from scrambling to get last-minute data into the case with the appropriate medical review, quality control, and so forth. In such a situation, two versions of a case may be open at the same time. Most computer systems are able to handle these versioning issues. In occasional situations, additional data may indeed be added to the case at the last minute if deemed critical (e.g., death outcome has just arrived).

■ Case Distribution and Transmission

Cases are next distributed to those in the company who need to see them (e.g., clinical research, legal) and to other companies with whom safety exchange agreements are in place. Cases are also submitted directly to the health agencies via E2B or other direct means (e.g., certified mail, courier) or distributed to others in the company, such as the regulatory department, for submission to the health authorities. Cases may also be sent to subsidiaries or affiliates worldwide for their submission to local agencies—often with a cover letter in the local language and, in some instances, with a translation of the case itself into the local language if English is not accepted. If cases are submitted in the European Union, whether clinical trial or postmarketing, they must also be submitted to EudraVigilance.

■ Tracking

It is critical to have markers in the database to track cases through the processing system. Each drug safety specialist and manager should be aware of all pending cases, their status in the trip toward completion/closure, and, in particular, the deadlines for each case. It is critical

that all 7- and 15-day reports be tracked so that none is submitted late to the health authorities, subsidiaries, or business partners. The manager can reallocate cases or other work to ensure that the time-critical cases are handled appropriately in case of absence, vacation, staff overload, or maldistribution of caseloads.

Similarly, nonexpedited cases that need to be completed for aggregate reports should be tracked so that they are completed by the time of data lock. This can be as frequent as every 3 months for NDA periodic reports or every 6 months for PSURs. The dates of the periodic reports are known in advance, so there is no excuse for a case's missing the report.

In general, tracking should be done electronically and generated automatically from the drug safety database unless there are so few cases that manual tracking is practical. Most modern drug safety databases have a tracking function with customizable reports. Manual tracking on spreadsheets is time consuming and usually unsatisfactory once AE volume grows and the staff becomes large.

The question often arises in a small company about whether it should have a safety department or a database. In regard to a safety department, if a drug is in clinical trials or marketed, the answer is yes. That department may be one person supervising the outsourced CRO or partner handling the safety. Such a situation may be satisfactory for small companies with few AE cases. Once the volume and complexity grow (e.g., marketing in multiple countries), the need for an in-house safety function and database becomes more compelling. Although it is explicitly stated by some regulatory authorities that an electronic safety database is not necessarily obligatory, all the appropriate (templated) reporting (e.g., PSURs) must still be done and, without a database, this may not be feasible or practical. The question then becomes whether it is practical for both business and safety reasons to rely on a CRO or partner for all safety functions with the subsequent benefits and costs (both monetary and not) of such an arrangement. For some companies, this may be worthwhile, but not so for others.

In addition to tracking the AEs that arrive and are processed, track the following key performance indicators:

- Total number of AEs
- SAEs
- Non-SAEs
- Clinical trial AEs/SAEs
- Spontaneous AEs/SAEs
  - Expedited reports from clinical trials (e.g., to the IND) and postmarketing (NDA, MA):

- Those submitted on time
- Those submitted late, by how much, why, and corrective actions taken
- Cases submitted to business partners and others
- Time to process cases, depending on case type (expedited, serious nonexpedited, nonserious, etc.)
- Time to submission to each health agency (FDA, EMA, etc.)
- Tracking by drug or class of products or drug safety teams, depending on how the drug safety group and the company are organized
- Annual reports, postmarketing reports (PSURs, NDA Periodic Reports)

It is useful periodically to graph and publish these metrics ("key performance indicators," or "KPIs") for the entire drug safety staff. Such data can also be used for resource allocation, budgeting, projection of future work (e.g., AEs for allergy drugs peak twice a year and more staff may be needed then), and justification for more resources. The metrics may aid in identifying problems, or "rough spots," and help to institute changes to prevent recurrence of such problems. Publicly posted data should not identify individuals or point out "nonproducers" to shame them into speeding up. Praise should always be done publicly, but chastisement should be done privately.

The timing, sequence, and duration of each step in processing an AE should be clearly spelled out in a measurable and auditable SOP or working document. If the company determines that, say, all SAEs will be completed within 10 calendar days and all nonserious cases within 30 calendar days, this timing should be built into each case. This should be done automatically in the database workflow system with a tickler, e-mail, or similar reminders to the concerned individual, telling him or her of the timing and due date for each case. The due dates would be updated as needed (e.g., it is determined to be or not to be a 15-day expedited report, or a case is upgraded from nonserious to serious). Attention must be paid to weekends and holidays in calculating due dates.

Each person in the workflow must know when his or her task is due, and the manager must be able to track the case through each step to ensure its completion. Other companies have "pools" of people handling each step rather than having one drug safety specialist "own" the case. In the pool situation, the first available "pool" member handling that step processes the case.

■ Investigator Notification

The concept of investigator notification of expedited clinical trial reports used to be simple but has now become somewhat more complicated.

The ICH proposals in E6 are somewhat ambiguous:

- The sponsor should promptly notify all concerned investigator(s)/institution(s) and the regulatory authority(ies) of findings that could affect adversely the safety of subjects, impact the conduct of the trial, or alter the IRB/IEC's approval/favorable opinion to continue the trial (5.16.2).
- The sponsor should expedite the reporting to all concerned investigator(s)/institutions(s), to the IRB(s)/IEC(s), where required, and to the regulatory authority(ies) of all adverse drug reactions (ADRs) that are both serious and unexpected (5.17.1).

The EU is more explicit:

- The sponsor shall inform all investigators concerned of findings that could adversely affect the safety of study subjects.
  - The information can be aggregated in a line listing of SUSARs accompanied by a summary of the evolving safety profile of the product.
  - In the case of blinded trials, the line listing should present data on all SUSARs, regardless of the medication administered (e.g., active/placebo), maintaining the blind.
- If a significant safety issue is identified, either on receipt of an ICSR or on review of aggregate data, the sponsor should immediately notify all investigators.
- A safety issue that affects the course of the clinical study or development project, including suspension of the study program or safety-related amendments to study protocols, should also be reported to the investigators (Volume 10).

Note: No time frame specified. Many companies use the 15-day requirement used in the United States.

The U.S. regulations are also somewhat ambiguous, particularly in terms of format:

- All IND Safety Reports (expedited reports) must go to the FDA and "all participating investigators" in a written form (21CFR312.32(c))... in 15 calendar days.

- 21CFR32(B)(ii) requires that "the sponsor shall identify all safety reports, previously filed with the IND concerning a similar adverse experience, and shall analyze the significance of the adverse experience in light of the previous, similar reports."

As of March 2011 FDA updated its clinical trial safety regulations. In regard to investigator notification, FDA indicated that

- All participating investigators in open INDs (including investigator initiated trials) should be notified in an IND safety report of potential serious risks.
- Follow-up reports should be sent to investigators to inform and update them about an important suspected adverse reaction if it significantly affects the care of the subjects or conduct of the study.
- Minor refinements that do not significantly affect care of subjects or conduct of the study need to be sent to FDA but need not be sent to investigators.
- Such information may be communicated to investigators in a routine update of the investigator brochure.

These requirements have been interpreted in various ways. "Participating Investigators" is ambiguous. Many companies take a conservative view and report all expedited reports to all investigators in all phase I, II, and III trials, as well as to investigators in investigator-initiated trials using this study drug whether for this indication or not. Some sponsors will also send spontaneous reports for this drug to investigators if it is also on the market. The drug safety group prepares the analysis of similar cases from the safety database and sometimes from the clinical trial database if cases are present there that are not in the drug safety database.

■ 15 Calendar Days and Day 0 Versus Day 1

The FDA in its draft guidance "Post-Marketing Safety Reporting for Human Drug and Biological Products Including Vaccines" of March 2001 (Web Resource 41-2), refers to the completion of box G4 on the MedWatch 3500A form as the date the company has knowledge of the four criteria for a valid AE (reporter, patient, event, drug) and that this is day 0 of the 15-day time clock. This then gives 16 calendar days for a case. The document also notes clearly that the case must be submitted by day 15, which means it will be received at the FDA in a few days if sent by mail or the next day if sent by overnight courier. If the 15th calendar day is a weekend or a U.S. federal holiday, the report may be submitted on the first working day after the weekend or holiday. However, if a company has submission obligations in countries outside the United States, the federal holiday (and possibly even the weekends) should not be allowed to permit a delay in submission.

The EU is more explicit and states in Volume 9A (Section 4.2 Reporting Time Frames): "The date the Marketing Authorisation Holder becomes aware of a case which fulfils the minimum information should be considered day 0. The same applies if new information on the case is received by the MAH i.e. the reporting time clock begins again for the submission of the follow-up report from the day the MAH receives relevant follow-up information....The clock for expedited reporting starts (day 0) as soon as the minimum information has been brought to the attention of any personnel of the Marketing Authorisation Holder or an organisation holding a contractual agreement with the MAH including medical representatives."

The Safety Department's Role in Clinical Research, Marketing and Sales, Labeling, Regulatory, Due Diligence, and Legal Issues

■ Clinical Research

The clinical research (or medical research) department is the section of a company (or CRO) that does clinical trials and studies. There are many ways to structure such departments. Some companies have their research department do only phase II and III (developmental) trials, with a separate group handling phase I (clinical pharmacology and early safety studies mainly) and another group handling phase IV (postmarketing) studies and commitments. Alternatively, there may be separate groups handling different types of products: biologics, drugs, devices, or over-the-counter products. Other structures are by country or geographic region: U.S. studies, European Union studies, and "rest of the world" studies. Multiple hybrids of these models exist with and without outsourcing of some of the functions.

Whatever the structure of the clinical research division may be, the drug safety department must play a continuous role in these groups' day-to-day activities because clinical studies almost always produce adverse events (AEs). The drug safety group must ensure that it receives all appropriate AEs from all trials. "Appropriate" usually means all serious AEs (SAEs), some or all

non-SAEs, and all pregnancy cases (not AEs, of course, but in practice handled like AEs from a logistic point of view; see Chapter 15). In most countries of the world, there is a requirement to report certain clinical trial SAEs to the health authorities in either 7 or 15 days (expedited reports) or periodically (e.g., yearly). Unless the clinical research divisions are able to receive and process such AEs themselves, these cases must be sent to the drug safety department.

The clinical research and drug safety groups must establish a process to ensure that all SAEs are reported to the company within 24 to 48 hours after occurrence at a clinical site. This allows the company to process them and report the cases to the appropriate health authorities, particularly for the 7- or 15-calendar-day SAEs.

The investigators must be trained and sensitized (on a continual basis) to report SAEs. Usually, this means reporting all SAEs on an expedited basis, and reporting the nonserious AEs weekly, monthly, or only at the end of the study. Note that the obligation of the investigator to report SAEs to the sponsor is clearly stated in the FDA regulations: "An investigator must immediately report to the sponsor any SAE, whether or not considered drug related, including those listed in the protocol or investigator brochure and must include an assessment of whether there is a reasonable possibility that the drug caused the event" (21CFR312.64(b)). Similar obligations apply in other countries.

The process involves the capture of the AE on the case report form or in the electronic data capture (EDC) system, with transmission of the information to the company or CRO. Transmission to the company or CRO is done either electronically in the EDC system or by the older means of written case report forms or dedicated SAE collection forms that are faxed or e-mailed. This information must contain all the data necessary for the SAE case to be entered into the safety database and for preparation of an E2B transmission or a MedWatch or CIOMS I form for submission to the concerned health authorities, the clinical investigators, and IRBs/Ethics Committees when required. This process often involves queries to the investigator (done either by drug safety directly or via the clinical research department, or CRO). Care must be taken to avoid having multiple company departments sending repetitive questions to the investigator; usually a single point of contact is best from the company. This process can become exceedingly complex if SAE volume is very high, if multiple worldwide sites are involved, if a clinical research organization or other intermediaries are involved, if a cooperative group is involved (e.g., in oncology studies), or if a governmental agency (e.g., National Institutes of Health) is involved.

Some studies generate very large numbers of SAEs, such as oncology studies in very ill patients receiving toxic study drugs. If studies run long enough, just about every patient (whether on study drug, comparator, or placebo) will have an AE (though not necessarily an ADR) at some point during the trial. Normally, all SAEs are transmitted to the company within 1 or 2 days. However, for some studies, various protocol customizations may be done to ensure that the critical and important SAEs (those that are unexpected or related to the study drug) reach the company within 1–2 days and the health agencies within 7–15 days, though all SAEs should be sent to the sponsor immediately. Nonserious AEs may be reported to the company in a less urgent fashion (e.g., monthly or even at the end of the study) and to the agencies in the annual or special periodic reports.

In some cases, arrangements may be made with the health agencies overseeing a study to report certain expected SAEs periodically rather than as expedited reports. Most health agencies (including the FDA and European Union agencies) are willing to negotiate such arrangements. For large multinational trials, this may require negotiations with multiple national health authorities to reach a workable consensus that meets all needs. For example, a protocol might state that, because drug X in previous trials has been shown to produce mild gastrointestinal, urinary, and pulmonary hemorrhage in this patient group, these cases will not be reported until the end of the trial unless the patient dies or the patient requires a transfusion (for example). Hemorrhage from other body sites would be SAEs and reported to the company in 1–2 days.

Many companies, especially the larger ones, maintain two "safety databases." One very common model has a safety database maintained by the drug safety department and a clinical trial database maintained by the clinical research/statistics groups. The drug safety database holds two sets of data: (1) the SAEs from clinical trials and (2) all spontaneous serious and nonserious reports; that is, nonserious clinical trial AEs are not kept in this safety database. This database is used for the regulatory reporting of spontaneous and clinical trial SAE expedited reports, Periodic Safety Update Reports (PSURs), and annual clinical trial safety reports (e.g., IND annual reports). The clinical research department maintains the other database that holds all safety and efficacy data from clinical trials (but no spontaneous reports) and is used in preparing the final clinical study report for each study as well as safety sections for Marketing Authorization dossiers and integrated safety summaries for New Drug Application (NDA) submissions.

The data in the two databases for any given clinical trial patient may (unfortunately) be different. One reason is due to different mechanisms of data collection. In paper-based (non-EDC) trials, the drug safety database usually receives data from the investigator using a dedicated SAE reporting form rather than multiple pages from the case report form. The clinical trial database receives the data on the pages in the CRF that are used for SAE/AE data collection. The data may differ if the SAE collection form is not filled in at the same time or by the same person as the CRF. Thus, the same SAE information is collected in two different places for each patient and may not be reconciled at the investigator site. Also, follow-up information may be entered into the CRF and not sent on the separate SAE collection form or vice versa. In addition, the drug safety group receives a clinical trial SAE within 24–48 hours after the investigator first notes it. The clinical trial database may not receive the CRF data for several weeks if the CRFs are "harvested" only every 6 weeks or so by the medical monitor. The use of EDC usually alleviates this problem if all the safety data are collected in the EDC and transmitted to the drug safety group. If the EDC system only collects safety data and notifies the company by an e-mail alert that a new SAE has been collected, the investigator may still end up sending a separate SAE sheet to the company, which could differ from the EDC data. So unless the safety data are collected and transmitted in only one place and manner, there is the risk of differing and incorrect or out-of-date information being present in the two company safety databases.

Other differences between the databases may occur if different people (one person in the drug safety department and one in the clinical research department) code each case differently. Follow-up information or corrected data may reach one database and not the other. More subtle differences may arise in the data that are collected. For example, for the clinical research department, the drug compliance (what percentage of the study drug was actually taken by the patient and which doses were missed) is critical. To the safety department, it is less important that the patient took 75% of the study drug versus 85% or 95%. To drug safety, it is a much more binary (yes/no) question of whether or not the drug was ingested at all (though, of course, dose-related effects may occur). Drug safety usually spends less time clarifying the dosing schedule followed by the patients than the clinical research department does.

It is thus necessary to reconcile the cases within the two databases to ensure that the data, or at least the key data, are identical. This can be done at the end of the trial or during the trial as each patient or groups of patients complete the study. This can be a very time-consuming procedure requiring detailed case review by the drug safety and clinical research groups. Differences must be ironed out, and sometimes new queries to the investigative sites are generated from the reconciliation. Another vexing problem that occurs occasionally for 15-day alert cases concerns important follow-up information that arrives in clinical research and is not sent to the drug safety group for submission to the health authorities as a follow-up alert report. This produces a late alert report because the data were in-house for weeks or months before the 15-day alert was sent to the health agencies.

The drug safety group may be involved in the creation by clinical research of the final study report for each individual study as well as the final integrated safety summary for the submission dossier (e.g., MA or NDA). This includes data reconciliation as well as supplying the "narrative" (or "capsule summary") or other data sets prepared for each case to clinical research to aid them in preparing their final study reports. If there are postmar-

keting data held by drug safety, these will usually need to be supplied to the dossier as well.

The clinical research and drug safety groups usually collaborate when a signal is being worked up or an ad hoc health authority question is received. For example, if a health agency asks about a particular AE or groups of AEs (e.g., acute pancreatitis or all pancreatic AEs), it is usually necessary to pull the non-SAEs from the clinical research database and the SAEs from the drug safety database to capture all the AEs in question. Because of the way data are entered into the clinical research database (either at the end of the study or when batches of data arrive at the data entry site), the drug safety database is usually more up to date for SAEs at any one time because drug safety usually enters data immediately upon receipt, and clinical research may enter data periodically, when a group of CRFs arrives, or even at the end of the study. If EDC is used and the data are efficiently collected and distributed to both databases, this problem may be largely alleviated.

The use of electronic data capture, where each investigator enters data into a database in real time, making them available immediately to clinical research, statistics, drug safety, and others involved in the study, has changed to some degree the way data are handled and analyzed by companies and health authorities. The concept of a single (or distributed) central database (or data warehouse) holding all information that can be viewed by any party that needs to see it can now be created fairly easily. Thus, an investigator could enter a patient's study data into the study database by simply logging on to a personalized, secure URL. The efficacy and safety data would go ("be pushed") to a central server (perhaps somewhere in the "cloud") and would be immediately accessible to the clinical research department, the drug safety group, operations, senior management, CROs, partners, accounting (to pay investigators after a certain number of patients are enrolled), and any other groups or individuals who need access. Various limits on the amount of data that is viewable can be used, allowing access only to the data needed. Alternatively, all the data can go into one central site, and each department can "pull" the data it needs when it needs them. From the drug safety point of view, anything that prevents data entry into two databases at different times, by different people using different forms or data entry screens, is a significant virtue. Setting up such systems requires much thought and work up-front before the study starts. It is hoped that drug safety is involved in creating the system, processes, and data rules from the beginning.

The clinical research department and the safety department also interact at development, project planning, and risk management meetings as well as on signaling, training sessions, preparation of annual reports, investigator brochure updates, and so on. The drug safety group is also frequently charged with sending blinded or unblinded safety information to drug safety monitoring committees or data monitoring boards. These are outside groups that evaluate the safety profile and status of a study on an ongoing basis during the study to ensure patient safety and data integrity. This may become tricky if the drug safety group breaks individual patients' blinding codes to report the case unblinded to the health agencies and data committees but, at the same time, endeavors to maintain the blind for the clinical research and biostatistics departments (see Chapter 37 on E2A). Drug safety may also assist the clinical research department in preparing data for meetings with health authorities, health agency advisory committee meetings, responses to ad hoc queries, and so forth.

Sometimes the dealings between the two departments may become strained. The clinical research physicians and staff dealing with the drug in question often feel it is "their baby" and become protective and defensive about it. This may be because they "believe" in the drug and want to give it the benefit of the doubt as well as for potential financial reasons: bonuses and rewards are better for drugs that succeed in clinical trials and get approved for marketing. They also may feel (sometimes correctly) that they are much more familiar with the drug, its activity, safety, and behavior, than the drug safety group, which may handle a whole array of drugs and must, of necessity, devote less time to the drug in question. In addition, the clinical research group deals with both safety and efficacy and may feel they have a better appreciation of the balance between risk and benefit compared with the drug safety folks, who tend to see the risk side and rarely are involved in the benefit side. However, the drug safety personnel usually have better understanding of seriousness, labeledness, and (perhaps) causality, because they have more experience across many drug classes. From a practical point of view, a system of adjudication and resolution of disagreements (e.g., serious vs. nonserious) must exist and must function rapidly. In most, but not all situations, drug safety tends to have the final say on reportability of cases to the health authorities. The company does not want to be in a position where clinical research does not want a case reported as a 7- or 15-day report and drug safety does. A paper trail showing that the company did not take the most conservative position

(i.e., reporting the case when there is some doubt) may be embarrassing at best and harmful at worst.

CROs

If the sponsor is using one or more CROs for various clinical research (or safety or regulatory functions), the safety department should be in close and continued touch with the external CRO(s). If the CRO is handling some or all of the safety functions for the company, one or more internal groups should track, both in real time and with periodic audits and quality reviews, how the safety work is being handled. Although outsourced, the pharmaceutical company still has the legal (and moral) responsibility for the safety of its drug.

■ Marketing and Sales

Drug safety and marketing/sales interact in various ways. At some level in each company, a medical group (sometimes drug safety, sometimes medical affairs, sometimes regulatory, sometimes another group) must review advertising and promotional copy for drugs to be sure that the medical and safety claims are correct. That is, the claims made by the company must correctly reflect the information contained in the official labeling (the approved Package Insert in the United States).

Marketing will often ask drug safety for information on AEs for their own uses (to help sell more product). Although it is hard to refuse to supply such data, drug safety should remind the marketers that spontaneous drug safety data cannot, as a rule, be used for promotional activities or safety claims.

Drug safety may also be asked to supply data that the customer relations department (often within marketing, where technical and scientific questions are directed) uses to prepare responses to patients' or healthcare professionals' medical queries ("Have you ever seen pulmonary emboli with this drug in young women? If yes, how did the patients do and how were they treated?"). Some companies might make the safety data available to more groups in the company than drug safety. This may be a dangerous course to take if the data are used for inappropriate (if not flat-out illegal) purposes. It is a wise policy to let the drug safety group be the gatekeeper for the drug safety data.

In the evaluation of signals and in the production of certain reports, including PSURs and other required reports for regulatory agencies, it is necessary for drug safety to obtain drug use data, such as sales data, patients using the drug, tonnage shipped, or prescriptions written, to estimate a reporting frequency of AEs. These data are usually obtained and kept by the marketing and sales departments. Sometimes they are generated internally and sometimes they are purchased from outside vendors who track prescriptions and sales. This is another area of interaction between drug safety and marketing/sales.

Drug safety often does training of sales representatives, advertising copywriters, and others in the marketing and sales departments in regard to the reporting of AEs. Although the sales force generally believes that its job is to sell drugs and not collect AEs, it is now generally understood by all parties that sales representatives (as well as all company employees, agents, etc.), when they hear of AEs on their products, have an obligation to report them to the safety department for follow-up and regulatory reporting.

In a more subtle way, drug safety must also influence and reinforce its ethical and legal role with marketing and sales. Many salespeople, particularly those handling over-the-counter products, do not fully comprehend that the pharmaceutical industry, along with the financial and nuclear power industries, is among the most regulated industries in the world. The limitations, reporting obligations, and safety issues are often not in the mind-set of marketers and salespeople, whose job and pay depend on product sales. It is drug safety that often must set the limits on what marketing and sales can and may do. For this reason, the marketers often call the drug safety department the "sales prevention department" and the head physician "Dr. No." If the company management does not appreciate this and does not ensure that safety is handled properly, the company may suffer severe regulatory, legal, and sales consequences, particularly if a safety issue arises.

The drug safety department is a cost center that never produces revenue and profit for a company. This tends to produce, in some drug safety people, a siege mentality because they carry little weight in the corporate hierarchy and are continually "fighting" to get their message out. The primary goal of the safety department, of course, is to prevent patient harm and to protect the public health. This viewpoint is sometimes not shared by others in the company who believe that the safety department's primary job is to protect the company's products at all costs. In fact, by doing correct and complete safety work, the safety department protects the company's products so that, at some point down the road, when the safety issues arise, they will not produce drug withdrawals, lawsuits, and patient harm. However, this is often a hard concept

to "sell to the sales department." Potential dollars not lost in the future do not appear on balance sheets or get people raises and bonuses.

■ The Labeling Department

The drug safety department will have some role in label creation and maintenance. Labeling is defined broadly and includes the marketed labeling (Package Insert, SmPC, PIL, CCSI, wording on the box or package, etc.) as well as the Investigator Brochure for drugs in clinical trials. At the simplest level, drug safety supplies AE information, particularly on treatment-emergent AEs for marketed products, to the department (e.g., regulatory affairs, medical writing, dedicated label departments) that creates and maintains the label. The safety department may also be charged with periodic or continuous label review to ensure that the label contains the latest scientific and medical information. This may mean that the safety department must notify the appropriate departments of new AEs worthy of being put into the label (usually with due process and prior approval by a labeling or safety committee), changes in the pregnancy status of a drug, new warnings, contraindications, and precautions both for the product and for the whole class of drugs ("class labeling"). It is also worthwhile for the drug safety or labeling department to scan the drugs labels of other companies' products for the appearance in these other drugs' labeling of a new drug interaction with other marketed drugs. The actual division of these duties is not clearly standardized and varies from company to company.

■ The Legal Department

The drug safety department may be involved with the legal department when AEs are reported in cases under litigation or when there is threat of litigation. In such instances, the lawyers usually forbid the drug safety department to have direct contact with the patient or healthcare providers. All contact to obtain further safety information is usually done through the company's legal department. In addition, one or more people from the drug safety department (usually physicians) may be subpoenaed to testify in cases involving the company and safety issues related to its products. This involves "witness training" for those at risk to be called on to testify in court or to give depositions.

It is also common, when a company is being sued, for the plaintiff's attorneys to request copies of safety information. This process is called "discovery." The safety department may be forced to stop work to prepare or assist in preparing paper or electronic copies of hundreds to thousands of pages of material needed in a very tight time frame. In the worst case, the drug safety department may have its paper or electronic files sealed to prevent any changes or the adding of new information. Drug safety is also heavily involved in preparing the company's defense in such cases and in evaluating claims that have not yet reached litigation.

In some companies, the legal department may have some say in review of the expedited reports, PSURs, submissions (MAs, NDAs), and other documents and reports produced by the safety department. This may be a two-sided coin, as the legal department will not want drug safety to indicate that the drug may have caused an AE. This can be very problematic as companies are expected to make judgments in signaling reports, expedited reports, PSURs, and other documents in regard to causality. The legal department may not want such "admissions" made that could come back to bite the company should a court case arise.

The legal department may be helpful in setting up safety data exchange agreements with other companies to ensure that the company receives all appropriate safety information.

In practice, when wisdom prevails, the drug safety group and the legal department are allies in the desire for the facts and the science to be handled correctly, transparently, and honestly. This is always the best policy for the company, the patients, the healthcare professionals, and the stockholders, though in the heat of battle and fog of war this may not be evident.

■ Regulatory Affairs Department

Although the drug safety department often reports to the clinical research department in a company, the drug safety department's function is primarily regulatory. In some companies, particularly small ones, the regulatory group may also handle drug safety functions.

Drug safety is responsible for the preparation and submission of expedited reporting (7- and 15-day reports, MedWatch/CIOMS I reports, E2B reports), PSURs, and NDA periodic reports and such to the health agencies and similar reports to business partners and others. The regulatory department may have a role in reporting cases to the health agencies (e.g., sometimes assigning a special number to each submission, such as a serial number for FDA reporting) or tracking such cases. This requires careful and detailed procedures to ensure that reports are

not lost or sent in late. Regulatory affairs is usually the intermediary in any direct contact between health agencies and the safety department and other departments in the company, because most companies prefer to carefully control and monitor all communications with health authorities. Most company employees are not permitted to contact the health agencies directly but must go through regulatory affairs, whether in the home office or in subsidiaries or affiliates.

The health authorities may approach the company and request that a labeling change be made. Such communications will usually go to the regulatory department (whether in the home office or in the local affiliate, partner, or subsidiary) as the point of entry into the company. This usually results in the company's invoking an SOP-defined process or setting up a task force, including drug safety, clinical research, regulatory, and animal toxicology, to respond to the request.

■ The Quality and Compliance Department

The drug safety group interacts with the quality group and the compliance group (which may be the same group or different groups) both in regard to the safety department's duties and in regard to assisting in technical matters when these groups are dealing with safety issues in other departments.

For drug safety functions, the quality/compliance group may assist and oversee preparation of SOPs, processes, and interactions within the company to be sure the group is handling its functions correctly. They may also audit the drug safety group periodically and assist in or oversee any Corrective Action/Preventive Action Plans (CAPAs) that might be the outcome of the audit. They will also assist in and sometimes take the operational lead in handling and responding to external audits and governmental inspections of the drug safety group. They may be involved in audits of investigator sites, vendors and contract research organizations, business partner standard operating procedures and safety data, and manufacturing safety issues. This is highly variable from company to company. As with legal, the quality and compliance group should, ideally, work as partners with the drug safety group rather than purely as overseers and "police."

■ New Business Due Diligence

When a company wishes to purchase or license in a drug product to develop or sell, it usually examines the entire data set for the drug to be purchased. This includes the review of manufacturing data, standard operating procedures, animal toxicology and pharmacology data, clinical data, regulatory correspondence with the health agencies, and so forth. The drug safety department may be called in during this "due diligence" review to examine the clinical safety data, including expedited reports (E2B, MedWatch and CIOMS forms), risk management plans, PSURs and NDA periodic reports, clinical trial annual reports and IND annual reports, health agency queries and other interactions, and all sorts of other safety data. Sometimes the data are available electronically, sometimes on paper, or both. Sometimes it is aggregate data primarily, and other times it is less well-organized individual patient safety information. For a drug that has not been tested in humans or only minimally so, the data may be sparse; for a marketed drug, it may be extensive.

In general, the safety evaluation of a drug should include all clinical trial and postmarketing safety data, regulatory correspondence, and animal toxicology data. Attention should be paid, in clinical trial data, to dropouts, deaths, lack of efficacy, and lost-to-follow-up cases and any other areas where safety data might be lurking. The safety department should take the view that the information supplied to them is data intended to "make the sale" and as such it will highlight favorable information and put less favorable data in the background. Although the outright hiding of safety data is rare, it is not unheard of, and the safety reviewer should approach the due diligence duty with healthy skepticism. The safety reviewer cannot say yes or no to the company's in-licensing a product but must spell out the safety and risk part of the "benefit–risk" analysis that the company performs.

■ Toxicology and Pharmacology

Drug safety will interact with these groups when animal and laboratory testing results are needed for safety evaluations and in ongoing drug life cycle risk management evaluations. Sometimes the drug safety group will need to go back to the animal data to analyze a signal or safety issue to see whether there were any early clues in the preclinical data. Other times, the toxicology group may call on drug safety should they find a striking safety concern in an animal study that may produce a 15-day expedited report. Usually, the drug safety group is called on to assist, as these reports are generally quite rare and the toxicology groups ask for assistance from drug safety and regulatory in preparation of the submissions.

■ Signaling and Epidemiology Groups

Drug safety will often interact on a very tight basis with these groups to supply data as well as to sit in on sessions that analyze, evaluate, and prepare further actions (e.g., clinical trials, epidemiology studies, registries). Coordination regarding signals noted in PSURs or other reports prepared by drug safety should be done with the signaling and epidemiology groups. Joint meetings are usually held periodically. This varies from company to company.

■ The Medical Information Department

Drug safety may interact with the internal or external groups handling communications into and out of the company. For incoming questions, this will include complaints, AEs, product quality issues, and queries from patients, consumers, and healthcare professionals. The safety group should ensure that SOPs are in place that will get AEs, particularly SAEs, to the drug safety group in a timely manner with all the appropriate information allowing follow-up by the safety group. The medical information department may also handle after-hours communications. That is, they may set up either internal or outsourced systems (e.g., phone centers, poison control centers) to receive after-hours AEs and complaints. Drug safety should be sure that all processes are in place to ensure that such AEs and complaints get to drug safety promptly.

Drug safety may also supply safety information for queries to the medical information department that go beyond the official labeling. That is, most companies do not allow their staff to make medical judgments or give clinical advice on their drugs. The usual responses follow the officially approved labeling and go no further. However, sometimes, physician-to-physician requests come into the company, asking certain questions that go beyond the labeling (e.g., "Have pulmonary emboli been seen with this drug and if so, what was the course and treatment?"). The drug safety group may be requested to supply data from its database to answer such questions.

■ Manufacturing (Product Quality Complaints)

In the signal analysis of a product, it is not sufficient to simply examine AE data. The signal reviewer must also review product quality complaints. It is entirely possible that the AE is due to a problem in the manufacturing process that produced an impurity, an unstable product, an excipient issue, a manufacturing process, a counterfeit product, or a vendor change that produced unforeseen bad effects. This is surprisingly common, as companies change vendors frequently for raw materials and product

containers and make process changes when efficiencies or new machines are available. These are all done under appropriate change control (or should be), but unintended consequences can occur. For this reason, the signal review must include product quality complaints and drug safety must communicate frequently with colleagues in the manufacturing area when issues arise.

43

SOPs, Working Documents, Manuals, Guidelines

United States, European Union, and other health authority regulations require that companies have written standard operating procedures (SOPs) to handle drug safety and pharmacovigilance. These documents in the aggregate are known as "procedural documents." These are documents that describe the general or specific steps to be done in a process, job, or function to ensure that the result is obtained in a complete, reproducible fashion and delivers what is sought. The procedure should be descriptive and may be used for training and as a reference document.

The following is from the U.S. Food and Drug Administration's (FDA's) document for inspectors conducting adverse event (AE) audits (Chapter 53: Post-Marketing Surveillance and Epidemiology: Human Drugs, Enforcement of the Post-Marketing Adverse Drug Experience Reporting Regulations, September 30, 1999, Field Reporting Requirements. See Web Resource 43-1):

The regulations (21 CFR 211.198) require that... manufacturers...have written procedures for complaint files including provisions for determining whether a complaint represents a serious and unexpected ADE. The regulations (21 CFR 211.25) also require that qualified personnel investigate and evaluate ADEs. If serious deficiencies are found during the inspection, obtain copies of the procedures and determine personnel qualifications and staffing, especially if the firm utilizes computerized reporting. Effective April 6, 1998, any person subject to the ADE Reporting regulations, including those that do not have approved applications, shall develop written procedures for the surveillance, receipt, evaluation, and reporting of postmarketing adverse drug experiences to FDA (21 CFR 314.80(b) and 21 CFR 310.305(a)).

In the European Union, Volume 9A specifies that written procedures exist and goes on to list those that are required (at a minimum).

An essential element of any pharmacovigilance system is that there are clear, written procedures in place. Care should be taken to ensure that quality control and review are appropriately addressed in the various processes and reflected in the relevant procedures:

- The activities of the QPPV and the back-up procedure to apply in their absence;
- The collection, processing (including data entry and data management), quality control, coding, classification, medical review, and reporting of ICSRs:
- Reports of different types:
  - Organized data collection schemes (solicited), unsolicited, clinical trials, literature
  - The process should ensure that reports from different sources are captured:
    - EEA and third countries, healthcare professionals, sales and marketing personnel, other Marketing Authorization Holder personnel, licensing partners,
    - Competent Authorities, compassionate use, patients, others;
- The follow-up of reports for missing information and for information on the progress and outcome of the case(s);
- Detection of duplicate reports;
- Expedited reporting;
- Electronic reporting;
- Periodic Safety Update Reports (PSURs):
  - The preparation, processing, quality control, review (including medical review) and reporting;
- Global pharmacovigilance activities applying to all products: Continuous monitoring of the safety profile of authorized medicinal products
  - Signal detection and review;
  - Risk-benefit assessment;
  - Reporting and communication notifying Competent Authorities and healthcare professionals of changes to the risk-benefit balance of products, etc.;
- Interaction between safety issues and product defects;
- Responses to requests for information from regulatory authorities;
- Handling of urgent safety restrictions and safety variations;
- Meeting commitments to Competent Authorities in relation to a Marketing Authorization;
- Global pharmacovigilance activities applying to all products (signal detection, evaluation, reporting, communication, etc.);
- Management and use of databases or other recording systems;
- Internal audit of the pharmacovigilance system;
- Training;
- Archiving.

A list and copies of the global and EEA procedures should be available within 24 hours on request by the Competent Authorities. Any additional local procedures should be available to respond to specific requests.

One of the first requests that an inspector from the FDA, the Medicines and Healthcare Products Regulatory Agency (MHRA), or European Medicines Agency (EMA) will make at the beginning of a drug safety inspection is for copies of the drug safety SOPs and related documents (such as guidelines, working documents, manuals, etc.). Usually, the company has an index or listing of these documents that is given to the inspector, who then chooses which ones to examine. Companies then must expect that the government inspectors, corporate auditors, vendors doing due diligence, and others will read the SOPs in detail and expect those people in the company governed by the SOPs to follow them scrupulously. Auditors will also look at working documents, manuals and guidelines, and other documents (see below) that groups prepare to aid in their work in addition to SOPs. The auditors also expect the staff to adhere to these guidelines too, especially if they are approved by some formal or semiformal company mechanism. Note that putting a process or requirement in a working document rather than in the SOP does not free the staff from adhering to the requirement. Thus, it is not a good strategy to relegate certain requirements to a working document or guideline in the hope that the inspector will not examine them or hold the staff responsible for these requirements too. All procedural documents are "fair game."

Companies or health agencies may create multiple levels of procedures. For a large company, there may be a very high-level (or "global" or "corporate") SOP that states the scope, mission, and broad outlines of the safety policy. Then, each division within the scope may develop its own localized policy, and subdivisions may then develop theirs. Usually, two to three layers are the practical limit of this hierarchy. For example, for a large multinational company, one way to approach this is to create three levels of SOPs:

1. High-level corporate policy that applies to all divisions of the company: This is the corporate policy to collect, analyze, and report to the appropriate health authorities and internal and external clients all AEs, product quality complaints, and medication errors that the company learns about its products that occur in humans and animals.

2. Division level: Each division of the company then prepares a more detailed version of the high-level policy that applies only to that division:

   ■ Human products division: Creates a broad policy to put the high-level policy into effect. This would cover all research and marketing in the home country and abroad (directly or via subsidiaries or affiliates) and directs them to prepare their own local SOPs (in their local language with a translation into English for review by the quality group).

3. Subdivision level: Each section (e.g., the French affiliate) within a division then creates its own SOPs to put the policies noted above into place in their local language. There may be multiple policies needed to accomplish this, and they should specifically cover such things as responsibility by job title (e.g., the medical monitor is responsible for...), timing (e.g., all serious AEs from investigational sites sent to the company within one working day of occurrence by electronic transmission, fax, e-mail...), and so on.

For example, the following units could create one or more SOPs to cover the following:

■ The drug safety unit SOPs would cover the specific details of the handling of spontaneous serious AEs, spontaneous nonserious AEs, literature AEs, clinical trial AEs from phase I–IV studies, clinical trial AEs from investigator-initiated trials, AEs from business partners, or AEs from consumers, periodic reporting, signal detection, and so forth.

■ The clinical research unit SOPs would cover instructions to investigators and monitor what and when to send AEs using a particular written form, or how to handle the case in the electronic case report form (EDC system).

■ The animal toxicology/pharmacology unit(s) should have SOPs covering how and when animal findings regarding safety and toxicity should be

reported and to whom, because in many jurisdictions, animal findings that may result in safety issues in humans must be reported within 15 calendar days as expedited reports.

Other documents at any level can also be created. At any point, a unit may create documents to assist staff in doing their daily jobs. These documents might be manuals (e.g., a data entry manual explaining screen by screen how to enter AE cases into the safety database), guidelines, guidances, "cheat sheets" (e.g., a table of all AEs listed in a drug's Package Insert to aid in the rapid determination of whether an AE is labeled/listed), process guides, and various other work aids. Ideally, these should be done somewhat formally with version control and verified to be correct and consistent from person to person within a group.

SOPs must be kept in tight control because they represent the "bible" and contain instructions to the employees that must be followed. Only the latest version of the SOP should be used and available to all employees. In theory, keeping only the latest versions of SOPs online ensures that employees do not use older, outdated versions. However, in practice, especially if there are many SOPs, employees print out copies rather than looking online every time they have a question (e.g., they might have to log out of a case they are entering into the database to look up an SOP question). This tends to defeat the purpose of SOPs but is probably unavoidable. In that case, the printed version should contain a statement to the effect: "This printed copy does not necessarily represent the latest in-force version of this SOP. The current in-force copy may be found online at [give link or URL]." Alternatively, the SOP group may issue to every employee covered printed copies of the SOPs that are numbered, dated, and version controlled. When a new version of an SOP is published, a member of the SOP group should update each binder, replacing the old version with the new version.

Clearly, very tight version control must be maintained. This should be spelled out in the SOP that governs SOP creation and maintenance. It should cover how and by whom it is determined that an SOP is needed and its creation, review, approval, and updating. A system of version control and numbering should be described. It should also mandate training appropriate employees on the new procedures.

Copies of older, outdated SOPs should be retained, as a health agency inspector may wish to see the SOP in force at the time when a case that is months or even years old is examined. The company may avoid a citation by showing that a particular SOP requirement that is in place now was not in place when the case was actually received and processed.

Training on SOPs is obligatory. Training should not be simply distribution of the SOPs and having each person read them. Efforts should be made using professional, dedicated trainers (e.g., employees who have some skills in teaching and training) to develop a methodology to ensure that training is effective. This includes setting up training and retraining schedules and curricula and using effective technology (interesting presentations, video, web-based training, etc.). Many companies will conduct testing after the training to ensure that the content was absorbed. This is somewhat controversial, though most companies will test manual data entry, as this critical function must be done correctly. Many companies have training departments that "certify" trainers ("train the trainers") within divisions of the company. The trainers themselves may not train on all SOPs but may enlist subject-matter experts to do the actual training. The trainers may review and approve the training materials. In addition, detailed records of training must be kept. They should be at the employee level and at the group level so that it can be easily demonstrated (with written records) to an auditor that every employee was successfully trained. Copies of the training materials (such as PowerPoint decks) must also be retained.

It is not sufficient to write and publish SOPs. They must be followed. The quality department should review (audit) SOPs on several levels:

- Do the SOPs meet the mission and standards they set? For example, if a safety SOP requires adherence to U.S. and European Union expedited reporting requirements, the SOP should be audited against the U.S. and European Union regulations, laws, and guidelines. This is often a difficult job for an auditor, because it requires that he or she must be familiar with these laws and regulations. Historically, the groups doing pharmacovigilance audits also did clinical research audits as well as, in some cases, financial, Good Laboratory Practice, and Good Manufacturing Practice audits. This would often mean that the auditors had only a superficial knowledge of safety requirements and best practices. The trend now is for developing specialized drug safety auditing units that have employees with detailed knowledge of PV—often former case processors or staff from the drug safety unit who wish to move out of the "firing line." Thus, the auditor is able to make a learned judgment on

whether the SOP meets the appropriate regulatory requirements and is best (or at least acceptable!) practice.

- The second level of review is the more common and, in general, easier level to audit: Are employees adhering to the requirements of the SOP? If the SOP is clear and prescriptive, the auditor is easily able to verify whether the procedures are done appropriately. For example, if the SOP requires that each AE report coming into the safety department is manually or electronically date-stamped immediately on receipt and then entered into the database within 2 working days, it is relatively straightforward for the auditor to check the date stamp and compare it with the date of data entry.

Another level of review is internal consistency. If each subsidiary in the countries where a multinational company sells the drug has a safety SOP, these SOPs should be reviewed for consistency with the higher level SOP and, if desired and appropriate, with each other.

Although CIOMS and ICH (see Chapters 36 and 37, respectively) have done much work to harmonize requirements and regulations, there are still significant differences between and among each country's requirements, particularly in clinical trials, where there is less harmonization than in the marketed drug arena. These differences, on the working level, can be substantial and difficult for companies to work out in a manner satisfactory to all parties.

In our age of globalization, it is now common for companies to work with many other companies (either pharma/biotech companies or CROs) in codevelopment, comarketing, and other joint arrangements. Some of these can involve multiple companies throughout the world. Such situations require that some level of coordination and agreement is reached on how SOPs and processes will be handled.

The specific requirements of SOPs may also present problems in such situations. If one company uses only E2B case submission and the other company uses MedWatch or CIOMS I forms, there will be issues to resolve. Or, if two companies agree to exchange with each other completed CIOMS I forms for all serious AEs and one company bases its procedure on completing the forms by calendar day 7 and the other by calendar day 11, there may be significant timing and process issues, forcing one of the companies to alter its procedure to accommodate a shortened preparation schedule. One company may require a legal review of each case and the other may not. At some point, most companies harmonize as much as they can and "agree to disagree" on the remainder of the issues. Generally, the larger the company, the less flexible it is.

Although it would be ideal to have only one set of SOPs in place for a study or drug on the market, it is often the case that each company uses its own SOPs. Differences in case handling, processing, medical review, and so forth, must be ironed out before the study is begun or the drug marketed. There is no one correct or ideal way to do this. Each situation is usually customized, and compromise may be required by one or all parties. This can be difficult for large companies with rigid systems in place that do not wish to make exceptions or "one-offs." Sometimes companies may not permit their (highly proprietary) SOPs to leave their building. The other company may see them but only by physically visiting the site where the first company keeps the SOPs. This can make harmonization of SOPs between the companies rather difficult. See Chapter 47 on safety exchange agreements.

The listing of European Union SOPs that should be present is fairly complete. In addition to those, it is usually wise to have SOPs that cover other areas, including:

- Handling AEs in clinical research, including investigator-initiated trials as well as phase I–IV studies
- Handling AEs from marketing and sales, legal, telephone operators, webmasters, and the mailroom
- Reporting requirements for employees not normally involved in safety, specifying that all AEs must be sent to drug safety within certain time frames (i.e., if an accounting department employee hears from a neighbor over the weekend that one of the company's products made him sick, that AE should be reported to drug safety)
- Handling of AEs in animals
- The mechanics of the drug safety department:
  - Receipt of AEs from trials, spontaneous reports, consumers, electronic data capture, logging, database entry, quality review, narrative preparation, the Medical Dictionary for Regulatory Activities coding conventions, drug naming conventions, breaking the blind in clinical trials, literature review, medical review, querying, and follow-up
  - Handling of 7-day expedited reports
  - Handling of 15-day expedited reports (clinical trial and postmarketing)
- How to develop safety agreements with partners; handling of reports sent to business partners and internal clients
- E2B reporting
- Preparation of Investigational New Drug Application annual reports, Annual Safety Reports, New Drug Application periodic reports, Periodic Safety Update Reports, and other aggregate reports
- Contacts with government agencies
- Crisis management and disaster recovery
- Database management and access
- How to handle an audit
- Archiving and filing; record retention
- Signaling
- Life cycle risk management and preparation of risk documents (e.g. REMs and RMPs)
- Medication error handling
- Product quality handling
- Quality assurance and quality compliance
- SOP preparation and maintenance
- Litigation
- Training

This list is not complete and will be tailored by each organization. Some organizations will be "lumpers" and others will be "splitters," creating fewer or more SOPs.

All SOPs, working documents, manuals, and such should be reviewed periodically (at least yearly and more frequently if appropriate) to be sure they are still applicable and up to date. They should, in particular, be compared with regulations and requirements in force, best practices, and what is really happening in the organization they apply to. It may surprise that what is written in the SOP may not be what is really happening "in the trenches." Adjustments in process and SOP should be made. All changes in the documents should be carefully documented and noted in the "changes in the new version" section of the document. Training should be performed as necessary.

For a good review of SOPs in the pharma industry, see Gough, Hamrell, Standard Operating Procedures (SOPs): How to write them to be effective tools. *Drug Inf J.* 2010;44:463–468.

44

Training

Two broad and related areas are addressed here: (1) training of the drug safety staff and (2) training of the other employees in the organization who need to know something about drug safety.

In any organization, there are two broad areas of training required. The first includes the corporate/organizational requirements and includes such things as using the computer systems, corporate ethics, behavior and mission, equality in the workplace, getting along with coworkers, safety in the workplace, filling out needed forms for payroll and benefits, and other corporate level matters that everyone in the organization needs to know. These programs are usually taught to all employees by the corporate-level training group. These are not addressed further here.

The other area of training, discussed in detail in this chapter, involves job-specific drug safety training. Nearly all drug safety groups now have a training function, and many groups now have full-time dedicated trainers whose job it is to handle all the aspects of training and instruction. This group sets up a training system with tailored curricula, depending on the personnel and jobs being trained. Usually a fair amount of customization is required to train the right people on the right things.

For live training, the training group sets up schedules for training and makeup sessions for those who missed the first session. Although they may do much of the training themselves, especially on high-level or more general subjects, the training group will create a roster of subject-matter experts who will be called on to train in highly specialized or technical areas that the trainers cannot teach. The training group works with the quality and compliance groups as well as with the drug safety group to determine which employees should be trained in which areas. They determine which training can be "one shot" and which requires updating or refresher training. Some groups with high turnover require frequent training sessions for new employees (e.g., the sales force), whereas others are often more stable and do not require training sessions as frequently.

The training job may require significant travel if training is done at various sites around the home country or the world. This is particularly true for multinational organizations and those that have employees working at home or off-site. The levels of training for full-time employees versus consultants should also be taken into account. Consultants, part-timers, interim employees, and other non-full-time employees still need training for their jobs. Issues of training of non-English-speaking employees need to be addressed, especially now that English is often required for international communications in drug safety and international business in general.

Much training now is being done as "distance learning," using electronic resources such as live or recorded webinars, teleconferences, and software that allows personal study at the time and pace that the trainee desires. The training group should have a good understanding of these newer technologies. The use of consulting and outsourcing in the appropriate circumstances should also be considered.

The training group should set up a record-keeping system, both for the training department to document globally who was trained and for employee-specific training files, which usually remain within each employee's human resources or departmental dossier. Copies of the training materials (e.g., PowerPoint slides) should also be retained in the master file. Thus, during an inspection by the health agency, the training group can demonstrate that training of a particular function (e.g., handling 7-day expedited reports) was done to the appropriate groups (e.g., drug safety, clinical research, regulatory affairs), with the training documentation (slides, handouts) on file. In addition, the training group can go to each employee's file and show the record, indicating that that employee was trained on this function on this particular date. All of this documentation can be kept electronically.

The training group should work with the departments to be trained as well as with drug safety to prepare a matrix of which employees (by title or function) need which training modules and at what frequency. They should determine which employees, consultants, and interim workers need refresher training even if the standard operating procedures (SOPs) and processes have not changed.

Many companies now have a general corporate policy that requires all employees and agents of the company (including consultants and temporary employees) to report AEs to the drug safety group if they hear about them during and outside of work. This usually refers to marketed drugs and covers such items as when a neighbor or relative casually notes that he or she took your company's drug XX and had a bad reaction. The policy requires the employee to report the AE to the drug safety group by the next business day with sufficient contact information to allow drug safety to follow up on the report and to get the details of the case. This should be routinely done (with periodic reminders) in all companies with marketed products with an e-mail blast, memo, or company newsletter.

On drug safety issues, it is necessary to train several groups ("feeder groups") within the company on their duties in regard to sending AEs to drug safety and then the handling and distribution of the cases. Groups that require training include the marketing and sales groups, the legal department, the mailroom staff, the telephone operators, senior corporate management and their administrative staff (who often receive complaint letters addressed to the Chief Executive Officer or President), all clinical research and support groups, medical affairs, the product complaint department, the quality and compliance groups, regulatory affairs, medical information/services, the new business development group, the library, IT and webmasters, and any other groups identified as being involved with AE or safety reports.

Outside groups needing training include clinical or contract research organizations doing work with or for the company as well as all other contractors and outsourcers (e.g., hired sales forces, such as rent-a-reps), investigators doing clinical research who need to report AEs to the company, outside legal counsel, and other business partners who, by contract, need to adhere to the company's SOPs. This may sometimes be difficult to determine.

As the training needs of the organization increase because of new hires, expansion, and changes in regulations and requirements, it is unlikely that the personnel and travel budget in the training department will increase proportionately. This forces the group to increase productivity and to "work smarter." There are many ways to do this, including web-based training or simply recording a training session as a video and posting it online with required viewing and some level of assurance that the employee actually viewed the information, such as a test of the material. The issue of testing arises frequently. It is generally accepted that it is not sufficient to simply train people by having them read materials or attend live classroom sessions or one-on-one training. Some determination of whether the material has been absorbed is usually required. This can be done by formal testing at the end of training or at some point after training is completed (e.g., yearly at the same time each year). The testing may be anonymous or the results made known only to the person being tested and not the trainer or supervisor. Retraining and retesting for people who fail may be required. In all cases, good pedagogic techniques must be followed, such as "praise publicly, reproach privately." The training group typically prepares modules covering each section or subsection listed below and can thus pick out which modules should be used to train which employees as a function of the employee's job and experience. For example, internal hires may need less training than new hires.

Organizational Structure and Site Information

Training should cover:

- New employee orientation (usually done by human resources)
- Introduction to staff and organization
- Review of training curriculum
- Site information
- Telephone, password, voice mail, computer and web functions
- Safety department overview—structure and functions, teams, support staff
- Subsidiary, affiliate, and country operations
- Duties and responsibilities of the position
- Performance objectives and measures; goal setting
- Support groups
- Training from other divisions (e.g., as provided by clinical research, legal, regulatory affairs, informatics)
- Emergency procedures if the site is not accessible or the computers are down

Computer, Forms, Electronic, and Print Resources

- Computer and internet accounts and password
- Applications
- Help desk
- E-mail policies
- Storage drives
- Corporate website and portals
- Services accessible online: library, benefits, forms
- Wi-Fi use and security issues
- Logging on from off-site
- Smartphone (e.g., Blackberry, Android, iPhone, Tablets)

What Is Pharmacovigilance?

- Governing U.S., European Union, and other country or region regulations, laws, guidelines, directives
- SOPs, manuals, job aids, guidelines

- Terminology
- Functioning and duties of the health agencies (competent authorities) governing the company's products: U.S. FDA, European Union EMA, MHRA, and so forth
- Mission of drug safety
- Labeling—Summary of Product Characteristics (SmPC), Package Insert, Investigator Brochure, Company Core Safety Information and Data Sheet

Corporate and Drug Safety SOPs, Working Documents, Guidelines, and Manuals

- High-level corporate SOPs
- Divisional SOPs
- Drug safety SOPs
- Other departments' SOPs that touch on drug safety
- International Organization for Standards (ISO) requirements if applicable (This group produces SOPs and standards that are accepted and followed in many fields, including device manufacture in the United States. See Web Resource 44-1.)

Medical Dictionary for Regulatory Activities (MedDRA) and Other Dictionaries

- Introduction to MedDRA
- The MedDRA browser
- Coding AEs: Maintenance and Support Service Organization and FDA conventions
- Requesting new codes and periodic updates
- Drug dictionary
- Other dictionaries (e.g., abbreviations) and conventions

Safety Database

- Access to the database: IDs and passwords
- Screen-by-screen training on data entry
- Pregnancy cases, mother–child cases, and other special situations
- Data privacy

- Laboratory data
- Source documents and scanning
- Archiving and deleting cases
- Clock start date and other date issues
- Duplicates
- Transmission of expedited reports to the FDA or other regulatory agencies
- Transmission of cases to business partners
- Workflow
- Quality checks (QA and QC)
- Requesting follow-up information from the reporter/investigator
- Preparing reports, cover letters, investigator letters
- Ad hoc queries, structured query language, query by example
- Device, combination product, vaccine, biologics, blood product issues
- E2B import and export

Workflow

- Handling 7-day clinical trial expedited reports
- Handling 15-day clinical trial (IND) expedited reports
- Handling 15-day expedited reports (postmarketing and clinical trial)
- Global expedited reports
- Electronic data capture (EDC) safety handling in clinical trials
- E2B and non-E2B report submission
- Eudravigilance submission
- Nonexpedited serious reports
- Nonserious reports
- Pregnancy cases
- Literature reports

- Stimulated reports and investigator-initiated study reports
- Medication errors
- Product quality reports
- Medical (physician) review
- Quality checks
- Aggregate reports: PSURs, Annual Safety Reports, IND annual reports, NDA periodic reports, PADERs
- Interactions with other departments (e.g., clinical research, regulatory)
- Breaking the blind in clinical trials: individual cases and at the end of the trial for all cases

Partner and CRO Interactions

Signaling and Pharmacovigilance

- Signal generation, handling, and workup
- Risk management and preparation of REMs and RMPs
- Crisis management
- Drug withdrawal, protocol changes, stopping studies, tampering, and other urgent issues
- Label changes
- Media training

Outside Training

There are now many organizations (both profit-making and nonprofit) around the world that now offer training in drug safety and pharmacovigilance. They are of variable quality and depth. Some are quite useful and accurate. Others are incomplete, contain incorrect information, or are high on opinion and low on fact. They are usually quite expensive and the buyer should be wary (caveat emptor).

45

Vaccinovigilance

Lisa Beth Ferstenberg, MD

Vigilance for vaccines is different from vigilance for drugs. We will review the difference between vaccinovigilance and pharmacovigilance—the U.S. Initiative: VAERS, the European Initiative: GACVS, and the European Commissions, Vaccine Adverse Event Reporting, and sources of additional information.

■ Differences Between Vaccinovigilance and Pharmacovigilance

Adverse event reporting, whether associated with a drug or a vaccine, captures information on known or suspected reactions to administered substances; however, in the case of a drug, the substance is usually administered as an intervention for an existing illness or condition, and in the case of a vaccine, it is given to prevent an illness. This critical difference, between intervention and prevention, affects the entire analysis, interpretation, and implications of vigilance data.

In general, severe adverse events to vaccines are rare. Approximately 85% of reported adverse events are mild and self-limiting and usually involve local reactions, such as pain or itching at the site of administration, or systemic reactions, such as fever or irritability. The 15% of reported severe adverse events may include seizures, high fevers, life-threatening illnesses, or death (Web Resource 45-1).

The notable difference between vaccine-related adverse events, whether minor or severe, and those associated with drugs is that vaccine-related adverse events are usually immunologic and signal immune response (Web Resource 45-2). For drugs, however, adverse events more frequently indicate organ toxicity. Since the vaccine's objective is to elicit an immune response to a target antigen, the emergence of an immunologic or inflammatory response can indicate that the patient is developing a desirable immune response, whereas in drug-related toxicity, the reaction almost invariably indicates an undesirable effect.

The contextual differences between intervention and prevention affect the interpretation of data derived from adverse event reporting. For a drug-related adverse event, the patient presents to the health professional with an array of symptoms, and if new symptoms develop following treatment, there is a reasonable likelihood that the provider following the patient will be informed of their occurrence and will be able to assess them in the context of the illness. Vaccines, however, are often administered en masse to large populations not seeing a provider for a specific complaint. When an adverse event occurs, the patient is less likely to have access to the provider who administered the vaccine, and the provider is less likely to know the patient's history of prior health or underlying conditions. In addition, little to no information may be available about how many doses of the vaccine have been administered in the population, to whom, and with what results (Hanslik, Boelle, *Med Sci [Paris]* 2007;23[4]: 391–398).

In addition to safety, establishing vaccine effectiveness requires recognizing the epidemiologic pattern of the disease to be prevented. Ideally, efficacy is expressed as a reduction in the incidence of the infectious disease in vaccinated subjects as compared with the unvaccinated population. In reality, disease reporting in populations is frequently incomplete in both vaccinated and unvaccinated populations; hence, patients who report adverse events to vaccines frequently represent the richest source of data obtainable about the epidemiology of both an infectious disease and its prevention.

Why is this safety and efficacy information not available from clinical trials done before approval? Despite the large sample sizes enrolled in phase I–III clinical trials (patient numbers can be in the tens of thousands), most preapproval clinical trials are designed to limit the number of confounding variables that would make it difficult to interpret the data. Hence, much older and much younger patients may not be enrolled, and patients with a wide variety of comorbidities may have been excluded. Typically, when a new vaccine is first introduced to the market, little may be known about vaccination risks in immunocompromised patients, pregnant women, cancer patients, and patients with serious underlying diseases.

■ The United States Initiative: VAERS

The Vaccine Adverse Event Reporting System (VAERS) used in the United States is the postmarketing safety surveillance program created by the Centers for Disease Control and Prevention (CDC) and the U.S. Food and Drug Administration (FDA) in response to the National Childhood Vaccine Injury Act (NCVIA) of 1986. This law requires health professionals and vaccine manufacturers to report to the Department of Health and Human Services (HHS), of which both CDC and FDA are divisions, specific adverse events that occur following vaccines. The objectives of the program are as follows:

1. To detect new, unusual, or rare adverse events associated with vaccine administration
2. To monitor increases in the incidence of known adverse events
3. To identify potential patient-associated risk factors that may predispose individuals to vaccine-associated adverse events
4. To identify vaccine lots that may be associated with an unusually high rate of adverse events
5. To assess the safety of newly licensed vaccines in large diverse populations once they have been released to market

Anyone can report an adverse event through VAERS, including patients and health professionals. The system is a passive surveillance program, which means that it suffers from the following limitations:

1. Underreporting of adverse events
2. Differential reporting, which is a pattern of increased reporting when a vaccine is new that falls off with time
3. Stimulated reporting, which occurs when a new adverse event is first recognized and a flurry of similar or alleged events are then reported
4. Coincidental events, which occurs when an unrelated temporal event is reported as being associated with receipt of a vaccine
5. Poor data quality, with a great deal of missing information and lack of patient follow-up
6. Lack of denominator data, when information on the number of doses of a vaccine administered in the population is not available

Nevertheless, approximately 30,000 adverse events are reported to VAERS annually, of which only 13% are severe, i.e., associated with disability, hospitalization, life-threatening illnesses, or death (Web Resource 45-1).

■ GACVS and the European Commissions

The Global Advisory Committee on Vaccine Safety (GACVS) was established by the World Health Organization (WHO) to address issues of vaccine safety throughout Europe. They established their directives around two general issues regarding Adverse Events Following Immunization (AEFI). The first issue is monitoring vaccine safety. The committee called for prompt data transmission by member countries, assurance of data quality, and the processing and analysis of data for timely signal detection and implementation of action as required.

The second issue focuses on using data collected for detailed examination of pressing questions that affect the efficacy of vaccination programs. This includes an understanding of the safety of preservatives and other nonantigenic ingredients used in manufacturing and formulating vaccines (such as adjuvants, stabilizers), and residuals such as formaldehyde, toxins, viral growth media substrates, and vectors (Lankinin, Pastila, Kilpi, et al., *Bull World Health Organ* 2004;82(11):811–890).

Preventing loss of confidence in vaccine programs is a major objective of understanding their safety. Lack of immunization and subsequent risk of disease has generally proved to be of far greater risk than risk of toxicity from either the antigenic or the nonantigenic materials in vaccines. GACVS has worked with manufacturers to analyze detailed information concerning complexity of the vaccine formulation and manufacturing processes, storage and handling processes, administration procedures, and host-related factors. Other researchers have also analyzed their institutional databases to identify antigenic and nonantigenic components that can be specifically related to vaccine-associated adverse events (Nakayama, Onoda, *Vaccine* 2007;25[3]:570–576).

Issues related to specific vaccines have become major subjects of study for GACVS in answer to their mission of vaccine safety and public protection. For example, understanding the association between the genetic characteristics of mumps vaccines and their association with neurovirulence has resulted in the development of more precise and consistent neurovirulence assays. These may be particularly important in understanding the potential of specific strains of vaccine to cause aseptic meningitis. Another example has been identifying specific strains of BCG, the vaccine for tuberculosis (TB), that cause systemic infections, termed *bcgosis* in young children and infants who are HIV positive.

The Euvax Project, the VENICE Inventory (Vaccine European New Integrated Collaboration Effort), the Uppsala Monitoring Centre, and similar programs in Europe are other useful initiatives established by the Commission of European Communities to respond to better standards in program monitoring and collaboration on safety issues. They grew out of recognizing that efforts around pediatric immunization programs were fairly satisfactory but that a number of special target groups required greater attention. The objective was to create databases on all aspects of immunization programs, including planning, administration, funding, and monitoring. Populations targeted included immigrants, especially illegal immigrants who easily escape the healthcare system and frequently carry new strains of disease across borders; refugees, who are not covered by legislation; military recruits and staff, who may cross in and out of foreign countries and who routinely receive as many as 18 different immunizations; occupational risk groups, such as prison workers and healthcare professionals; and travelers.

■ Vaccine Adverse Event Reporting

The value of postmarketing vaccinovigilance as the key to understanding the role of vaccines in protecting individuals from contracting disease and protecting communities from the spread of disease is clear. The differences inherent in studying a vaccine in otherwise healthy patients in clinical trials and learning about vaccines when they are delivered widespread in a population make it imperative that effective vaccinovigilance systems are established and maintained (Mayans, Robertson, Duclos, *Bull World Health Organ* 2000;78[9]:1167). VAERS and the European MedDRA-based databases are essential for tracking, documenting, and elucidating safety signals in complex settings but are only as good as the data that enters the system. Through multiple websites, such as FDA, CDC, MedDRA MSSO, and others, data can be entered by anyone familiar with an adverse event that occurs in association with a vaccine. The following list can be used as a guideline for information that should be gathered before accessing these websites so that information will be as complete and as reliable as possible.

Information Checklist for Vaccine Adverse Event Reporting

1. Case description
2. Patient age
3. Patient medical history
4. Time interval from receipt of vaccine to adverse event
5. Trade name of vaccine
6. Lot number of vaccine dose
7. Dosage administered
8. Date of administration
9. Vaccination site/route of administration
10. Concomitant vaccines administered

11. Concomitant medications taken

12. Rechallenge data if patients have had this or other vaccines before

13. Outcome information

In the United States, AEs to vaccines should be reported to the FDA. Full reporting information is available at Web Resource 45-3. Reports may be submitted online, by fax, or by regular mail.

The European Union System

It is also useful to recognize what the European system has classified as Adverse Events of Special Interest (AESI), which are believed to be particularly significant as potentially serious adverse events that may be associated with vaccine administration (Greenberg, et al., *New Engl J Med* 2009;361[25]:2405–2413). The AESI include:

- Neuritis
- Convulsions
- Severe allergic or anaphylactic reactions
- Syncope
- Encephalitis
- Thrombocytopenia
- Vasculitis
- Guillain-Barré syndrome
- Bell's palsy

Further information concerning vaccine adverse events, data about relatedness of particular adverse events with vaccines, and links for reporting adverse events are offered in the next section.

Sources of Additional Information

Useful links can be found at the websites for FDA, CDC, WHO, National Institutes of Health, and HHS. Other useful sources of information include the following:

- Immunization Action Coalition (Web Resource 45-4)
- Clinicaltrials.gov: Vaccine Adverse Reactions (Web Resource 45-5)
- Institute for Vaccine Safety (Johns Hopkins University School of Public Health) (Web Resource 45-6)
- National Network for Immunization Information (NNii) (Web Resource 45-7)

- VAERS (Web Resource 45-1)

The last two sites are particularly useful for submitting VAERs.

In the European Union, the EMA's Vaccine Working Party (VWP) (Web Resource 45-8) was established to provide recommendations to the Committee for Medicinal Products for Human Use (CHMP) on all matters relating directly or indirectly to vaccines.

The VWP's tasks include the following:

- Preparing, reviewing, and updating guidelines to ensure that vaccine-specific issues are fully addressed
- Supporting dossier evaluation of new Marketing Authorization applications for vaccines and of any postmarketing submission (e.g., variations, follow-up measures)
- Providing to the CHMP and European Commission scientific advice on general and product-specific matters relating to the pharmaceutical and biological aspects of vaccines, as well as the development and clinical use of vaccines in children and adults
- Liaising with interested parties (e.g., trade organizations, pharmaceutical industry, academia, and patients' organizations)
- European cooperation on vaccine-specific issues
- International cooperation, for example with the WHO
- Contributing to and organizing vaccine-related workshops and training
- On request of the CHMP, constituting a rapid-acting crisis group to take on board-specific issues relating to vaccines, with the objective of exchanging information at the European level and of coordinating responses to the public in a timely manner, for example in relation to an influenza pandemic, vaccines for emerging or reemerging diseases (including against pathogens potentially used for bioterrorism), and other public health issues
- Supporting the conduct of vaccine-specific epidemiological studies
- Supporting the implementation of the Vaccine Identification Standards Initiative (VISI) for recording vaccine usage at the European level to ensure effective pharmacovigilance activities and to facilitate epidemiological investigations
- Monitoring the development of new vaccine technologies (e.g., DNA-based vaccines, cancer vaccines, AIDS vaccines) and the development of new adjuvants

■ Monitoring and providing input for developing new centralized vaccines, with a view to gradually fostering harmonization of immunization schedules in such a way that flexibility is maintained for local, specific public health needs.

In the United Kingdom, the MHRA monitors vaccine safety as they do drugs. See their website (Web Resource 45-9).

In Canada, the Public Health Agency of Canada handles vaccine safety (Web Resource 45-8). They have established the Canadian Adverse Events Following Immunization Surveillance System (CAEFISS). See their website (Web Resource 45-10) for further information on submission of postimmunization AEs.

Toxic Effects of Immunogenicity to Biopharmaceuticals

Ana T. Menendez, PhD

■ Introduction

Biopharmaceuticals developed by recombinant DNA technology are delivering their great promise in therapeutics because of their excellent targeting and their ability to mimic endogenous protein counterparts. Such drugs have been successfully marketed for years, and currently dozens of novel biopharmaceuticals are undergoing clinical trials.

The advantage of biopharmaceuticals is tempered with the danger of inducing immune responses that can lead to serious adverse events (AEs) because the biopharmaceutical is recognized as "non-self." Although classic small molecule drugs can induce immunologic responses that produce AEs, these incidents are far more common with biopharmaceuticals. The immune response principally involves generating antibodies to the biopharmaceutical with the potential to induce acute life-threatening anaphylactic Type I reactions (if IgE antibodies are generated) or less dangerous but more common infusion reactions, consisting of symptoms such as headache, nausea, fever, chills, dizziness, flushing, pruritus, and chest or back pain. Nonacute consequences are generated from delayed T-cell hypersensitivity and immune complexes, which result in myalgia, arthralgia with fever, skin rash, pruritus, and other symptoms. The worst immunological

safety situation occurs when patients begins to produce antibodies to their own endogenous proteins, in which case all treatment needs to be halted and immunosuppressive lifesaving support must be given.

All antibodies bind the therapeutic drug and can cause antibody–drug immune complexes that are cleared quickly from the serum and decrease efficacy. Immune complexes may also produce toxicity by producing renal damage in sensitive populations. A subset of these antibodies is called neutralizing because they can also directly block the interaction of the drug with its therapeutic target. Neutralizing antibodies have a clear effect on efficacy and may also be responsible for toxicity if they obliterate the endogenous protein.

Various external factors, such as the patient population, the disease being treated, the dose, the administration route, etc., can play a role in the immunogenicity of the drug. Product quality issues, such as inappropriate impurity clearance processes and improper handling of the vial, can also induce aggregation or abnormal forms of the biopharmaceutical before it is administered to the patient. Deviations from the recommended instructions for storing and preparing the biopharmaceutical can also produce safety problems. U.S. Food and Drug Administration (FDA), European Medicines Agency (EMA), and other agencies require that immunogenicity issues be characterized as best as possible during development as well as after marketing begins. A Risk Evaluation and Mitigation Strategy/Risk Management Plan (REMS/RMP) is also required in most cases with the marketing application. This document is project-specific and must contain a communication strategy covering any immunogenicity issues previously identified, expected, or discovered after commercialization. Risk minimization and mitigation efforts, in addition to communication measures, include specific investigation tools like antibody testing assays. Case studies on various biopharmaceuticals follow, illustrating the varied immunologic consequences seen with biopharmaceuticals.

■ Granulocyte-Colony Stimulating Factor (G-CSF): Minimal Antibody Production

Recombinant G-CSF is used to boost neutrophil production in patients undergoing chemotherapy. The binding antibody rate was low (3%) during clinical trials, as expected in an immunosuppressed population, and the antibodies were not neutralizing. Infusion reactions were rare. A biosimilar was recently approved that demonstrated no sign of immunogenicity.

■ Thrombopoietin (TPO): Major Immunogenic Toxicity

Endogenous TPO is required for the growth of megakaryocytes, the precursor of platelets found in bone marrow. Clinical trials with exogenous TPO or pegylated TPO demonstrated a high immunogenic incidence of neutralizing antibodies to endogenous TPO. The treatment caused severe thrombocytopenia in both healthy volunteers and cancer patients due to marked reduction of megakaryocytes. Elevated levels of inactive TPO were also observed. TPO has the potential to be an important therapeutic protein, but despite many clinical trials, currently no approved forms of TPO are on the market because of its high immunogenicity risk.

■ Insulin: Antibodies Without Significant Clinical Toxicity

Insulin was one of the first biopharmaceuticals developed (first available in 1922), using extracts of porcine and bovine pancreas. Some patients who developed antibodies to insulin not only exhibited allergic reactions and became resistant to insulin but also had more frequent hypoglycemic events. This counterintuitive effect occurred because the insulin-antibody immune complex acted as a slow release depot for the insulin. Thus, the patient received insulin from the immediate injection and from the insulin released later from the immune complex. Preparations that were not properly cleaned of pancreatic residue produced a significant number of AEs.

The development of recombinant insulin greatly reduced the immunogenic response. Antibody expression with these new preparations remains stable or decreases over time, with few AEs or loss of efficacy. An immunogenic response, when it does happen, does not seem to impact the glycemic index or produce significant AEs. Inhaled recombinant insulin produced significant binding and neutralizing antibodies, but interestingly, they did not affect efficacy or safety. Thus, immunogenicity is not considered a significant safety concern with the current recombinant insulin preparations.

■ Natalizumab: Short-Term, Self-Limited Adverse Reactions

This product is a monoclonal antibody that belongs to a new class of drug called selective adhesion molecule inhibitors. It binds to the cell surface to reduce the inflammatory response in multiple sclerosis patients.

Natalizumab induces two types of immunogenic responses in 3–4% of multiple sclerosis patients: (1) a persistent response that remains steady over treatment and (2) a transient response that peaks at about 3 months posttreatment and resolves by 6 months.

1. The persistent population experienced a complete loss of efficacy caused by rapid clearance of natalizumab and the presence of neutralizing antibodies. About three quarters of persistent patients also suffered infusion-related AEs.

2. The transient population (~1/3 of the patients that exhibited an immune response) experienced equivalent efficacy and infusion-related reactions compared to patients that did not express antibodies.

Infusion reactions consisted of hypersensitivity, urticaria, rigors, nausea, vomiting, flushing, myalgia, hypertension, dyspnea, anxiety, and tachycardia. A pharmacovigilance plan was developed, and it was concluded that patients who experience disease progression or continued infusion reactions must be evaluated for the presence of antibodies, with repeat testing after 3 months to confirm persistent antibody status. As most patients do not develop antibodies, routine monitoring is usually not required of patients undergoing treatment. Natalizumab has been noted to produce a rare but sometimes fatal adverse reaction: progressive multifocal leukoencephalopathy (PML) as well as immune reconstitution inflammatory syndrome (IRIS).

Although some of the manifestations of these AEs implicate the immune system, the direct mechanisms and causes are still undergoing investigation.

Infliximab: Additional Immunosuppressive Therapy Needed

Patients who suffer from inflammatory diseases (rheumatoid arthritis, psoriasis, etc.) are routinely treated with biopharmaceuticals that block tumor necrosis factor-a. Infliximab is a humanized mouse antibody that was the first anti-TNF-α biopharmaceutical. Numerous postapproval studies clearly demonstrated that patients who produce antibody have more infusion reactions, less likelihood of clinical remission, and faster relapse. Patients also required additional concomitant treatment, such as azathioprine, mercaptopurine, methotrexate, or mesalamine, to achieve maximal benefit. The presence of pretreatment antinuclear antibodies predicted an increased immunogenicity risk and infusion reactions. Interestingly, a fully humanized monoclonal antibody to TNF-α did not demonstrate a significantly different immunogenic profile.

Enzyme Replacement Therapy: Endogenous Protein Is Absent

Several rare diseases consist of a genetic enzymatic deficiency that results in faulty lysosomal storage. The lack of expression of a particular protein in a patient presents a unique risk since the patient's immune system recognizes the protein as "non-self." In some cases, constant exposure to the biopharmaceutical can induce tolerance. The use of immunosuppressive regimens usually allows continued efficacy.

Fabry disease is an X-linked lysozome storage disorder characterized by deficient expression of a-galactosidase, resulting in renal, cardiologic, skin, and eye problems. Recombinant α-galactosidase is the

principal treatment. Males with this disease have a higher rate of antibodies against the enzyme because the protein is unknown to the immune system, whereas antibody production in female carriers is low because they have some residual α-galactosidase production. More than 50% of the male patients develop IgG-related infusion reactions with chills, fever, acroparesthesias, and dyspnea.

Pompe disease is a progressive glycogen storage disease due to the lack of a-glucosidase, which produces muscle weakness with cardiac, pulmonary, and other symptoms. It is seen in infants, children, and adults. The presence of antibodies to recombinant a-glucosidase therapy poses a serious obstacle to successful treatment. Specific protocols that increase immune tolerance of the treatments (e.g., rituxan, methotrexate, cyclosporine) have produced better clinical outcomes.

Gaucher's disease is a lipid storage disease caused by a deficiency of glucocerebrosidase producing various symptoms, including bone pain, fractures, cognitive impairment, easy bruising, hepatosplenomegaly, cardiac and lung problems, and seizures. Treatment is recombinant glucocerebrosidase. Since the approval of the drug in 1994, an intensive 10-year pharmacovigilance study focusing on immunogenicity was performed. The immunosurveillance summary data indicated a trend of variable antibody response during the early period, which became less variable with more mature manufacturing processes. The patients developed IgG to recombinant glucocerebrosidase within the first 6 months of treatment and rarely developed antibodies after 12 months. The most frequently reported AEs were nonserious infusion reactions that were predominantly self-limiting and were managed by decreasing the rate of infusion or pretreatment with antihistamines or anti-inflammatory drugs.

Erythropoietin (EPO): Formulation Change Producing Immunotoxicity

EPO is an endogenous protein required for the growth of erythrocytes. Various genetically modified variants and formulations of recombinant erythropoietin have been widely used since 1989 to treat renal and nonrenal anemia. Reports of antibodies were rare. In 1999, a sharp increase of pure red cell aplasia (PRCA) was observed due to neutralizing antibodies to endogenous EPO. This increased incidence was only found in patients treated with Eprex brand in prefilled syringes containing the product in polysorbate 80 instead of the previous formulation containing human serum albumin. Most of the cases required immunosuppressive therapy after cessation of

EPO treatment to stop antibody development to endogenous EPO. The PRCA incidence in Eprex was decreased by 83% after procedures were adopted to ensure appropriate storage, handling, and administration. No clear cause of the immunogenicity was found, though there is some suggestion that the formation of aggregates was the most likely explanation in the new formulation. This history resulted in stringent immunogenicity requirements in the regulatory guidances for EPOs.

■ Conclusions

Biopharmaceuticals can produce many different types of immunologic effects. They range from minimum antibody production (G-CSF) to major toxicity, precluding further development and use (TPO). In certain situations, antibodies were produced but did not significantly affect the therapy (recombinant insulin). Other biopharmaceuticals can either demonstrate a short-term, self-limited reaction or a persistent response that leads to cessation of therapy only for the persistent population (natalizumab), while others require additional immunosuppressive intervention to block antibody formation (infliximab, enzyme replacement therapy). Finally, changes in manufacturing processes (recombinant glucocerebrosidase) and formulation (EPO) can alter or produce immunogenicity. As with all therapies, each biopharmaceutical should be treated as a novel substance, and a carefully thought-out RES/RMP with an immunogenicity plan should be done and is usually obligatory.

One should also keep in mind that all of the classic toxicity (similar to small molecule drugs) may be seen as well as idiosyncratic adverse reactions. Product-quality issues may also be greater than those seen with small molecule drugs, as the manufacturing processes are often far more complex with biological products. Poor storage, packaging problems, or process changes or errors can make a "clean" protein immunogenic. As with other drugs, changes in route of administration may produce increased toxicity.

Business Partners and Exchange of Safety Data

Development costs for a new chemical entity from creation to marketing range from $400 million to $2 billion (depending on how one calculates these costs) (see Frank, *J Health Econ.* 2003;325:330; Web Resources 47-1 and 47-2). In addition, patents are now being challenged and generics are proliferating. One response to these phenomena includes the development and marketing of a product by multiple partner companies. No matter which side of the argument one is on regarding the appropriateness of some drug development, these costs and risks are high and companies look for ways to protect themselves from the risks of failure.

One response is partnerships. The goal is to speed up development, share costs and risks, and use the additive or synergistic strengths of each partner. Codevelopment often is limited to two partners, but combinations of three or more partners are common, especially when expanding into areas (e.g., Japan, China) where language, laws, and customs are often a challenge for U.S. and European

Union companies or small start-ups. The current trend in the pharmaceutical world is for codevelopment and co-promotion/marketing of products as expenses skyrocket and simultaneous rather than sequential international development occurs. We are now seeing large, small, and midsized companies creating contractual arrangements with one or multiple other pharmaceutical companies, contract research organizations (CROs), and other vendors to handle development, sales, marketing, safety handling, regulatory matters, phone centers, manufacturing, and just about every other possible function except senior management. These contracts may be short-term or long-term and involve companies all over the world.

Whenever two or more companies join forces for whatever reason, a written contract must be developed between or among them. Normally, these contracts are developed by the "business development" or "licensing group" with input from the legal department and other groups on a "need-to-know" basis. Often they are developed under great secrecy (for competitive reasons), and others in the company are not informed of the situation until the last minute, when their input and/or approval is requested, often with a minimal amount of lead time. ("The CEO wants to sign this contract tomorrow morning. Please approve your section now.")

The safety group (unless involved in due diligence) may be one of those groups learning about the agreement at the last minute and asked to review a document with a minimal or even nonexistent safety section. Sometimes when the safety section is present, it is incorrect and would not keep the company in compliance with regulations in countries where the partners are working or help protect the company from litigation and other pitfalls.

When such a situation occurs, the immediate acute step is to ask that the safety section, if inadequate, be removed and replaced with one or both of the following:

1. A "generic" or "one-size-fits-all" safety section (see below).

2. A statement that a safety section is needed and will be developed by the safety groups of the respective signatory companies to cover safety data issues within, say, 90 days. It will be appended to the agreement or will act as a stand-alone agreement (whichever the lawyers prefer). This time frame may need to be shortened if the sales or studies start in a shorter time. Often, however, studies or sales will not begin for several months, giving all parties sufficient time to develop a safety section.

Why a Written Safety Exchange Agreement Is Needed

There are multiple reasons to have safety agreements:

- To remain in compliance with health authority requirements (e.g., FDA: 21CFR314.80(b); EU: Volume 9A Sections 1.3 and 2.2.3.e)

- To give guidance and instructions to all involved parties with regard to their responsibilities for drug safety

- To ensure that all parties receive the safety documents they need to remain in full compliance with all regulatory and legal requirements in their jurisdictions of sale or study

- To ensure that adequate signaling is done and that a benefit-to-risk analysis incorporates as complete a database as possible

- To produce the best product labeling possible to protect the public health

- To have data ready for a corporate audit or health authority inspection

- To have data available for litigation should that situation arise

Telling the Safety Department About a New Contract or Arrangement

The safety department should be informed of any agreement being negotiated early on in the process so it can review the document and determine what is needed concerning safety. This should be included in all company standard operating procedures (SOPs) on the negotiation of agreements with other parties where drug products (either finished products or components) are involved. Agreements for non-product-related items do not need to be included (e.g., raw chemical products, supplying vending machines, or ordering furniture).

Many types of arrangements must have safety agreements. They include but are not limited to agreements on licensing-in or licensing-out; manufacturing; comarketing; codevelopment, including preclinical or clinical development; advertising; clinical study research; consultants; contract sales forces; distribution; disease management programs; patient support programs; promotion and copromotion; speakers bureau consultants; master vendors; other vendors; and other services. These contracts may cover all possible permutations: prescription drugs, over-the-counter drugs, drugs that are prescription in one country and over the counter in another, biologics, blood products, devices, nutraceuticals, cosmetics, foods, and combination products (a device with a drug in it, such as a prefilled syringe, a drug-impregnated gauze pad, or two drugs in one tablet).

The Generic, Boilerplate, or Template Agreement

Even before any agreement is on the table, the drug safety and the legal groups (at least) should develop a "boilerplate," "generic," or template agreement approved by management and general enough to be inserted into almost any type of contract anywhere in the world, either in the body of the contract or as an appendix, until a customized agreement is made to replace it. Multiple regional versions and languages might be necessary. The agreement should, at the very least, specify the following:

- Exchange between the parties of all serious adverse events (SAEs) from clinical trials, spontaneous reporting, solicited reporting, literature, special arrangements (e.g., named patient or compassionate use) and health authorities. Cases should be exchanged as either MedWatch/CIOMS I forms or E2B files within a specified time frame from first receipt by anyone in the companies or their agents. They should be exchanged in sufficient time to meet expedited reporting rules (usually 15 calendar days) so that exchange should, in general, be no later than 10 or so calendar days. Deaths and life-threatening SAEs from trials should be exchanged in time to meet 7-day reporting requirements (e.g., 5 calendar days) for deaths and life-threatening events. If this is too difficult to distinguish from other SAEs, then all SAEs should be exchanged in 5 or so calendar days.

- All regulatory submissions (Periodic Safety Update Reports [PSURs], NDA Periodic Reports, Annual Reports, and their local equivalents) should be exchanged between the parties within a specified time (e.g., 1 week) after submission to the health authorities.

- A formal and detailed safety agreement will be completed by the two drug safety groups within, say, 90 days of the signing of the contract.

The above generic agreement should suffice in almost all cases until the formal safety document is created. Additions, of course, may be added to the generic agreement if the specific case warrants it and if there is sufficient time to get agreement internally and from the other contractual partner. This could include exchange of communications with the health authorities, including safety reviews of PSURs, literature searches, and a data dump (e.g., a paper printout or an electronic file of all AEs in the safety database) from the partner holding the safety database.

Developing a Safety Agreement with the Safety Department

As soon as the type of contract is determined and the safety department is brought into the discussions, the area of involvement should be ascertained: geographic territories (e.g., United States only, United States and the European Union, Canada, Poland, etc.), regulatory and marketing status indications (MA/NDA approved, in clinical trials only), labeling, etc. This allows the tailoring of the specific agreement to ensure that all needs are met.

At this point the safety and regulatory departments will be able to determine what is needed. If the drug has never been marketed, for example, there will not be an issue of postmarketing spontaneous SAE reports, and this may not need to be included in the agreement (though a clause indicating that the agreement will be revised, say, 60 days before a marketing request is submitted anywhere in the world does). If more than one other partner is involved, this also allows the signatories to determine various responsibilities and negotiate any new or altered requirements.

Again, there is no "one-size-fits-all" safety arrangement that can simply be dropped into a contract to take care of everything. Each agreement must be negotiated individually. Usually, face-to-face contacts between the two (or more) safety departments facilitate the successful preparation of a safety agreement. As always, contrary to the saying, business is personal, and it is always easier to develop a successful working relationship of trust and confidence if personal contact has been established rather than relying only on e-mails, video conferences, and telephone calls. A meeting should be set up at the earliest reasonable time after preliminary negotiations are started to hammer out the final document. The safety department needs to be given sufficient authority to negotiate such an agreement (pending, of course, final management and legal approval on both sides). The complexity of these agreements increases exponentially if multiple companies and CROs are involved. In such situations, it is usually worthwhile for one of the companies or partners to take the lead in safety matters.

The Safety Agreement Database

For companies that make many agreements worldwide, it is imperative that a database containing the key points of the safety agreements (and if possible the imaged agreements themselves) be maintained. Multinational companies may have tens of thousands of such agreements, in multiple countries, in multiple languages, often with differing products, durations, responsibilities, and territories. The agreements will become out of date rapidly as new terms are made, new products launched, new formulations made, and new partners (or distributors or sales forces, etc.) brought in or terminated. A database will help track this. The database may start as a spreadsheet, but it may be necessary to develop (with the IT department) or purchase a database to track and report on agreements. As always, the database must have the appropriate security, testing, validation, and change control.

Historically, the legal and new business departments will not keep sufficiently detailed records to ensure regulatory compliance regarding safety matters (a sad fact). Thus, it falls on the drug safety department to do its best to ensure that all revisions to agreements are transmitted to the central (or designated) safety department. A dedicated person must be designated and have the responsibility to track and revise such agreements and changes to them. Any new conditions (new INDs, NDAs, Marketing Authorizations, new products, new regulations, new PSUR dates, etc.) must be transmitted to the drug safety groups involved (e.g., the processing group, the PSUR group). In the European Union, the QPPV is responsible for ensuring that this occurs. Periodic reports of contracts in force, dates of expiration (where they exist), and obligations should be issued to the parties who need them.

The Safety Agreement Contents

Ideally, all agreements should be in English or available in English, especially in companies that work or sell across borders. This is not always the case. If not, they should be translated into English for all parties involved to be able to know and adhere to their obligations. The contents should cover the following:

The Regulatory Status

A table by country with approval date, license holder, companies marketing the product, and name should be included. A copy of the regulatory table in a PSUR is usually acceptable. It should contain:

- IND or equivalents
- MAs, NDAs/BLAs, or equivalents (in the European Union, type of approval: central, mutual recognition, etc.)
- Other: named patient/compassionate use, restrictions on use
- REMS/RMPs in place

The Regulatory Responsibilities

The regulatory status of the products may not be the same in each territory or country. It may be a marketed product in one and in clinical trials in the other. All this must be tracked. It should be clarified what regulatory status and responsibilities are to be held by each party and in what country (if multiple countries are involved). Particular attention should be paid to assignment of regulatory responsibilities in countries where each contractual party has a regulatory office or physical presence. The actual

names and contact information for the responsible parties should be listed in an appendix (allowing easy updating of changes in personnel, phone numbers).

It should be clarified who reports in each country, who makes contact with health authorities, who answers questions (and if consultation with the other party is obtained or not within X number of days, etc.), and how REMS/RMPs or special conditions are handled. The qualified person(s) in the European Union should be clearly stated. A mechanism should be outlined for the obtaining of any waivers or changes to routine procedures that may be desired by the clinical teams, such as reporting certain SAEs monthly or quarterly rather than as expedited reports.

For the European Union, the Qualified Person must be clearly specified. If there are two (one in each company), duties must be agreed on and the competent authorities so notified.

Regulatory Documents

The owner and maintainer of documents should be specified for the Investigator Brochure, the SmPC/PI/PIL, all other labeling (CCSI), the Package Insert, the product monograph, the investigational and clinical core safety documents, and protocols. Any consultation and approval for each should be specified. The timing and format of exchange should be spelled out for all documents. There should be an assurance that the latest documents in force will be sent out to all parties automatically on update or revision.

Health Authority Queries and Requests

It should be stated clearly how health authority requests and queries are to be handled. Usually, the company in the country where the request is made must do the physical answering (in the local language), but the content of the response needs to be done by agreed-on methods, particularly if it is a critical medical question involving stopping of studies, drug withdrawal, or labeling change. Case-specific questions of minor import may usually be answered locally, but anything more important should be resolved by the appropriate groups in each company (usually through a joint operating committee). A method of dispute resolution must be specified so that senior management can make the final determination in the appropriate time frame. This usually involves the regulatory and safety departments as well as the clinical research groups in each company. Any "pass through" situations (e.g., by a CRO to the sponsor) should be spelled out. The mechanism of answering questions and requirements from health agency reviewers of PSURs should also be made clear, particularly if questions are received from multiple authorities for each PSUR.

■ Regulatory Submissions

Who submits which documents in which countries should be clearly noted. This includes individual cases (7- and 15-day cases) whether by paper or E2B. Whether copies of submissions should be exchanged (even though the identical MedWatch or CIOMS I form has already been exchanged by the drug safety groups already) should be stated. This might be necessary if the other party wishes to know the serial number (in IND submissions) or date of submission. EudraVigilance submissions should also be clarified.

Similarly, all other regulatory submissions (investigator brochures, labeling changes, PSURs, NDA periodic reports, annual reports, IND annual reports, information amendments, desk copies, postmarketing commitments, REMS/RMPs, etc.) should be spelled out and exchange methodology noted. It is critical to specify whether the other parties have review and approval privileges or are merely given information copies of such documents.

■ Investigator and Investigational Review Board/Ethics Committee Notifications: Blinding and Unblinding, Data Safety Management Boards

The mechanism and responsibilities for the preparation of the investigator notification of expedited reports (also called the investigator letter), new IB versions, and changes in the benefit–risk analysis need to be detailed. In addition, in those countries where the sponsor must inform the Ethics Committees/Investigational Review Boards, this should be spelled out. It should be clarified whether the same exact letter is to be used worldwide, and if so, whether a mechanism for its preparation (within the same 15-calendar-day time frame required for the alert report) must be specified.

Most regulatory agencies prefer or require that all expedited reports be submitted unblinded (the code broken). If this is done, the companies must agree on a mechanism for unblinding and the transmission of the unblinded cases (or just the unblinding code) to the other party(ies). This can be difficult if companies want to keep the clinical research team and statisticians blinded.

If one or more Data Safety Management Boards are involved either in clinical trials or even (as some companies now do) after marketing, the responsibilities of the partners in regard to these committees should be spelled out, including the powers and functions of the boards and the interactions with the various partners.

■ Safety Databases

The parties should agree on who will keep and maintain what data in their respective databases. It should be agreed by all parties that one party (often the largest company or the originating company) maintains the "official" database that will be used as the definitive one for preparing all regulatory reports.

It is nearly impossible, if not totally impossible, to maintain up-to-date, fully reconciled databases when each party has its own database. The maintenance of reconciled, separate databases by each company (even if the same brand of commercial database) produces differences between or among the databases. Problems arise if there are different drug dictionaries, different ways of handling data (e.g., laboratory), different coding conventions, different MedDRA versions, different narrative writing styles, and so on.

All parties should "agree to disagree" and accept that each will maintain a database but that one agreed-on database will be the "official" one. In the European Union, the Qualified Person for PV must be physically present in Europe with direct access to the database (per Volume 9A), making this database the "official" one for the European Union at the very least.

As an alternative, only one database is maintained by one company with access to the data for the drug in question by the other companies. This has been problematic in the past but newer technologies, with the database remaining in the "cloud" on the internet in a single database, can go a long way to resolve this if all parties agree. The major difficulties are usually political and corporate rather than technical or IT.

The parties must agree on whose SOPs, guidelines, manuals, and so forth, apply where, when, and to whom. In some cases, one or more new SOPs will be created for that partnership only. In other cases, each party uses its own SOPs and reconciliations or changes are made as needed.

Definitions

Either in the body of the agreement or as an appendix, the parties should agree on the definitions of terms used, including serious, nonserious, medically significant (important), labeling, expedited, expected, unexpected, labeled, unlabeled, listed, unlisted, and causality (relatedness). This may be a contentious issue because there are no international standards for causality, and the parties need to agree on definitions, particularly for ambiguous terms such as "unlikely related," the four criteria for the minimal data set, clock start date, and so on. The language of exchange should be specified as well, and how documents not in English will be handled (full translations or not).

The clock start date is sometimes an area of controversy. The United States and the European Union largely agree that the clock start day is day zero and it starts when anyone anywhere in any company, agent, distributor, and so forth, receives sufficient detail to make the case a valid ICSR (patient, drug, reporter, AE). Not all countries agree on this, however, and some start the clock at a later date (when the case is received by the company in that country from a foreign source). The most conservative and usually wisest course is to start the clock when the first person anywhere has enough detail for the case to be valid.

Data and Mechanisms of Data Exchange

The physical exchange method must be specified:

- Paper copies versus E2B.
- "Push versus pull," that is, does party A send ("push") data to party B or does party B go onto a website or portal to obtain ("pull") it. How are confirmations handled? It is not enough for party A to send a case; party B must actually receive it. This needs to be verified with acknowledgment of receipt mechanism built in.
- Mechanism of transmission: fax, e-mail with attached PDF files, source documents.
- Documents in which a signature copy is needed to be maintained on file.
- Privacy and anonymization issues to ensure data security and privacy.

Documents to be exchanged must be specified. This is particularly critical for individual case reports. Will MedWatch forms, CIOMS I forms, an SAE data collection form, source documents or an E2B file be exchanged? If CIOMS I or MedWatch forms are exchanged, will they be complete or in draft and on what day after clock start? If source documents are exchanged initially, will finalized MedWatch or CIOMS I forms also be exchanged? Is it acceptable that each party creates its own narrative and coding, realizing that there will be differences between the two (or more) parties? If reconciliation is desired, how can this be done rapidly so that 7- and 15-day reports are consistent? How are follow-up data handled?

- In practice, it is common that the party that receives the case handles the full processing of the case (including follow-up) and sends a completed MedWatch or CIOMS I form or E2B to the other partner(s) by a particular calendar day (usually 8 to 10 days after clock start). This will allow the other parties to upload or enter the data into their database (unchanged) and transmit any expedited cases to the health authority. This will also allow them time to check the case against local labeling if the product is marketed with different labeling in the recipient company's territories.

- Once a sufficient volume of cases is attained (suggesting success in the clinical trial or marketing), a "well-oiled machine" must exist to process and transmit SAEs, particularly if the volumes are high. Reconciliation and "discussions" over particular cases must be the exception and not the rule if on-time regulatory reporting is to be maintained. Keep in mind that submission of a case as an expedited report does not admit that the drug caused the event.

- Seven-day expedited reports from clinical trials must be handled in a much more rapid time frame (usually 4–5 calendar days) to ensure regulatory compliance.

- Companies should reach agreement that the most conservative call on seriousness, expectedness, and causality carries the day for SAEs. That is, if one company believes a case is unlabeled or possibly related and the other does not, the case is considered unlabeled or possibly related. This may force a company to submit a case as an expedited report that it does not believe to be one because the other company does.

- If CROs are involved, the agreement must account for them in terms of timing and exchange method. Written agreements with the clinical research organizations are, of course, required. The regulatory agencies must be notified in writing of the duties devolved onto the clinical research organization(s).

- In the European Union, if there are several companies and thus several QPs, the single "designated" QP should be noted and the dealings between and among the other QPs clarified.

- Follow-ups are done by the party receiving the original SAE (or nonserious AE if follow-ups are done for these). The other parties may pose questions for the company doing the follow-up but usually follow-up is left to their discretion and medical expertise. It should be specified when it is done and how frequently. All follow-up information is handled in the same manner as initial information. It should be stated clearly who reviews the worldwide literature for SAEs and NSAEs and how they are handled when found. If the drug is marketed in the European Union, literature for the product should be searched weekly.

A method used by many companies is as follows:

- All SAEs are exchanged as CIOMS I/MedWatch forms or E2B files by calendar day 10 after clock start anywhere in the world at the first company (or agent) and used as-is, without changes to coding or narrative. Much less commonly, the SAE data collection form or source documents (from clinical trials and spontaneous cases) are exchanged by calendar day 5. In this case, each company writes its own narrative and does its own coding based on this "source document" to create an ICSR. Each company submits its own version to the regulatory agencies in its domain. Because these reports are created by each company on their own, they differ. If some documents are not in English, this should be noted and should not be a surprise to the company receiving untranslated documents.

- All clinical trial deaths or life-threatening SAEs are exchanged within 4 to 5 calendar days. Sometimes this is limited to the subset of unlabeled (unexpected) cases only; this requires that the receiving company trust the judgment of the sending company on labeledness. This covers 7-day expedited cases.

- All nonserious spontaneous cases are exchanged on a monthly basis (or twice monthly if the volume is very large). Line listings or MedWatch/CIOMS I forms/E2B files may be used.

- Nonserious clinical trial cases are not exchanged and are kept only in the clinical trial database of the company(ies) doing the trial.

- Follow-up is done for all SAEs, with at least two contacts attempted for spontaneous cases (more

if a critical case such as an alert report) and whatever is necessary for clinical trial cases (where the investigator should be accessible to give complete follow-up).

■ Signaling, Safety Reviews, and Risk Management

The agreement should specify how signaling is done by one or more parties and, if so, how disputes are resolved. It is common to form a safety review committee that meets periodically, usually by telephone, webinar, or video conference, to review the logistics and operational issues of safety handling as well as any SAEs and safety signals that arise. Usually, the logistics and operations dominate the initial meetings until all glitches are resolved. At that point, with operational issues minimal and with more SAEs arriving, the signal reviewers predominate. Meetings may be weekly to biweekly initially and then at a monthly or quarterly frequency if no safety or signaling issues arrive. Ad hoc meetings should be held, as needed, for urgent issues. It should be clear how risk management is handled and who prepares and approves any RMPs or REMS that might be needed.

■ Audits

A quality system procedure should be in place to ensure that all requirements for safety are in place. Audits should occur periodically to ensure this. The audits may be done by each company (or a third party) and should look at the contracts to be sure they are adequate and that their provisions are followed by all parties.

■ Other Issues

If not noted elsewhere, mechanisms for dispute resolution should be described in detail.

- Other product-specific issues relating to devices, vaccines, biologics, and nutraceuticals.

- Any specific regulatory requests (e.g., special reporting of certain SAEs) should be mentioned.

- An agreed-on time to review the safety exchange agreement should be specified. It is usually yearly but may be more or less frequently if circumstances warrant. Any change in regulatory status (e.g., a new trial, indication, MA/NDA approval) should trigger a review of the safety agreement.

- Agreement on who does medical literature searches should also be noted.
- Risk management agreements and postmarketing commitments with health agencies should also be exchanged and agreed on.
- Risk management/minimization issues and postmarketing commitments and promises.
- Inspections and audits of one another and by third parties (that is, health agencies). How are they handled? Who is present? How are issues resolved?
- All arrangements must be written down in the Summary (or Description) of PV Systems kept by companies with MAs or trials in the European Union.
- Duplicate submissions of cases to the same health authority must be avoided.
- A mechanism to track changes in safety regulations and requirements should be in place and the agreements updated as needed.
- Usual and unusual marketing arrangements and programs must be covered (e.g. patient support programs, local clinical or observational trials).
- If companies merge, acquire, or sell or transfer the MA, the safety responsibilities must still be done and accounted for.
- Any outsourcing or subcontracting should be agreed on by all parties.
- Training, particularly where differences in procedures produce different processes, must be done and coordinated as necessary.
- A mechanism to handle crisis management, recalls, withdrawals, and stopping trials must be developed and agreed on.
- Appendices.

The appendices should contain information that may change frequently, including names, addresses, contact information, territories in question, product names, and registration numbers.

Soft Points

- Do not underestimate cultural (both national and corporate) differences, language matters, business etiquette, communication, leadership, and logistics. Someone must be in charge and the maximum

in diplomacy and goodwill should be used to smooth and resolve the issues that will invariably arise.

- Keep in mind time zones when partners are on two or more continents. If Asia, North America, and Europe are involved, someone will always be up in the middle of the night for any teleconference!
- Particular difficulties may occur in "big pharma"–"small pharma" agreements. The "big" players should be particularly sensitive not to dictate a "know-it-all" attitude. There must be understanding that some things will be difficult politically and culturally in the other company because of politics, culture, stubbornness, and local legal matters. Small companies may not have the resources of big players and one person may have many responsibilities.
- It is wise to have at least one face-to-face meeting before the contract is in place and then periodically after the contract begins.
- Not everybody speaks, writes, or understands English well. This is particularly an issue between a large company located in a native-English-speaking country and a small firm in a non-English-speaking country. Again, sensitivity to such differences should be kept in mind.
- Management should be (where possible) sensitized to the criticality of safety exchange. Failure to get this right can produce enormously bad consequences for all parties (not to mention the patients!).

Comments

Health authorities and inspectors are now paying particular attention to safety exchange agreements as more complexity has been introduced into the pharmaceutical world, with more outsourcing, fragmentation, and specialization of functions.

Inspectors insist that all responsibilities be noted in contracts and agreements so that all PV obligations are fulfilled. In the European Union, the QP will be the focal point of this. The inspectors will expect the contracts and documents to be available and the appropriate parts to be in English so that they (and the drug safety department) are able to read them.

Audits and Inspections

The Basics

The U.S. Food and Drug (FDA), the European Medicines Agency (EMA), the United Kingdom's Medicines and Healthcare Products Regulatory Agency (MHRA), Health Canada, and many other national health authorities are permitted or required by law to perform inspections of companies to ensure that they comply with all safety reporting regulations.

■ The Basics

Although the terms often used interchangeably, audit and inspection are not quite the same. An inspection in the drug safety context generally refers to an inquiry, examination, and verification of processes, data, records, regulatory compliance and databases etc. by a government or official authority. An audit is the same but done by a nongovernmental entity, such as one's own company, or a partner, vendor, supplier, client, and so forth. Note: In this chapter, unless otherwise specified, the terms will be used interchangeably.

Government inspections are largely done to protect the public health: to verify compliance to the regulations, to monitor the industry, as part of normal business (e.g., a routine every 2 to 3-year inspection), for cause to investigate a problem. Audits are done primarily for business reasons: compliance to regulations; due diligence of a new or ongoing vendor, partner, client, supplier; investigation of a problem; routine as part of a quality management system, and so forth.

Such audits and inspections may be periodic and routine (e.g., yearly) covering one or more products, general or specific (e.g., look at a newly installed IT system) or they may be nonperiodic for cause, looking at a specific problem or issue. "Targets" of the audit include the pharma company (headquarters, regional or national offices, clinical research, monitors, legal, the CEOs office, telephone operators, websites and webmasters, regulatory, legal, sales, marketing, ad agencies, data entry, IT department, training department, medical writing, aggregate reporting group (PSURs), licensing group, compliance/quality group, manufacturing, product quality partners, distributors, codevelopers, licensees and licensors, vendors, contractors, CROs, data storage facilities, archiving, investigator sites, and anyone in the safety "chain." It may cover clinical research and unapproved drugs or marketed products or both.

Most agencies now are doing inspections on a risk basis. That is, they classify and inspect on a priority basis those companies perceived to be at higher risk of having safety issues. The agencies use either a formal risk rating system (MHRA; see below) or a more informal ranking (companies that just merged, have safety problems, launch a major new or toxic drug, etc.) to prioritize their inspections.

For inspections in the European Union, a very detailed document must be supplied some 6 to 8 weeks before the inspection. This document comes in several forms, depending on the country (called the Summary of PV Systems in the United Kingdom and the Detailed Description of PV Systems by the EMA). It must be prepared and submitted before an inspection (and in MA filings). It may run, with appendices, hundreds of pages, and is supplied on a CD or DVD. In addition, the United Kingdom also requests that firms supply a "Compliance Report," which measures a firm's "risk" and "control." See Chapter 45 for full details on these reports.

■ Scope of the Audit

Anything and anyone involved in AEs and safety are fair game. The audit will cover the processing and handling of safety information from all sources; SOPs; working documents, guidances, manuals; measurable and quantifiable data; follow-up; coding (MedDRA, drugs); literature review; medical information; queries and questions; expedited reporting (7-and 15-day reports); periodic reporting; risk management and epidemiology; safety agreements with partners, codevelopers, CROs, and so forth; handling of technical and product quality complaints; medication errors; registries; call centers; outsourcing and off-shoring; quality systems; IT; data privacy and security; data backup and archiving; training; off-hour and weekend/holiday coverage; crisis management; safety information communication; safety labeling; signaling; and problem escalation.

The auditors will likely ask for the following documents:

- General
  - Organizational charts to ascertain the personnel involved in handling AEs, complaints, and safety data
  - All procedural safety documents including standard operating procedures (SOPs), working documents, guidelines, manuals

  - All correspondence, meeting minutes, and notes relating to AE handling both internal and external (including health authorities)
  - A list of all products marketed in the country concerned along with their approved current labeling
  - A list of all collection sites, processing sites, and reporting units that handle cases
  - Copies of all contracts or safety agreements covering the receipt, handling, evaluation, and reporting of AEs to the health authorities
  - Job descriptions and training records
  - The quality system in place
  - How medical literature is searched (which databases) and handled
  - For European Union inspections, all information pertaining to the Qualified Person and his or her duties and function
- Specific Products
  - Drugs most likely to have unexpected SAEs
  - Drugs that could cause serious medical problems if they fail to produce their expected pharmacologic actions
  - Drugs most likely to have unexpected AEs are those meeting the following criteria:
    - Approved recently (e.g., last year or two)
    - New molecular entities
    - Known or suspected bioavailability or bioequivalence problems
  - REMS/RMPs, postmarketing safety commitments
- Specific Cases
  - A list of late expedited reports for the last year or two
  - Serious unlabeled AEs, particularly those involving death or hospitalization
  - Incomplete, serious, unexpected AEs or reports with unlabeled AEs and no outcome
  - Incomplete or nonvalid cases
  - "Non-cases"—that is, cases that do not have all four minimum criteria
  - Pregnancy listings

They will examine the cases for completeness and accuracy to ensure that all serious and unexpected spontaneous reports were submitted to the health agency within 15 calendar days:

- Was information on the form available at the time of submission?
- Was all relevant information included on the form?
- Was the initial receiving date supplied to the agency the same date as the initial receipt of information by the manufacturer?
- Was new follow-up information submitted to the agency?
- Where feasible, particularly when hospitalization, permanent disability, or death occurred, did the firm obtain important follow-up information to enable complete evaluation of the report?
- PSURs/PADERs
  - Copies of some or all of the reports for the drug(s) for the last year or two
  - Are all the appropriate reports and listings included?
  - Were the reports submitted in a timely manner?
  - Periodic reports that include unexpected SAEs that should have been submitted as 15-day reports
- IT Matters
  - Validation documents, change control SOP, disaster recovery procedures and results of testing, a system demonstration
- Clinical Trial Safety
  - Study protocol and amendments
  - IRB approvals, amendments, and yearly reapproval
  - Consent (including amendments)
  - Investigator brochure and updates
  - Investigator meeting presentations
  - Data safety monitoring board charter and meeting minutes
  - Investigator/IRB/ethics committee notifications for 15-day reports

The inspectors will request to meet with the appropriate people (both managers and staff) to go through the documents received. The company needs to make preparations (see below) to handle these requests. Questions may include the following:

- How does each type of AE come into the company and how are they handled?
- Are AEs being missed? Are all possible routes of entry into the company covered to ensure that cases are not missed?

- How are cases numbered and tracked?
- Case handling specifics: How are electronic (EDC, E2B), mail, and phone cases triaged and handled? How are AEs or potential AEs and complaints logged in?
- Are medical evaluations performed for each case and by whom and when?
- How and when is follow-up done?
- Who assesses seriousness and labeledness? Is the correct label used?
- Who determines whether a case is a 15-day alert report or is to be included in the PSURs/PADERs?
- Who sends the expedited reports and periodic reports to the health authorities? Where are these documents stored (paper or electronically) or archived?
- How is labeling handled and how does the company ensure that the labeling reflects the safety status of the drug?
- Are all the databases (commercial or custombuilt) used for drug safety functions in compliance regarding validation, change control, data security and privacy, audit trails, and so forth?

In general, the government inspectors can see everything, though in general they do not look at commercial and money issues. The question of whether to supply internal or external audits of a company's drug safety system often arises. The companies do not want to provide internal audit reports, arguing that they do not want to be "hanged by their own reports" and will avoid writing down anything problematic to avoid this. The FDA usually has not pressed for these reports, accepting a summary or the CAPA rather than the report itself. The European Union generally asks for and receives the reports.

■ How an Inspection Flows

There are different methodologies from agency to agency and from company to company. Broadly speaking, inspectors arrive (announced or unannounced; see below) and should be immediately welcomed and brought to a well-equipped workroom. The drug safety group and the "host" (usually someone from the company compliance or auditing group who handles the logistics and flow) decide on the agenda. If governmental, the inspectors may or may not reveal all the reasons for the audit (routine, for cause, etc.).

The inspectors will ask for various documents (SOPs, line listings, organization charts, late expedited reports and PSURs, labeling, IT documents, etc) either up-front or as the inspection unrolls. They may request copies of some to take with them. The company must be able to provide these rapidly, usually within 24 hours, no matter where in the world they are stored. The inspectors will then read the documents, interview personnel, and visit the drug safety group (and others), the server area, and so forth. Company staff should take copious notes and minutes. Informal or formal summary closeouts may occur at the end of each day. Ideally, inspectors give continual feedback.

On the last day, there is a formal, scheduled closeout meeting, which senior management usually attends. The inspectors sum up their findings and issue a report. Usually, a short written summary is handed to the company at that meeting and a more formal report issued later on. In situations where very serious problems are found, the mechanisms for escalation within the health agency may be invoked (leading to severe public chastisement and other penalties) and this may be revealed at the closeout meeting. The company must then prepare a CAPA Plan (corrective action, preventive action) and put it into force.

Many agencies, particularly in the European Union, charge the company being examined for the inspection. Fees may be upward of $25,000 and more, depending on the length of the inspection. Travel expenses must also be covered. Inspections usually last a week or so at the minimum and, in egregious cases, may run months.

■ Findings

There are usually three categories of findings: (1) critical, (2) major, and (3) minor (other). The definitions vary slightly:

FDA

- Critical: Regulatory Compliance Affected. A finding that impacts the validity/usability of the data or has a significant subject protection/safety implication. This includes fraud, repeated and deliberate lack of obtaining informed consent, nonreporting/submission of a reportable adverse event.
- Major: Violation of a requirement, which individually would not directly impact data usability/validity or patient safety or regulatory compliance, but if repeated consistently, could become critical.
- Minor: Nonadherence to internal procedure or requirement.

EMA

- Critical: A deficiency in pharmacovigilance systems, practices, or processes that adversely affects the rights, safety, or well-being of patients, that poses a potential risk to public health, or that represents a serious violation of applicable legislation and guidelines.
- Major: A deficiency in pharmacovigilance systems, practices, or processes that could potentially adversely affect the rights, safety, or well-being of patients, that could potentially pose a risk to public health, or that represents a violation of applicable legislation and guidelines.
- Minor: A deficiency in pharmacovigilance systems, practices, or processes that would not be expected to adversely affect the rights, safety, or well-being of patients.

■ Penalties

These vary by country and region. For example, in the United States, several levels of penalties are possible. One or more may be imposed:

- FDA 483: A report of deficiencies following an FDA inspection. Requires a response and an action plan for correction of deficiencies.
- Establishment Inspection Report (EIR): Prepared by the inspectors, giving a very detailed account of the findings.
- Warning Letter: A letter to the CEO following repeated violations. Requires an urgent response and plan. Publicized on FDA's website.
- Seizure of product: Cessation of sales, termination of the NDA.
- Consent decree: An agreement with FDA before a federal judge on action steps and penalties.
- Criminal prosecution: willful and repeated violations.

■ Common Inspection Findings

- Failure to submit or late expedited and periodic reports
- Inaccurate or incomplete reports to agency questions and requests
- Failure to do follow-up for serious and unexpected AEs
- Lack of or inadequately written SOPs

- Failure by the company to follow its own SOPs
- Database issues, including inadequate validation and security
- European Union Qualified Person deficiencies (training, coverage, oversight, etc.)
- Technical issues: incorrectly formatted submissions and reports, poor quality
- Safety signals missed, ignored, or poorly assessed
- Lack or inadequate metrics and performance measures
- No or poor-quality management system
- Labeling problems (CCSI, SPC, Package Insert)
- Problems and CAPAs from previous inspections not corrected and promises not kept

■ The Response to the Inspection or Audit

A written response is required to the findings in most inspections by governments. The response should address each point in the inspectors' report. In most cases, the company agrees with the issues cited and responds with high-level commitments to correct the issues. The document must be well thought-out and agreed to fully by the company management as it represents a formal and written commitment to the government(s) in question.

Responses to findings from nongovernmental audits are a business decision, but if the findings are violations of governmental requirements that an agency inspector would cite also, then they should be corrected. The findings should be prioritized, with the critical ones acted on first. The document must be specific and detailed (responding to each point made by the inspectors), with clearly assigned responsibilities, action steps, and time frames for completion. For inspections that have critical or major findings, expect a reinspection within 6 months to a year.

■ The Corrective Action Preventive Action Plan (CAPA)

Separate from the initial response letter, a CAPA plan must be set up to deal with the specific findings of an inspection by a health agency. This is an internal company document and usually does not have to be sent to the health authority or auditor. It should specifically be a series of actions to correct and prevent the findings of the inspection or audit. It should be "owned" and tracked by someone in the company. Action items should be clear and discrete with a specific person named as the responsible party its completion. Each item should have a due date. In severe cases, a summary or periodic progress report of the CAPA may be sent to the health agency to show good faith and progress.

■ FDA Inspections

In the United States, the FDA does two types of safety inspections: (1) routine surveillance inspections, and (2) "for cause" or "directed" inspections. The selection criteria include simple routine surveillance, looking at all companies on a periodic basis (e.g., every 1–2 years), or some sort of trigger at FDA, such as a history of violations (late expedited reports or periodic reports, significant recalls, etc.) or the recent launch of a major new chemical entity. Inspections may be done in the United States or abroad, and all drugs marketed in the United States are "fair game." If the inspection is for cause, the inspectors have specific information, including MedWatch forms or other information they may or may not reveal to the company under inspection. The inspector may have reviewed previous FDA inspections of the company as well as AE lists from the FDA database (Adverse Event Reporting System) and periodic reports.

The inspectors (usually one or two per inspection) are often from the local FDA office and are sometimes accompanied by inspectors with a particular specialty from other offices or the main office. They are guided by an inspection manual that summarizes what the inspectors should examine. Obviously, it behooves the company to review this document and to ensure that the areas scrutinized in an FDA inspection are handled correctly.

The high-level goals of the inspection are to ensure that the company adheres to all appropriate federal regulations regarding safety data collection, analysis and storage (both paper and electronic), reporting to the FDA, and product labeling, and that drug risks are recognized rapidly and handled in an appropriate manner to protect the public health. Areas inspected include AEs, medical errors, and product-quality complaints.

Inspections are usually unannounced, and the FDA inspector or inspectors simply arrive at the offices of the company. They present their credentials and documentation for the company to sign, acknowledging their arrival and the review of credentials. Applicants, manufacturers, packers, and distributors are subject to AE inspections.

The FDA has increased the number of inspections it is performing. It is hiring more inspectors and other personnel and has established offices outside the United States, in Asia and in South America. The commissioner has noted that some FDA enforcement efforts have been weak and that this is changing in order to deter other potential violators, communicate the issues to the public, create a level playing field for industry, and increase public confidence in the FDA. Vigilance is expected by companies in regard to how they handle safety problems with their products. They are expected to act quickly and thoroughly to correct problems. Failure to act will produce enforcement and penalties. Warning letters will be sent quickly, and action is expected immediately. The receipt of a Warning Letter is a very serious matter. It is addressed to senior management (usually the chief executive officer of the corporation) and requires a detailed written response within a short time (usually 15 working days), indicating the corrective actions to be taken.

Comments on EMA and MHRA Inspections

Inspections by the European Union and other governments around the world usually follow the same general principles noted above. Some differences do apply. European Union inspections are usually announced in advance, and both parties agree on a mutually acceptable date. The company being inspected must supply to the competent authority a key document describing their PV system as well as most of the documents to be reviewed during the inspection. This may be massive, and the documents are sent on a CD or DVD many weeks before the inspection. Thus, the inspectors walk in knowing the company's PV situation rather well, as they have reviewed the documents before arriving (see Chapter 49, "Summary/Description of PV Systems and Risk-Based Inspections").

In European Union inspections, the Qualified Person for PV plays a critical role. He or she may be the lead for the drug safety group in the audit response. At the very least, he or she must answer for the entire system, actions, effectiveness, and handling of drug safety for the company (see Chapter 23 on the QPPV).

Quality Systems and Inspection Preparation in Companies

It is highly recommended that companies set up within their quality or compliance groups a regular schedule for inspections of the company's PV functions, covering pre- and postmarketing situations and paralleling

the type of audit done by the health agencies. PV is now so specialized that dedicated, PV-experienced auditors should be used. These should be done at least yearly, especially if the company's products (new or old) have significant safety issues. Every company, whether selling or doing trials in the European Union, should have an up-to-date Summary/Description of PV Systems on file, ready to use for an inspection or audit (see Chapter 49 on this document). If a company does not have a quality or compliance group it should outsource this function but should still ensure that someone in the company has the responsibility for quality and compliance and oversees all outsourced functions.

Every company should have an SOP in place on how to handle outside audits. It should cover the following:

- A procedure should be in place to alert the receptionist at all company sites on what to do when inspectors show up, particularly unannounced FDA inspections. Whom to call (immediately) to greet the inspectors and then who will handle all logistics during the inspection.

- An "escort," "host," or "facilitator" should be designated who will accompany all inspectors at all times. The host handles all the logistics and ensures that meeting rooms and refreshments (usually limited to no more than coffee and cake) are available, and that the appropriate company representatives are available to meet with the inspectors. If there is more than one inspector (as there usually is), the company should ensure that there are sufficient hosts to accompany all inspectors should they split up. These are often company representatives from the quality, compliance, or regulatory sections. It is generally not wise to have company attorneys present unless the inspectors also have an attorney present.

- A minute-taker ("scribe") must be present at all meetings to record all issues brought up, to note all promises made by the company, and to ensure that all promised deliverables are delivered. The minute-taker should write up the minutes of the meeting (including listing all documents delivered) at the end of each day's audit.

- A system to have copies made of documents that are requested by the inspectors must be in place. Copies should be done on special paper marked (or watermarked) "confidential" or the equivalent. Duplicates of everything handed to the inspectors should be retained in the company's inspection files.

- The meeting room should be separate from the drug safety section. It is generally not wise to have the auditor wandering around the section being inspected unless this is arranged in advance or officially requested. Obviously, the drug safety section should ensure that all documents are in their appropriate places and that the staff is aware the inspectors are present.

- Never lie. Always tell the truth. Answer the questions posed. Do not volunteer information. Do not guess. If you do not know the answer to a question, say so. Try to find (with the help of the facilitator) someone who can answer it. If you do not understand a question, ask for it to be repeated or clarified.

Key Documents

U.S. FDA

- 7353.001 Chapter 53—Postmarketing Surveillance and Epidemiology: Enforcement of the postmarketing adverse drug experience reporting regulations (Web Resource 48-1)
- Regulatory Procedures Manual March 2008 (Web Resource 48-2)
- Office of Regulatory Affairs, Compliance References (Web Resource 48-3)
- Guidance for Industry Good Pharmacovigilance Practices and Pharmacoepidemiologic Assessment (Web Resource 48-4)

United Kingdom MHRA

- Summary of PV Systems (Web Resource 48-5)
- Good Pharmacovigilance Practice (Web Resource 48-6)
- Chart of MHRA PV Inspection Process (Web Resource 48-7)

- FAQs on Good PV Practices (Web Resource 48-8)

EMA

- Volume 9A—Guidelines on Pharmacovigilance for Medicinal Products for Human Use. Part 2.4 PV Inspections (Web Resource 48-9)
    - Sections 2.2–2.4 Detailed Description of the PV System, Compliance Monitoring by the Competent Authorities and Pharmacovigilance Inspections
- Volume 10—Guidelines on Clinical Trials (Web Resource 48-10)
    - Inspections—Good Clinical Practice (Web Resource 48-11)

■ Summary and Comments

Audits and inspections are now a requisite fact of life in the pharmaceutical industry, and drug safety is no exception. High quality work must be done, and it must be monitored through formal systems. The health authorities are now inspecting companies (pharma companies, vendors, licensors, IT companies, etc.), and the ability to "withstand and survive" such inspections is obligatory. Internal PV audits must be done and must become a routine part of life.

Many issues remain to be resolved as more countries are starting to do inspections and are getting tougher and better at it. One can easily envision the day when dozens of countries do inspections, producing "an audit a week," as one health authority arrives as soon as the last one leaves. Obviously, international coordination to avoid duplicative efforts will likely occur. However, as inspections seem to be either revenue-neutral or actual profit centers for health agencies, it may be difficult for the agencies to give up such lucrative sources of income. How this plays out remains to be seen.

49

Summary/Description of PV Systems and Risk-Based Inspections

Companies doing business or clinical trials in the European Union must prepare and have on file a critical document known as the Detailed Description of Pharmacovigilance Systems. It is described in Volume 9A. The equivalent in the United Kingdom is the Summary of PV Systems.

- Summary of PV Systems (Web Resource 49-1)
- Volume 9A—Guidelines on Pharmacovigilance for Medicinal Products for Human Use. Part 2.4 PV Inspections (Web Resource 49-2)
  - Section 2.2 Detailed Description of the PV System, Compliance Monitoring by the Competent Authorities and Pharmacovigilance Inspections

These documents are usually required in Marketing Authorizations submitted to the European Medicines Agency (EMA) or member states for approval of a drug and must be on file. They will be required for pharmacovigilance (PV) inspections by European Union-competent authorities. Companies not doing business or trials in the European Union do not need this document, as it is not required (yet) by other agencies. Nonetheless, it is a wise idea to prepare this document and update it periodically. By preparing it, the company will have a good idea of the status and quality of its PV systems. Some companies require this as part of their quality management systems.

■ The Detailed Description of the PV System (Volume 9A Section 2.2)

The key parts of the DDPVS are noted here:

- 2.2.1 A detailed description of the pharmacovigilance system, including the proof of the availability of the services of the QPPV and the proof that the Marketing Authorization Holder has the necessary means for the collection and notification of any adverse reaction. It should contain an overview of the PV system with information on the key elements.
- 2.2.2 A signed statement from the MAH and the QP that the qualified person is available and responsible for pharmacovigilance and has the necessary means for the collection and notification of any adverse reaction occurring everywhere in the world.
- 2.2.3a) The name and contact information of the QPPV (24/7), with a CV, job description, and backup information.

- 2.2.3b) Location and identification of where the main EEA and global PV are done—particularly ICSRs and PSURs. Where PV data are accessible in the European Union. Organization charts and descriptions of the global and European PV units and their relationships. Licensing partnerships should be noted in an addendum. Flow diagrams showing how safety reports are processed.

- 2.2.3c) SOPs should be in place to cover the following processes and quality control to ensure their correct functioning:
  - QPPV and backup activities
  - The collection, processing, data entry, quality control, coding, classification, medical review, and reporting of ICSRs from solicited and unsolicited mechanisms, clinical trials, literature, healthcare professionals, sales and marketing, and other MAH, compassionate use, consumer reports, health agencies, and so forth, worldwide
  - Follow-up, detection of duplicates, electronic reporting, expedited reporting, PSURs
  - Global pharmacovigilance activities. Continuous monitoring of the safety of authorized products, signal detection, risk benefit assessment, reporting and communication to authorities, and medical professionals
  - Interaction between safety issues and product defects
  - Responses to requests for information from regulatory authorities
  - Handling of urgent safety restrictions and safety variations
  - Meeting commitments to agencies
  - Database handling and management
  - Internal auditing of the PV system
  - Archiving
  - Training

- 2.2.3d) Databases: A listing and description of the main PV databases used (compilation of safety reports, expedited and electronic reporting, signaling, sharing and accessing global data), a statement on their validation status, status of compliance with requirements for electronic reporting, a copy of the registration of the QPPV with EudraVigilance and identification of the process used for electronic reporting to competent authorities, who is responsible for operation of the databases and their location.

- 2.2.3e) Contractual agreements with outside organizations or persons, Including comarketing agreements and contracting out of PV activities, with a description of the nature of the agreements. Product-specific agreements may be listed in an appendix.

- 2.2.3f) Training: A description of the training systems and where the training records, CVs, and job descriptions are filed.

- 2.2.3g) Documentation: A description of the locations of PV source documents, including archiving arrangements.

- 2.2.3h) Quality Management System: A description of the system cross-referencing the functions noted in the other sections of the Description of PV Systems. Roles and responsibilities for the activities and documentation, quality control and review, and CAPAs should be noted.

- 2.2.3i) Supporting Documentation: Documentation on the PV system should be available during the pre- and postauthorization period.

■ The MHRA Summary of PV Systems (SPS)

This document is required by the United Kingdom's MHRA. It is very similar to the European Union Description document described above. Key points and differences include:

- Companies should view the SPS as a living document and it should be kept up to date.
- Companies will have 6 weeks or so to prepare/update it when an inspection is due to occur.
- It should be no more than 25 pages (excluding appendices).
- Large companies with several divisions that are very different and have very different PV systems may need to prepare more than one SPS.
- The main focus is on the United Kingdom functioning.

The various sections of the document include:

- Section 1: Contacts and Licenses
  - Main United Kingdom contacts, where PV is done, QP contact information, company names and addresses if more than one product licenses are held in the United Kingdom under different company names.

- Number of National and Centralized licenses held.
- Section 2: Company Structure
  - Company structure: holding/parent company, global subsidiaries, therapeutic areas and product portfolio, recent mergers or acquisitions
  - An overview of how PV is done.
- Section 3: PV Activities
  - A summary of the PV activities by the main PV site(s) in the United Kingdom and globally: "who, what, when, where, how, and why." It should include but is not limited to: a summary of the PV activities performed by other departments (e.g., Medical Information, Regulatory Affairs, and Product Quality), the process for spontaneous and clinical trial ADR management—from receipt to data entry, review, and expedited reporting with flow diagrams(s), compliance monitoring activities, management and monitoring of clinical trial drug safety (including data reconciliation), PSUR preparation and submission, QP activities, processes for signal generation, trend evaluation and labeling changes, Risk Management Plans produced.
- Section 4: IT
  - The currently used local and global systems. Details of the databases/computerized systems used to collect, collate, and evaluate information about suspected ADRS (spontaneous, solicited, and trials), to include: whether the system was developed in-house or commercially and whether the system has been configured or customized following purchase; and validation status, location of the validation documentation, version details; who is responsible for system maintenance and support.
  - Historic situation: A summary of the legacy database used to collect, collate, and evaluate information over the last 5 years.
- Section 5: Quality Management System
  - If the Company intends to change the system within the next 6 months, provide a summary of the planned changes.
  - Indicate who is responsible for auditing the PV system and provide a description. How long audit reports are kept and where they are stored.

- Section 6: Training Records
  - Description of the United Kingdom training record system and the location of the records, CVs, and job descriptions.
- Section 7: Archiving
  - A description of the archiving activities for PV documents and if outsourced details of the company(ies) doing so.
- Section 8: Comments and Questions
  - Any additional assumptions, issues, etc., that are applicable.
- Appendices
  - Key personnel: organization charts for the United Kingdom and global PV and Medical Information (and contractors) departments, with names and job titles. CV and job description for QP and deputy.
  - Portfolio: All licensed products in the United Kingdom
    - Active ingredient(s), United Kingdom trade name; State if the product is not marketed in the United Kingdom; Method of approval (national, mutual recognition, centralized); Reference Member State (for mutually recognized products); Black triangle products; the five products that generated the greatest number of ADR reports in the last year.
  - Studies: A list of all ongoing phases I–III company-sponsored clinical trials that have at least one site in the European Union/EEA. A global list of all ongoing postauthorization clinical studies, including interventional clinical studies and noninterventional studies of United Kingdom-licensed products.
  - Quality Management System: Details of the global SOPs describing the content, format, approval, and review procedures for all levels of procedural documentation (i.e., SOP on SOPs), list of titles of all global, regional, and local PV procedural documents (e.g., policies, SOPs, and working instructions). A list of all other local documents that relate to PV (e.g., from Medical Information, Product Quality, Regulatory Affairs).
  - Regulatory Reporting—Compliance Statistics
    - For spontaneous expedited reports to the MHRA for the last 2 years, a monthly breakdown of: total ADR reports (nonserious and serious) received globally, total expedited

ADR reports submitted to MHRA, total late reports submitted to MHRA, late reports as a percentage of the total number of expedited submissions to MHRA.

- For clinical trial expedited reports to the MHRA for the last 2 years, expedited SUSARs submitted to MHRA, late SUSAR reports, number of late reports as a percentage of the total number of expedited submissions to MHRA.
- PSUR reporting for last 2 years of PSURs to be submitted within 60 days of data lock-point: product, data lock-point, date submitted.

- Third-Party Agreements (e.g., licensing, marketing, distribution, and CROs and other service providers of PV): A list of all United Kingdom and global agreements with third parties concerning marketed products and products not yet marketed/under development. Details of any activities/functions related to PV that are outsourced by the global PV group or in the United Kingdom (e.g., medical information, regulatory affairs, sales force, PSUR preparation, expedited reporting).

- Product-Related Safety Issues: Details of any EEA products withdrawn from any global market in the last 5 years due to safety issues. Details of all Urgent Safety Restrictions in the last 2 years.

- Document Requests to be Submitted with the SPS: Include a copy of the SOPs for:
    - Case processing of spontaneous adverse drug reaction reports
    - Case processing of clinical trial SAE reports
    - Follow-up of individual cases
    - Regulatory reporting of expedited reports to MHRA and EMEA
    - Monitoring of regulatory compliance with 7- and 15-day requirements
    - PSUR preparation and submission
    - Signal detection/trend analysis
    - Enquiry-handling by medical information function in the United Kingdom

Comments: Clearly, this is a major document with multiple appendices and data that must be obtained from many sources within the company that might not be handy or readily available to the PV department (e.g., holding company, global trials). This document should be prepared as a matter of routine, updated periodically, and kept on file. To prepare this in 6 weeks upon notification of an MHRA inspection can be a prodigious 24/7 effort.

■ The Compliance Report (MHRA)

The MHRA has introduced a report that it is requesting firms to fill in. It is known as a Compliance Report, which the MHRA will use to determine an organization's risk, previous inspection history, and organization change to determine the organization's control of its risk.

A score is calculated with the amount of control subtracted from the amount of risk; both are scored between 0 and 100 (highest), so the risk assessment consequently has values from -100 to +100, with -100 being the best possible score.

The assessments will be ranked by the MHRA and inspections of firms will be prioritized based on greatest risk. Companies are not obliged to fill in a compliance report, but "failure to submit a Completed Report will be assessed as a high-risk answer to all questions, with a subsequent risk score of 100 being assigned," thus increasing the likelihood of an inspection. Further details on the report and templates are available at Web Resource 49-3.

The report covers the following activities/functions: QPPV, Medical Information, Quality Complaint Handling, Literature Searching, Spontaneous Case Processing, Regulatory Authority Case Processing, Literature Case Processing, Other Noninterventional Study Case Processing, PSUR Production, Signal Detection, Signal Evaluation, Variation submission, and Database Maintenance and Support. The scope is United Kingdom receipt for medical information and quality complaints, United Kingdom submission for variations, and worldwide for all of the other activities.

Outsourcing information for the activities listed above is requested: Is the function outsourced? To Whom, At What Location, Have they been audited?

Information on Quality Management Systems in place for each of the activities is requested, including the procedure in place, training performed, whether the process has been audited and whether the outputs are archived.

For each of the above categories, the following is stated: Who performs the task, where it is done, the number of people doing the task, and the number of activities in the last year.

Compliance with expedited reporting and PSUR time frames is measured by supplying the number of expedited cases (United Kingdom, European Union, and global) and PSURs done and the percent submitted on time.

Staff turnover in the last year in Medical Information, Case Processing, PSUR Production, and Signal Detection and Review is requested.

The number of agreements for in-licensing, out-licensing, distribution, comarketing, and colicensing is requested.

Details of all risk management plans (internal and health authority-approved) as well as Risk Minimization Plans are requested.

Details on product-related safety issues are requested, including:

- How many products have been withdrawn for safety reasons (anywhere in the world) in the previous calendar year?
- How many products have had urgent safety restrictions in the previous calendar year?
- How many products have been formally referred to the CHMP for safety reasons in the previous calendar year?
- How many variations were submitted that included a change to the safety information contained in United Kingdom SPCs in the previous calendar year?
- How many of these were initiated by the company in the previous calendar year?

■ Comment

Clearly this document has been well thought out by the MHRA and asks the questions that will show whether a company has control over each of the key areas in drug safety as well as the turnover ("churn") of personnel, the number of outsourced functions, the number of safety issues, the number of outside business agreements, and label (SPC) changes for safety and late reporting. Obviously the higher each number is, the worse the risk is. Whether a company has an MA in the United Kingdom or not, it is worth filling in this document as a tool for risk estimation within a company.

CHAPTER 50

Ethical Issues and Conflicts of Interest

The ethical issues of business and medicine have become complex and difficult. Years ago, before medicine was thought of as "big business," the ethics of medicine were somewhat cleaner (at least on paper). Physicians adhered to the Hippocratic Oath, which said, in regard to drugs, "I will neither give a deadly drug to anybody who asked for it, nor will I make a suggestion to this effect." It is not so simple now that we know almost all drugs can be deadly. See "The Hippocratic Oath Today: Meaningless Relic or Invaluable Moral Guide?" at Web Resource 50-1.

The physician's obligation for most of the years since Hippocrates was primarily to the individual patient. The physician had little in his or her armamentarium that was effective in diagnosis or treatment. Diagnosis relied on the physician's brain, without laboratory tests or other investigations. Real medications were few, and often useless, adulterated, or impure. Clinical research dates only to the eighteenth century and serious use of clinical research to the nineteenth century. Surgery was, at least until anesthesia was developed also in the nineteenth century, crude and painful at best and fatal at worst. The physician comforted and predicted and often did little else.

How that has changed! Physicians (plus nurses, physician assistants, nurse practitioners, midwives, and many other healthcare providers) now have an extraordinary array of diagnostic and therapeutic choices available. There are far more choices than the practitioner is able to keep up with and use appropriately.

But the cost of this great improvement in diagnosis and therapeutics has been the introduction of complexity and conflicting agendas, as healthcare professionals now have obligations to society, employers, governments, insurance companies, partners, and hospitals. The days when the patient paid his or her $5 cash for an office visit (and $8 for a home visit) are long gone. The world of big business has now caught up with big medicine. Costs of physician and other healthcare provider services, procedures, surgeries, laboratory tests, medications, and devices have skyrocketed. The entire dynamics of medicine and health care have changed. The next frontier will be how to handle the rationing that will occur (it's here already, in fact) as the population of baby boomers ages and resources are unable to keep up with the demand for healthcare services.

The question of what is a pharmaceutical company's responsibility should be addressed. There are, broadly speaking, two schools of thought on corporate responsibility. The first is the one of "fiduciary responsibility," which states roughly that a company's role is to maximize profitability and shareholder/stockholder value while staying within the law. The second view holds that companies have additional moral obligations to their "stakeholders" above and beyond simply making as much money as possible for the stockholders (owners) of the company. The stakeholders include the patients and their families, healthcare personnel, employees, the communities where the company is located, the public at large, and vendors. America and other parts of the world have shifted from the first view toward the second one or some combination thereof. There is currently a major and ongoing debate on corporate ethics and responsibilities, with one side saying that "corporate ethics" is a contradiction in terms, or an oxymoron, and the other that we are moving to a new view of corporate behavior. This debate then tempers the view one takes regarding the behavior of companies and their individual employees, regulators, customers, bystanders, and others. The debate is not unique to the pharma world and has been seen with BP and the Gulf oil spill, Union Carbide and Bhopal, and many other tragedies. Business ethics is now a hot topic in business schools.

Accompanying the changes in the structure of medicine have been changes in the roles and obligations of physicians and other healthcare providers. For example, the physician's role in clinical research is ambiguous. By doing clinical research, the physician is experimenting on patients (or even normal subjects) with new medications that may not help the individual patient but that may help humankind (if the new product represents a real breakthrough) and definitely will help the drug company involved. This is a concept not envisioned in Hippocrates' time. An excellent review of the issues appears in the Stanford (University) Encyclopedia of Philosophy (Web Resource 50-2). The multiple views and conflicts are discussed relating to a basic philosophical question: "Clinical research poses a very practical and practically vital example of one of the most fundamental concerns in moral theory. When is it acceptable to expose some to risks of harm for the benefit of others?"

The specific ethical obligations and considerations in regard to the pharmaceutical industry is a topic of lively discussion, and many websites offer opinions. A Google search on "ethics" and "pharmaceuticals" produced more than 1.6 million hits, and a search on "ethics" and "drug safety" produced more than 100,000 hits.

For an excellent review of the ethical issues in the pharmaceutical world, see M. D. B. Stephens's superb section entitled, "Ethical Issues In Drug Safety," in Stephens's *Detection of New Adverse Drug Reactions*, 5th ed. (Wiley, Hoboken, NJ, 2004, pp. 591–648). This article covers clinical trials, the use of placebo, ethics committees, conflicts of interest, informed consent, patient protection, publications, symposia, advertising and promotion, labeling, and relations with government.

Companies are set up, as noted above, to make money. They do so by selling various drug/device/biologic products that have known faults or defects listed in the labeling as adverse events (AEs), warnings, and precautions. For all new products, the complete risk profile is not completely known until well after marketing begins and exposure to much larger and heterogeneous populations than during clinical trials occurs.

For just about all drugs, the safety of use in pregnancy has not been studied. The company has invested enormous amounts of money in the development and then promotion of the products that have a finite (financial) life span due to patent expiration and new and better products coming along. When a drug is approved, it is judged by health authorities to have a benefit profile greater than its risk profile, translated by the public into the shorthand of "safe and effective," although it really means "relatively safe and relatively effective and hopefully more of the latter than the former."

Companies will do everything within their power to promote and protect their products. The drug safety group (along with the product quality department if separate) is the department that receives only bad news about product use. This department must determine, in very short time frames, whether the serious or fatal problems reported are due to the drug. Some of the cases must be reported to the government within a week or two and others tallied up in summary reports as signals for internal corporate review and, sometimes, submission to the health authorities. Real-time, online tracking of AEs and drug safety issues are coming but are not here yet.

The primary duty of the drug safety group is to protect the public health. A secondary duty is to protect the company's products only insofar as this does not conflict with the primary protection of the public health. It is always interesting to read the introduction to the corporate standard operating procedure or mission statement for the drug safety group to see whether this distinction is respected. It usually is, at least on paper.

It is interesting to note that large universities in the United States, for the past 20-plus years, have had the right to patent and make profit from pharmaceutical discoveries from their labs. This has led to some phenomenal successes, with hundreds of millions of dollars of royalties from drug sales coming into the university treasuries. Not surprisingly, the universities are reacting just like for-profit pharmaceutical companies when their monetary stream is threatened or interrupted. They sue one another and drug companies to protect their interests.

The next sections address some of the areas of controversy that touch drug safety.

■ Dynamics in Play in Regard to Drug Safety and Companies

- Corporations are rarely run by physicians or clinicians and more often by non-medically trained marketers, sales personnel, lawyers, and accountants. Such managers, who work their way up the corporate ladder, usually do not do a stint in the drug safety department. It is thus understandable that the senior corporate view on drug safety is sometimes vague and often ill-defined.

- The rules governing drug safety are arcane, highly technical, and very difficult to understand (even for those in the business). Management rarely wants details but rather prefers "executive summaries" of data that may not capture the nuances of the clinical judgment involved in drug safety decisions. In addition, there is legal discouragement about writing down real or potential "bad things" about the drug products in e-mail or memos. Management may work on the MEGO ("my eyes glaze over") or MITIN ("more information than I need") principles regarding drug safety.

- The drug safety group is a "cost center" and not a profit center. Pharmacovigilance professionals often argue that their approach saves the company money and shame by preventing safety problems from becoming safety crises, resulting in crisis management procedures, patient harm, litigation, restrictions on use, or even withdrawal from the market. This argument, of theoretical future dollars saved by the safety department, usually carries little weight.

- The drug safety function is not glamorous and usually not well funded—at least not as well funded as the clinical research and sales organizations. The same holds true, by the way, in most drug regulatory authorities: there is more staff studying dossiers in view of approving new products

than studying adverse drug reaction reports. And in medical schools, pharmacovigilance is not even part of the curriculum. As the saying goes, drug safety is the "poor stepchild." This may be changing somewhat, as various "scandals" and the public awareness that drug safety really does matter may increase funding and resources available.

- In many companies, the drug safety group is scattered at several sites around the world and often away from the main campus or headquarters of the company ("out of sight, out of mind").

- Delivering bad news up the corporate ladder is, in the best of times, accepted but not welcomed. In the worst of times, it is actively discouraged and punished. It is hard to "speak truth to power." The messengers are indeed sometimes "killed." The mechanism of reporting on signals that could drastically reduce sales, if confirmed or made known, is often convoluted, requiring the safety message to work its way up the corporate chain before it reaches someone with decision-making power.

- Delivering bad news is generally not as well paid as delivering good news (completing clinical trials, selling more drug, etc.) in companies. No one is compensated more for sending in additional 15-day alert reports.

- Rightly or wrongly, the reputation for honesty of drug companies (including their drug safety groups) is not high in the eyes of health authorities, regulators, consumer groups, and the public. This tends to produce a mentality within the companies of "circling the wagons." Companies, again rightly or wrongly, put little trust or credence into AE reports from certain groups such as consumer groups, disease groups, and attorneys, and react defensively.

- The drug safety group ("the sales prevention department") is usually grudgingly accepted as a "necessary evil" by other groups in the company.

- The group handling business negotiations for in-licensing new products often do not think of drug safety or bring it into play at the very last minute.

- It is often very difficult to convince sales and marketing departments of the need to train both new and current salespeople on AE reporting ("The job of the sales force is to sell."). Training is often relegated to giving out reading material, or if an actual physical presentation is permitted, it is often done at 4:30 PM on a Friday afternoon.

- Drug safety often reports into the medical research department. Less commonly, it reports into the legal or regulatory departments. It should never report to a marketing or sales function. The drug safety organization may report to a nonempowered, low-level, relatively junior employee with little organizational voice or influence and no internal "champion."

- There are few ways for management to measure drug safety performance. Clearly, measuring the on-time reporting performance for 15-day Periodic Safety Update Reports, New Drug Application periodic reports, and Investigational New Drug Application annual reports is the most common metric used, but this simply captures mechanical performance and not the medical protection and risk management aspects of pharmacovigilance. Softer measures such as "the health authority's satisfaction with our performance" are nearly impossible to measure.

- Pharmaceutical companies are asked to present statistically significant efficacy data to prove that a drug should be approved by the health authorities to market a product. Thus, many in senior management assume that safety data work the same way. They do not.

- Management often takes the view that a serious safety issue must be proven with hard data. There must be clear causality associated with the drug and no alternate explanations for the safety problem. Thus, some managers will not accept drug safety physicians' views that a particular serious and severe medical problem is probably or possibly due to the drug and that a change in the product labeling is warranted. Clear proof in several or many patients is demanded.

- Alternative explanations are often presumed to be the cause of the problem: "This patient smokes, drinks, is hypertensive and both parents have heart disease. How can you say our drug caused this patient's heart attack?" Sometimes the drug truly is the cause of the problem even though there are other possible causes (see also the fialuridine story in Chapter 52).

- The problem may be reduced to a more simple question: is the drug innocent until proven guilty of a safety problem or is the drug guilty of a safety problem until proven innocent? In the past, the "innocent until proven guilty" view predominated. Now, the pendulum is swinging toward early notification of the public of potential safety issues even

if events are not clearly due to the drug. Whether this will prove to be good for the public health (moving people off dangerous drugs) or bad for the public health (moving people to other more toxic or costly alternatives) remains to be seen. People feel better about warning the public and medical providers of possible issues. Whether this improves health outcomes has not been proven.

- The "level playing field" argument is often made by nonmedical personnel in regard to reporting and acting on safety issues. The argument for this runs roughly as follows: "If we as a company have to report that our drug X seems to be causing ventricular fibrillation, then our competitors' products, which also cause ventricular fibrillation (as evidenced by Freedom of Information Act or medical literature reports), should also be obliged to change their labeling." This then puts pressure on the drug safety department either to not report or to minimize such events until they are "proven." Companies thus sometimes try to make deals with the agencies ("We'll change our label if you make our competitors also change theirs," or "This should be class labeling"). This rarely works.

- Interestingly, physicians are now found more and more commonly in marketing departments, where they tend to take on the coloration of marketers and lose the coloration of physicians. They then may take on an adversarial ("devil's advocate") role in relation to the drug safety physicians.

- In a similar vein, physicians working in the medical research department (phases II and III) often become quite "protective and possessive" about the drugs they are studying and may take a doubting view that "their" drug could produce such serious AEs and, thus, that these serious AEs are "unrelated" to the study drug. This is one reason the final determination of causality, labeling, and reportability should rest with the drug safety group.

- Physicians and, to a lesser degree, other healthcare professionals working in industry (including drug safety) are/were often looked down on by physicians and healthcare workers "out in the real world." Some consider pharmaceutical professionals to have "sold out."

- There are few formal training programs for drug safety personnel either in medical, nursing, or pharmacy schools. There are courses on drug safety lasting from a day to a week or two (usually by nonacademic institutions), and there is a scarcity of textbooks. Training tends to be similar to an apprenticeship. This is slowly changing, with universities in North America (University of Medicine and Dentistry of New Jersey, Eastern Michigan University, University of Montreal, McGill University) and others in Europe and elsewhere beginning to develop programs in "industrial pharmacology." It is also hoped a better term will be found.

- Drug safety officers, unless they worked previously for health agencies, really do not have a good feel for how the drug safety agency works (and vice versa). Although there are contacts between industry and the agencies through the International Conference on Harmonization, Council for International Organizations of Medical Sciences, Drug Information Association, CIOMS, and other venues, such contact is usually at a distance and defensive because of perceived conflicts of interest and different "agendas."

- Drug safety personnel, as with any other company personnel, receive performance bonuses and may own stock or stock options. Hence, pay is tied to company performance as well as to the individual's work.

- Drug safety units are under continued scrutiny by the health agencies (particularly in the form of inspections) and internal auditors.

- There are significant pressures on drug safety personnel in regard to work volume and time allocated to complete tasks (especially those time frames regulated by law), difficulty in finding experienced safety officers, and difficulty in training safety officers.

- Outsourcing and off-shoring are moving many drug safety jobs out of Europe and North America, forcing a larger pool of workers in these venues to compete for fewer and fewer jobs. Drug Safety is now a "buyer's market."

- The upward corporate career mobility for personnel in drug safety groups is limited usually to that group or related (epidemiology, signaling) functions. Rarely do employees move high up in the corporate hierarchy unless they leave the drug safety unit.

There are clear and obvious potential conflicts evident in such a situation. Drug safety personnel are paid by the company and will, in general, receive better pay and more rewards if the company does well and sells more drugs. However, enlightened companies tend to realize increasingly that they cannot "play games" with the drug safety units. Drug safety personnel tend to be somewhat defensive and "paranoid," lacing their worldview with dark humor. Whether the job produces such character traits or rather attracts people with such traits from the beginning is unclear.

■ Data Safety Management Boards and Ethics Committees/IRBs

Another interesting area is DSMBs (see Chapter 32), which are generally hired and paid by pharmaceutical companies to review safety data in ongoing clinical trials. Board members, usually external physicians and drug safety experts, must make medically correct and honest judgments on patient safety and trial integrity independent of the company. The inherent conflicts here are clear: board members are paid by the company but must make decisions that may adversely affect the company (and the board members' income if the trials end early).

Similarly, ethics committees are usually paid to approve and monitor trials. Some ethics committees are "for-profit" companies, and even nonprofit university ethics committees may bring in a stream of income for the institution.

■ Dynamics in Play in Regard to Drug Safety and Health Agencies

- Health workers in the health and drug safety agencies are not involved in the fiduciary aspects of profit-making companies. Their job is more clearly that of protecting the health of the public, though they are no more free from outside political, financial, and other influences than are pharma company personnel.

- In the United States, the Food and Drug Administration and the personnel in the FDA have multiple masters to answer to (either formally in the organization structure or informally), including the senior management of the FDA, the cabinet department to which they report (Health and Human Services), the president, Congress, and various other overseers, including the Justice Department and the Public Health Service. Funding is not always dispersed at a level perceived to be necessary for adequate functioning. Similar multiple masters may be seen in other countries, although in many instances the reporting line is much cleaner through the Ministry of Health only.

- The agencies are heavily scrutinized by the media (at least in the United States), more so than safety departments in pharmaceutical companies.

- Employees at the agencies tend to make less money than corresponding personnel in pharmaceutical companies, though this differential may be narrowing in some countries.

- The agencies tend to be underfunded and understaffed compared with the resources in pharmaceutical companies if one looks at the number of AEs received and the drugs under scrutiny. Some multinational companies' drug safety departments are bigger than the health agency's safety staffs.

- The perception is that the agency is not expected or "allowed" to make mistakes. Bad outcomes, serious outcomes, and patient deaths are not supposed to occur in drugs approved by the health agency. Others feel, however, that the agencies (especially FDA, where a 6-month review period is now the norm), approve drugs "too quickly or too slowly," according to one's point of view.

- The FDA and other agencies are going through a turbulent period (short-term leadership, loss of experienced personnel, reorganizations, criticism from the outside, drug withdrawals, etc.).

- Many agencies have been accused of being in bed with the industry, and critics point to the large number of people who move from health agency to industry jobs and vice versa. The claim here is that an agency person will not be tough on industry if he or she expects to want a job in industry in the next couple of years.

- Duplicative and, in a sense, competitive pharmacovigilance is done by other major health authorities around the world. If a drug is removed from the market or the labeling is changed in one country or region, particularly a "major" one like the United States or the European Union, the other agencies often feel obliged to follow suit.

- Health agency workers often feel they are doing "God's work," and are "purer" than those folks in industry who are just interested in making money.

- Many agencies have limited regulatory powers. For example, there is limited regulatory power to force label changes and regulate neutraceuticals and old over-the-counter products. It is also difficult and time consuming to change the regulations. Member states in the European Union have devolved certain functions and decisions to the European Medicines Agency and other bodies in London or Brussels.

- Government safety officers, unless they previously worked in industry, often do not have a good feel for how corporate decisions and governance occur.

Similarly, company employees do not always have an understanding of how government functions (though many will say they do, having fought battles to get a driving license or resolve a tax dispute).

- It is not clear how the lower-level safety officers are able to get their views brought up the line in health agencies. Whistle-blowing is a dangerous action.

Dynamics in Play in Regard to Drug Safety and Academia and Nonacademic Healthcare Facilities

- In the United States, and to a lesser degree in Canada, the role of the universities and medical, nursing, and pharmacy schools in drug safety training, surveillance, and research is minimal. These schools train healthcare practitioners but offer minimal training in drug safety, interactions, and so forth. Courses tend to focus on the concepts of pharmacology and the clinical use of medications.

- Occasionally, industry physicians hold academic positions at medical schools, often in the clinical research or pharmacology units and occasionally in the clinics (seeing patients, though malpractice insurance issues tend to prevent this in the United States). Thus, there is little "cross-fertilization" among colleagues. Similarly, medical personnel in health agencies rarely hold academic positions at medical institutions, also minimizing cross-fertilization. In contrast, France, for example, has a very tight relationship between the regulatory agency and the regional university hospitals in handling drug safety.

- Academics perform heavily paid consultation and clinical research for the pharmaceutical industry. Physicians and other scientists in academia perform clinical trials and postmarketing trials, give lectures in speakers' bureaus funded by the industry, and so on. They are sometimes referred to as "key opinion leaders (KOLs)." They may own stock in pharmaceutical companies. This has produced a wave of scandals in the United States and elsewhere, as it is revealed that some academics have created for-profit companies to develop, research, and market products or receive hundreds of thousands or even millions of dollars from pharma companies. Although this is not forbidden in most cases, these ventures and endeavors were not declared to the universities as required in their rules.

This is an evolving situation, and with more and more transparency, it is likely that rules and standards will change.

- Academics sit on health agency advisory committees in the United States, Europe, Canada, and elsewhere, where they play key roles. Ideally, they should have no conflicts of interest. If any exist, they must be declared. It is sometimes hard to find an expert in a drug or disease who has not, at some point in his or her career, worked with the industry to study new products or uses.

- Academics may sit on hospital formulary committees and have a major say in which products are used (and sold) in that institution, even when they have been paid to study these products.

- Some academic research units receive some funding from industry, and clinical trials in academic units usually charge industry significant "university overhead" to allow the trials to be done at their institutions. Thus, industry becomes a significant source of academic funding at some institutions. In addition, some institutions in the United States now make significant money from drug sales for which they hold patents and receive royalties. There are virtually no medical or pharmacy faculties that do not receive direct or indirect grants, awards, scholarships, speakers' fees, unrestricted educational grants, continuing medical education (CME) grants, expenses, professorships (chairs), and so forth, from industry. Some companies go so far as to install a pharmaceutical research center or an endowed chair on the campus of prestigious medical faculties. This entire situation is now being questioned, but given that governments seem to have less money and companies more money, it is not clear how this will evolve.

■ Dynamics in Play in Regard to Drug Safety and Consumer Groups, Disease Groups, and the Internet (Blogs, Websites, Social Media, etc.)

- These are usually nonprofit organizations created by patients with common diseases or medication use.

- There are occasional organizations or sites set up with other goals in mind. See http://www.adrugrecall.com/html/about.html, which states this is "an extensive website intended to provide readers with important information about dangerous drugs, which cause serious side effects and adverse events. Our main objective is to give our readers the resources and support necessary to handle legal issues that arise from defective pharmaceutical products."

- Also see Worst Pills, Best Pills (Web Resource 50-3), run by the Public Citizen's Health Research Group. This group notes that it gives an "expert, independent second opinion for prescription drug information."

- A common view among some patient groups (and even some medical groups) is that the industry is monolithic and "bad." The groups often believe (sometimes quite rightly) that the industry regards them as adversaries. They often believe industry cannot police itself and do not trust industry drug safety conclusions.

- There are now many blogs, websites, RSS feeds, podcasts, webinars, tweets, and all sorts of other internet-based sources on drugs, drug safety, and related issues. Some are polemical and have "aggressive" points of view; others are more "balanced;" some are academic; some are for-profit groups; some are from pharmaceutical companies (though this is not always evident) and more. Social media (Twitter, Facebook, etc.) are now being used for drug safety information both by companies and health agencies. As always, a healthy skepticism is necessary when reading these sites, especially when their provenance and funding are unclear.

- Drug safety issues sell newspapers and draw eyes to websites, blogs, and television.

- Such stories do not need to be based on scientific data but may rather rest on accusations or human-interest issues.

- Safe drugs do not make good stories. Dangerous ones or potentially dangerous ones do.

- There is no obligation to present both sides of a story.

- There is little obligation to correct stories that turn out to be incorrect or overblown ("A lie can travel halfway around the world while the truth is putting on its boots."—Mark Twain).

- Experienced reporters and television personalities are far more skilled at communicating on television and in the media than drug safety personnel (even those who have had "media training") and can make a non-media-savvy interviewee look quite silly or foolish.

- Data presented in the media may be "precise" but not "accurate." Data may also be presented that are of little clinical meaning or that represent a hypothesis or a "study" based on a handful of patients ("coffee linked to pancreatic cancer").

■ Dynamics in Play in Regard to Drug Safety and Lawyers/Litigation

- Few people in the medical profession want to have anything to do with lawyers or litigation. Drug safety personnel in the industry and government are no different and generally do not like to testify in court and try to avoid lawyers and litigation.

- Dealings with lawyers and litigation tend to take enormous amounts of time and offer little in return to the safety personnel involved.

- Law and litigation involve, usually, adversarial procedures and are very different from the collegial, consensual, and scientific approach most safety officers have from medical training, experience, and affinity. There is no obligation to be even-handed or to present both sides of the story.

- Testimony, whether in court or at depositions, is usually highly stressful and time-consuming.

- There are monetary goals involved in lawsuits in addition to the claimed goals of fairness and justice.

■ Codes of Conduct

Various groups have put out codes of conduct (usually voluntary) for marketing and detailing drug information to physicians and other healthcare professionals. See, for example, the codes put out by the American pharmaceutical industry association PhRMA at Web Resource 50-4. Strict codes putting limits on detailing have been put forth by hospitals and medical centers. There is a lively debate ongoing about the best way to convey information on pharmaceuticals to physicians and other healthcare providers as well as patients. Similarly, direct-to-consumer advertising in the United States has elicited strong and sometimes angry discussions. The use of social media and the internet is likely to play a large role in this now rapidly changing area.

■ Comments and Summary

The entire field of drug safety is chock full of conflicts of interest and personal or institutional agendas, some of which are obvious and some less so. No one owns the truth. Trust but verify. All statements should be questioned and skepticism is a virtue. Safety profiles of products are incredibly dynamic and change almost daily. What is true today may not be so tomorrow. Beware of statements such as those listed below. They may not all be false, but they should be viewed with skepticism until proven otherwise:

- "Of course I've consulted for XX, Inc., or received speakers' bureaus fees, but they do not influence my judgment in any way."
- "Of course I see drug reps, but they are not my sole source of information and I make independent judgments."
- "I've never received a dime from industry. (But I own a lot of their stock. Or my wife or children do.)"
- "This drug is (perfectly) safe."
- "Our only interest is the public health."
- "I only do what is right for the patient, not the clinical trial or company."
- "This drug has not been proven to produce atrial fibrillation" (or some other serious AE). "The cases we do have are under investigation and all the patients had risk factors." "The serious AE was due to the patient's lifestyle and risk factors."
- "We have no reports that this drug caused atrial fibrillation." (But someone else might and we haven't looked).

But all is not lost, nor does cynicism reign everywhere. The current system, which is made up of multiple competing forces sometimes pulling in different directions and sometimes in the same direction, has tended to arrive at the truth after all is said and done. It arguably takes too long and some people are hurt and some even die. We have nothing better yet but many people in the health agencies, the industry, and elsewhere are searching assiduously for better methodologies in the world of drug safety. That will probably arrive sooner rather than later. The conflicts of interest, however, will likely continue. The history of science suggests we will get better and better, though slowly, asymptotically, and with pain along the way.

51

Vigilance of Natural Health Products

Mano Murty, MD, CCFP, FCFP,* Kevin Bernardo, ND, BHsc,* and Alison Ingham, PhD**

*Marketed Health Products Directorate, Health Canada
   (contact: mano_murty@hc-sc.gc.ca)
**Natural Health Products Directorate, Health Canada

This chapter is an introduction to the science of natural health products (NHPs) and related vigilance activities. For simplicity, the term *natural health products* (NHP) will be used to denote a wide variety of substances, as defined in Canada's regulatory definition (see Table 51.1).

Studies show that the use of NHPs is increasing in the general population, including among children, pregnant women, and seniors. The perception is that "natural" means safe and, therefore, not able to cause adverse reactions (ARs) (Brulotte and Vohra 2008; Chiu et al. 2009; Ernst 1999; Forster et al. 2006; Kelly et al. 2005; Vohra et al. 2009; Woodward 2005). These products are being used to maintain health and to prevent and treat various medical conditions. Although most NHPs are considered low-risk, serious ARs associated with NHPs continue to be reported (Furbee et al. 2006). An element related to safety is direct-to-consumer advertising, which may lead to misuse by consumers, some of whom may have chronic or serious illness, increasing the risk of adverse interaction (Torok and Murray 2008). Self-diagnosing an ailment and self-selecting a treatment can lead to

serious ARs, masking a serious illness or causing a delay in receiving necessary treatment (Lapi et al. 2008).

Labeling is another concern because it may or may not reflect actual product ingredients and indications for appropriate use. While Canada has implemented labeling standards of authorized NHPs, many unauthorized NHPs

Table 51.1	Health Canada's Definition of a Natural Health Product
Substance	■ Plants, algae, bacteria, fungi, nonhuman animal materials ■ Extracts or isolates of the above ■ Vitamins and minerals ■ Amino acids and essential fatty acids ■ Synthetic duplicates of natural ingredients ■ Probiotics ■ Traditional and homeopathic medicines
Function	■ Diagnosis, treatment, mitigation, and prevention of disease ■ Restoring or correcting organic function to maintain and promote health

Source: Health Canada Website. Overview of natural health products regulations. http://www.hc-sc.gc.ca/dhp-mps/prodnatur/legislation/docs/regula-regle_over-apercu-eng.php. Accessed September 1, 2010

available worldwide have minimal or misleading labels (Web Resource 51-1).

These and other emerging safety issues have raised awareness within the scientific and medical communities about including NHPs in the pharmacovigilance framework.

As many of the NHPs on the international market do not undergo premarket studies, safety data are sparse. This is the main challenge not only to the regulators but also to all relevant stakeholders, such as healthcare practitioners, consumers, and the NHP industry (Murty 2007).

Special considerations and expertise are required to collect quality data, identify and assess signals, and implement risk mitigation strategies with NHPs. A dedicated vigilance program for NHPs is imperative for promoting public safety. Such a program will need to consider some of the following key factors: (a) prevalence of NHP use and safety issues; (b) data sources and Adverse Reaction Reporting (ARR); (c) ARs and causality assessment; (d) safety analysis: signal evaluation; (e) NHP interactions and medical relevance; (f) international collaboration: methods to address regulatory diversity; (g) initiatives to strengthen vigilance of NHPs. This chapter will give an overview of these factors and associated challenges. The Canadian Regulatory framework for NHPs will be used to exemplify some methods to strengthen vigilance of NHPs.

■ Prevalence of NHP Use and Safety Issues

Canada and the United States report more than 70% of their population use NHPs (IPSOS Reid 2005; Loman 2003). Use by children in some countries has been estimated to be 17–33% (Brulotte and Vohra 2008). NHPs are readily available without prescription in grocery stores, retail pharmacies, health food stores, and on the internet. It is now well known that NHPs can exhibit pharmacological and physiological activities and, in some cases, can cause harm (McFarlin et al. 1999; Menniti-Ippolito et al. 2008). As the use of botanical medicines increases, consumers expose themselves to potential ARs, many of which go undetected, as a medical consultation is not always sought. Interactions between NHP–drugs, NHP–NHPs, and NHP–food leading to clinically relevant events have been reported (De Smet 2006; MacDonald et al. 2009). These form some of the safety issues that need to be considered when reviewing these products.

Even when safety studies are available on individual ingredients, the multitude of ingredients used in combi-

nation are poorly studied, and risk cannot be excluded. As accurate data on exposure to NHPs and their consumption are often unknown, estimating a safety issue and the affected population remains a challenge. Lack of guidelines and international regulation of the NHP ingredients and the limited number of human clinical studies on safety and efficacy are some additional factors contributing to potential health risk (Foster et al. 2005).

■ Data Sources and Adverse Reaction Reporting (ARR)

The role of healthcare practitioners (HCPs) in the overall vigilance of NHPs is critical in obtaining quality data. They are in a unique position to promote disclosure of NHP use and potential ARs at the time of every patient encounter. The reliability of the information connected to the NHP (e.g., quality of the product and assurance of the correct species and part of the plant), is pivotal in evaluating ARs associated with the use of NHPs (Farah et al. 2006). Most NHPs consist of multiple ingredients, the identification of which may be difficult. Safety and efficacy of NHPs depend on the quality of source materials used in production. Several factors determine the quality of source material, including environmental conditions, cultivation, harvesting, collection, transport, and storage. Adulteration of NHPs with pharmaceutical drugs or with other NHP ingredients is a major issue associated with safety and pharmacovigilance of NHPs (Mahady et al. 2008). Another concern with all health products, including NHPs, is counterfeiting. The risk with counterfeit products is that they may not contain the active ingredients that consumers would normally expect in authorized health products

Most countries regulate NHPs as foods or dietary supplements, which are not monitored through AR reporting systems. In Canada, NHPs are regulated according to the NHP Regulations, which allow voluntary, spontaneous ARs to be collected by Health Canada. However, such systems have limitations, such as underreporting and poor quality data. Underreporting is common for all health products; it is estimated to be 10% for pharmaceuticals and <1% for NHPs (Woo 2007).

Some factors that contribute to underreporting include consumers' and HCPs' lack of awareness that ARs can be associated with NHPs. Furthermore, many NHPs are regulated in a manner that does not facilitate AR reporting. In addition, many consumers are unaware that they can report ARs. Clinicians often do not have access to toxicity profiles of many NHPs; therefore, they are challenged in recognizing the link to the NHP and reporting the AR.

ARs and Causality Assessment

ARs are considered suspicions, and causality must be verified, which is challenging for many NHPs. Key issues in evaluating adverse events in a spontaneous reporting system include limited medical information, limited manufacturer information, limited ability to analyze trends, and lack of premarket safety and effectiveness information. ARs can be Type A or Type B (WHO 2004). Type A reactions are mostly pharmacological and dose-related, with predictable toxicity (e.g., aristolochic acid-induced nephrotoxicity; St. John's wort (*Hypericum perforatum*) altering therapeutic levels of multiple drugs). Type B refers to idiosyncratic reactions (not dose-related, not predictable), such as allergy/hepatitis and anaphylaxis. From our experience, most of the ARs associated with NHPs relate to idiosyncratic reactions (Type B) unless there is an ingredient that has been demonstrated to have inherent toxicity (Vivekanand 2010; Wai et al. 2007).

Acute ARs associated with NHPs are easily detected but may not be immediately attributed to the NHP. However, subtle symptoms of toxicity or long-term detrimental effects, such as carcinogenic, mutagenic, or teratogenic effects, may be easily missed (Singhuber et al. 2009). ARs associated with NHPs relate to multiple factors, such as product pharmacological activity/

misidentification or adulteration, consumer use, or interaction with drugs, foods, or other NHPs (see Table 51.2).

Interaction with pharmaceuticals becomes critical if the pharmaceutical, such as warfarin, has a narrow therapeutic index. ARs can be misinterpreted and attributed to a conventional drug or to the disease process. This can lead to inappropriate or delayed management. Causal relationships can be evaluated using several algorithms (Jordan et al. 2010; Naranjo et al. 1981). However, there are challenges and limitations with these tools, as they were mostly designed for single-ingredient products.

The following criteria aid in the causality evaluation of an AR case report: (a) core information (reporter, patient, suspect product, and AR) along with additional information; (b) medical information (age, gender, history, diagnosis, dose, and duration of use, time between product administration and adverse reaction, dechallenge/rechallenge information, concomitant medical conditions and health products, lab analysis, social history, medical intervention); (c) product information (label contents, brand name and ingredient, type of extract, concentration, lot number, expiration date); and (d) Market Authorization Holder (MAH) info (contact name/address). A single botanical may contain multiple constituents, and a botanical combination product may contain several times that number. Variability in active ingredients, some with possible inherent toxicity, and the vast number of ingredients included in some products, limit the ability to assess or attribute to a single NHP ingredient the cause of the AR.

Table 51.2	Examples of Product-Related Factors That Impact on the Safety Evaluation of NHPs
Product Factors	**Potential Impact on Safety**
Multi-ingredients/Not Standardized Among Different Companies	Some have >100 ingredients; different companies can offer different formulations and combinations of ingredients; also variability in active ingredients
Multiple chemical substances within each product ingredient	Each chemical substance (e.g., alkaloids) may have either inherent toxicity or interaction potential.
Claim/Label Accuracy	Label claims may not always reflect the actual ingredients or botanical species; some traditional products may have language not understood by all consumers
Quality of Product: Manufacturing Practices	Failure of Good Manufacturing Practices, such as misidentification, contamination with microbials, heavy metals, adulteration with pharmaceuticals, substitution
Product Classification	Food-NHP classification for risk mitigation strategies.
Nomenclature	Not standardized worldwide for specific ingredients.
Product Name	Look-alike and sound-alike products may contain different ingredients and indications.

Note: NHP, natural health products.

Safety Analysis: Signal Evaluation

Causality assessment combined with the totality of evidence can enable the separation of a potential "signal" from what appears to be background noise. Reliable data sources (see Table 51.3), published literature, and population exposure information can clarify the trend of the signal and perhaps aid comparison of regulatory actions taken in various jurisdictions, such as risk communication, enhanced labeling, restriction on use, or withdrawal of the product. Product laboratory analysis, when available, can strengthen the signal and differentiate between harms related to adulteration or contamination and those related to NHP constituents and their potential interaction with other NHPs, drugs, or foods.

Table 51.3	Examples of Reliable Data Sources for NHPs

- Health Canada: Licensed Natural Health Products Database
  http://webprod.hc-sc.gc.ca/lnhpd-bdpsnh/start-debuter.do?language-langage=english
- Health Canada: Natural Health Products (information on current regulations, licensing, and safety)
  http://www.hc-sc.gc.ca/dhp-mps/prodnatur/legislation/docs/regula-regle_over-apercu-eng.php
- Health Canada: Natural Health Products Ingredient Database Online Solution system, which allows looking up various ingredients and licensing information for products sold in Canada
  http://webprod.hc-sc.gc.ca/nhpid-bdipsn/search-rechercheReq.do
- National Centre for Complementary and Alternative Medicine
  http://nccam.nih.gov/htdig/search.html
- Natural Standard database
  http://www.naturalstandard.com/
- Medline Plus (from the U.S. National Library of Medicine)
  http://www.nlm.nih.gov/medlineplus/
- CAMline
  http://www.camline.ca/naturalhealthprod/naturalhealthprod.php
- Mayo Clinic
  http://www.mayoclinic.com/
- Natural Medicines Comprehensive Database
  http://www.naturaldatabase.com

Note: NHP, natural health products.

NHP Interactions and Medical Relevance

As with drugs, the mechanism of toxicity and interactions is not clear. One NHP that has been well studied is St. John's wort. It is often recommended to treat anxiety or depression and is well known for its interaction with any drug that is metabolized by the CYP450 cytochrome 3A4 system (Cvijovic et al. 2009 (paper); Cvijovic et al. 2009 (interaction grid); De Smet et al. 2008). Both conventional and complementary practitioners will need to be aware of the potential interactions between NHPs and drugs. It is therefore critical to encourage patients to disclose all health products they take.

International Collaboration: Methods to Address Regulatory Diversity

Most NHP-related ARs reported tend to be low in number and lacking in detailed information. A strong collaboration with international regulatory agencies is essential in collecting quality data related to NHP trends, such as evolving safety signals.

However, challenges occur when comparing data and implementing regulatory actions, mainly due to a general lack of standardization in the way countries "regulate" NHPs. Table 51.4 lists the framework used in several countries to regulate NHPs. Many countries use a multiple class system to define and regulate natural health products. Some classify vitamins and minerals as foods (e.g., the United States and the United Kingdom) and herbal medicines as a subset of drugs, and some classify according to traditional forms of medicines such as traditional Chinese medicines (TCM).

Initiatives to Strengthen Vigilance of NHPs

Listed below are initiatives under way or being considered in the NHP sector:

1. Further national and international collaboration among regulators and others (such as the NHP industry):

   - "Vigimed" is an e-mail discussion forum for national pharmacovigilance centers. It provides real-life data and is maintained by the

Table 51.4   Regulatory Practices in Several Countries as They Relate to NHPs

Product Classification Categories

	Canada	Australia	United States	European Union	China	India	Japan
Vitamin/Mineral Supplements	Premarket authorization as per the NHP Regulations	Complementary medicines regulations include GMP and AR reporting	DSHEA [a] Regulations include GMPs and AR reporting	Food Supplements Directive 2002/46/EC.	Interim Administrative Measures for Health Food Registration (2005) premarket registration.	Food Safety and Standards Act Products are considered to be foods. Regulations do not include GMPs or pharmacovigilance, and there are no specific regulations for supplements or fortified foods.	FOSHU, Regulations include premarket review [b]
Fortified Foods	Requirements under the Food and Drug Regulations allow for limited addition of vitamins and minerals to certain foods; individual products do not undergo premarket review	Foods	Foods	Currently in process of drafting Fortified Foods Regulation. [c]	Interim Administrative Measures for Health Food Registration (2005).	Food Safety and Standards Act	FOSHU
Traditional Herbal Medicines	Premarket authorization as per the NHP Regulations	Complementary medicines	DSHEA	Directive on traditional herbal medicinal products (2004/24/EC). Simplified registration scheme. Products have to meet the same standards for safety and quality as conventional pharmaceuticals, but efficacy is demonstrated by traditional use.	Regulated by the State Drug Administration under the same laws as conventional pharmaceuticals. Special requirements of traditional use without demonstrated harmful effects. [d]	Drugs and Cosmetics Act	Pharmaceutical Affairs Law, Regulations include GMP, premarket authorization, and adverse-effect monitoring

Continued

Table 51.4   Regulatory Practices in Several Countries as They Relate to NHPs (cont.)

Product Classification Categories

	Canada	Australia	United States	European Union	China	India	Japan
Herbal Products	Premarket authorization as per the NHP Regulations	Complementary medicines	DSHEA	Traditional herbal medicinal products are regulated as conventional pharmaceuticals. Many are sold without restriction in individual countries (i.e., unlicensed).	Regulated by the State Drug Administration under the same laws as conventional pharmaceuticals.	Food Safety and Standards Act or Drugs and Cosmetics Act	Pharmaceutical Affairs Law
Drugs Derived from Plants	If drug requires a prescription, it is under the Food and Drug Regulations; otherwise, it is under NHP regulations	Drugs	Drugs	Regulated as conventional pharmaceuticals.	Regulated as conventional pharmaceuticals.	Drugs and Cosmetics Act	Pharmaceutical Affairs Law

Note: AR, adverse reaction; GMP, Good Manufacturing Practice; NHP, natural health products.
a.) DSHEA, Dietary Supplement Health and Education Act of 1994.
b.) FOSHU, Foods for Specified Health Use, Japanese Ministry of Health and Welfare. http://www.mhlw.go.jp/english/topics/foodsafety/fhc/02.html. Accessed August 1, 2010.
c.) Nutraceutical and Functional Food Regulations in the United States and Around the World. D Bagchi, ed. (2008).
d.) National Policy on Traditional Medicine and Regulation of Herbal Medicines: Report of a WHO global survey (WHO 2005).

WHO Uppsala Monitoring Centre (Johansson et al. 2007).

- International Regulatory Cooperation for Herbal Medicines (IRCH), a global network of regulatory agencies that handle botanical medicines, was established in 2006 under the coordination of the World Health Organization (WHO) and currently has 23 member countries. Participation is through annual plenary meetings and a series of working groups on particular topics (e.g., Vigilance of Herbal Products).

- Work-sharing initiatives are also being set up with countries to compare specific reports, such as Periodic Safety Update Reports (PSURs). Health Canada has recently set up a work-sharing initiative, Quadrilateral Consortium, with HSA Singapore, TGA Australia, and Swiss Medic, to advance this initiative.

- International harmonization efforts also include the Forum on Harmonization of Herbal Medicines (FHH), a network of several countries (China/Hong Kong, Australia, Japan, Korea, Singapore, and Vietnam) that have established regulations on herbal medicines. There are three subcommittees within this network, one of which focuses on ARs and Vigilance of Herbals. Canada has recently joined this forum.

- Standardization in botanical nomenclature is conducted by Health Canada, Australia's Therapeutic Goods Administration, International Conference on Harmonization of Technical Requirements for Registration of Pharmaceuticals for Human Use, and the Uppsala Monitoring Centre to standardize the botanical names and to create an herbal Anatomical Therapeutic Chemical (ATC) Classification System for international use. This can facilitate the collating of data about ARs to a species or product.

- Methods are being implemented by countries whereby good manufacturing practices for NHPs can be enforced. In Canada, since the NHPR have been introduced in 2004, a process has been ongoing to license and regulate NHPs, a large number of which were already on the market. Recently (August 2010), Canada has developed additional regulations, Natural Health Products–Unprocessed Product License Application Regulations (NHP-UPLAR), to address this issue (Web Resources 51-2 and 51-3).

2. Educating conventional and complementary practitioners, healthcare practitioners, and consumers on AR reporting ("Health Canada's Educational Module for Naturopathic Doctors"; "Health Canada's Educational Module for Healthcare Practitioners and Consumers") (Web Resources 51-4 and 51-5).

3. Requiring the NHP industry to track and report ARs by submitting PSURs or Annual Summary Reports, providing a worldwide safety experience of the product (Web Resource 51-6).

4. Using other sources of ARs, such as active surveillance programs, targeting HCPs and Poison Control Centers.

5. Promoting NHP research, specifically human clinical studies, to elicit direct evidence of toxic effects or ARs.

6. Using risk evaluation, assessment, minimization, and communication programs with impact analysis throughout the life cycle of the product.

7. Harmonizing and standardizing of product labeling for NHPs.

■ Summary

NHP safety data are sparse. To improve both quantity and quality of data, general principles of surveillance need to be applied throughout the product life cycle in regulating NHPs. Chemical complexity, multiple ingredients, limited clinical data, and lack of standardized products are some of the key challenges in safety evaluation of these products. ARs are used to identify areas of concern warranting further investigation and to initiate regulatory actions based on the totality of the evidence. There is a need for healthcare practitioners and other relevant stakeholders to work together to increase AR reporting. As novel products with new combinations of ingredients are manufactured, a strong vigilance program for NHPs is critical so that the benefits outweigh the potential risks. Safety surveillance of health products, including NHPs, is a continuous process throughout the product life cycle and is a shared responsibility, among the regulator who reviews and monitors the health product, the manufacturer who makes the health product and is responsible for monitoring it through its life cycle, the health professional who provides advice to the patient, and the informed consumer who uses it. The issue of how to get sparse data accepted as valid evidence remains an ongoing challenge for the regulatory and legal realms.

■ Acknowledgments

We would like to thank Dr. Duc Vu, Dr. Robin Marles, and Dr. Vicky Hogan for helpful comments and Terry Chernis for library services.

■ References

Brulotte J, Vohra S. Epidemiology of NHP-drug interactions: identification and evaluation. *Curr Drug Metab*. 2008;9:1049–1054.

Chiu J, Yau T, Epstein RJ. Complications of traditional Chinese/herbal medicines (TCM)—a guide for perplexed oncologists and other cancer caregivers. *Supportive Care Cancer*. 2009;17:231–240.

Cvijovic K, Boon H, Barnes J, et al. A tool for rapid identification of potential herbal medicine–drug interactions. Can Pharmacists J. 2009;142:224–227. (Paper: http://www.cpjournal.ca/doi/pdf/10.3821/1913-701X-142.5.224)

Cvijovic K, Boon H, Barnes J, et al. A tool for rapid identification of potential herbal medicine–drug interactions. *Can Pharmacists J*. 2009. (Grid: http://www.cpjournal.ca/doi/pdf/10.3821/1913-701X-142.5.224a)

De Smet PAGM. Clinical risk management of herb–drug interactions. *Br J Clin Pharmacol*. 2006;63:258–267.

De Smet PAGM, Floor-Schreudering A, Bouvy ML, Wensing M. Clinical risk management of interactions between natural products and drugs. *Curr Drug Metab*. 2008;9:1055–1062.

Ernst E. Prevalence of CAM for children: a systematic review. *Eur J Paediatr*. 1999;158(1):7–11.

Farah MH, Olsson S, Bate J, et al. Botanical nomenclature in pharmacovigilance and a recommendation for standardisation. *Drug Safety*. 2006;29:1023–1029.

Forster DA, Denning A, Wills G, Bolger M, McCarthy E. Herbal medicine use during pregnancy in a group of Australian women. *BMC Pregnancy Childbirth*. 2006;200(6):21.

Foster BC, Arnason JT, Briggs CJ. Natural health products and drug disposition. *Annu Rev Pharmacol Toxicol*. 2005;45:203–226.

Furbee RB, Barlotta KS, Allen MK, Holstege CP. Hepatotoxicity associated with herbal products. *Clin Lab Med*. 2006.26(1):227–241.

Health Canada's educational module for naturopathic doctors. http://www.hc-sc.gc.ca/dhp-mps/medeff/centre-learn-appren/nd-dn_ar-ei_module-eng.php. Accessed on September 1, 2010.

Health Canada's educational module for healthcare practitioners and consumers. http://www.hc-sc.gc.ca/dhp-mps/pubs/medeff/_guide/2008-ar-ei_guide-ldir/index-eng.php. Accessed on September 1, 2010.

IPSOS Reid. Baseline NHP survey among consumers. http://www.hc-sc.gc.ca/dhp-mps/pubs/natur/eng_cons_survey-eng.php. 2005. Accessed September 1, 2010.

Johansson K, Olsson S, Hellman B, Meyboom RHB. An analysis of vigimed, a global e-mail system for the exchange of pharmacovigilance information. *Drug Safety*. 2007;30:883–889.

Jordan SA, Cunningham DG, Marles RJ. Assessment of herbal medicinal products: challenges, and opportunities to increase the knowledge base for safety assessment. *Toxicol Appl Pharmacol*. 2010;243;198–216.

Kelly JP, Kaufman DW, Kelley K, Rosenburg L, Anderson TE, Mitchell AA. Recent trends in use of herbal and other natural products. *Arch Intern Med*. 2005;165(3):281–286.

Lapi F, Gallo E, Bernasconi S, et al. Myopathies associated with red yeast rice and liquorice: spontaneous reports from the Italian Surveillance System of Natural Health Products. *Br J Clin Pharmacol*. 2008;66:572–574.

Loman DG. The use of complementary and alternative healthcare practices among children. *J Paediatr Health Care*. 2003;17:58–63.

MacDonald L, Murty M, Foster BC. Antiviral drug disposition and natural health products: risk of therapeutic alteration and resistance. *Exp Opin Drug Metab Toxicol*. 2009;5(6):563–578.

Mahady GB, Dog TL, Barrett ML, et al. United States Pharmacopeia review of the black cohosh case reports of hepatotoxicity. *Menopause*. 2008;15:628–638.

McFarlin BL, Gibson MH, O'Rear J, Harman P. A national survey of herbal preparation use by nurse-midwives for labor stimulation: review of the literature and recommendations for practice. *J Nurse Midwifery*. 1999;44:205–216.

Menniti-Ippolito F, Mazzanti G, Vitalone A, Firenzuoli F, Santuccio C. Surveillance of suspected adverse reactions to natural health products: the case of propolis. *Drug Safety*. 2008;31:419–423.

Murty M. Postmarket surveillance of natural health products in Canada: clinical and federal regulatory perspectives. *Can J Physiol Pharmacol*. 2007;85(9):952–955.

Naranjo CA, Busto U, Sellers EM, et al. A method for estimating the probability of adverse drug reactions. *Clin Pharm Ther*. 1981;30:239–245.

Singhuber J, Zhu M, Prinz S, Kopp B. *Aconitum* in traditional Chinese medicine—a valuable drug or an unpredictable risk? *J Ethnopharmacol*. 2009;126:18–30.

Torok CB, Murray TH. Wielding the sword of professional ethics against misleading dietary supplement claims. *Glycobiology*. 2008;18:660–663.

Vivekanand JHA. Herbal medicines and chronic kidney disease. *Nephrology*. 2010;15:10–17.

Vohra S, Brulotte J, Le C, Charrois T, Laeeque H. Adverse events associated with paediatric use of complementary and alternative medicine: results of a Canadian Paediatric Surveillance Program survey. *Paediatr Child Health*. 2009;14(6):385–387.

Wai C, Tan B, Chan C, et al. Drug-induced liver injury at an Asian center: a prospective study. *Liver Int*. 2007;27(4):465–474.

WHO guidelines on safety monitoring of herbal medicines in pharmacovigilance systems. 2004. http://apps.who.int/medicinedocs/index/assoc/s7148e/s7148e.pdf.

Woo JJY. Adverse event monitoring and multivitamin-multimineral dietary supplements. *Am J Clin Nutr*. 2007;85:323S–324S.

Woodward KN. The potential impact of the use of homeopathic and herbal remedies on monitoring the safety of prescription products. *Human Exp Toxicol*. 2005;24:219–233.

52

Real-World Issues: Fialuridine

Fialuridine (FIAU) was a drug used to treat hepatitis B virus (HBV) in the early 1990s. Its use in one clinical trial in particular produced seven cases of severe hepatic toxicity (including five deaths) in 15 patients. This trial produced major fallout in the world of clinical research in the United States. The events are briefly reviewed here, and a few comments are made in regard to the drug safety aspects of the study.

FIAU is a pyrimidine nucleoside analogue believed to be a promising treatment for HBV patients. It had previously been studied in a major cancer hospital against other viral infections, including cytomegalovirus (CMV) and various herpes viruses, with some promising results. Animal studies revealed vomiting, diarrhea, mild cardiac toxicity at high doses, and bone marrow toxicity. No liver toxicity was noted in any of the animal models (rat, mouse, and monkey).

In 1989, a small pharmaceutical company, together with the National Institutes of Allergy and Infectious Diseases, did a phase I/II dose escalation trial in human immunodeficiency virus (HIV) patients with positive CMV

cultures using fiacitabine (FIAU is an active metabolite of fiacitabine). The study of 12 patients did not show an effect on the CMV. Adverse events (AEs) reported were nausea, fatigue, and an increased creatine phosphokinase in one patient. No one died during the study. Follow-up showed four deaths, including one patient who had hepatitis B about 6 months after the end of the study. His death was believed to be due to the underlying hepatitis and other hepatotoxic medications he was taking.

In 1990, a short-term treatment (2 weeks) study of FIAU was done on HIV patients. During the study, it became clear that there was a significant effect on HBV but probably little CMV efficacy. The protocol was amended to allow HBV patients to enter also. Investigators at the National Institutes of Health (NIH) joined the study team. Significant decreases in HBV DNA were noted. Some patients also developed doubling or tripling of serum transaminase levels. It was unclear whether the transaminase elevations were AEs due to the drug or due to the so-called flare phenomenon of elevated transaminases seen when HBV viremia drops with other drug treatment (e.g., interferon).

In 1991, the positive results from this trial led to a trial of 4 weeks of FIAU therapy. The trial showed excellent results in groups receiving the highest dosages, with major reductions in HBV DNA. No AEs producing dropout or dose modification occurred. "Flares" and HBV DNA rebound were noted in several patients, but three of nine patients had continued suppression of HBV DNA and normal liver tests and were HBV-antigen negative. One patient developed abdominal pain (but with normal liver and pancreas tests) that resolved 4 months after the trial. One patient was diagnosed with cholelithiasis, and another had an episode of peripheral neuropathy. One patient died. He had chronic hepatitis B and had a good result with FIAU in the trial as judged by his HBV DNA level. He had nausea and fatigue during the trial. One month after the last dose of FIAU, his transaminase was noted to be four times normal, and he complained of nausea, fatigue, and abdominal pain. A nonstudy physician recommended cholecystectomy, which was done under general anesthesia. Liver biopsy revealed chronic active hepatitis and steatosis. He deteriorated after surgery and died a few months later. An autopsy revealed steatosis. His death was attributed primarily to the anesthesia drugs administered.

On the basis of these results, the NIH and Eli Lilly, Inc. (now developing the drug) began a study in 1993 of carefully selected hepatitis B patients with a planned treatment period of 6 months of FIAU. Within the first few weeks of the study start, some patients complained of fatigue, nausea, cramps, and diarrhea. Some patients had dose interruption. No abnormal laboratory tests were noted. However, all patients had decreases in HBV DNA, and 6 of 10 became HBV DNA negative. The data were reviewed at about 6 weeks into the trial, and because of the positive results, the investigators opted to continue.

A few days later one patient who had discontinued the drug 2 weeks previously presented to an emergency room with nausea, weakness, and hypotension. The transaminases were normal, but the bilirubin and lactic acid levels were elevated. The patient went on to develop liver and renal failure and died, despite liver transplantation. The autopsy revealed pancreatitis, glomerulonephritis, esophageal varices, and pneumonia. The liver showed micro- and macrovascular steatosis, cholestasis, and chronic active hepatitis.

Within 2 or 3 days of the patient's first showing up at the emergency room, the study was stopped, and all patients still on FIAU were told to stop the drug. All patients (15) were admitted to the NIH Clinical Center for observation. Despite stopping the drug, seven patients developed hepatic failure, pancreatitis, neuropathy, and myopathy and were to have liver transplantation. Five died (some after transplantation) and two survived. Eight of the 15 patients had no AEs.

As a result of this disaster, several inquiries were set up. The U.S. Food and Drug Administration (FDA) established an internal task force and issued a report in November 1993. It was believed that there were many episodes of "missed toxicity" and that the AEs were attributed to the disease rather than to the study drug. The task force also felt that the informed consents and the study monitoring and oversight were not adequate. The FDA issued warning letters to the investigators charging, among other things, failure to immediately report serious AEs to the sponsor and investigational review boards, failure to reduce or terminate dosing in subjects with moderate toxicity, failure to describe all foreseeable risks in the informed consent, failure to follow up on serious AEs, failure to include complete and accurate safety data in the investigator brochure, and failure to adequately monitor by not ensuring that all AEs were reported in the case report forms.

NIH did its own investigation and concluded that the rationale for the studies was strong, especially in light of the lack of other (oral) therapy for the disease in question. The NIH investigators believed the protocols were "meticulously" prepared and implemented and that fatal outcomes could not have been predicted from the AEs. They also noted that the AEs were adequately reported. Thus, NIH and the FDA investigations reached opposite conclusions.

Next, an investigation was done by the Institute of Medicine (IOM) at the request of the secretary of health and human services. The IOM, a private, nonprofit, nongovernmental organization, is part of the National Academy of Sciences. Its review largely agreed with that of the NIH. It concluded that excellent attention was paid to safety monitoring and that there were no significant violations of study conduct or informed consent. They concluded that rapid action to stop the study actually saved lives and prevented an even worse tragedy.

These events were extensively discussed and criticized. Press coverage was vivid and lurid, and a congressional investigation in 1994 occurred with strong charges thrown about. Further work revealed that the FIAU toxicity was due to mitochondrial damage by the drug.

Much has occurred since then in regard to tightening and harmonizing regulations and clinical trial oversight. It is not the intent here to review the issues in clinical trial regulation, oversight and monitoring, or politics. Instead, the drug safety implications are discussed.

■ Serious and nonserious AEs due to (study or marketed) drugs may occur that mimic the disease being treated. The implications of this are important.

It is not adequate to attribute serious AEs to the disease or condition being treated, background medical conditions, intercurrent problems, or other nondrug causes without a careful consideration of a drug-related etiology. A very high level of suspicion that the drug produced the serious AE must be maintained at all times when evaluating whether a drug has produced a particular AE. The drug is not "innocent until proven guilty."

- Clinical trial safety oversight by the company (sponsor) and the investigator must be "meticulous." All regulatory requirements (protocol design, investigator qualification, AE collection, reporting and review, consent forms, investigational review board oversight, safety data review committees, etc.) must be followed strictly and completely.

  - A data safety plan (risk management) must be drawn up and in place before the study starts.

  - Prestudy signals (from animal data or other clinical trials or class drugs) must be followed carefully.

  - Investigator (and sponsor, and monitor) training must be done before the study starts and during the study if new personnel become involved. The training should be of high quality, customized to the study, and done by a training specialist (not simply printed material).

  - A sponsor physician must be designated as clearly in charge of the ongoing safety review. Qualified investigational review boards with high-quality experienced personnel who have sufficient time to review safety data must be used. Sponsors and investigators must supply the investigational review boards with easily reviewable data sent at frequent periods.

- Companies and institutions doing clinical trials must have a crisis management plan in place to do a preliminary investigation and to take appropriate actions on critical safety issues within a few hours.

- Larger political and governmental solutions should also be considered (presumably they are), including full-time dedicated national safety monitoring committees, a separate safety organization within the federal government, involvement of academia in ongoing safety monitoring (as in France), limitation of proprietary secrets, an AE reporting system in a federal database for clinical trial AEs combining the safety efforts put into case report form safety reporting with those for regulatory serious AE reporting (this refers to duplication of reporting in clinical trials: to the drug safety group and in the case report form), continued research into trend analysis and early signaling, and so on.

See an excellent review on the FIAU safety issues:

Nickas J. Clinical trial safety surveillance in the new regulatory and harmonization environment: lessons learned from the "Fialuridine crisis." *Drug Inform J.* 1997;31:63–70.

An excellent review of the situation is available:

Saag M. A review of the FIAU tragedy and its effect on clinical research. *J Clin Res Practice.* 1999;1:21–32.

Also see the IOM report:

Manning FJ, Swartz M, eds. Review of the Fialuridine (FIAU) clinical trials. Committee to Review the Fialuridine (FIAU/FIAC) Clinical Trials. Division of Health Sciences Policy. Institute of Medicine. Washington, DC: National Academy Press, 1995.

53

Real-World Issues: Fen-Phen

What is now called the "fen-phen" issue refers to the combination of fenfluramine and phentermine. Both products had long been approved (in 1973 and 1959, respectively) by the U.S. Food and Drug Administration (FDA) as appetite suppressants.

Reports in the literature of pulmonary hypertension and fenfluramine appeared in the 1980s and 1990s. Reports of headache, insomnia, nervousness, irritability, palpitations, tachycardia, and elevations in blood pressure were seen with phentermine. Few long-term data were available for the use of these drugs at the time.

The combination of fenfluramine and phentermine was never approved by the FDA, and their use was "off-label." However, millions of prescriptions for their use were written (Diet pills redux [editorial]. *N Engl J Med.* 1997;337:629–630).

After this increased use, reports of toxicity started to appear. One report cited the death of a 29-year-old woman after only 23 days of the combination (Mark, Patalas, Chang, et al., N Engl J Med. 1997;337:602–606). Also in 1997, the Mayo Clinic reported 24 women who

developed valvular heart disease (mitral, aortic, and tricuspid, sometimes more than one valve) after a mean of 12 months of combination therapy (with one woman using the drugs for only 1 month). One third had pulmonary hypertension, and several required valve surgery (Connolly, Crary, McGoon, et al., N Engl J Med. 1997;337:635). Valvular disease with only fenfluramine or only dexfenfluramine was also reported.

By November 1997, the Centers for Disease Control and Prevention reported 144 spontaneous cases of fenfluramine or dexfenfluramine with or without phentermine producing valvular disease. Reports of abnormal echocardiograms in fen-phen or dexfen-phen patients were received by the FDA. They noted 30% abnormal echocardiograms in 291 asymptomatic screened patients, primarily with aortic regurgitation. Many of the patients were women.

Fenfluramine and dexfenfluramine were withdrawn from the market in late 1997. Phentermine was not withdrawn because no cases were reported to the FDA with this drug alone (as of September 1997).

The FDA noted in its Q&A of September 1997 (Web Resource 48-1) that because valve disease is not usually associated with drug use, it was not screened for in patients and no cases were detected in 500 patients in a 1-year clinical trial. It noted that the link between symptoms and drug use was not "obvious." In addition, there were few animal data to suggest this toxicity, and early on most patients and physicians did not give too much thought to pulmonary toxicity with these drugs.

After this publicity, not surprisingly, many new cases were noted and lawsuits were filed. In October 1999, the manufacturer agreed to a class action settlement of up to $4.75 billion. A trust was established by the manufacturer by order of the U.S. District Court to administer the claims and payments of benefits to registered class members, providing for benefits including refunds for the costs of Pondimin and Redux, medical monitoring and some medical treatment or payment for monitoring and treatment, and compensation for specifically defined valvular heart conditions. Several safety lessons were learned:

- Untested combinations of approved products may be quite dangerous even if the individual products are not—and especially if the individual products are.

- Old products are not always "well known" or studied.

- Old safety lessons or safety clues may be minimized or forgotten.

- Unintended consequences (AEs) may occur at any time (see fialuridine, Chapter 52, and diethylstilbestrol, Chapter 6) in an unexpected organ system or patient.

- Dose matters. But sometimes it does not.

- "Absence of evidence is not evidence of absence." That is, just because there is no finding of a particular AE or disease in clinical trials or patients treated with a drug does not mean that it was sought. And if it was sought, it might not have been sought in the right patients at the right time with the proper diagnostic tools and tests.

- Companies, physicians, and regulators should be very careful about off-label use, and better ways to monitor their effects need to be developed. There are many valid medical reasons for certain off-label uses, especially in oncology, but extreme care must be exercised, particularly when there is no clear clinical or scientific basis for such use.

- Intelligent and clever clinicians can still discover serious drug AEs in the course of their daily practice. Such serious AEs should indeed be reported to the health authority or company.

- Drug usage, when popular and extrapolated to the populations of North America, Europe, Japan, and elsewhere, can produce enormous benefits to individuals, healthcare practitioners, and society. It can also produce major disasters.

Real-World Issues: Nomifensine

Nomifensine (Merital) was first used as an antidepressant in Germany in 1976, in the United Kingdom in 1977, and in the United States in 1985. From 1978 to 1985, some 165,000 to 251,000 prescriptions were written each year. Between 1978 and 1979, the manufacturer received four reports of hemolytic anemia. A case report was published in the medical literature in 1979. From 1981 to 1982, three more cases in the United Kingdom were reported. From 1979 to 1980, the company did immunologic studies of some 300 patients. In 1981, the United Kingdom labeling was changed to indicate that rare cases of hemolytic anemia were reported.

At this time, the labeling also stated that rare cases of liver enzyme elevation were noted. In the 1980s, the use of nomifensine increased, and by 1986, 296 adverse event (AE) reports were received by the manufacturer, including 16 positive Coombs' tests and 45 hemolytic anemias, as well as 27 jaundice reports, 12 abnormal liver function tests, 6 hepatitis reports, and 1 hepatic necrosis

report. The first United Kingdom fatalities were reported in 1985. Further case reports were published from 1980 to 1985, noting hemolytic anemia (with and without renal failure), thrombocytopenia, hepatitis, fatal alveolitis, a systemic lupus erythematosus-like fatal reaction, and fatal immune hemolysis. By June 1985, the estimated incidence of hemolytic anemia was 1 in 20,000. Further reports were received, and by November, the estimated rate was 1 in 4,000.

"Dear Doctor" letters were sent out in 1985 in the United Kingdom, and the drug was withdrawn from all worldwide markets in January 1986 (Stonier, Pharmacoepidemiology Drug Safety. 2002;1:177–185; Stonier, Edwards, Nomifensine and haemolytic anemia, in *Pharmacovigilance*, Wiley, Hoboken, NJ, 2002).

During this time (late 1970s to the 1980s), the state of drug safety and pharmacovigilance reporting was markedly different from today. The International Conference on Harmonization, European Medicines Agency, and MedWatch were not yet in existence, and many countries had disparate or nonrigorous AE reporting systems.

The drug was approved by the U.S. Food and Drug Administration (FDA) in 1984 (after some 6 years reviewing the dossier), and marketing began in the United States in July 1985. Up to 10,000,000 patients were exposed to the drug by then. The drug was withdrawn from all markets (including the United States) in January 1986.

In the United States, the question then arose regarding how the FDA could have approved the product and then permitted marketing while the crescendo of cases was building up, especially in 1984–1985. Hearings in the U.S. House of Representatives (Congress) were held in early 1986, and the FDA launched an investigation in August 1986.

A summary report was issued by the FDA (Kurtzweil, FDA Consumer, September 1991, p. 42). The FDA investigation revealed that two deaths, an Italian in 1980 and a French woman in 1984 (before the approval in the United States), were known to the company but not reported to the FDA until 1986, months after the drug was withdrawn from the market. Nine other deaths, including three in the United States, also occurred. As the FDA notes in its report: "The investigation, which lasted a year and a half, was lengthy because officials of the US company refused to allow personnel who had been directly involved in analyzing and reporting adverse drug reactions to speak to FDA investigators. In addition, months often passed before they provided written answers to investigators' questions."

The FDA was able to gather evidence showing that the company, Hoechst AG in Germany, and a former medical director of the clinical research division "had been aware of the deaths of the two European women shortly after they had occurred but had failed to report them to FDA as required." The FDA found no evidence that the U.S. division of the company (Hoechst-Roussel) had withheld information from the FDA. In December 1990, the U.S. federal attorney in New Jersey charged Hoechst AG and the medical director by name with failing to report the two European deaths. No charges were filed against Hoechst-Roussel. In April 1991, Hoechst AG and the medical director pleaded guilty to the charges and were

fined the maximum amount allowed by law. Nomifensine became something of a worldwide cause célèbre.

Several safety lessons were learned:

- Always do the right thing.
- Do not withhold safety data from the FDA and other health authorities.
- The company should speak with one voice and say the same (correct) thing to all health authorities at the same time.
- Report all data in a proper and timely manner and document it with meticulously kept records.
- Proper written procedures must be in place to ensure that all safety data are reported to all branches of the company (especially multinational companies) that need these data. The company should perform periodic internal audits to ensure that this is happening. Any deficiencies should be remedied immediately, and data that should have been reported must be reported to the health authorities as soon as the issue is discovered (painful though this may be).
- Cooperate with all health authority investigations.
- The senior officers of the company must understand the significance of the drug safety function and put their full weight, support, and resources into ensuring that safety is done correctly.
- Maintain a high index of suspicion that AEs may be due to the drug and not to other causes.
- Physicians and those in positions of senior responsibility in the company should be aware that they may be held personally liable (criminally and civilly) if they do not do their safety duties.

Ensure that safety information is reported to the health authorities as required before, during, and after Marketing Authorization submission.

Web Resources

Ref.	URL	Notes
3-1	http://www.fda.gov/AboutFDA/CentersOffices/CDER/ucm169921.htm	FDA Office of Drug Safety Annual Report 2004
3-2	http://www.who-umc.org/DynPage.aspx	The Uppsala Monitoring Centre
3-3	http://www.who-umc.org/DynPage.aspx?id=13140&mn=1514#1	WHO Programme for International Drug Monitoring
3-4	http://ec.europa.eu/health/documents/eudralex/vol-9/index_en.htm	EudraLex—Volume 9 Pharmacovigilance Guidelines
3-5	http://www.tga.gov.au/docs/html/adrguide.htm	Australian Government Guidelines on the reporting of adverse drug reactions by drug sponsors
3-6	http://www.hc-sc.gc.ca/dhp-mps/pubs/medeff/_guide/2009-guidance-directrice_reporting-notification/index-eng.php#sect21	Health Canada Guidance Document for Industry—Reporting Adverse Reactions to Marketed Health Products
4-1	http://www.fda.gov/AboutFDA/WhatWeDo/History/Overviews/ucm056044.htm	FDA Story of the Laws Behind the Labels
4-2	http://www.accessdata.fda.gov/scripts/cdrh/cfdocs/cfCFR/CFRSearch.cfm	CFR—Code of Federal Regulations Title 21
4-3	http://www.accessdata.fda.gov/scripts/oc/ohrms/index.cfm	FDA Federal Register
4-4	http://www.fda.gov/RegulatoryInformation/Legislation/FederalFoodDrugandCosmeticActFDCAct/default.htm	Federal Food, Drug, and Cosmetic Act (FD&C Act)

Ref.	URL	Notes
4-5	http://www.fda.gov/Drugs/ResourcesForYou/Industry/default.htm	FDA Information for Industry (Drugs)
4-6	http://www.fda.gov/MedicalDevices/ResourcesforYou/Industry/default.htm	FDA Industry (Medical Devices)
4-7	http://www.fda.gov/BiologicsBloodVaccines/ResourcesforYou/Industry/default.htm	FDA Industry (Biologics)
4-8	http://www.fda.gov/Food/DietarySupplements/default.htm	FDA Dietary Supplements
4-9	http://www.fda.gov/RegulatoryInformation/Guidances/default.htm	FDA Guidances
4-10	http://www.fda.gov/Safety/MedWatch/default.htm	MedWatch: The FDA Safety Information and Adverse Event Reporting Program
4-11	http://www.fda.gov/Safety/MedWatch/ucm228488.htm	46 MedWatch e-mail notification system
4-12	www.fda.gov/downloads/Drugs/GuidanceComplianceRegulatoryInformation/Guidances/ucm071981.pdf	Guidance for Industry: Postmarketing Adverse Experience Reporting for Human Drug and Licensed Biological Products: Clarification of What to Report
4-13	http://www.fda.gov/BiologicsBloodVaccines/GuidanceComplianceRegulatoryInformation/Guidances/Vaccines/ucm074850.htm	Draft Guidance for Industry: Postmarketing Safety Reporting for Human Drug and Biological Products Including Vaccines
4-14	http://www.fda.gov/Drugs/GuidanceComplianceRegulatoryInformation/Surveillance/ucm129115.htm	Staff Manual Guide: Chapter 53; Postmarketing Surveillance and Epidemiology: Human Drugs
4-15	http://www.fda.gov/ScienceResearch/SpecialTopics/RunningClinicalTrials/ProposedRegulationsandDraftGuidances/default.htm	21 CFR Parts 310, 312, et al.—Safety Reporting Requirements for Human Drug and Biological Products; Proposed Rule
4-16	http://eudravigilance.emea.europa.eu/human/euPoliciesAndDocs02.asp	EudraVigilance Community legislation and guidance documents
4-17	http://ec.europa.eu/enterprise/sectors/pharmaceuticals/documents/eudralex/index_en.htm	EU Legislation—Eudralex
4-18	http://www.ema.europa.eu/ema/index.jsp?curl=pages/contacts/CHMP/people_listing_000019.jsp&murl=menus/about_us/about_us.jsp&mid=WC0b01ac580028d92&jsenabled=true	Pharmacovigilance Working Party (PhVWP)
4-19	http://ec.europa.eu/enterprise/sectors/pharmaceuticals/documents/eudralex/vol-9/index_en.htm	EurdraLex—Volume 9 Pharmacovigilance guidelines
4-20	http://ec.europa.eu/enterprise/sectors/pharmaceuticals/documents/eudralex/vol-10/index_en.htm	EudraLex—Volume 10 Clinical trial guidelines
4-21	http://www.fda.gov/Drugs/GuidanceComplianceRegulatoryInformation/Surveillance/AdverseDrugEffects/ucm070434.htm	FDA Reports Received and Reports Entered into AERS by Year
4-22	http://clinicaltrials.gov/ct2/home	U.S. National Institutes of Health Clinical Trials
4-23	http://www.fda.gov/Safety/FDAsSentinelInitiative/default.htm	FDA's Sentinel Initiative
4-24	http://www.hc-sc.gc.ca/dhp-mps/medeff/advers-react-neg/index-eng.php#a3	Health Canada Adverse Reaction Information

Ref.	URL	Notes
4-25	http://www.mhra.gov.uk/Safetyinformation/Howwemonitorthesafetyofproducts/Medicines/Pharmacovigilance/index.htm	UK's MHRA Pharmacovigilance
4-26	http://www.pfizer.com/health/medicine_safety/medicine_safety.jsp	Pfizer Medicine Safety
4-27	http://www.merck.com/corporate-responsibility/safety-products/approach.html	Ensuring Confidence in the Safety and Quality of Our Products (Merck)
4-28	http://www.corporatecitizenship.novartis.com/patients/patient-safety.shtml	Citizenship@Novartis Patient Safety
5-1	http://www.fda.gov/safety/MedWatch/default.htm	MedWatch: The FDA Safety Information and Adverse Event Reporting Program
5-2	http://www.hc-sc.gc.ca/dhp-mps/medeff/index-eng.php	MedEffect Canada
5-3	http://yellowcard.mhra.gov.uk/	YellowCard
5-4	http://www.afssaps.fr/Activites/Pharmacovigilance/Signalements-et-declarations/%28offset%29/3	French Health Authority
5-5	http://www.ipecamericas.org/	International Pharmaceutical Excipients Council of the Americas
5-6	http://www.ich.org/products/guidelines/quality/article/quality-guidelines.html	ICH document Q8
5-7	http://www.ct-toolkit.ac.uk/_db/_documents/Joint_Project_Guidance_on_Pharmacovigilance.pdf	UK Department of Health/Medical Research Clinical Trials Toolkit
5-8	http://www.fda.gov/Drugs/DevelopmentApprovalProcess/HowDrugsareDevelopedandApproved/ApprovalApplications/InvestigationalNewDrugINDApplication/default.htm.	
5-9	http://www.fda.gov/NewsEvents/Newsroom/PressAnnouncements/2009/ucm171632.htm	FDA Draft Guidance for Industry on Drug Anticounterfeiting Focus on physical chemical indentifiers
5-10	http://www.fda.gov/downloads/Drugs/GuidanceComplianceRegulatoryInformation/Guidances/UCM171575.pdf	Guidance for Industry Incorporation of Physical-Chemical Identifiers into Solid Oral Dosage Form Drug Products for Anticounterfeiting
5-11	http://www.fda.gov/Drugs/ResourcesForYou/Consumers/BuyingUsingMedicineSafely/BuyingMedicinesOvertheInternet/default.htm	FDA Guide to Buying Medicine over the Internet
5-12	http://www.mhra.gov.uk/Safetyinformation/Generalsafetyinformationandadvice/Adviceandinformationforconsumers/Counterfeitmedicinesanddevices/index.htm	MHRA Counterfeit medicines and devices
5-13	http://www.who.int/mediacentre/factsheets/fs275/en/index.html	WHO Medicines: Counterfeit Medicines
5-14	http://www.fda.gov/NewsEvents/Newsroom/PressAnnouncements/ucm149532.htm	FDA press release on sahib plant in India
5-15	www.fda.gov/downloads/Safety/SafetyofSpecificProducts/UCM184049.pdf	FDA's Approach to Medical Product Supply Chain Safety
5-16	http://www.fda.gov/ICECI/CriminalInvestigations/ucm206314.htm	March 25, 2010: Two Arrested for Illegally Trafficking Counterfeit Weight Loss Medication

Ref.	URL	Notes
6-1	www.fda.gov/downloads/BiologicsBloodVaccines/CellularGeneTherapyProducts/UCM150110.pdf	Gene Therapy Patient Tracking System
6-2	www.fda.gov/downloads/Drugs/GuidanceComplianceRegulatoryInformation/Guidances/ucm070968.pdf	Guidance for Industry Antiretroviral Drugs Using Plasma HIV RNA Measurements—Clinical Considerations for Accelerated and Traditional Approval
6-3	http://www.desaction.org/ DES Action	
6-4	http://www.cdc.gov/DES/consumers/third/index.html	DES Third Generation
6-5	http://www.nap.edu/openbook.php?record_id=9269&page=18	Research Strategies for Assessing Adverse Events Associated with Vaccines: A Workshop Summary (1994)
7-1	www.fda.gov/downloads/Safety/MedWatch/UCM168505.pdf	The Clinical Impact of Adverse Event Reporting (October 1996)
8-1	http://www.fda.gov/Drugs/GuidanceComplianceRegulatoryInformation/Surveillance/AdverseDrugEffects/default.htm	FDA Adverse Event Reporting System (AERS)
8-2	http://www.fda.gov/RegulatoryInformation/FOI/HowtoMakeaFOIARequest/default.htm	How to Make a FIOA Request
8-3	http://www.accessdata.fda.gov/scripts/cder/pmc/index.cfm	FDA Postmarket Requirements and Commitments
8-4	http://www.fda.gov/Drugs/GuidanceComplianceRegulatoryInformation/Surveillance/AdverseDrugEffects/ucm082196.htm	Potential Signals of Serious Risks/New Safety Information Identified from the Adverse Event Reporting System (AERS)
8-5	http://www.fda.gov/Drugs/DrugSafety/PostmarketDrugSafetyInformationforPatientsandProviders/ucm111350.htm	Approved Risk Evaluation and Mitigation Strategies (REMS)
8-6	http://www.fda.gov/Drugs/DrugSafety/PostmarketDrugSafetyInformationforPatientsandProviders/ucm103457.htm	Postmarketing Safety Evaluation of New Molecular Entities: Final Report
8-7	http://clinicaltrials.gov/	ClinicalTrials.gov
8-8	http://www.accessdata.fda.gov/scripts/cder/drugsatfda/index.cfm	Drugs@FDA
8-9	http://www.umc-products.com/DynPage.aspx?id=73590&mn1=1107&mn2=1132	VigiBase™
8-10	http://www.umc-products.com/DynPage.aspx?id=73567&mn1=1107&mn2=1132&mn3=6052	How to order ADR information from VigiBase™
8-11	http://www.umc-products.com/DynPage.aspx?id=73566&mn1=1107&mn2=1132&mn3=6050	VigiBase™ Web Access
8-12	http://www.sickkids.ca/Learning/PatientsandFamilies/Motherisk/index.html	Motherisk (University of Toronto/Sick Kids)
8-13	http://www.motherisk.org/women/drugs.jsp	Motherisk Drugs During Pregnancy
8-14	http://www.mhra.gov.uk/Onlineservices/Medicines/Druganalysisprints/index.htm	MHRA Download Drug Analysis Prints (DAPs)
8-15	http://depts.washington.edu/terisweb/teris/index.html	Teratogen Information System (TERIS)

Ref.	URL	Notes
8-16	http://www.gprd.com/home/	The General Practice Research Database
8-17	http://www.bridgetodata.org/	B.R.I.D.G.E. TO_DATA
8-18	http://www.hl7.org/about/index.cfm	HL7 International
9-1	http://www.fda.gov/regulatoryinformation/legislation/federalfooddrugand cosmeticactfdcact/default.htm	Federal Food, Drug, and Cosmetic Act (FD&C Act)
9-2	http://www.gpo.gov/fdsys/	Federal Register
9-3	http://www.gpo.gov/fdsys/browse/collectionCfr.action?collectionCode=CFR	Code of Federal Regulations (CFR)
9-4	http://www.fda.gov/Drugs/GuidanceComplianceRegulatoryInformation/ Guidances/default.htm	FDA Guidances (Drugs)
9-5	http://www.fda.gov/Drugs/GuidanceComplianceRegulatoryInformation/ Guidances/ucm064993.htm	FDA Drug Safety
9-6	http://www.fda.gov/ScienceResearch/SpecialTopics/RunningClinicalTrials/ GuidancesInformationSheetsandNotices/default.htm	FDA Guidance Documents (Including Information Sheets) and Notices
9-7	http://www.fda.gov/downloads/Drugs/ GuidanceComplianceRegulatoryInformation/Guidances/ucm079645.pdf	Center for Drug Evaluation and Research List of Guidance Documents
9-8	http://europa.eu/documentation/legislation/index_en.htm	EU Legislation
9-9	http://www.ema.europa.eu/htms/human/raguidelines/pharmacovigilance.htm	EU Pharmacovigilance: Regulatory and Procedural Guidance
9-10	http://www.ema.europa.eu/ema/index.jsp?curl=pages/contacts/ CHMP/people_listing_000019.jsp&murl=menus/about_us/about_ us.jsp&mid=WC0b01ac0580028d92	Pharmacovigilance Working Party (PhVWP)
9-11	http://www.fda.gov/RegulatoryInformation/Legislation/ FederalFoodDrugandCosmeticActFDCAct/SignificantAmendmentstotheFDCAct/ ucm148035.htm	FDA Dietary Supplement and Nonprescription Drug Consumer Protection Act
9-12	http://www.fda.gov/downloads/Drugs/ GuidanceComplianceRegulatoryInformation/Guidances/UCM171672.pdf	Guidance for Industry Postmarketing Adverse Event Reporting for Nonprescription Human Drug Products Marketed Without an Approved Application
9-13	http://www.hc-sc.gc.ca/dhp-mps/pubs/medeff/_guide/2009-guidance-directrice_ reporting-notification/index-eng.php	Health Canada Guidance Document for Industry— Reporting Adverse Reactions to Marketed Health Products
9-14	http://www.isoponline.org/drug-safety.html	Drug Safety, ISoP Official Journal
9-15	http://adisonline.com/drugsafety/pages/default.aspx	Drug Safety, ISoP Official Journal
9-16	http://informahealthcare.com/loi/eds	Expert Opinion of Drug Safety
9-17	http://www.pharmacoepi.org/publications/journal.cfm	Pharmacoepidemiology and Drug Safety (PDS)
9-18	http://onlinelibrary.wiley.com/journal/10.1002/%28ISSN%291099-1557;jsessioni d=E768BD0EEAEA7336D45EA020BB56558D.d02t01	Pharmacoepidemiology and Drug Safety

Ref.	URL	Notes
9-19	http://www.diahome.org/en/Resources/Publications/JournalsandMagazines	Drug Information Journal
9-20	http://appliedclinicaltrialsonline.findpharma.com	Applied Clinical Trials Online
9-21	http://www.raps.org/personifyebusiness/MemberCenter/BenefitsandServices/tabid/177/Default.aspx	Regulatory Affairs Professionals Society
9-22	http://www.diahome.org/en/FlagshipMeetings/ConferencesandMeetings	Drug Information Association Annual Conferences and Meetings
9-23	http://www.peri.org/	PERI
9-24	http://www.who-umc.org/DynPage.aspx	The Uppsala Monitoring Centre
9-25	http://www.dsru.org/trainingcourses/index.html?PHPSESSID=116de8de63389ab2016bd54c40432929	Drug Safety Research Unit
9-26	http://www.isoponline.org/training.html	The International Society for Pharmacovigilance Meetings and Training Courses
9-27	http://www.pharmacoepi.org/resources/index.cfm	International Society for Pharmacoepidemiology Conferences, Meetings, and Training Courses
9-28	http://www.raps.org/personifyebusiness/ConferencesTraining/tabid/161/Default.aspx	The Regulatory Affairs Professionals Society
9-29	http://dia.custombriefings.com/	DIA Daily
9-30	http://www.diahome.org/DIAHOME/Resources/FindPublications.aspx?pubid=DISPTCH	DIA Dispatch
9-31	http://www.diahome.org/en/Resources/Publications/eNewsLetters.htm	DIA Global Regulatory Activity Digest
9-32	http://www.fiercepharma.com	Fierce Pharma
9-33	www.pharmalot.com	Pharmalot
9-34	http://www.google.com/alerts	Google Alerts
10-1	http://www.ich.org/products/guidelines/efficacy/article/efficacy-guidelines.html	Guidance on Clinical Investigation of Medicinal Products in the Pediatric Population
10-2	www.fda.gov/ohrms/dockets/ac/03/briefing/3927B1_05_1998%20Pediatric%20Rule.pdf	Regulations Requiring Manufacturers to Assess the Safety and Effectiveness of New Drugs and Biological Products in Pediatric Patients
10-3	www.fda.gov/downloads/Drugs/GuidanceComplianceRegulatoryInformation/Guidances/UCM080558.pdf	Guidance for Industry Qualifying for Pediatric Exclusivity Under Section 505A of the Federal Food, Drug, and Cosmetic Act
10-4	http://www.fda.gov/downloads/Drugs/GuidanceComplianceRegulatoryInformation/Guidances/ucm072034.pdf	Guidance for Industry Recommendations for Complying With the Pediatric Rule (21 CFR 314.55(a) and 601.27(a))
10-5	http://www.fda.gov/AdvisoryCommittees/CommitteesMeetingMaterials/PediatricAdvisoryCommittee/default.htm	FDA Pediatric Advisory Committee

Ref.	URL	Notes
10-6	http://www.fda.gov/ScienceResearch/SpecialTopics/PediatricTherapeuticsResearch/ucm123229.htm	FDA Pediatric Advisory Committee Safety Reporting
10-7	http://www.fda.gov/ScienceResearch/SpecialTopics/PediatricTherapeuticsResearch/ucm107519.htm	FDA New Pediatric Information in Labeling
10-8	http://www.fda.gov/ForConsumers/ConsumerUpdates/ucm048515.htm	FDA Using Over-the-Counter Cough and Cold Product in Children
10-9	http://www.fda.gov/Drugs/DrugSafety/InformationbyDrugClass/ucm096273.htm	FDA Antidepressant Use in Children, Adolescents, and Adults
10-10	http://www.ema.europa.eu/pdfs/human/referral/SSRIs/12891805en.pdf	European Medicines Agency finalises review of antidepressants in children and adolescents
10-11	http://eur-lex.europa.eu/LexUriServ/site/en/consleg/2006/R/02006R1901-20070126-en.pdf	Regulation (EC) No 1901-2006
10-12	http://www.ema.europa.eu/ema/index.jsp?curl=pages/regulation/general/general_content_000023.jsp&murl=menus/regulations/regulations.jsp&mid=WC0b01ac05800240cd	Pediatric Medicine Development
10-13	http://www.mhra.gov.uk/Howweregulate/Medicines/Medicinesforchildren/index.htm	MHRA Medicines for Children
10-14	http://www.merck.com/mmpe/sec23/ch341/ch341d.html#CHDJHFCC	Merck Drug Categories of Concern in the Elderly
10-15	www.fda.gov/downloads/Drugs/GuidanceComplianceRegulatoryInformation/Guidances/ucm075062.pdf	Guidance for Industry Content and Format for Geriatric Labeling
10-16	http://www.fda.gov/Drugs/ResourcesForYou/ucm163959.htm	FDA Medicines and You: A Guide for Older Adults
10-17	http://www.ema.europa.eu/pdfs/human/opiniongen/49892006en.pdf	Adequacy of Guidance on the Elderly Regarding Medicinal Products for Human Use
10-18	http://www.ema.europa.eu/htms/human/elderly/elderly_patients_special_population.htm	EMA Medicines for the Elderly
10-19	http://medicine.iupui.edu/clinpharm/ddis	Cytochrome P450 drug interactions
10-20	http://www.netwellness.org/healthtopics/aahealth/tuskegee.cfm	African American Health Clinical Trial Diversity: The Need and the Challenge
10-21	http://www.fda.gov/RegulatoryInformation/Guidances/ucm126340.htm	FDA Collection of Race and Ethnicity Data in Clinical Trials
11-1	http://medicine.iupui.edu/clinpharm/ddis/table.asp	P450 Drug Interaction Table
11-2	http://www.fda.gov/ForConsumers/ConsumerUpdates/ucm096386.htm	FDA Avoiding Drug Interactions
11-3	http://www.ema.europa.eu/pdfs/human/ewp/12521110endraft.pdf	EMA Guideline on the Investigation of Drug Interactions
11-4	http://www.pharmacists.ca/content/consumer_patient/resource_centre/working/pdf/Expanding_the_Role_of_Pharmacists.pdf	Canadian Pharmacists Association Expanding the Role of Pharmacists
12-1	http://www.fda.gov/Drugs/GuidanceComplianceRegulatoryInformation/Surveillance/AdverseDrugEffects/ucm070093.htm	FDA Adverse Event Reporting System (AERS) Statistics

Ref.	URL	Notes
12-2	www.fda.gov/Drugs/GuidanceComplianceRegulatoryInformation/Surveillance/ucm129115.htm	FDA Staff Manual Guide: Chapter 53; Postmarketing Surveillance and Epidemiology: Human Drugs
12-3	http://www.mhra.gov.uk/Howweregulate/Medicines/Inspectionandstandards/GoodPharmacovigilancePractice/Frequentlyaskedquestions/index.htm#2	MHRA Frequently asked questions for Good Pharmacovigilance Practice
12-4	http://www.ec.europa.eu/health/documents/eudralex/vol-4/index_en.htm	EudraLex—Volume 4 Good Manufacturing Practice (GMP) Guidelines
12-5	http://www.fda.gov/ICECI/EnforcementActions/BioresearchMonitoring/ucm135196.htm	FDA Guidance for Industry—Computerized Systems Used in Clinical Trials
13-1	http://www.fda.gov/BiologicsBloodVaccines/GuidanceComplianceRegulatoryInformation/Guidances/Vaccines/ucm074850.htm	Draft Guidance for Industry: Postmarketing Safety Reporting for Human Drug and Biological Products Including Vaccines
13-2	http://www.meddramsso.com/subscriber_smq.asp	Standardized MedDRA Queries (SMQs)
13-3	http://www.lareb.nl/documents/njm2005_1993.pdf	The Netherlands Journal of Medicine—Is this reaction caused by this drug?
13-4	http://www.fda.gov/downloads/RegulatoryInformation/Guidances/UCM126834.pdf	Guidance for Industry Good Pharmacovigilance Practices and Pharmacoepidemiologic Assessment
13-5	http://ec.europa.eu/health/files/eudralex/vol-10/21_susar_rev2_2006_04_11_en.pdf	Detailed guidance on the collection, verification, and presentation of adverse reaction reports arising from clinical trials on medicinal products for human use
13-6	http://www.who-umc.org/DynPage.aspx?id=22682	Causality Assessment of Suspected Adverse Reactions
14-1	http://www.umc-products.com/DynPage.aspx?id=73589&mn1=1107&mn2=1664	Adverse Reaction Terminology WHO-ART
14-2	http://www.meddramsso.com	MedDRA MSSO
14-3	http://www.meddramsso.com/public_aboutMedDRA_regulatory.asp	MedDRA MSSO Regulatory Information
14-4	http://www.meddramsso.com/wbb/wbb_index.html	MedDRA Web-Based Browser
14-5	http://www.meddramsso.com/subscriber_library_ptc.asp	MedDRA Points to Consider
14-6	http://www.fda.gov/downloads/RegulatoryInformation/Guidances/UCM126958.pdf	Guidance for Industry Premarketing Risk Assessment
14-7	http://www.meddramsso.com/subscriber_smq.asp	Standardised MedDRA Queries (SMQs)
14-8	http://www.meddramsso.com/subscriber_download.asp	MedDRA Downloads
14-9	http://www.ihtsdo.org	International Health Terminology Standards Development Organization (IHTSDO)

Ref.	URL	Notes
14-10	http://ctep.cancer.gov/protocolDevelopment/electronic_applications/ctc.htm#ctc_40	Common Terminology Criteria for Adverse Events (CTCAE) and Common Toxicity Criteria (CTC)
14-11	http://evs.nci.nih.gov/ftp1/CTCAE/About.html	CTCAE Files
14-12	http://www.fda.gov/NewsEvents/Newsroom/PressAnnouncements/2006/ucm108575.htm	FDA Cautions Consumers Against Filling U.S. Prescriptions Abroad
14-13	http://www.ama-assn.org/ama/pub/physician-resources/medical-science/united-states-adopted-names-council.shtml	American States Adopted Names
14-14	http://www.who.int/medicines/services/inn/en/index.html	WHO International Nonproprietary Names
14-15	http://www.hc-sc.gc.ca/dhp-mps/brgtherap/applic-demande/guides/drugs-drogues/lasa_premkt-noms_semblables_precomm-eng.php	Health Canada Guidance for Industry: Drug Name Review: Look-alike Sound-alike (LA/SL) Health Product Names
14-16	http://www.mhra.gov.uk/Howweregulate/Medicines/Namingofmedicines/CON009668 MHRA	Naming of medicines
14-17	http://www.emea.europa.eu/pdfs/human/regaffair/032898en.pdf	EU Guideline on the Acceptability of Names for Human Medicinal Products Processed Through the Centralised Procedure
14-18	http://www.ismp.org/	Institute for Safe Medication Practices
14-19	http://www.ismp.org/Tools/confuseddrugnames.pdf	ISMP's List of Confused Drug Names
14-20	http://www.umc-products.com/DynPage.aspx?id=73588&mn1=1107&mn2=1139	WHO Dictionary Enhanced
14-21	http://www.umc-products.com/DynPage.aspx?id=73551&mn1=1107&mn2=1139&mn3=6040	WHO Dictionary Samples
14-22	http://eudravigilance.emea.europa.eu/human/evMpd01.asp	EudraVigilance Medicinal Product Dictionary
15-1	http://www.fda.gov/BiologicsBloodVaccines/GuidanceComplianceRegulatoryInformation/Guidances/Vaccines/ucm074850.htm	FDA Draft Guidance for Industry: Postmarketing Safety Reporting for Human Drug and Biological Products Including Vaccines
15-2	http://www.cancer.gov/cancertopics/pdq/supportivecare/nausea/HealthProfessional/page5	Acute/Delayed Nausea and Vomiting (Emesis) Etiology
15-3	http://ec.europa.eu/health/documents/eudralex/vol-10/index_en.htm	Volume 10 Clinical trials guidelines
15-4	http://ec.europa.eu/health/files/eudralex/vol-10/21_susar_rev2_2006_04_11_en.pdf	Detailed guidance on the collection, verification and presentation of adverse reaction reports arising from clinical trials on medicinal products for human use (April 2006)
15-5	http://www.hc-sc.gc.ca/dhp-mps/compli-conform/clini-pract-prat/reg/1024-eng.php	Health Canada Regulations amending the food and drug regulations (1024—clinical trials)

Ref.	URL	Notes
15-6	http://www.hc-sc.gc.ca/dhp-mps/compli-conform/clini-pract-prat/docs/gui_68-eng.php	Health Canada Guidance for Records Related to Clinical Trials (GUIDE—0068)
16-1	http://www.fda.gov/Drugs/DrugSafety/PostmarketDrugSafetyInformationforPatientsandProviders/default.htm	Postmarket Drug Safety Information for Patients and Providers
16-2	http://www.fda.gov/ScienceResearch/SpecialTopics/RunningClinicalTrials/GuidancesInformationSheetsandNotices/default.htm	Guidance Documents (Including Information Sheets) and Notices
16-3	http://www.fda.gov/Drugs/GuidanceComplianceRegulatoryInformation/Surveillance/ucm090394.htm	Regulation and Policies and Procedures for Postmarketing Surveillance Programs
16-4	http://www.fda.gov/Drugs/GuidanceComplianceRegulatoryInformation/Guidances/default.htm	Guidances (Drugs)
16-5	http://www.fda.gov/BiologicsBloodVaccines/GuidanceComplianceRegulatoryInformation/default.htm	Guidance, Compliance & Regulatory Information (Biologics)
16-6	http://www.fda.gov/BiologicsBloodVaccines/ResourcesforYou/Industry/default.htm	Industry (Biologics)
16-7	http://www.fda.gov/Drugs/GuidanceComplianceRegulatoryInformation/Surveillance/ucm129115.htm	Staff Manual Guide: Chapter 53; Postmarketing Surveillance and Epidemiology: Human Drugs
16-8	http://www.fda.gov/Drugs/GuidanceComplianceRegulatoryInformation/Surveillance/AdverseDrugEffects/UCM082196 Potential Signals of Serious Risks/New	Safety Information Identified from the Adverse Event Reporting System (AERS)
16-9	http://www.fda.gov/Safety/MedWatch/default.htm	MedWatch: The FDA Safety Information and Adverse Event Reporting Program
16-10	http://www.fda.gov/Drugs/GuidanceComplianceRegulatoryInformation/Surveillance/AdverseDrugEffects/default.htm	Adverse Event Reporting System (AERS)
16.11	http://www.fda.gov/AboutFDA/CentersOffices/CDER/ucm106368.htm	Over-the-Counter (OTC) Related Federal Register Notices, Ingredient References, and Other Regulatory Information
16-12	http://www.fda.gov/Drugs/DevelopmentApprovalProcess/SmallBusinessAssistance/ucm069962.htm	Small Business Assistance: Frequently Asked Questions for New Drug Product Exclusivity
16-13	http://www.fda.gov/Safety/MedWatch/HowToReport/ucm166910.htm	MedWatch to Manufacturer Program
16-14	http://www.fda.gov/AboutFDA/CentersOffices/CDER/ucm082071.htm	Drug Quality Reporting System (DQRS)
16-15	http://www.foiservices.com/index.cfm	FOI Services
16-16	http://www.fda.gov/Safety/MedWatch/HowToReport/DownloadForms/ucm149238.htm	Instructions for Completing Form FDA 3500A
16-17	http://www.fda.gov/downloads/Safety/MedWatch/HowToReport/DownloadForms/UCM082725.pdf	Healthcare Professional MedWatch Form
16-18	http://www.fda.gov/Drugs/GuidanceComplianceRegulatoryInformation/Surveillance/AdverseDrugEffects/ucm115894.htm	Adverse Events Reporting System (AERS) Electronic Submissions

Ref.	URL	Notes
16-19	http://ec.europa.eu/health/documents/eudralex/vol-9/index_en.htm	EudraLex—Volume 9 Pharmacovigilance Guidelines
16-20	http://www.pharmpress.com/shop/pdf/good_pharm_PG.doc	Good Pharmacovigilance Practice Guide
16-21	http://www.hc-sc.gc.ca/dhp-mps/pubs/medeff/_guide/2009-guidance-directrice_reporting-notification/index-eng.php	Health Canada Guidance Document for Industry—Reporting Adverse Reactions to Marketed Health Products
16-22	http://www.tga.gov.au/adr/pharmaco.pdf	Australian Guidelines for Pharmacovigilance Responsibilities of Sponsors of Registered Medicines Regulated by Drug Safety and Evaluation Branch
17-1	http://www.fda.gov/Drugs/GuidanceComplianceRegulatoryInformation/Guidances/default.htm	Guidances (Drugs)
17-2	http://www.fda.gov/downloads/Drugs/GuidanceComplianceRegulatoryInformation/Guidances/UCM071981.pdf	Guidance for Industry Postmarketing Adverse Experience Reporting for Human Drug and Licensed Biological Products: Clarification of What to Report
17-3	http://www.fda.gov/BiologicsBloodVaccines/GuidanceComplianceRegulatoryInformation/Guidances/Vaccines/ucm074850.htm	Draft Guidance for Industry: Postmarketing Safety Reporting for Human Drug and Biological Products Including Vaccines
18-1	http://www.pharmacoepi.org/	International Society for Pharmacoepidemiology
18-2	http://www.pharmacoepi.org/about/index.cfm	International Society for Pharmacoepidemiology About Pharmacology
18-3	www.dictionary.com	
18-4	http://www.un.org/Pubs/CyberSchoolBus/special/health/glossary	Glossary for Fighting Disease: Health at the End of the Millennium
18-5	http://www.medicine.ox.ac.uk/bandolier/band25/b25-6.html	Swots Corner: What is an odds ratio?
18-6	http://www.medicine.ox.ac.uk/bandolier/index.html	Bandolier
19-1	http://www.who-umc.org/DynPage.aspx?id=22676#signaldef	Side Effect—Adverse Reaction
19-2	http://www.fda.gov/Drugs/GuidanceComplianceRegulatoryInformation/Surveillance/AdverseDrugEffects/UCM082196	Potential Signals of Serious Risks/New Safety Information Identified from the Adverse Event Reporting System (AERS)
19-3	www.dsru.org/	Drug Research Safety Unit
19-4	http://www.gprd.com/home	The General Practice Research Database
19-5	http://www.bridgetodata.org	B.R.I.D.G.E. TO_DATA

Ref.	URL	Notes
19-6	http://www.phaseforward.com/products/safety/default.aspx	Empirica Signal (Oracle/Phase Forward) TM
19-7	http://spotfire.tibco.com/products/clinical-development.aspx	TIBCO Spotfire®
19-8	http://www.i-review.com/index.php?option=com_content&task=view&id=26&Itemid=35	Integrated Review TM and J Review®
19-9	http://www.arisglobal.com/products/agsignals.php	agSignalsTM
19-10	http://www.mhra.gov.uk/Howweregulate/Medicines/Inspectionandstandards/GoodPharmacovigilancePractice/Frequentlyaskedquestions/CON2030417	MHRA Frequently asked questions for Good Pharmacovigilance Practice
19-11	http://www.meddramsso.com/subscriber_smq.asp	MedDRA Standardised MedDRA Queries (SMQs)
20-1	http://www.arisglobal.com/products/arisg.php	ArisG by ArisGlobal®
20-2	http://www.oracle.com/us/industries/health-sciences/027631.htm	Argus by Oracle, Inc.
20-3	http://www.phaseforward.com/products/safety/aer/default.aspx	Empirica Trace by Phase Forward, Inc.
20-4	http://search.oracle.com/search/search?start=1&nodeid=&fid=&keyword=AERS&group=Oracle.com	AERs by Oracle, Inc.
20-5	http://www.hl7.org/about/index.cfm?ref=nav	Health Level 7 (HL-7)
20-6	http://www.fda.gov/MedicalDevices/DeviceRegulationandGuidance/PostmarketRequirements/ReportingAdverseEvents/ucm127951.htm	Health Level Seven (HL7) Individual Case Safety Reporting (ICSR) Files
20-7	http://www.cdisc.org	CDISC
21-1	http://www.osaka-info.jp/en/search/detail/sightseeing_1919.html	Sukunahikona Shrine
21-2	http://www.fda.gov/AboutFDA/CentersOffices/OrganizationCharts/ucm135674.htm	Center for Drug Evaluation and Research
21-3	www.fda.gov/cder	U.S. Food and Drug Administration—Drugs
21-4	http://www.fda.gov/AdvisoryCommittees/default.htm	FDA Advisory Committees
21-5	http://www.fda.gov/AboutFDA/CentersOffices/CDER/ucm082129.htm	Drug Safety Oversight Board
21-6	www.fda.gov/downloads/AboutFDA/CentersOffices/CDER/ManualofPoliciesProcedures/ucm073564.pdf	Manual of Policies and Procedures
21-7	http://www.fda.gov/AboutFDA/Basics/default.htm	FDA Basics
21-8	http://www.fda.gov/Drugs/DrugSafety/PostmarketDrugSafetyInformationforPatientsandProviders/ucm111085.htm	Index to Drug-Specific Information
21-9	http://www.fda.gov/Drugs/DevelopmentApprovalProcess/default.htm	Development & Approval Process (Drugs)
21-10	http://www.fda.gov/Drugs/GuidanceComplianceRegulatoryInformation/default.htm	Guidance, Compliance, & Regulatory Information
21-11	http://www.fda.gov/Drugs/ResourcesForYou/Industry/default.htm	Information for Industry (Drugs)
21-12	http://www.fda.gov/Safety/MedWatch/default.htm	MedWatch: The FDA Safety Information and Adverse Event Reporting Program
21-13	http://www.accessdata.fda.gov/scripts/cder/drugsatfda/index.cfm	Drugs@FDA
21-14	http://www.fda.gov/Safety/Recalls/default.htm	Recalls, Market Withdrawals, & Safety Alerts

Ref.	**URL**	**Notes**
21-15	https://www.safetyreporting.hhs.gov	The Safety Reporting Portal
21-16	https://www.safetyreporting.hhs.gov/fpsr/FAQ.aspx	The Safety Reporting Portal FAQs
21-17	http://www.fda.gov/Drugs/GuidanceComplianceRegulatoryInformation/Surveillance/AdverseDrugEffects/UCM082196	Potential Signals of Serious Risks/New Safety Information Identified from the Adverse Event Reporting System (AERS)
21-18	http://www.fda.gov/Drugs/DrugSafety/PostmarketDrugSafetyInformationforPatientsandProviders/ucm111350.htm	Approved Risk Evaluation and Mitigation Strategies (REMS)
21-19	http://www.fda.gov/Drugs/GuidanceComplianceRegulatoryInformation/Guidances/default.htm	Guidances (Drugs)
21-20	http://www.fda.gov/Drugs/DrugSafety/PostmarketDrugSafetyInformationforPatientsandProviders/ucm112911.htm	Postmarket Drug Safety Information for Patients and Providers: Selected Safety Regulations
21-21	http://www.fda.gov/ICECI/EnforcementActions/WarningLetters/default.htm	Warning Letters
21-22	http://www.fda.gov/Drugs/DevelopmentApprovalProcess/DevelopmentResources/Labeling/ucm093307.htm	Pregnancy and Lactation Labeling
21-23	http://www.fda.gov/ForIndustry/UserFees/PrescriptionDrugUserFee/default.htm	Prescription Drug User Fee Act (PDUFA)
21-24	http://www.fda.gov/AboutFDA/CentersOffices/CDER/ucm106491.htm	Office of Surveillance and Epidemiology (OSE)
21-25	http://www.fda.gov/Drugs/GuidanceComplianceRegulatoryInformation/Surveillance/AdverseDrugEffects/default.htm	Adverse Event Reporting System (AERS)
21-26	http://www.fda.gov/Safety/MedWatch/HowToReport/ucm166910.htm	MedWatch to Manufacturer Program
21-27	http://www.mhra.gov.uk/Safetyinformation/Reportingsafetyproblems/Reportingsuspectedadversedrugreactions/InformationforthePharmaceuticalIndustry/AnonymisedSinglePatientReports/CON2025406	MHRA Anonymised Single Patient Reports
21-28	http://dailymed.nlm.nih.gov/dailymed/about.cfm	DailyMed
21-29	http://www.fda.gov/Drugs/DrugSafety/ucm085729.htm	Medication Guides
21-30	http://www.fda.gov/Drugs/DrugSafety/MedicationErrors/default.htm	Medication Errors
21-31	http://www.fda.gov/Drugs/DrugSafety/ucm187806.htm	Safe Use Initiative
21-32	http://www.fda.gov/Safety/SafetyofSpecificProducts/ucm180582.htm	Federal Risk Management Framework
21-33	http://dailymed.nlm.nih.gov/dailymed/about.cfm	DailyMed
21-34	http://www.fda.gov/Safety/MedWatch/HowToReport/ucm085568.htm	Reporting By Health Professionals
21-35	https://www.accessdata.fda.gov/scripts/medwatch/medwatch-online.htm	MedWatch Online Voluntary Reporting Form (3500)
21-36	http://www.fda.gov/Safety/MedWatch/	Reporting Serious Problems to FDA
21-37	http://www.fda.gov/Safety/MedWatch/HowToReport/ucm085680.htm	OTC Products and Dietary Supplements
21-38	http://www.fda.gov/Safety/MedWatch/HowToReport/ucm085692.htm	Drug/Biologic/Human Cell, Tissues, and Cellular and Tissue-Based Product Manufacturers, Distributors, and Packers

Ref.	URL	Notes
21-39	http://www.fda.gov/BiologicsBloodVaccines/SafetyAvailability/ReportaProblem/ucm152576.htm	Human Cell & Tissue Products (HCT/P) Adverse Reaction Reporting
21-40	http://www.fda.gov/Drugs/InformationOnDrugs/ucm135151.htm	Adverse Event Reporting System (AERS)
21-41	http://www.fda.gov/Drugs/GuidanceComplianceRegulatoryInformation/Surveillance/AdverseDrugEffects/ucm082193.htm	The Adverse Event Reporting System (AERS): Latest Quarterly Data Files
21-42	http://www.fda.gov/Drugs/InformationOnDrugs/ucm142931.htm	Postmarket Requirements and Committees
21-43	http://www.fda.gov/BiologicsBloodVaccines/SafetyAvailability/ReportaProblem/VaccineAdverseEvents/Overview/default.htm	VAERS Overview
21-44	http://www.accessdata.fda.gov/scripts/cdrh/cfdocs/cfMAUDE/search.cfm	MAUDE—Manufacturer and User Facility Device Experience
21-45	http://www.clinicaltrials.gov/	ClinicalTrials.gov
21-46	http://www.accessdata.fda.gov/scripts/plantox/index.cfm	FDA Poisonous Plant Database
21-47	http://www.fda.gov/Drugs/DrugSafety/PostmarketDrugSafetyInformationforPatientsandProviders/default.htm	Postmarket Drug Safety Information for Patients and Providers
21-48	http://www.fda.gov/RegulatoryInformation/Guidances/default.htm	Guidances
21-49	http://www.fda.gov/AboutFDA/CentersOffices/CDER/ucm093452.htm	Regulation of Nonprescription Products
21-50	http://www.fda.gov/RegulatoryInformation/Legislation/FederalFoodDrugandCosmeticActFDCAct/SignificantAmendmentstotheFDCAct/FoodandDrugAdministrationAmendmentsActof2007/default.htm	Food and Drug Administration Amendments Act (FDAAA) of 2007
21-51	http://www.fda.gov/Drugs/GuidanceComplianceRegulatoryInformation/EnforcementActivitiesbyFDA/WarningLettersandNoticeofViolationLetterstoPharmaceuticalCompanies/default.htm	Warning Letters and Notice of Violation Letters to Pharmaceutical Companies
21-52	http://www.fda.gov/InternationalPrograms/Agreements/ucm131179.htm#intlorg	International Organizations and Foreign Government Agencies
21-53	http://www.fda.gov/Food/DietarySupplements/default.htm	Dietary Supplements
21-54	http://www.accessdata.fda.gov/scripts/cdrh/cfdocs/cfcfr/cfrsearch.cfm	CFR—Code of Federal Regulations Title 21
21-55	http://www.fda.gov/AboutFDA/CentersOffices/CBER/default.htm	About the Center for Biologics Evaluation and Research
21-56	http://www.fda.gov/BiologicsBloodVaccines/default.htm	Vaccines, Blood & Biologics
21-57	http://www.fda.gov/BiologicsBloodVaccines/SafetyAvailability/ReportaProblem/VaccineAdverseEvents/default.htm	Vaccine Adverse Events
21-58	http://vaers.hhs.gov/index	Vaccine Adverse Event Reporting System
21-59	http://vaers.hhs.gov/esub/index	Report an Adverse Event
21-60	http://wonder.cdc.gov/vaers.html	VAERS Request
21-61	http://www.fda.gov/MedicalDevices/default.htm	FDA Medical Devices
21-62	http://www.fda.gov/MedicalDevices/Safety/default.htm	Medical Device Safety
21-63	http://www.fda.gov/MedicalDevices/Safety/ReportaProblem/default.htm	How to Report a Problem (Medical Devices)

Ref.	URL	Notes
21-64	http://www.fda.gov/MedicalDevices/DeviceRegulationandGuidance/default.htm	Device Advice: Device Regulation and Guidance
21-65	http://www.fda.gov/downloads/Drugs/GuidanceComplianceRegulatoryInformation/Guidances/UCM071982.pdf	Guidance for Industry Postmarketing Adverse Event Reporting for Nonprescription Human Drug Products Marketing Without an Approved Application
21-66	http://www.fda.gov/AboutFDA/CentersOffices/CDER/ucm209187.htm	Drug Safety Oversight Board Meeting, March 18, 2010
21-67	http://www.fda.gov/ForIndustry/UserFees/PrescriptionDrugUserFee/ucm118934.htm	Prescription Drug User Fee Act Five-Year Plans
21-68	http://www.fda.gov/Safety/FDAsSentinelInitiative/default.htm	FDA's Sentinel Initiative
21-69	http://edocket.access.gpo.gov/2003/03-5204.htm	Safety Reporting Requirements for Human Drug and Biological Products
21-70	www.fda.gov/downloads/Drugs/GuidanceComplianceRegulatoryInformation/Guidances/ucm071981.pdf	Guidance for Industry Postmarketing Adverse Experience Reporting for Human Drug and Licensed Biological Products: Clarification of What to Report
21-71	http://www.fda.gov/Drugs/NewsEvents/ucm130958.htm	What's New (Drugs)
21-72	http://www.fda.gov/AboutFDA/ContactFDA/StayInformed/GetEmailUpdates/default.htm	Get Email Updates
21-73	https://service.govdelivery.com/service/action/multiSubscribe Email Updates	
21-74	http://www.fda.gov/Drugs/ucm181556.htm	Drug Information on Twitter
22-1	http://www.ema.europa.eu/ema/index.jsp?curl=/pages/home/Home_Page.jsp European Medicines Agency	
22-2	http://www.ema.europa.eu/ema/index.jsp?curl=pages/about_us/general/general_content_000112.jsp&murl=menus/about_us/about_us.jsp&mid=WC0b01ac0580028c2c	European Medicines Agency: Agency Structure
22-3	http://www.ema.europa.eu/ema/index.jsp?curl=pages/about_us/general/general_content_000095.jsp&murl=menus/about_us/about_us.jsp&mid=WC0b01ac0580028c7a&jsenabled=true	European Medicines Agency: CHMP: Overview
22-4	http://eudravigilance.emea.europa.eu/human/ichAndEtransmission03.asp	ICH Guidelines referring to electronic reporting in pharmacovigilance
22-5	http://ec.europa.eu/health/documents/eudralex/vol-9/index_en.htm	EudraLex—Volume 9 Pharmacovigilance guidelines
22-6	http://get.adobe.com/reader/	Adobe Reader
22-7	http://ec.europa.eu/enterprise/sectors/pharmaceuticals/documents/eudralex/vol-9/index_en.htm	EudraLex—Volume 9 Pharmacovigilance guidelines
22-8	http://ec.europa.eu/enterprise/sectors/pharmaceuticals/documents/eudralex/vol-10/index_en.htm	EudraLex—Volume 10 Clinical trials guidelines
22-9	http://www.ema.europa.eu/ema/index.jsp?curl=pages/medicines/landing/vet_epar_search.jsp&mid=WC0b01ac058008d7a8&murl=menus/medicines/medicines.jsp&jsenabled=true	European Public Assessment Reports (EPARs)

Ref.	URL	Notes
22-10	http://www.ema.europa.eu/ema/index.jsp?curl=pages/regulation/document_ listing/document_listing_000164.jsp&murl=menus/regulations/regulations. jsp&mid=WC0b01ac0580029754	Inspections procedures
22-11	http://www.ema.europa.eu/ema/index.jsp?curl=pages/regulation/document_ listing/document_listing_000306.jsp&murl=menus/regulations/regulations. jsp&mid=WC0b01ac058017e7fc	European Risk Management Strategy (ERMS)
22-12	http://www.ema.europa.eu/ema/index.jsp?curl=pages/partners_and_networks/ general/general_content_000212.jsp&murl=menus/partners_and_networks/ partners_and_networks.jsp&mid=	Partners & networks
22-13	http://www.ema.europa.eu/ema/index.jsp?curl=pages/news_and_events/ document_listing/document_listing_000198.jsp&mid=WC0b01ac0580033aa1& murl=menus/about_us/about_us.jsp&jsenabled=true	Monthly reports of the CHMP Pharmacovigilance Working Party
22-14	http://www.afssaps.fr	Agence française de sécurité sanitaire des produits de santé
22-15	http://www.cbg-meb.nl/CBG/en/human-medicines/actueel/default. htm?cat={EF3056BC-2A32-4688-ABE5-3F46C55524EE}	MEB
22-16	http://www.bfarm.de/cln_028/nn_1237712/EN/vigilance/vigilance-node-en. html__nnn=true	Bundesinstitut für Arzneimittel und Medizinprodukte
22-17	http://www.ema.europa.eu/ema/index.jsp?curl=pages/about_us/general/general_content_000292.jsp&murl=menus/about_us/about_ us.jsp&mid=WC0b01ac05800293a4	Roadmap to 2015
22-18	http://www.ema.europa.eu/ema/index.jsp?curl=pages/news_and_events/landing/ rss_feed.jsp&murl=menus/news_and_events/news_and_events.jsp&mid=WC0b0 1ac058007c0e8&jsenabled=true	RSS Feeds
24-1	http://www.mhra.gov.uk/index.htm	Medicines and Healthcare Products Regulatory Agency (MHRA)
24-2	http://www.mhra.gov.uk/Howweregulate/Medicines/index.htm	MHRA: How we regulate medicines
24-3	http://www.mhra.gov.uk/Safetyinformation/Reportingsafetyproblems/ Reportingsuspectedadversedrugreactions/Patientreporting/index.htm#5	MHRA: Patient reporting of suspected adverse drug reactions
24-4	http://www.mhra.gov.uk/Safetyinformation/Reportingsafetyproblems/ Reportingsuspectedadversedrugreactions/Healthcareprofessionalreporting/index. htm	MHRA: Healthcare professional reporting of suspected adverse drug reactions
24-5	http://www.mhra.gov.uk/Onlineservices/Medicines/Druganalysisprints/index.htm	MHRA: Download Drug Analysis Prints (DAPs)
24-6	http://www.mhra.gov.uk/Howweregulate/Medicines/ Overviewofmedicineslegislationandguidance/Pharmacovigilance/index.htm	MHRA: Overview of medicines legislation and guidance: Pharmacovigilance
24-7	http://www.mhra.gov.uk/Howweregulate/Medicines/Medicinesregulatorynews/ CON091186	MHRA: Draft consolidated UK medicines regulations
24-8	http://www.mhra.gov.uk/Howweregulate/Medicines/Inspectionandstandards/ GoodPharmacovigilancePractice/Riskbasedinspections/index.htm	MHRA: Good Pharmacovigilance Practice: Risk-based inspections
24-9	http://www.mhra.gov.uk/Pharmaceuticalindustry/index.htm	MHRA: Pharmaceutical industry: A one-stop resource
24-10	http://www.mhra.gov.uk/Pharmaceuticalindustry/SafetyandPharmacovigilance/ index.htm	MHRA: Pharmaceutical industry: Safety and pharmacovigilance

Ref.	URL	Notes
24-11	http://www.mhra.gov.uk/Safetyinformation/Howwemonitorthesafetyofproducts/Medicines/TheYellowCardScheme/YellowCarddata/Druganalysisprints/CON024109	MHRA: Download Drug Analysis Prints (DAPs)
24-12	http://www.mhra.gov.uk/Safetyinformation/Reportingsafetyproblems/Reportingsuspectedadversedrugreactions/InformationforthePharmaceuticalIndustry/AnonymisedSinglePatientReports/CON2025406	MHRA: Anonymised Single Patient Reports
24-13	https://subscriptions.mhra.gov.uk/service/multi_subscribe.html?origin=&code=UKMHRA	MHRA Email Alerting Service
24-14	www.pharmpress.com	Pharmaceutical Press
25-1	http://www.hc-sc.gc.ca/index-eng.php	Health Canada
25-2	www.healthcanada.gc.ca/medeffect	MedEffect Canada
25-3	http://www.hc-sc.gc.ca/dhp-mps/medeff/advers-react-neg/index-eng.php	Adverse Reaction Information
25-4	http://www.hc-sc.gc.ca/dhp-mps/pubs/medeff/_guide/2009-guidance-directrice_reporting-notification/index-eng.php	Guidance Document for Industry—Reporting Adverse Reactions to Marketed Health Products
25-5	http://www.hc-sc.gc.ca/dhp-mps/compli-conform/gmp-bpf/docs/pol_41_tc-tm-eng.php	Inspection Strategy for Post-Market Surveillance (POL-0041)
25-6	http://www.hc-sc.gc.ca/dhp-mps/prodpharma/applic-demande/guide-ld/vigilance/index-eng.php	Product Vigilance
25-7	http://www.hc-sc.gc.ca/dhp-mps/medeff/databasdon/index-eng.php	Canada Vigilance Adverse Reaction Online Database
25-8	http://www.hc-sc.gc.ca/dhp-mps/pubs/medeff/index-eng.php#a2	Reports and Publications—MedEffect Canada
25-9	http://www.hc-sc.gc.ca/dhp-mps/compli-conform/clini-pract-prat/reg/index-eng.php	Regulations
25-10	http://www.hc-sc.gc.ca/dhp-mps/medeff/subscribe-abonnement/index-eng.php	Stay Informed—MedEffect Canada
26-1	http://www.tga.gov.au/adr/bluecard.htm	Australian Government Report of suspected adverse reaction to medicines/vaccines
26-2	http://www.tga.gov.au/safety/monitoring.htm#devices	Monitoring the safety of therapeutic products in Australia
26-3	http://www.tga.gov.au/docs/html/adrguide.htm	Guidelines on the reporting of adverse drug reactions by drug sponsors
26-4	http://www.tga.gov.au/adr/pharmaco.htm	Australian guideline for pharmacovigilance responsibilities of sponsors of registered medicines regulated by Drug Safety and Evaluation Branch
26-5	http://www.tga.gov.au/adr/pmsguide.htm	Joint ADRAC-Medicines Australia guidelines for the design and conduct of company-sponsored post-marketing surveillance (PMS) studies

Ref.	URL	Notes
26-6	http://www.tga.gov.au/docs/html/ich37795.htm	Note for guidance on clinical safety data management: definitions and standard for expedited reporting
26-7	http://www.tga.gov.au/ct/index.htm	Clinical Trials in Australia
26-8	http://www.tga.gov.au/docs/html/euguideh.htm	European Union Guidelines
26-9	http://www.tga.gov.au/legis/index.htm	Australian therapeutic products legislation
26-10	http://www.tga.gov.au/pmeds/rmplans.htm	Risk management plans for prescription medicines
26-11	http://www.tga.gov.au/alerts/index.htm#medicines	TGA advisories
26-12	http://www.tga.gov.au/new/subscribe.htm#msu	TGA Email Updates Subscription
27-1	http://www.who-umc.org/DynPage.aspx?id=13140&mn=1514	WHO Programme for International Drug Monitoring
27-2	http://www.who-umc.org/DynPage.aspx?id=13136&mn=1512	UMC Publications
28-1	http://www.hhs.gov/ocr/privacy/hipaa/understanding/index.html	HIPAA Privacy Rule
28-2	www.fda.gov/downloads/RegulatoryInformation/Guidances/UCM126834.pdf	Guidance for Industry Good Pharmacovigilance Practices and Pharmacoepidemiologic Assessment
28-3	http://www.fda.gov/Safety/MedWatch/HowToReport/ucm085589.htm	HIPAA Compliance for Reporters to FDA MedWatch
28-4	http://www.fda.gov/Safety/FDAsSentinelInitiative/ucm089474.htm	The Sentinel Initiative: A National Strategy for Monitoring Medical Product Safety
28-5	http://eur-lex.europa.eu/LexUriServ/LexUriServ.do?uri=CELEX:31995L0046:en:HTML	Directive 95/46/EC
28-6	http://ec.europa.eu/justice_home/fsj/privacy/guide/index_en.htm	Data Protection
28-7	http://ec.europa.eu/justice_home/fsj/privacy/index_en.htm	Data Protection
28-8	http://www.export.gov/safeharbor/eg_main_018236.asp	Safe Harbor Overview
28-9	http://www.galexia.com/public/research/assets/safe_harbor_fact_or_fiction_2008/safe_harbor_fact_or_fiction-Introduc.html	The U.S. Safe Harbor—Fact or Fiction? (2008)
28-10	http://www.priv.gc.ca/fs-fi/02_05_d_15_e.cfm	Office of the Privacy Commissioner of Canada Resources
28-11	http://www.hc-sc.gc.ca/hcs-sss/pubs/ehealth-esante/2005-pancanad-priv/index-eng.php	Pan-Canadian Health Information Privacy and Confidentiality Framework
29-1	http://www.fda.gov/Drugs/GuidanceComplianceRegulatoryInformation/EnforcementActivitiesbyFDA/WarningLettersandNoticeofViolationLetterstoPharmaceuticalCompanies/default.htm	Warning Letters and Notice of Violation Letters to Pharmaceutical Companies
29-2	http://www.who.int/medicines/publications/essentialmedicines/en/	WHO Model Lists of Essential Medicines
29-3	www.clinicaltrials.gov	ClinicalTrials.gov
29-4	http://www.fda.gov/NewsEvents/Newsroom/PressAnnouncements/ucm212528.htm	FDA Transparency Task Force Unveils Draft Proposals on Agency Disclosure Policies

Ref.	**URL**	**Notes**
29-5	http://www.mhra.gov.uk/CrownCopyright/index.htm	MHRA Crown Copyright
29-6	http://www.fda.gov/AdvisoryCommittees/default.htm	FDA Advisory Committees
29-7	http://www.fda.gov/AdvisoryCommittees/CommitteesMeetingMaterials/Drugs/DrugSafetyandRiskManagementAdvisoryCommittee/default.htm	Drug Safety and Risk Management Advisory Committee
29-8	http://www.worstpills.org/	Worst Pills, Best Pills
29-9:	http://www.phrma.org/	PhRMA
29-10	http://www.efpia.org	European Federation of Pharmaceutical Industries and Associations
29-11	https://www.canadapharma.org/en/default.aspx	R&D—Canada's Research-Based Pharmaceutical Companies
29-12	http://www.diahome.org/DIAHome/Home.aspx	Drug Information Association
29-13	http://www.pharmacoepi.org/index.cfm	International Society for Pharmacoepidemiology
29-14	http://www.isoponline.org/about.html	International Society of Pharmacovigilance
29-15	http://www.raps.org/PersonifyEbusiness/Portals/_default/Skins/RAPS_V2Skin/home.aspx	Regulatory Affairs Professionals Society
29-16	http://www.appinet.org/default.aspx	Academy of Pharmaceutical Physicians and Investigators
29-17	http://pipaonline.org/	Pharmaceutical Information & Pharmacovigilance Association
29-18	http://www.emtrain.eu/index.php/imi-eat-programmes/eu2p	Eu2P
29-19	http://www.ismp.org/default.asp	Institute for Safe Medication Practices—PAGE 19
29-20	http://en.wikiquote.org/wiki/Daniel_Patrick_Moynihan	
30-1	http://www.ich.org/home.html	International Conference on Harmonisation of Technical Requirements for Registration of Pharmaceuticals for Human Use (ICH)
30-2	http://www.fda.gov/downloads/RegulatoryInformation/Guidances/ucm126958.pdf	Guidance for Industry Premarketing Risk Assessment
30-3	http://www.fda.gov/ohrms/dockets/ac/05/briefing/2005-4136b1_03_Risk%20Minimization%20Action%20Plans.pdf	Development and Use of Risk Minimization Action Plans (RiskMAPs)
30-4	http://www.fda.gov/ohrms/dockets/ac/05/briefing/2005-4136b1_02_Good%20Pharmacovigilance%20Practices.pdf	Good Pharmacovigilance Practices and Pharmacoepidemiologic Assessment
30-5	http://www.fda.gov/downloads/Drugs/GuidanceComplianceRegulatoryInformation/Guidances/UCM184128.pdf	Guidance for Industry Format and Content of Proposed Risk Evaluation and Mitigation Strategies (REMS), REMS Assessments, and Proposed REMS Modifications

Ref.	URL	Notes
30-6	http://www.fda.gov/Drugs/DrugSafety/PostmarketDrugSafetyInformationforPatientsandProviders/ucm111350.htm	Approved Risk Evaluation and Mitigation Strategies (REMS)
30-7	http://www.fda.gov/Drugs/DrugSafety/InformationbyDrugClass/ucm163647.htm	Opioid Drugs and Risk Evaluation and Mitigation Strategies (REMS)
30-8	www.ema.europa.eu/ema/pages/includes/document/open_document.jsp?webContentId=WC500006326	Guideline on Safety and Efficacy Follow-Up—Risk Management of Advanced Therapy Medicinal Products
31-1	http://www.fda.gov/downloads/RegulatoryInformation/Guidances/ucm126958.pdf	Premarketing Risk Assessment
31-2	http://www.fda.gov/ohrms/dockets/ac/05/briefing/2005-4136b1_03_Risk%20Minimization%20Action%20Plans.pdf	Development and Use of Risk Minimization Action Plans (RiskMAPs)
31-3	http://www.fda.gov/ohrms/dockets/ac/05/briefing/2005-4136b1_02_Good%20Pharmacovigilance%20Practices.pdf	Good Pharmacovigilance Practices and Pharmacoepidemiologic Assessment
31-4	http://ohsr.od.nih.gov/guidelines/helsinki.html	World Medical Association Declaration of Helsinki
31-5	http://www.nice.org.uk/	National Institute for Health and Clinical Excellence (UK)
32-1	www.fda.gov/RegulatoryInformation/Guidances/ucm127069.htm	The Establishment and Operation of Clinical Trial Data Monitoring Committees for Clinical Trial Sponsors
32-2	www.emea.europa.eu/pdfs/human/ewp/587203en.pdf	Guideline on Data Monitoring Committees
32-3	http://www.ich.org/products/guidelines/efficacy/article/efficacy-guidelines.html	ICH Harmonised Tripartite Guideline—Guideline for Good Clinical Practice E6(R1)
32-4	http://ec.europa.eu/health/documents/eudralex/vol-10/	Volume 10 Clinical trials guidelines
32-5	http://ec.europa.eu/health/files/eudralex/vol-10/12_ec_guideline_20060216_en.pdf	Detailed guidance on the application format and documentation to be submitted in an application for an Ethics Committee opinion on the clinical trial on medicinal products for human use (February 2006)
32-6	http://www.fda.gov/ScienceResearch/SpecialTopics/RunningClinicalTrials/GuidancesInformationSheetsandNotices/ucm113709.htm	Information Sheet Guidance for Institutional Review Boards (IRBs), Clinical Investigators, and Sponsors
32-7	http://www.fda.gov/downloads/RegulatoryInformation/Guidances/UCM197347.pdf	Guidance for IRBs, Clinical Investigators, and Sponsors

Ref.	URL	Notes
33-1	http://www.ich.org/home.html	The International Conference on Harmonisation of Technical Requirements for Registration of Pharmaceuticals for Human Use (ICH)
33-2	http://www.ema.europa.eu/Inspections/GMPhome.html	Good manufacturing practice/GDP compliance
33-3	http://www.mhra.gov.uk/Howweregulate/Medicines/Inspectionandstandards/GoodManufacturingPractice/Guidanceandlegislation/index.htm	MHRA Good Manufacturing Practice: Guidance and legislation
33-4	http://www.hc-sc.gc.ca/dhp-mps/compli-conform/gmp-bpf/docs/index-eng.php	Health Canada Guidance Documents
33-5	http://www.fda.gov/ICECI/EnforcementActions/WarningLetters/2003/ucm147897.htm	Kos Pharmaceuticals, Inc., December 29, 2003
33-6	http://www.fda.gov/Safety/Recalls/default.htm	Recalls, Market Withdrawals, & Safety Alerts
33-7	http://www.fda.gov/BiologicsBloodVaccines/SafetyAvailability/Recalls/default.htm	Recalls (Biologics)
33-8	http://www.fda.gov/downloads/Drugs/GuidanceComplianceRegulatoryInformation/Guidances/UCM171575.pdf	Guidance for Industry Incorporation of Physical-Chemical Identifiers into Solid Oral Dosage Form Drug Products for Anticounterfeiting
33-9	http://www.who.int/mediacentre/factsheets/fs275/en/	WHO Medicines: counterfeit
34-1	http://www.ich.org/home.html	The International Conference on Harmonisation of Technical Requirements for Registration of Pharmaceuticals for Human Use (ICH)
34-2	http://www.cioms.ch/	Council of International Organizations of Medical Sciences
34-3	http://edocket.access.gpo.gov/cfr_2002/aprqtr/21cfr1.3.htm	Title 21—Food and Drugs
34-4	http://www.fda.gov/Drugs/DrugSafety/ucm085729.htm	Medication Guides
34-5	http://www.fda.gov/ForIndustry/DataStandards/StructuredProductLabeling/default.htm	Structured Product Labeling Resources
34-6	http://www.accessdata.fda.gov/scripts/cdrh/cfdocs/cfcfr/CFRSearch.cfm?fr=201.57	CFR—Code of Federal Regulations Title 21
34-7	http://www.fda.gov/downloads/Drugs/GuidanceComplianceRegulatoryInformation/Guidances/ucm075082.pdf	Guidance for Industry Labeling for Human Prescription Drug and Biological Products—Implementing the New Content and Format Requirements
34-8	http://www.fda.gov/Drugs/GuidanceComplianceRegulatoryInformation/Guidances/ucm065010.htm	Labeling

Ref.	URL	Notes
34-9	http://www.fda.gov/downloads/Drugs/ GuidanceComplianceRegulatoryInformation/Guidances/ucm075057.pdf	Guidance for Industry Adverse Reactions Section of Labeling for Human Prescription Drug and Biological Products—Content and Format
34-10	http://pi.lilly.com/us/zyprexa-pi.pdf	Highlights of Prescribing Information: Zyprexa®
34-11	http://www.accessdata.fda.gov/scripts/cder/drugsatfda/index. cfm?fuseaction=Search.Label_ApprovalHistory	Drugs at FDA
34-12	http://www.accessdata.fda.gov/scripts/cder/drugsatfda/index.cfm	Drugs@FDA
34-13	https://www.pdrbookstore.com/ProdDetails.asp?ID=9781563637483&mlc= F8606PH01&cmpid=BAC-pdrhealth-house&attr=2010-PDR-160	2010 Physicians' Desk Reference at PDR Bookstore
34-14	http://www.pdrhealth.com/drugs/drugs-index.aspx	PDRhealth
34-15	http://ec.europa.eu/enterprise/sectors/pharmaceuticals/files/eudralex/vol-2/c/ smpc_guideline_rev2_en.pdf	A Guideline on Summary of Product Characteristics (SmPC) September 2009
34-16	http://ec.europa.eu/health/files/eudralex/vol-2/c/smpc_guideline_rev2_en.pdf	A Guideline on Summary of Product Characteristics (SmPC) September 2009
34-17	http://www.mhra.gov.uk/Publications/PublicAssessmentReports/CON038633	MHRA olanzapine Pliva SPC Public Assessment Report
34-18	http://www.pharmacists.ca/function/shopper/ProductDetail.cfm? ProdCompanyPassed=cpa&ProdCdPassed=cpa-2011E-W&PriceCategPassed =std&indexstart=1	Compendium of Pharmaceuticals and Specialties
34-19	http://www.vidal.fr/	Vidal
34-20	http://www.rote-liste.de/	Rote Liste
34-21	http://www.medicines.org.uk/EMC/default.aspx	electronic Medicines Compendium (eMC)
34-22	http://www.ema.europa.eu/htms/human/raguidelines/post.htm	Postmarketing authorisation: Regulatory and procedural guidance
35-1	http://www.fda.gov/Drugs/DevelopmentApprovalProcess/DevelopmentResources/ Labeling/ucm093307.htm	Pregnancy and Lactation Labeling
35-2	http://www.marchofdimes.com/peristats/	March of Dimes Birth Defect Foundation: PeriStats®
35-3	www.emea.europa.eu/pdfs/human/phvwp/31366605en.pdf	Guideline on the Exposure to Medicinal Products during Pregnancy: Need for Post-Authorisation Data
35-4	http://ec.europa.eu/enterprise/sectors/pharmaceuticals/files/eudralex/vol-2/c/ spcguidrev1-oct2005_en.pdf	A Guideline on Summary of Product Characteristics October 2005
35-5	www.fda.gov/downloads/Drugs/GuidanceComplianceRegulatoryInformation/ Guidances/ucm072133.pdf	Guidance for Industry Pharmacokinetics in Pregnancy—Study Design, Data Analysis, and Impact on Dosing and Labeling
35-6	http://www.who.int/child_adolescent_health/documents/55732/en/index.html	WHO Breastfeeding and maternal medication

Ref.	URL	Notes
35-7	http://www.pegintron.com/peg/application	PegIntron
35-8	http://www.perinatology.com/	Perinatology.com
35-9	http://www.motherisk.org/women/index.jsp	Motherisk
35-10	http://www.motherisk.org/women/drugs.jsp	Drugs in Pregnancy
35-11	http://www.otispregnancy.org/	Organization of Teratology Information Specialists (OTIS)
35-12	http://www.entis-org.com/	European Network Teratology Information Services (ENTIS)
35-13	http://www.eurocat-network.eu/	European Surveillance of Congenital Anomalies (eurocat)
35-14	http://www.socialstyrelsen.se/register/halsodataregister/medicinskafodelseregistret/inenglish	Swedish Medical Birth Registry
36-1	http://www.cioms.ch/	Council for International Organizations of Medical Sciences (CIOMS)
36-2	http://www.unesco.org/new/en/unesco/	United Nations Educational, Scientific and Cultural Organization (UNESCO)
37-1	http://www.ich.org/home.html	The International Conference on Harmonisation of Technical Requirements for Registration of Pharmaceuticals for Human Use (ICH)
37-2	www.fda.gov/downloads/Drugs/GuidanceComplianceRegulatoryInformation/Guidances/UCM071981.pdf	Guidance for Industry Postmarketing Adverse Experience Reporting for Human Drug and Licensed Biological Products: Clarification of What to Report
38-1	http://www.merriam-webster.com/netdict/commodity	Merriam-Webster Online Dictionary definition of commodity
39-1	http://www.gao.gov/cgi-bin/getrpt?GAO-03-536	Technology Transfer—Agencies' Rights to Federally Sponsored Biomedical Inventions, July 2003
39-2	http://www.emory.edu/EMORY_REPORT/erarchive/2005/August/August%201/drugsale.htm	Drug royalty sale fuels Emory resource, August 1, 2005
39-3	http://www.genomeweb.com/biotechtransferweek/royalty-pharma-northwestern-u-sloan-kettering-amgen-addrenex-pharmaceuticals-u-n	Royalty Pharma Buys Portion of NWU's Royalty Interest in Lyrica for $700M, December 31, 2007
39-4	http://www.cptech.org/ip/health/royalties/	CPT page on Royalties on patents for health care inventions
39-5	http://www.dailyprincetonian.com/2009/05/11/23681/	U. sues lab over cancer drug patent infringement, May 11, 2009
39-6	http://www.afssaps.fr/Activites/Pharmacovigilance/Centres-regionaux-de-pharmacovigilance/%28offset%29/4	AFSSAPS, in French
39-7	http://shrp.umdnj.edu/programs/biopharma/index.html	The Biopharma Educational Initiative

Ref.	URL	Notes
39-8	http://www.eu2p.org/	European Programme in Pharmacovigilance and Pharmacoepidemiology Programme
39-9	http://emtrain.spc.at/index.php?option=com_content&view=article&id=63&Itemid=47 EMTRAIN Eu2P	
39-10	http://www.imi.europa.eu/	Innovative Medicines Initiative
39-11	http://grants.nih.gov/grants/policy/coi/	Office of Extramural Research, National Institutes of Health
39-12	http://content.nejm.org/cgi/content/full/360/21/2160	Controlling Conflict of Interest—Proposals from the Institute of Medicine, May 21, 2009
39-13	http://www.phrma.org/principles_and_guidelines	PhRMA Principles and Guidelines
39-14	http://www.jointcommission.org/	The Joint Commission
39-15	http://www.cancer.northwestern.edu/research/research_programs/radar/sections/about.cfm	Robert H. Lurie Comprehensive Cancer Center of Northwestern University—RADAR Program
40-1	http://www.ihtsdo.org/snomed-ct/	International Health Terminology Standards Development Organisation
40-2	http://www.nlm.nih.gov/news/press_releases/paperlesspr03.html	HHS Launches New Efforts to Promote Paperless Health Care System
41-1	http://www.fda.gov/Safety/MedWatch/HowToReport/ucm166910.htm	MedWatch to Manufacturer Program
41-2	http://www.fda.gov/BiologicsBloodVaccines/GuidanceComplianceRegulatoryInformation/Guidances/Vaccines/ucm074850.htm	Draft Guidance for Industry: Postmarketing Safety Reporting for Human Drug and Biological Products Including Vaccines
43-1	http://www.fda.gov/Drugs/GuidanceComplianceRegulatoryInformation/Surveillance/ucm129115.htm	Staff Manual Guide: Chapter 53; Postmarketing Surveillance and Epidemiology: Human Drugs
44-1	www.iso.org/	International Organization for Standardization
45-1	http://vaers.hhs.gov/index	Vaccine Adverse Event Reporting System
45-2	http://dermnetnz.org/	DermNet NZ
45-3	http://vaers.hhs.gov/esub/index	Report an Adverse Event (VAERS)
45-4	www.immunize.org	Immunization Action Coalition
45-5	www.clintrials.gov	ClinicalTrials.gov
45-6	www.vaccinesafety.edu/	Institute for Vaccine Safety
45-7	www.immunizationinfo.org	National Network for Immunization Information
45-8	http://www.ema.europa.eu/htms/general/contacts/CHMP/CHMP_VWP.html	Vaccine Working Party (VWP)

Ref.	URL	Notes
45-9	http://www.mhra.gov.uk/Safetyinformation/Generalsafetyinformationandadvice/Product-specificinformationandadvice/Vaccinesafety/index.htm	MHRA Vaccine Safety
45-10	http://www.phac-aspc.gc.ca/im/vs-sv/caefiss-eng.php	Public Health Agency of Canada Vaccine Safety
47-1	http://www.cptech.org/ip/health/econ/frank2003.pdf	New estimates of drug development costs
47-2	http://content.healthaffairs.org/cgi/content/abstract/25/2/420	Estimating the cost of new drug development: Is it really $802 million?
48-1	http://www.fda.gov/Drugs/GuidanceComplianceRegulatoryInformation/Surveillance/ucm129115.htm	Staff Manual Guide: Chapter 53; Postmarketing Surveillance and Epidemiology: Human Drugs
48-2	http://www.fda.gov/ora/compliance_ref/rpm/pdftoc.html	Regulatory Procedures Manual
48-3	http://www.fda.gov/ora/compliance_ref/default.htm	Compliance Manuals
48-4	http://www.fda.gov/downloads/RegulatoryInformation/Guidances/UCM126834.pdf	Guidance for Industry: Good Pharmacovigilance Practices and Pharmacoepidemiologic Assessment
48-5	http://www.mhra.gov.uk/home/idcplg?IdcService=GET_FILE&dDocName=CON2018030&RevisionSelectionMethod=Latest	Part II: SPS Template
48-6	http://www.mhra.gov.uk/Howweregulate/Medicines/Inspectionandstandards/GoodPharmacovigilancePractice/Riskbasedinspections/CON044099	MHRA Good Pharmacovigilance Practice: Risk-based inspections
48-7	http://www.mhra.gov.uk/home/idcplg?IdcService=GET_FILE&dDocName=CON013899&RevisionSelectionMethod=Latest	Chart of MHRA PV Inspection Process
48-8	http://www.mhra.gov.uk/Howweregulate/Medicines/Inspectionandstandards/GoodPharmacovigilancePractice/Frequentlyaskedquestions/index.htm	Frequently asked questions for Good Pharmacovigilance Practice
48-9	http://ec.europa.eu/health/documents/eudralex/vol-9/index_en.htm	EudraLex—Volume 9 Pharmacovigilance guidelines
48-10	http://ec.europa.eu/health/documents/eudralex/vol-10/index_en.htm	EudraLex—Volume 10 Clinical trials guidelines
48-11	http://www.emea.europa.eu/Inspections/GCPgeneral.html	Good clinical practice compliance
49-1	http://www.mhra.gov.uk/home/idcplg?IdcService=GET_FILE&dDocName=CON2018030&RevisionSelectionMethod=Latest	Part II: SPS Template
49-2	http://ec.europa.eu/health/documents/eudralex/vol-9/index_en.htm	EudraLex—Volume 9 Pharmacovigilance guidelines
49-3	http://www.mhra.gov.uk/Howweregulate/Medicines/Inspectionandstandards/GoodPharmacovigilancePractice/Riskbasedinspections/index.htm#3	MHRA Good Pharmacovigilance Practice: Risk-based inspections
50-1	http://www.pbs.org/wgbh/nova/doctors/oath.html	The Hippocratic Oath Today
50-2	http://plato.stanford.edu/entries/clinical-research/	The Ethics of Clinical Research
50-3	http://www.worstpills.org/	Worst Pills, Best Pills
50-4	http://www.phrma.org/code_on_interactions_with_healthcare_professionals	PhRMA Code on Interactions with Healthcare Professionals
51-1	http://www.hc-sc.gc.ca/dhp-mps/prodnatur/legislation/docs/regula-regle_over-apercu-eng.php	

Ref.	URL	Notes
51-2	http://www.hc-sc.gc.ca/dhp-mps/compli-conform/info-prod/prodnatur/annex-complian-conform-pol-eng.php; http://www.hc-sc.gc.ca/dhp-mps/compli-conform/info-prod/prodnatur/questions-complian-conform-pol-eng.php	
51-3	http://www.healthcanada.gc.ca/exemption	
51-4	http://www.hc-sc.gc.ca/dhp-mps/medeff/centre-learn-appren/nd-dn_ar-ei_module-eng.php	
51-5	http://www.hc-sc.gc.ca/dhp-mps/medeff/centre-learn-appren/cons_ar-ei_module-eng.php	
51-6	http://www.hc-sc.gc.ca/dhp-mps/pubs/medeff/_guide/2009-guidance-directrice_reporting-notification/index-eng.php	

Abbreviations

Abbrev.	Meaning
AARP	American Association of Retired Persons
ADE	Adverse Drug Experience, Adverse Drug Event
ADME	Absorption, Distribution, Metabolism, and Excretion
ADR	Adverse Drug Reaction
AE	Adverse Event, Adverse Experience
AERS	Adverse Event Reporting System
AFSSAPS	Agence Française de Sécurité Sanitaire des Produits de Santé (French Health Agency)
AHA	American Hospital Association
AIDS	Acquired Immune Deficiency Syndrome
ALT	Alanine Transaminase
AMA	American Medical Association
ANDA	Abbreviated New Drug Application
APhA	American Pharmacists Association
AR	Adverse Reaction
AST	Aspartate Aminotransferase

Abbrev.	Meaning
BfArM	Bundesinstitut für Arzneimittel und Medizinprodukte (German Health Agency)
BLA	Biologic License Application
CANDA	Computer Assisted New Drug Application
CBER	Center for Biologics Evaluation and Research
CCA	Clear Cell Adenocarcinoma
CCDS	Company Core Data Sheet
CCSI	Company Core Safety Information
CDC	Center for Disease Control
CDER	Center for Drug Evaluation and Research
CDRH	Center for Devices and Radiological Health
CDS	Core Data Sheet
CEO	Chief Executive Officer
CERTS	Centers for Education & Research on Therapeutics
CFR	Code of Federal Regulations

Abbrev.	Meaning
CHF	Congestive Heart Failure
CHMP	Committee for Medicinal Products for Human Use
CIOMS	Council for International Organizations of Medical Sciences
CMC	Chemistry, Manufacturing Controls
CME	Continuing Medical Education
CNN	Cable News Network
CNS	Central Nervous System
CPK	Creatine Phosphokinase
CPS	Compendium of Pharmaceuticals and Specialties
CRC	Clinical Research Center
CRF	Case Report Form
CRO	Clinical Research Organization, Contract Research Organization
CRU	Clinical Research Unit
CSI	Core Safety Information
CTC	Clinical Trials Certificate
CTD	Common Technical Document
CTX	Clinical Trials Exemption
DAP	Drug Analysis Print (MHRA)
DCSI	Development Core Safety Information
DDMAC	Division of Drug Marketing, Advertising, and Communications
DDPVS	Detailed Description of Pharmacovigilance Systems
DES	Diethylstilbesterol
DIA	Drug Information Association
DMC	Data Monitoring Committee
DNA	Deoxyribonucleic Acid
DQRS	Drug Quality Reporting System
DRMP	Development Risk Management Plan
DS	Drug Safety
DSB	Drug Safety Oversight Board
DSMC	Data Safety Monitoring Committee
DSUR	Development Safety Update Report
DTD	Document Type Definition
ECG	Electrocardiogram

Abbrev.	Meaning
EDC	Electronic Data Capture
EDI	Electronic Data Interchange
EEA	European Economic Area
EMA	European Medicines Agency
EMEA	European Medicines Evaluation Agency—the old name for the European Medicines Agency
ENTIS	European Network of Teratology Information Services
ER	Emergency Room
EU	European Union
EUDRACT	European Clinical Trials Database
FAQ	Frequently Asked Questions
FD&C	Food, Drug, and Cosmetic Act
FDA	Food and Drug Administration
FIAU	Fialuridine
FMEA	Failure Mode and Effects Analysis
FOI	Freedom of Information
FTC	Federal Trade Commission
GCP	Good Clinical Practices
GLP	Good Laboratory Practice
GMP	Good Manufacturing Practice
GPRD	General Practice Research Database
GPVP	Good Pharmacovigilance Practices
GRAS	Generally Recognized as Safe
GRASE	Generally Recognized as Safe and Effective
HA	Health Authority
HBV	Hepatitis B Virus
HCV	Hepatitis C Virus
HHS	Department of Health and Human Services (US)
HIPAA	Health Insurance Portability and Accountability Act
HIV	Human Immunodeficiency Virus
HLGT	Higher Level Group Term
HLT	Higher Level Term
HMO	Health Maintenance Organization
IB	Investigator Brochure

Abbrev.	Meaning
IBD	International Birth Date
ICD	International Classification of Diseases
ICH	International Conference on Harmonization
ICSR	Individual Case Safety Report
ID	Identification
IFPMA	International Federation of Pharmaceutical Manufacturers and Associations
IIS	Investigator-Initiated Study
IIT	Investigator-Initiated Trial
IND	Investigational New Drug Application
INN	International Normalized Nomenclature
INR	International Normalized Ratio
IRB	Investigational Review Board
ISO	International Organization for Standards
ISPE	International Society of Pharmacoepidemiology
ISS	Integrated Summary of Safety
IT	Information Technology
JCAHO	Joint Commission on Accreditation of Healthcare Organizations now known as the Joint Commission
LFT	Liver Function Test
LLT	Lower Level Term
LOE	Lack of Efficacy
LSSS	Large Simple Safety Studies
LVEF	Left Ventricular Ejection Fraction
MA	Marketing Authorization
MAH	Marketing Authorization Holder
MAUDE	Manufacturer and User Facility Device Experience Database
MD	Medical Doctor (Physician)
ME	Medication Error
MedDRA	Medical Dictionary for Regulatory Activities
MHRA	Medicines and Healthcare Products Regulatory Agency
MMWR	Morbidity and Mortality Weekly Report

Abbrev.	Meaning
MSSO	Maintenance and Support Service Organization
NCE	New Chemical Entity
NDA	New Drug Application
NDS	New Drug Submission
NGO	Nongovernmental Organization
NIH	National Institutes of Health
NNH	Number Needed to Harm
NOS	Not Otherwise Specified
NP	National Formulary
NSAE	Nonserious Adverse Event
NSAID	Nonsteroidal Anti-inflammatory Drug
NY	New York
ODS	Office of Drug Safety
OTC	Over the Counter
OTIS	Organization of Teratology Information Services
PASS	Post Approval Safety Study
PD	Pharmacodynamics
PDF	Portable Document Format
PDR	Physicians' Desk Reference®
PDUFA	Prescription Drug User Fee Act
PERI	Pharmaceutical Education and Research Institute
PharmD	Doctor of Pharmacy
PhD	Doctor of Philosophy
PhRMA	Pharmaceutical Research Manufacturers of America
PI	Package Insert
PIL	Patient Information Leaflet
PK	Pharmacokinetics
PPA	Phenylpropanolamine
PRR	Proportional Reporting Ratio
PSUR	Periodic Safety Update Report
PT	Preferred Term
PV	Pharmacovigilance
PVP	Pharmacovigilance Working Party (EMA)

Abbrev.	Meaning
PVWP	Pharmacovigilance Working Party (EMA)
QA	Quality Assessment
QC	Quality Control
QP	Qualified Person
QPPV	Qualified Person for Pharmacovigilance
RCT	Randomized Clinical Trial
REMS	Risk Evaluation and Mitigation Strategy
RiskMAP	Risk Minimization Plan
RMP	Risk Management Plan
RN	Registered Nurse
RNA	Ribonucleic Acid
RR	Risk Ratio
RSI	Reference Safety Information
Rx	Prescription
SADR	Suspected Adverse Drug Reaction
SAE	Serious Adverse Event
SAR	Serious Adverse Reaction
SEC	Securities and Exchange Commission
SESAR	Suspected, Expected Serious, Adverse Reaction
SGML	Standard Generalized Markup Language
SGOT	Serum Glutamic Oxaloacetic Transaminase
SGPT	Serum Glutamic Pyruvic Transaminase
SLE	Systemic Lupus Erythematosis

Abbrev.	Meaning
SmPC	Summary of Product Characteristics
SMT	Safety Management Team
SNOMED	Systematized Nomenclature of Medicine
SOC	System Organ Class
SOP	Standard Operating Procedure(s)
SPC	Summary of Product Characteristics
SPL	Structured Product Labeling
SPS or SPVS	Summary of Pharmacovigilance Systems
SQL	Structured Query Language
SSRI	Selective Serotonin Reuptake Inhibitor
SUSAR	Suspected, Unexpected, Serious Adverse Reaction
UK	United Kingdom
UMC	Uppsala Monitoring Centre
UNESCO	United Nations Educational, Scientific, and Cultural Organization
URL	Uniform Resource Locator
US	United States
USAN	United States Adopted Name
USP	United States Pharmacopoeia
VAERS	Vaccine Adverse Event Reporting System
WD	Working Document
WP	Working Procedure
WHO	World Health Organization
XML	Extensible Markup Language

Index